The ELECTROCARDIOGRAM

A SELF-STUDY COURSE IN CLINICAL ELECTROCARDIOGRAPHY

EMANUEL STEIN

B.A., M.A., LL.B., M.D., F.A.C.P., F.A.C.C., F.C.C.P.

Medical Director, United States Public Health Service;
Cardiologist and Chief, Medical Education, United States
Public Health Service Hospital, Staten Island, New York

W. B. SAUNDERS COMPANY Philadelphia / London / Toronto

W. B. Saunders Company: West Washington Square
Philadelphia, PA 19105

1 St. Anne's Road
Eastbourne, East Sussex BN21 3UN, England

1 Goldthorne Avenue
Toronto, Ontario M8Z 5T9, Canada

Part of the royalties from this edition pledged to
the American College of Cardiology Heart House,
9111 Old Georgetown Road, Bethesda, Maryland 20014

The Electrocardiogram ISBN 0-7216-9893-X
ISBN 0-7216-8585-4

 Made in the United States of America. Press of W. B. Saunders Company. Library of Congress catalog card number 75-8186.

Last digit is the print number: 9 8 7 6 5 4 3 2

To my wife Bobbie
and our children
Cynthia Joy and Steven Gary

The program consists of this manual and ten sound tapes, and is a complete foundational course for the proper interpretation and full understanding of the clinical electrocardiogram. The manual can be used alone as a very concise introduction, a rapid review or a study guide. The tapes should be used in concert with the manual, as the author didactically examines the printed illustrations in a formal lecture sequence.

Explanation of the cover illustration

Original Cambridge electrocardiograph, manufactured in 1911 under agreement with Professor Willem Einthoven, the father of electrocardiography, and delivered to Dr. Thomas Lewis of the University College Hospital, London. (Photo shows Mr. Frost, the Cambridge chief inspector, acting as patient with the instrument prior to shipment to Dr. Lewis.)

Historical notes

During the second half of the 19th century, the association of an electrical potential with muscular contraction was investigated by physiologists. August Waller first recorded the potential variations generated by the human heart beat in 1887 in London. In 1903 Professor Willem Einthoven completed the first electrocardiograph. He used a string galvanometer in which a very fine quartz fiber, coated with silver to make it electrically conductive and stretched between the poles of a powerful electromagnet, underwent variable displacements when the unamplified currents arising from a patient passed through it. The string was illuminated by a very bright arc lamp beam and its shadow was focused onto a moving photographic plate. A rotary spoked wheel was used to interrupt the beam at regular intervals to provide timing marks on the plate. Einthoven communicated details of his invention to Horace Darwin (later Sir Horace Darwin, F.R.S.) of the Cambridge Scientific Instrument Company in England, and to the Messrs. Edelmann in Germany, with a suggestion that they should design and manufacture, under royalty agreement, an "electrocardiograph" that could be marketed. A disagreement between Einthoven and the Edelmanns resulted in Einthoven working exclusively with Cambridge, who manufactured their first machine in 1911 (see photo). Before 1916, 87 Cambridge electrocardiographs had been manufactured and shipped to 15 different countries as far distant as Japan, Australia, India and Russia. In 1911, Dr. Horatio B. Williams of the United States visited Einthoven and upon his return built an instrument with Charles Hindle, his mechanic. Hindle's design was good and he established a manufacturing company, in New York State, which merged with the British firm, Cambridge Instrument Company, Ltd., in 1922, changing its name to Cambridge Instrument Company, Inc. Since then, both American and British firms have benefited from their continuing exchange of new technologies. Early on, the electrocardiograph established its value in diagnostic medicine and today maintains itself as one of the most ubiquitous electronic instruments used in modern medicine.

PREFACE

Cassette Side 1

Welcome to our course in clinical electrocardiography. The aim has always been the practical, the clinical interpretation of the electrocardiogram. It is not all-inclusive; it is not encyclopedic, but a synthesis of vast amounts of material and, of necessity, reflects my ideas of the important and unimportant, with the time allotted accordingly.

I have found this course to be well balanced for a diverse group, including medical students, house officers, general practitioners, non-cardiologist internists, nurses and members of all other medical and surgical specialties. It is within the grasp of the allied health personnel in the coronary care unit, electrocardiography laboratory and emergency room. I have had enormous pleasure in teaching and satisfaction in watching my students learn and succeed.

Throughout the years there have been numerous requests for a recording of this course and copies of the slides. This undertaking is the result. It was a most difficult task to reduce the material in preparation for publication, from 2000 illustrations and more than 40 hours of taped lectures. All chapters were reduced, and the section devoted to pediatric electrocardiography was removed entirely. Many researchers may rightfully feel that their subject should have been included or given more weight and that other areas have been emphasized too much. I accept full responsibility for the allocation of priorities.

The spatial vector approach of Grant is emphasized in the instruction. Knowledge based on a maximum of concept and a minimum of pattern memorization is more easily acquired and more easily retained and applied. The electrocardiograms have been chosen with great care and confirmed, where possible, by clinical-pathological correlation, cardiac catheterization, X-ray and non-invasive techniques. Where appropriate, illustrations are repeated for the sake of continuity. When the question arose as to absolute accuracy versus ease of understanding in a given illustration, the decision generally was made in favor of ease of understanding.

This work was presented in the lecture hall and the tapes were meant to accompany the manual, which originally contained only the illustrations. However, enough text has been added to permit the manual to stand alone. Every effort was made to retain the flavor of the classroom in the manual and on the tapes. In this form the manual can be used as a concise review of electrocardiography after completion of the course.

The requirements for the mastery of this subject include diligence, application, patience and perseverance. This is one area of knowledge where you will learn by doing. The M.D. degree is not a categoric essential. Many, both physicians and non-physicians, have become proficient electrocardiographers. Paramount is the interest and determination of the individual. Philosophically,

It is the set of the sail,
And not the gale,
Which determines the way the ship goes.

It is the set of the soul
Which determines the goal
And not the calm or the strife.

For those who labor under the false assumption that to do anything with electrocardiography they must know everything about it, I wish to quote from the famed philosophical concept which may apply to any endeavor. "The day is short and the task is great. . . . It may not be upon you to complete the task, but neither should it be an excuse for you not to try."

My three great mentors were Drs. Robert P. Grant, John B. Schwedel and Sidney P. Schwartz. Drs. Grant and Schwedel are no longer with us. They were like brilliant comets that flew across the sky and were, all too quickly, no more. Their afterglow, however, has never failed to touch those who knew them. Dr. Schwartz has been interested in electrocardiography from his early interning days at Montefiore Hospital in New York City, and has made available, with characteristic grace, his dearly cherished and lovingly preserved collection of electrocardiograms dating back almost a half century. This work is the result of his successful teaching and keen interest in the young doctors who came under his guidance. I am deeply indebted to him. During my stay at Montefiore Hospital, for four years after medical school, the interest in all aspects of cardiology influenced most of us who were fortunate to have been there during that exciting period. My thanks also go to Drs. Doris J. W. Escher, Robert Eisenberg, Robert Rosenblum, Ira L. Rubin and Harry Gross.

For critical review and valuable suggestions I thank Drs. William Fox, Abner J. Delman, John W. Lister, Anthony N. Damato and Antonio R. Caracta. Dr. Fox also provided several excellent teaching electrocardiograms, as did Drs. Arnold B. Barr, Stephen P. Swersie and Mrs. Jo Ann Gassaway. To these I am very grateful.

I especially appreciate the help of my colleague, Dr. Anthony N. Damato, and of our co-workers in the laboratory at the United States Public Health Service Hospital, Staten Island, where the spirit of learning has been such that:

1. Time-honored "facts" have always been under challenge.
2. Many ideas, conceptualized before the sophistication of the modern laboratory was available, have been proved or disproved.
3. Principles, previously unknown, have come to light.

I should like to add appreciation to John J. Hanley, George W. Laurie and Paul E. Wayne for making the book and tapes possible. Special thanks are extended to Dr. Leo Weiner, former Chief of Medicine at St. Vincent's Hospital and Medical Center, Staten Island.

EMANUEL STEIN

CONTENTS

1

BASIC CONCEPTS AND THE NORMAL ELECTROCARDIOGRAM

Cassette Side 1—*Continued*

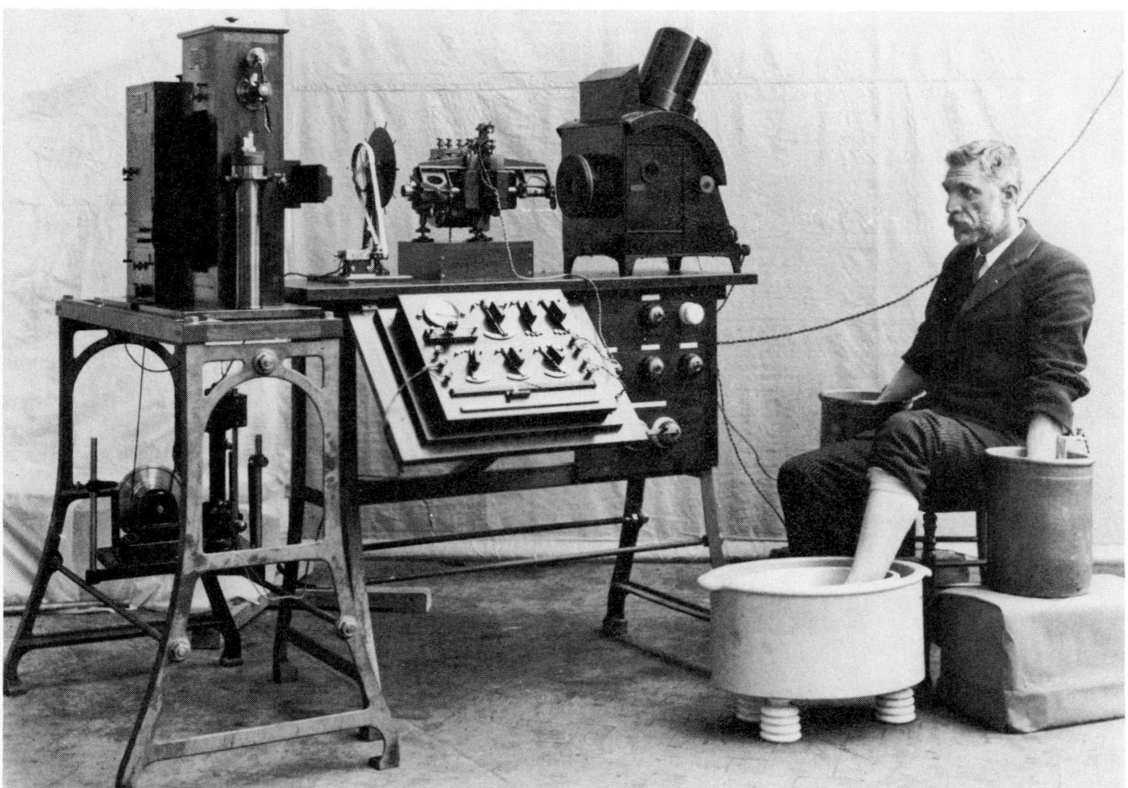

FIGURE 1-1. Original Cambridge electrocardiogram (1912), built for Sir Thomas Lewis. Produced under agreement with Prof. Willem Einthoven, the father of electrocardiography. (Courtesy of Cambridge Instrument Company, New York.)

It wasn't always easy to take electrocardiograms. Figure 1–1 illustrates what had to be done years ago. The gentleman whose electrocardiogram is being taken had to have both arms and his left leg in buckets of conducting solution. The recording was made on the large machine. In Figure 1–2, we see an electrocardiographic machine of a later date, still a far cry from the streamlined machines of today. However, this patient did not need buckets of conducting solution.

Willem Einthoven, who had worked with the string galvanometer, is known as the father of electrocardiography. The galvanometer, which is basic to all electrocardiographs, consists of a movable writing element within a magnetic field. A wire is connected to each end—one the positive electrode and the other the negative electrode. The difference in potential between the two poles can be measured by use of this instrument. When the two electrodes are placed on different positions on the body, the positive electrode on one extremity and the negative on another, they form what is known as a *lead.* The deflection which is recorded for each lead is a manifestation, at the body surface, of the electrical activity of the heart seen from the vantage point of that particular lead.

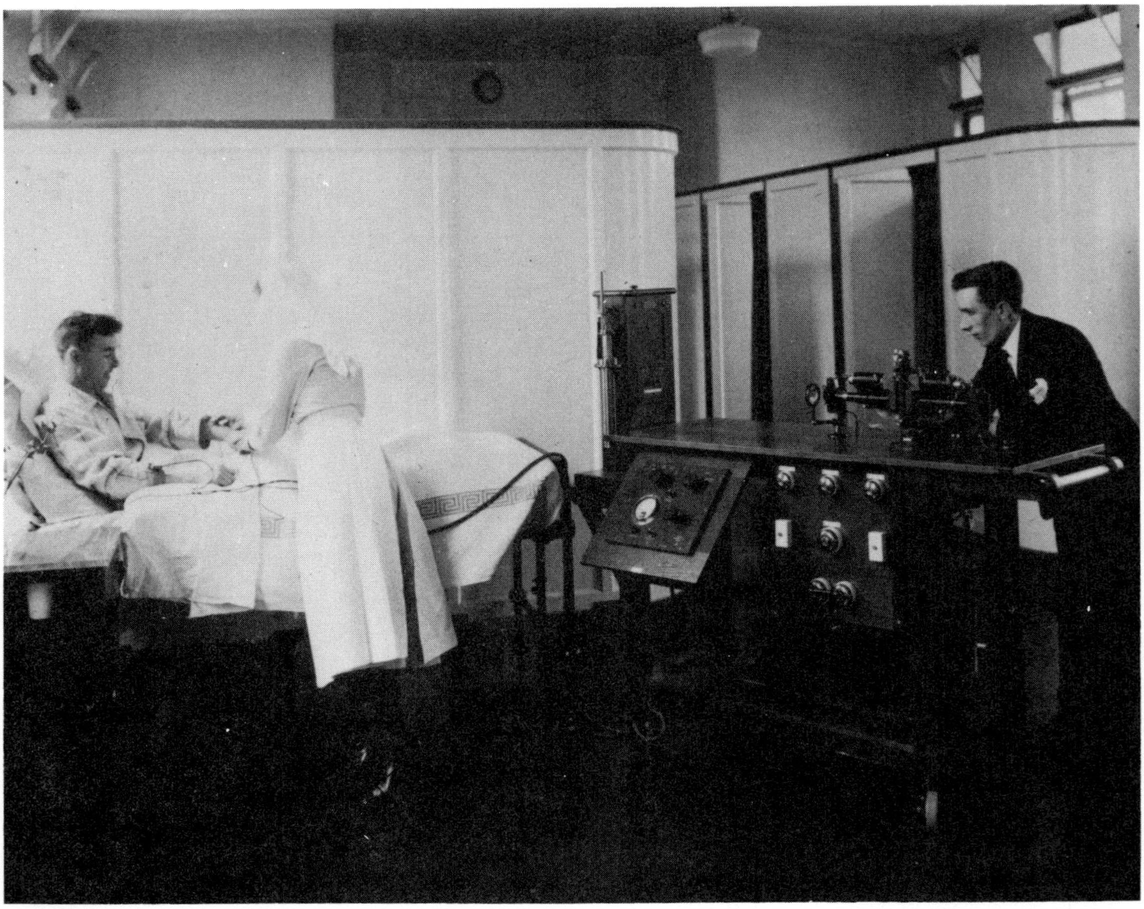

FIGURE 1–2. Early electrocardiographic equipment. (Courtesy of Cambridge Instrument Company, New York.)

FORMATION OF THE ELECTROCARDIOGRAPHIC LEADS

The Einthoven Triangle

Einthoven found that by connecting the right arm to the negative electrode and the left arm to the positive electrode, and inducing a current to flow, a certain deflection was recorded by the galvanometer; this is called lead I (Fig. 1–3).

By connecting the left arm with the left leg, the left arm to the negative electrode and the left leg to the positive electrode, Einthoven recorded another positive deflection with the galvanometer; this is known as lead III (Fig. 1–4).

FIGURE 1–3. Formation of lead I.

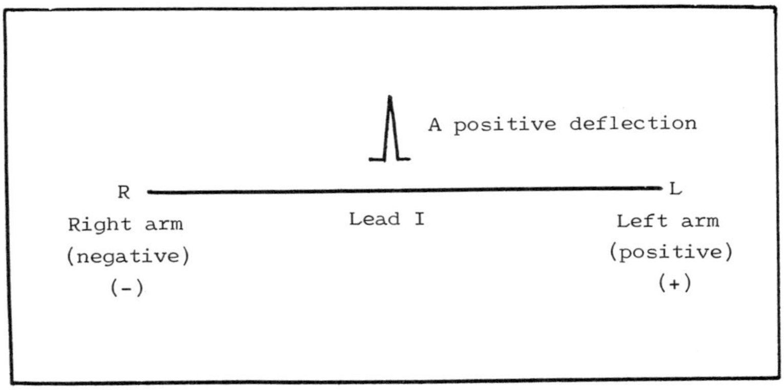

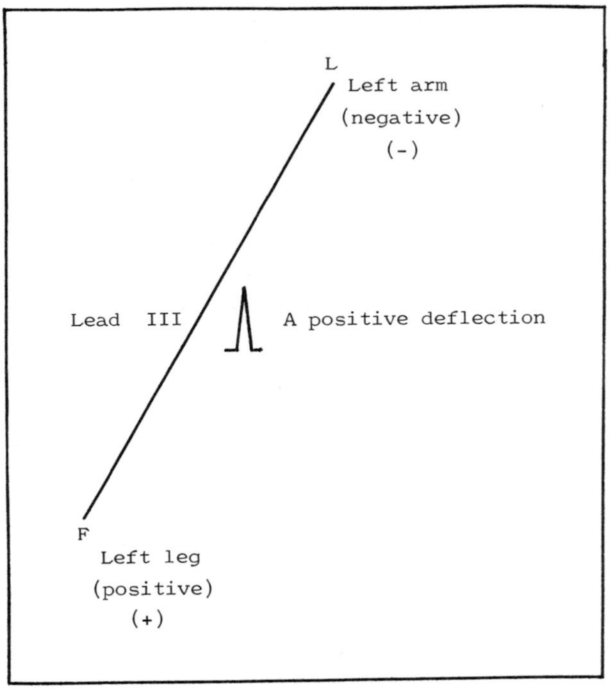

FIGURE 1–4. Formation of lead III.

In Figure 1–5 we see the *original* lead II. The information presented in Figures 1–5 and 1–6 is *not* correct today. It is included for basic understanding of the lead development.

By connecting the right arm and the left leg, the right arm to the positive electrode and the left leg to the negative electrode, Einthoven recorded a large negative deflection (Fig. 1–5).

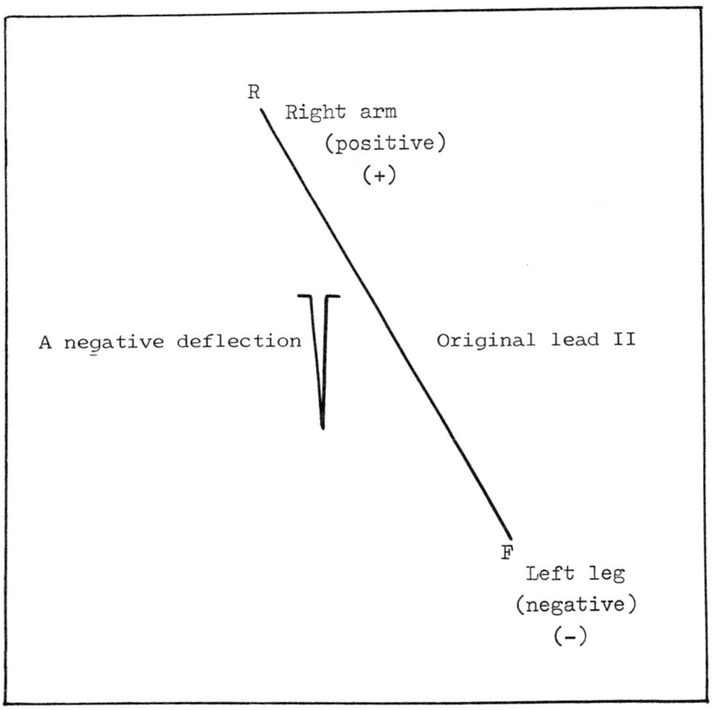

FIGURE 1–5. Formation of the original lead II. This was to be corrected later. See Figure 1–7.

In Figure 1–6*A*, Figures 1–3, 1–4 and 1–5 are brought together into a triangle, the *original* Einthoven triangle. Inspection of the triangle reveals a positive (+) charge and a negative (−) charge at each of the angles. The summation of the deflections also becomes apparent. If the triangle were to remain as indicated it should be noted that since:

a. the deflection in lead I = 5 mm.
b. the deflection in lead III = 5 mm.
c. the deflection in lead II = −10 mm.
the summation would be 0

and, therefore, leads I + III + II would equal 0.

A

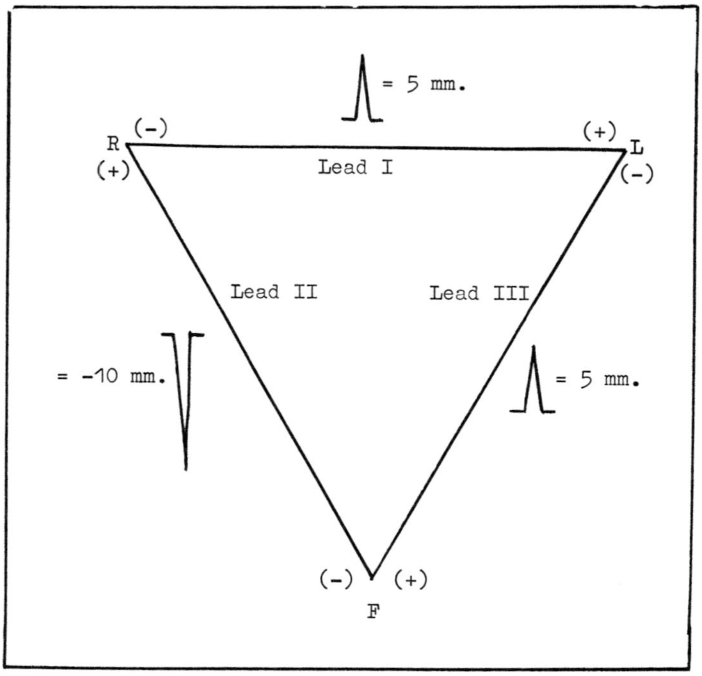

FIGURE 1–6*A*. The *original* Einthoven triangle.

Illustration continued on following page.

B

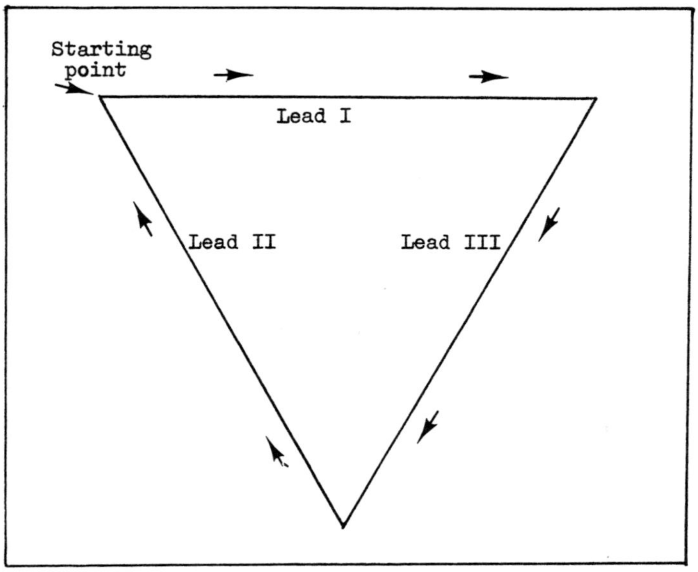

FIGURE 1–6*B*. Summation of the leads in the *original* Einthoven triangle.

In measuring the potentials, Einthoven originally started at the right arm, measuring first lead I, then lead III, then lead II, returning to the right arm (Fig. 1–6*B*). The vectorial sum of these potentials measured consecutively and returning to the point of origin equals 0. It would be as if you had travelled entirely around the world and returned to your point of origin. You would have travelled much but without any displacement. Einthoven, however, made a major change; he reversed the polarity of lead II (Fig. 1–7). According to Grant, it may be that he was not happy with a large negative deflection in lead II. By reversing the polarity of lead II—by making the right arm *negative* and the left leg *positive*—a positive deflection, of the same magnitude, resulted in lead II.

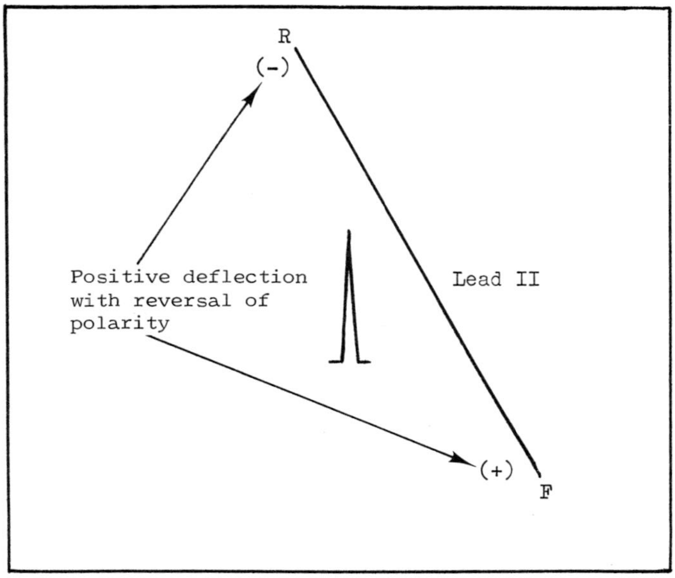

FIGURE 1–7. Lead II as known today, positive at the left leg and negative at the right arm, following reversal of polarity.

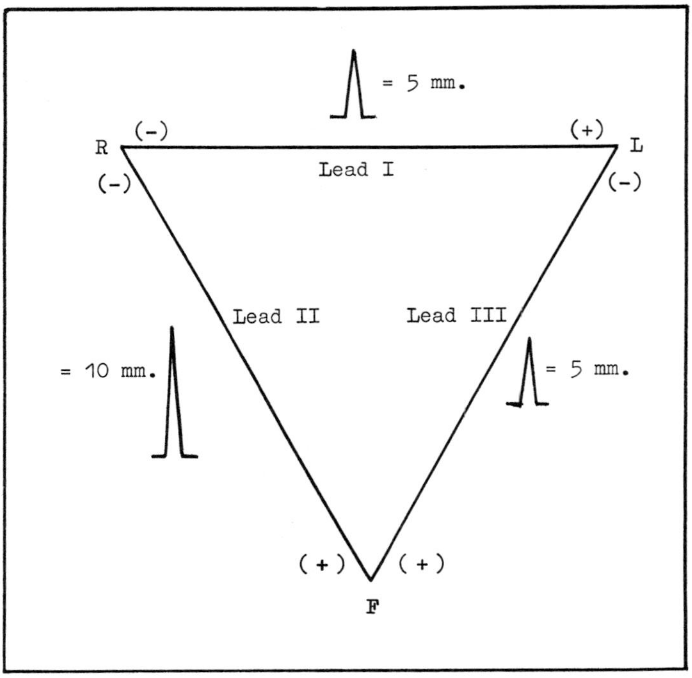

FIGURE 1–8. The Einthoven triangle as known today.

By reversing the polarity of lead II a new relationship was established (Figure 1–8). We no longer have the equation: leads I + III + II = 0. Note that since:

a. the deflection in lead I = 5 mm.
b. the deflection in lead III = 5 mm. and
c. the deflection in lead II = 10 mm.

the summation is as follows:

lead I + lead III = lead II

This is an electrical truth which always holds for the *areas* encompassed by each and every electrocardiographic deflection. We have used the heights and depths of the deflections as a good approximation.

Several assumptions are made in using the Einthoven triangle which are not strictly true. Note that:

a. The heart is not within a uniform volume conductor.

b. The leads do not form a true equilateral triangle.

c. The heart is not in the center of the triangle.

These, however, do not detract from the value of the Einthoven triangle in helping us to understand clinical electrocardiography.

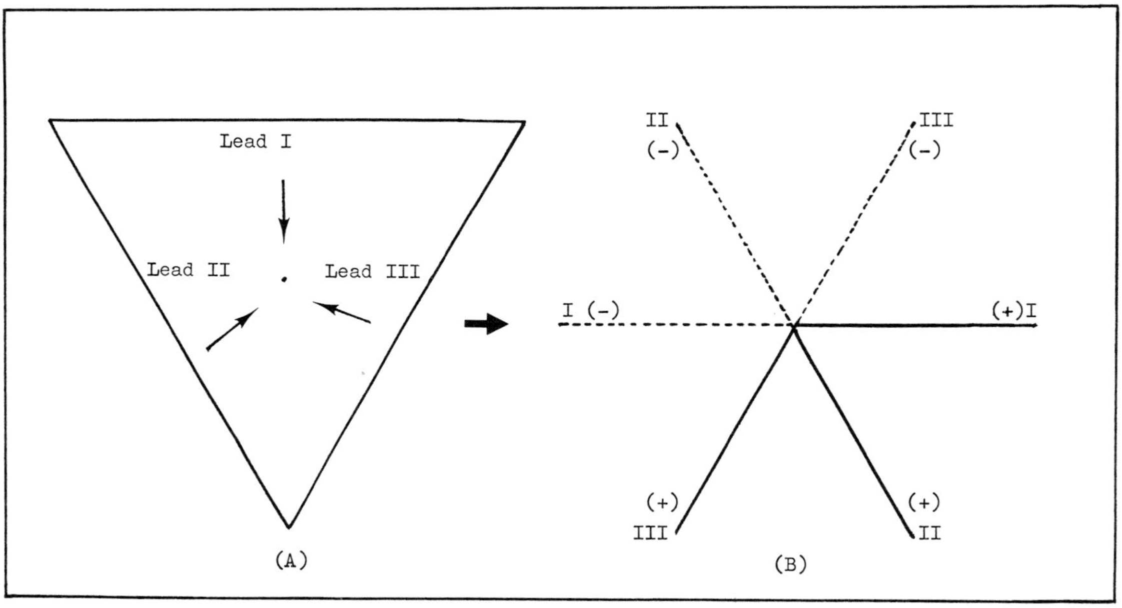

FIGURE 1–9. The Einthoven triangle (*A*) converted into a triaxial system (*B*).

Conversion of the Einthoven Triangle to a Triaxial System

In order to assign degrees, as presently used in electrocardiography, the Einthoven triangle (Fig. 1–9*A*) may be converted into a triaxial system (Fig. 1–9*B*) by bringing the sides of the triangle to the common center. The solid lines represent the positive half of each lead while the broken lines represent the negative half.

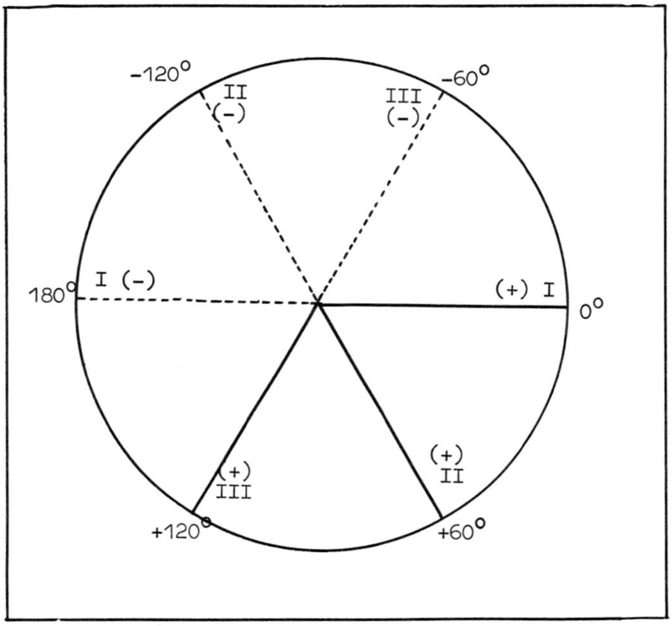

FIGURE 1–10. Indication of degrees. The solid line represents the positive half of each lead; the broken line represents the negative half.

In assigning degrees to the triaxial reference system the axes are 60° apart (Fig. 1–10). The positions of the positives and negatives remain as in the Einthoven triangle (Fig. 1–8).

In Figure 1–11 we have a further elaboration of the positive, negative and transitional zones of leads I, II and III. In Figure 1–11*A* positive lead I is indicated by the solid line at 0° and negative lead I by the broken line at 180°. Perpendicular to this line is the *transitional* zone of lead I. Lead I is most positive at the extreme left and most negative at the extreme right. As you approach the center from the positive and from the negative there is decreasing positivity and negativity, respectively. At the center of the circle, forming an angle of 90° with lead I, is the transitional zone, as noted above, the zone of null, which is neither positive nor negative (arrows); it divides the circle into two parts, one half positive and one half negative. The positive, negative and transitional zones of leads II and III are seen in Figure 1–11*B* and *C*, respectively.

Up to now we have been studying three leads, I, II and III. These are the *bipolar* extremity leads; each lead makes

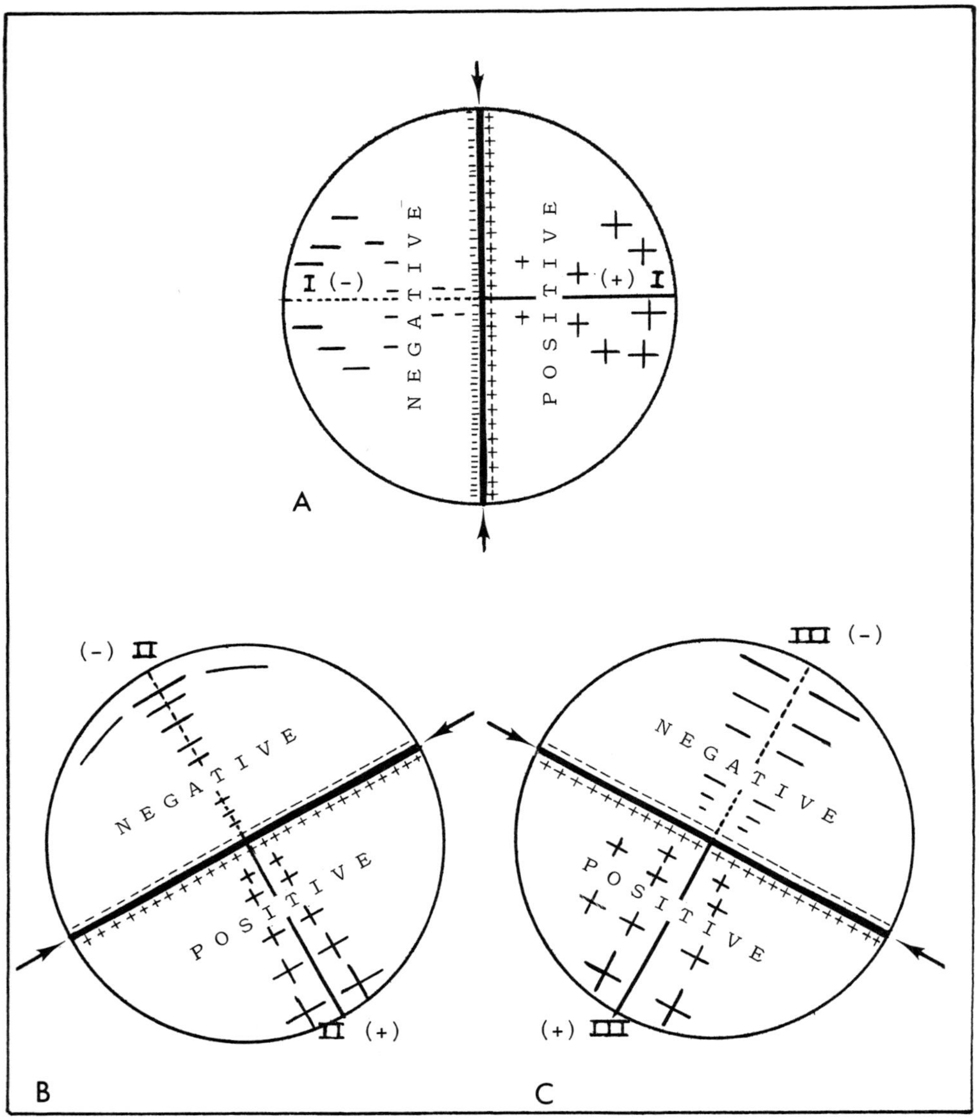

FIGURE 1–11. Positive, negative and transitional zones of leads I, II and III. The transitional zones are indicated by the arrows. Note the decreasing positivity and negativity as the transitional zone is approached.

use of *two* extremities, both arms for lead I, the right arm and left leg for lead II and the left arm and left leg for lead III. For many years these were the principal leads used in electrocardiography. In time other leads were added and became generally accepted. Among these were the *unipolar* extremity leads; only one pole, the *positive*, is attached to the right arm, left arm and left leg. The negative pole is attached to a central terminal. The letter V refers to these unipolar leads as well as to the precordial unipolar leads, to be studied later. The extremity unipolar leads were known as *VR* (right arm), *VL* (left arm) and *VF* (left leg). Following augmentation to produce larger deflections they are now known, respectively, as *aVR*, *aVL* and *aVF*. By adding these leads to the triaxial system (Fig. 1–10) a *hexaxial* system is formed. This is summarized in Figure 1–12. Each of the leads, *with the exception of aVR*, has its positive pole in the part of the circle from −30° to +120°. The positive pole of lead aVR is at −150°, which is outside the part

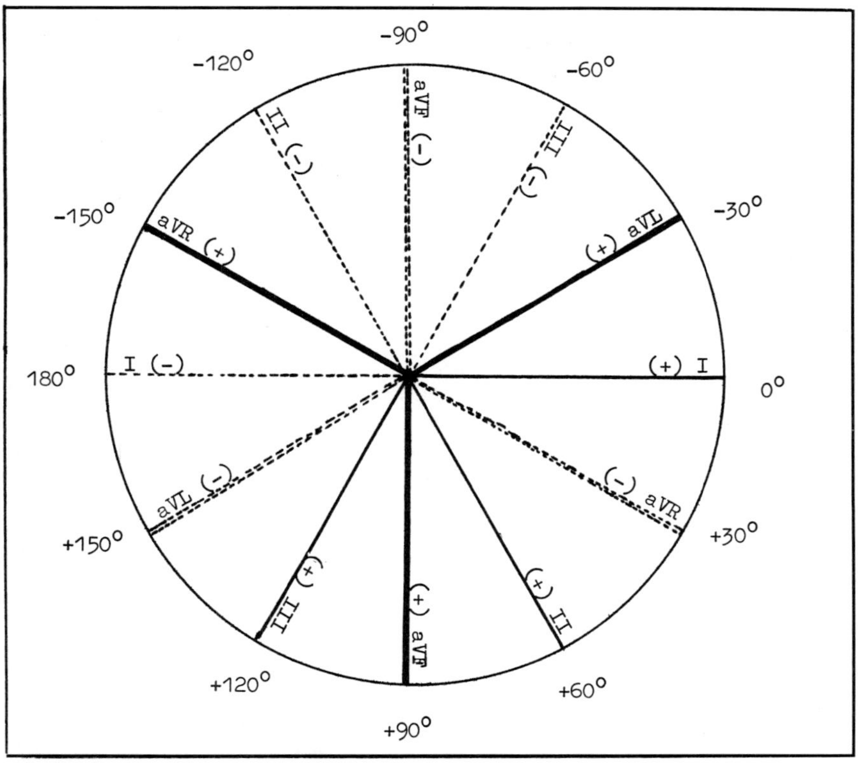

FIGURE 1–12. Formation of the hexaxial system. Addition of the three unipolar leads, aVR, aVL and aVF, with degrees assigned to all leads.* The solid line represents the positive half of each lead; the broken line represents the negative half. The part of the circle most frequently dealt with in clinical electrocardiography contains:

positive aVL	−30°
positive I	0°
negative aVR	+30°
positive II	+60°
positive aVF	+90°
positive III	+120°

Note that *negative* aVR at +30° is used. Positive aVR is at −150°, not in the part of the circle that is normally used.

Note: We have seen that *Leads I + III = Lead II.* The rule for Leads aVR, aVL and aVF is as follows: *Leads aVR + aVL + aVF = 0.* There was no reversal of polarity, as occurred in Lead II.

*By adding these leads to the triaxial system (Figure 1–10) a *hexaxial* system is formed, containing six leads.

of the circle normally utilized. *Negative aVR* at +30° is, therefore, frequently used in electrocardiographic evaluation.

In Figure 1–8 the summation for the bipolar extremity leads was shown to be

lead I + lead III = lead II

The summation for the unipolar extremity leads is as follows:

leads aVR + aVL + aVF = 0

Refer back to the discussion on the reversal of polarity in lead II. There was no such reversal of polarity for the unipolar extremity leads.

These relationships are of importance in the evaluation of every electrocardiogram and will be described in Figures 1–13 to 1–20.

PRACTICE ELECTROCARDIOGRAMS FOR ILLUSTRATION OF THE ELECTRICAL TRUTHS

Leads I + III = Lead II
Leads aVR + aVL + aVF = 0

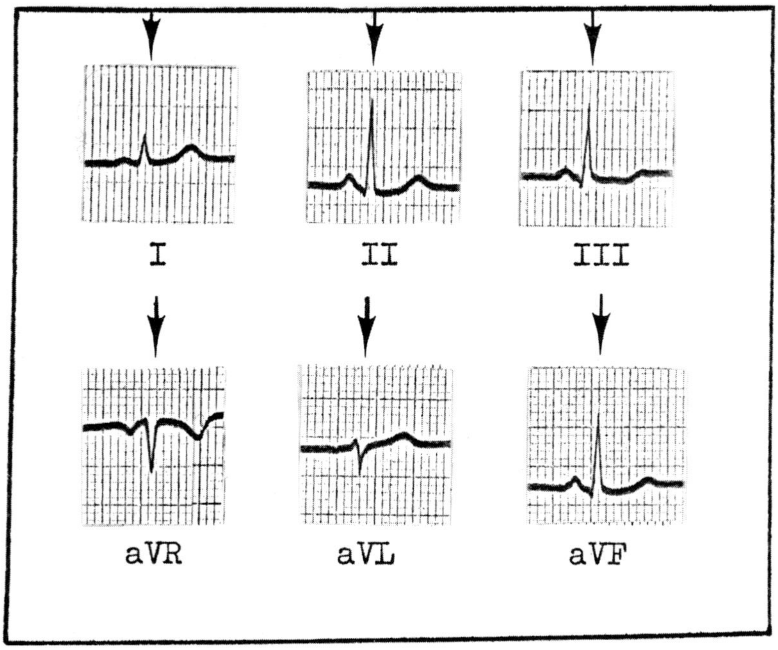

FIGURE 1–13. The deflection in lead I (arrow) is approximately 3 mm. tall and the deflection in lead III is 9 mm. tall. Using the rule that

leads I + III = lead II

the lead II deflection must be 12 mm. tall. Anytime you have two leads you should be able to solve for the third. The deflection in lead aVR is 6 mm. deep and the deflection in lead aVL is 4 mm. deep. Using the rule that

leads aVR + aVL + aVF = 0

the lead aVF deflection must be approximately 10 mm. tall.

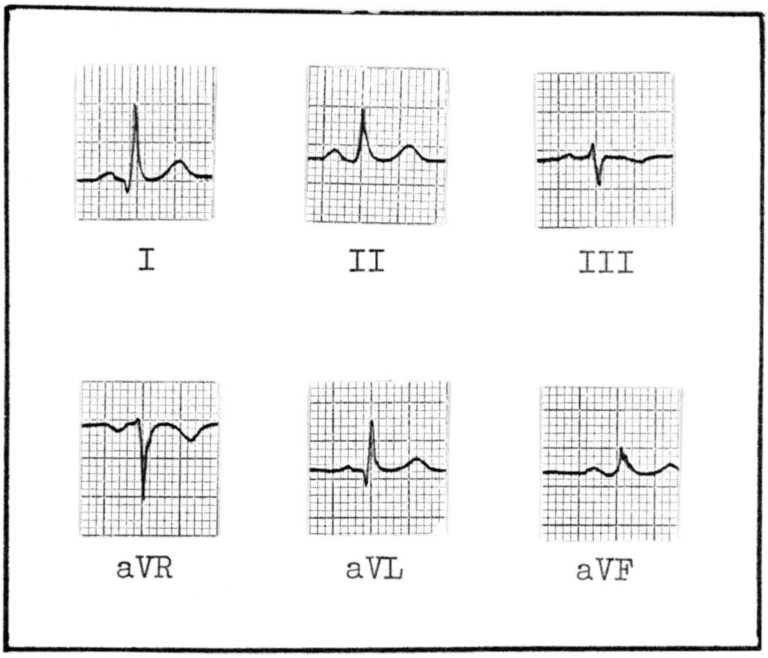

FIGURE 1–14. Lead I is taller than lead II, therefore lead III must be negative. Lead aVR is deeper than aVL is tall, therefore aVF must be small but positive.

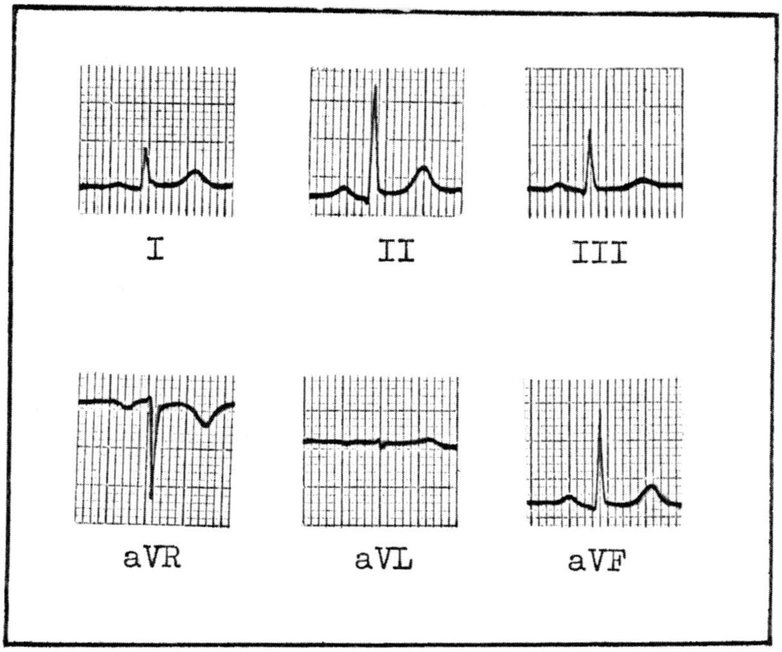

FIGURE 1-15. Leads I + III = lead II. Lead aVR is as deep as aVF is tall, therefore aVL must summate to 0, since leads aVR + aVL + aVF = 0.

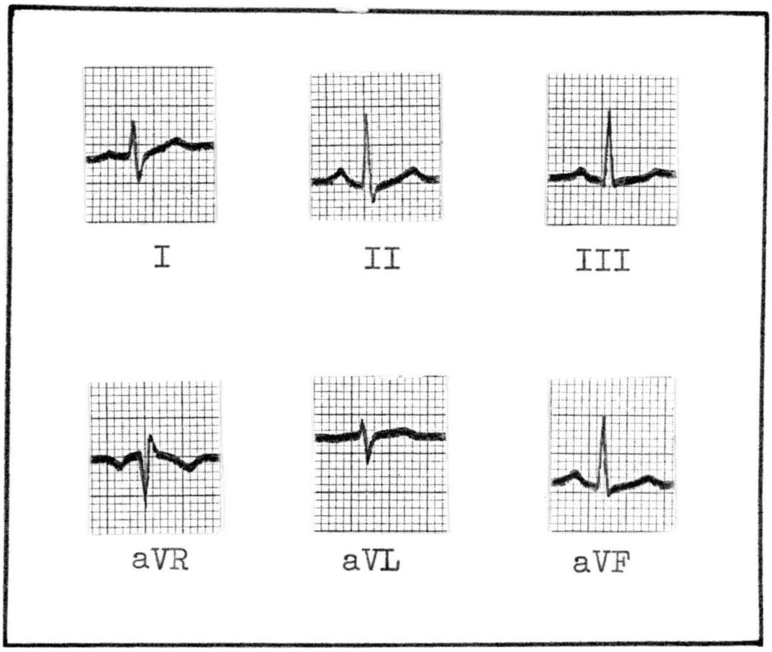

FIGURE 1-16. Lead II is approximately equal to lead III. Therefore, lead I must summate to approximately 0. Lead aVF is slightly taller than aVR is deep; therefore, aVL is slightly more negative than positive.

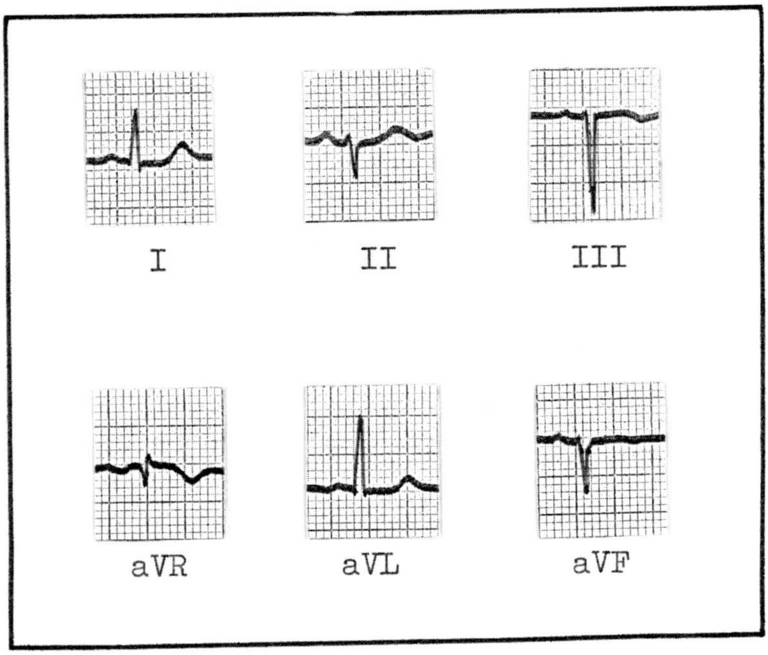

FIGURE 1–17. Lead I is less positive than lead III is negative. Lead II must then be negative. The negative aVR plus the negative aVF plus the positive aVL equal 0.

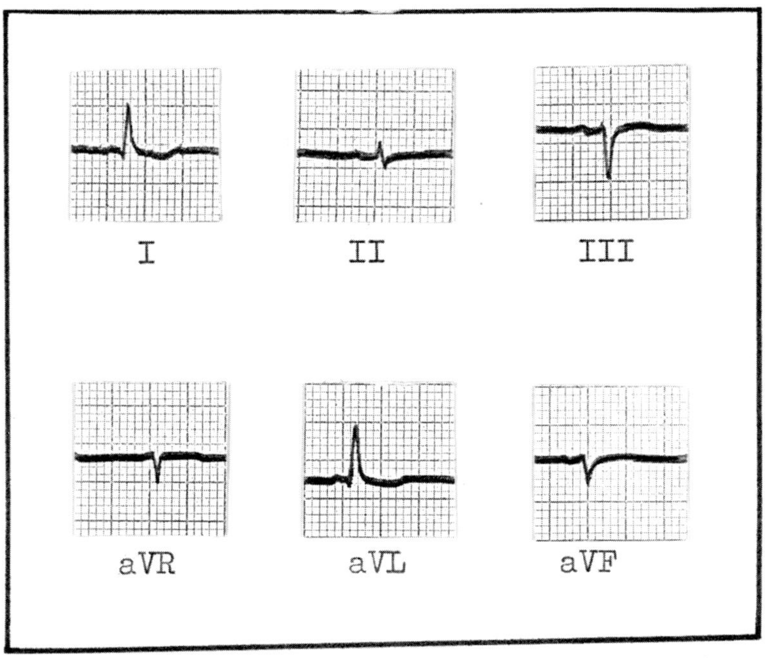

FIGURE 1–18. Lead II is small and equiphasic; lead I is then as positive as lead III is negative. Lead aVL is as positive as aVR plus aVF are negative.

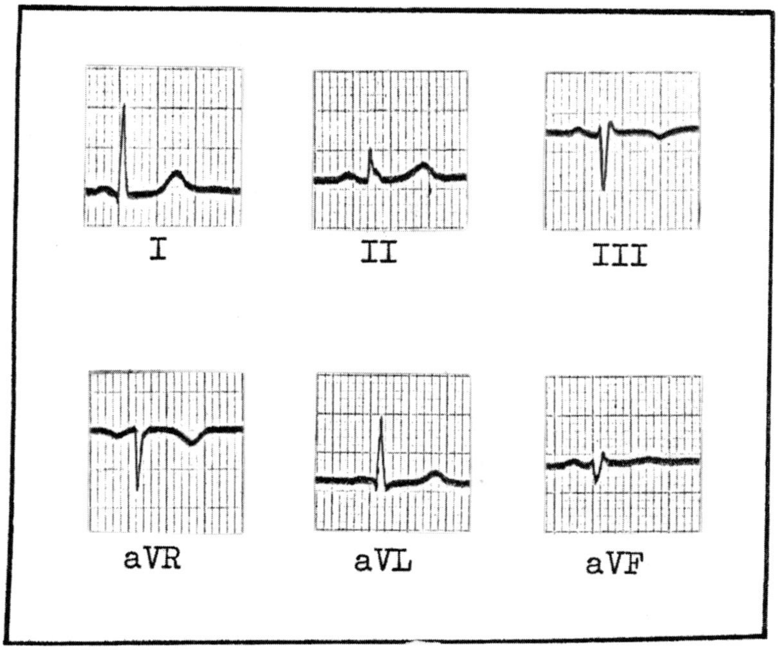

FIGURE 1–19. Lead III is less negative than lead I is positive. Lead II must then be smaller than lead I, but positive. The negative aVR plus the negative aVF plus the positive aVL equal 0.

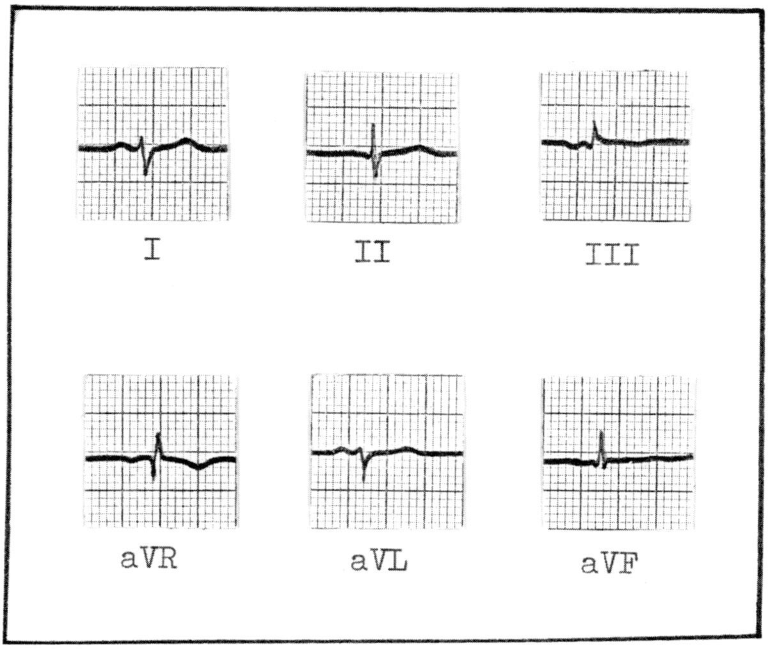

FIGURE 1–20. To reemphasize for convenience we have been using the height and depth of the deflections for summation; this gives a good approximation. Actually, for more accurate summation, the area encompassed by the deflections may be used. The rules again:

Leads I + III = lead II
Leads aVR + aVL + aVF = 0

Cassette Side 2

DEPOLARIZATION, REPOLARIZATION AND THE CONDUCTION SYSTEM OF THE HEART

Positive and negative ions line up on opposite sides of the semipermeable membrane which is found in all excitable tissue, including, of course, the heart. If a change occurs in the state of the semipermeable membrane, the ions then may cross. The state when the ions are lined up on their respective sides is the *polarized* state. *Depolarization* refers to the state when the ions have crossed the semipermeable membrane, and the process of restoring them to the proper side of the semipermeable membrane is the process of *repolarization*.

The normal site of impulse formation in the heart is the sinoatrial (S-A) node (Fig. 1–21). The atria are then depolarized, resulting in the P wave on the electrocardiogram. There is much ongoing research in the area of the specialized conduction system of the atria. The impulse then spreads through the atrioventricular (A-V) node and bundle of His to the left and right bundle branches and then to the ventricular muscle through the Purkinje network. The ventricular depolarization results in the inscription of the QRS complex on the electrocardiogram.

The S–T segment and T wave represent the repolarization of the ventricles (Fig. 1–22). Repolarization of the *atria* is usually obscured on the electrocardiogram by the small size of the waves and by the proximity of the QRS complex.

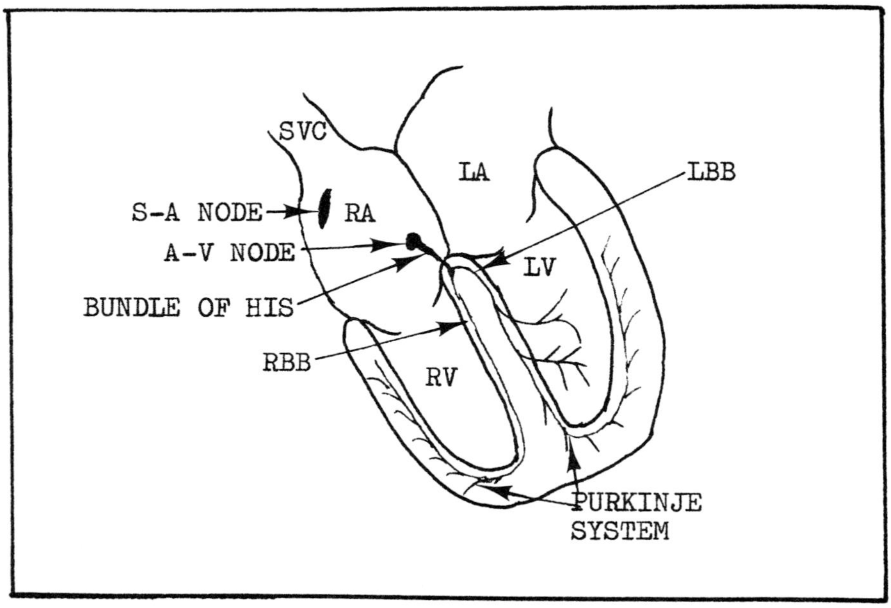

FIGURE 1–21. Conduction system of the heart. Abbreviations are as follows:

SVC	Superior vena cava
RA	Right atrium
LA	Left atrium
RV	Right ventricle
LV	Left ventricle
S–A	Sinoatrial (node)
A–V	Atrioventricular (node)
RBB	Right bundle branch
LBB	Left bundle branch

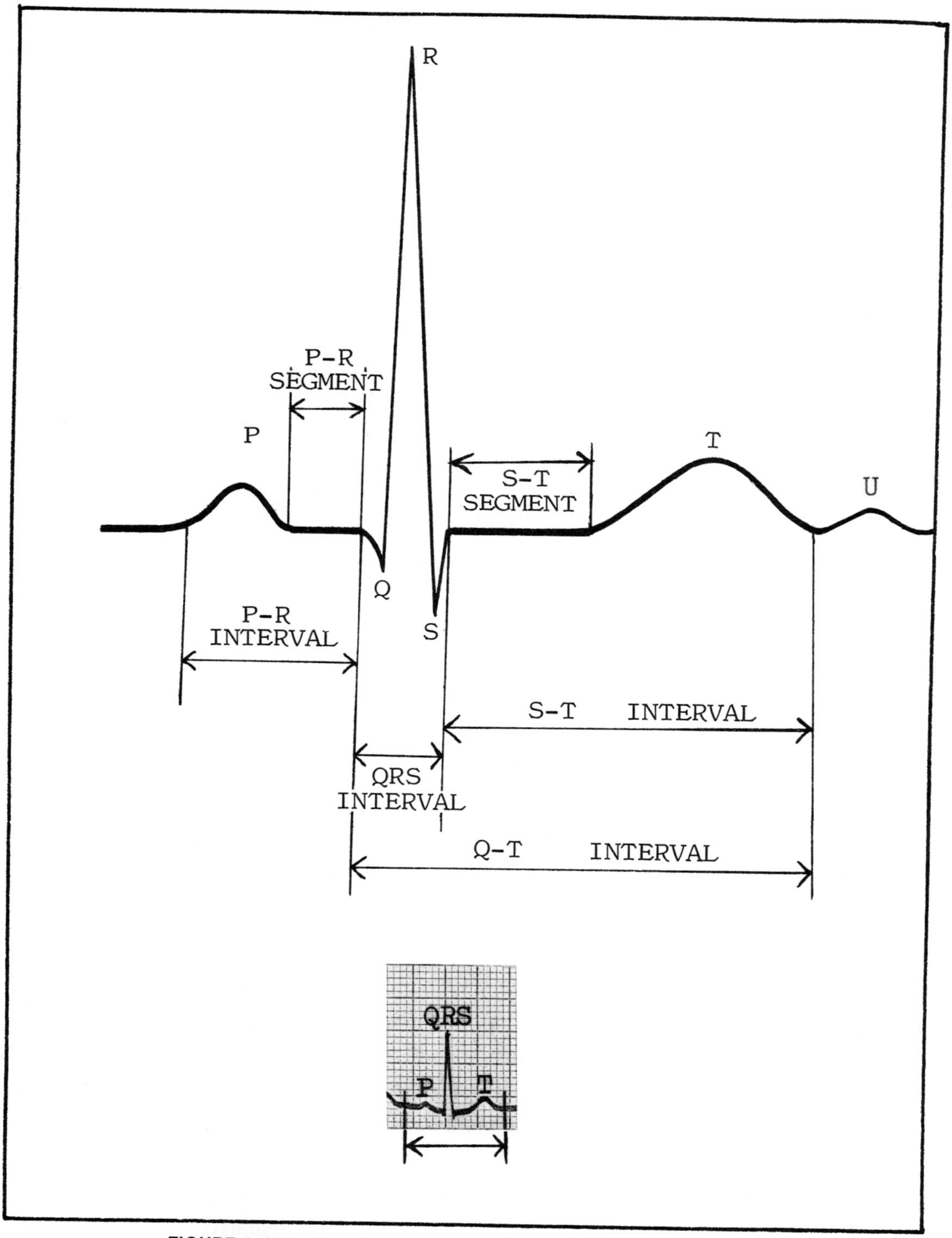

FIGURE 1–22. Electrocardiographic waves, intervals and segments.

TABLE 1–1. ELECTROCARDIOGRAPHIC WAVES, INTERVALS AND SEGMENTS (See Fig. 1–22)

P Wave. The P wave is produced by the depolarization of the atria.

QRS Complex. The QRS complex is produced by the depolarization of the ventricles.

Q Wave. The Q wave is the initial negative deflection of the QRS complex preceding the R wave.

R Wave. The R wave is the initial positive deflection of the QRS complex.

S Wave. The S wave is a negative deflection following the R wave and usually the terminal portion of the QRS complex. A second positive deflection (following the S wave) is called an R′ wave, which in turn may be followed by an S′ wave.

QS Complex. The QS complex means that there is no R wave. The entire ventricular complex is negative.

T Wave. The T wave is produced by the repolarization of the ventricles.

U Wave. The U wave follows the T wave. Its clinical significance will be illustrated in Chapter 4. It is not often seen in the normal electrocardiogram.

P–R Interval. From the beginning of the P wave to the beginning of the QRS complex. When a Q wave is present the interval may be called a P–Q interval.

P–R Segment. From the end of the P wave to the beginning of the QRS complex.

QRS Interval. From the beginning of the Q wave to the end of the S wave.

S–T Segment. From the end of the S wave to the beginning of the T wave representing the early phase of ventricular repolarization.

S–T Interval. From the end of the S wave to the end of the T wave representing the repolarization of the ventricles.

Q–T Interval. From the beginning of the QRS complex to the end of the T wave.

THE CARDIAC VECTORS

Electrical forces can be considered vector quantities. (The properties of a vector are magnitude, direction and sense.) A vector is represented by an arrow where both size and orientation are easily demonstrated. Let us relate this to the inscription of a single normal QRS complex on the electrocardiogram (Fig. 1–23*A*) within a period of 0.08 sec. (The normal QRS interval, from the beginning of the Q wave to the end of the S wave, does not exceed 0.10 sec.). Figure 1–23*B* illustrates the sequential instantaneous vectors generated during this single QRS cycle. The greater the muscle mass, the bigger will be the arrow. The magnitude and orientation of the vector will be determined from the position of the heart and the muscle mass, and the electrical and conductive properties of the heart. When we connect the arrows, which were drawn as if they arose from the same point of origin, we have what is known as the QRS loop (Fig. 1–23*C*). The *mean QRS vector* is the vectorial sum of all the instantaneous vectors within a single QRS cycle (Fig. 1–23*D*). We will often refer to the mean QRS vector, mean T vector and mean P vector in our study of electrocardiography. You may hear, because of common usage, the term "mean electrical axis" of the QRS, T and P when referring to the mean QRS, T and P vectors, respectively.

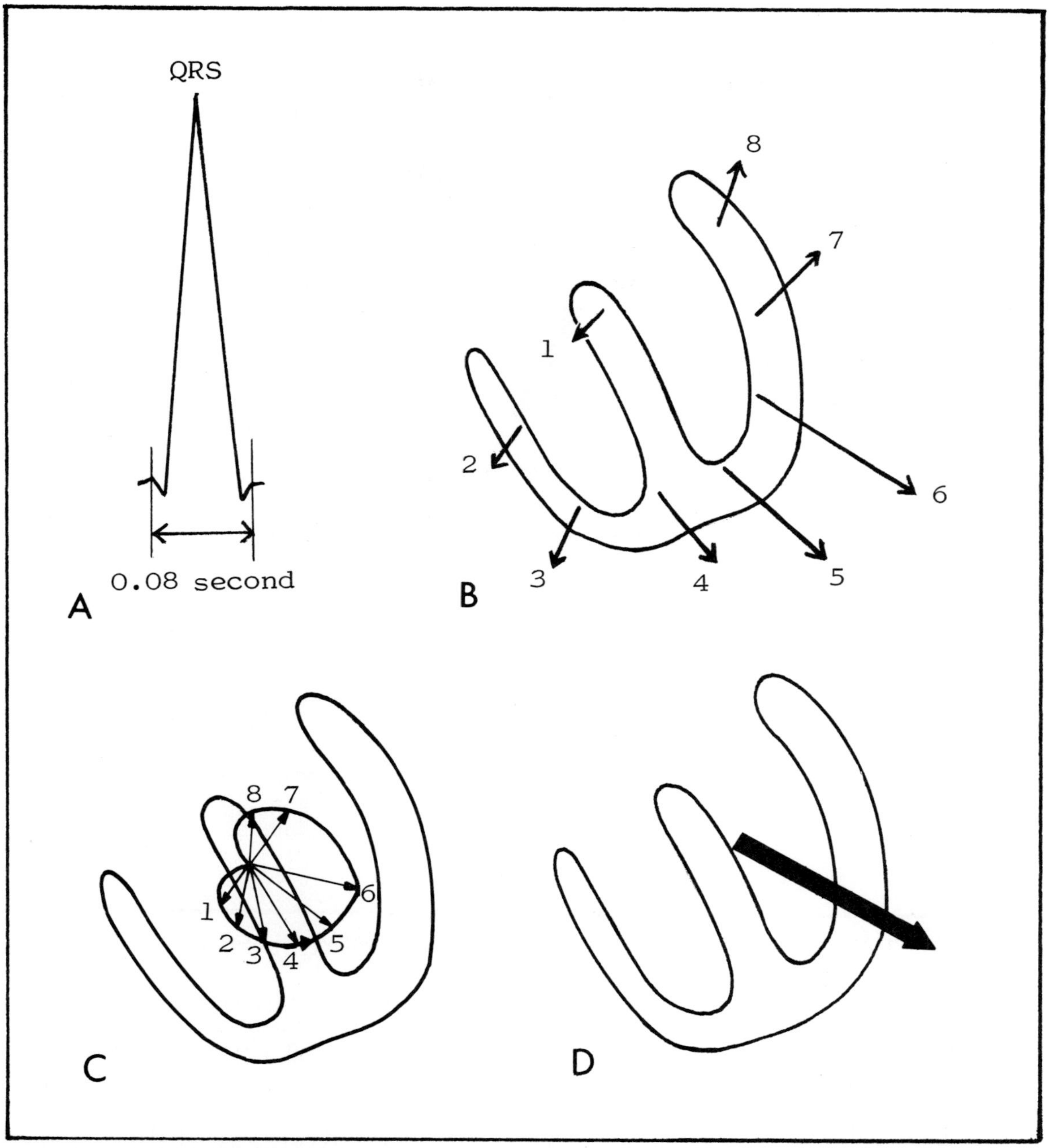

FIGURE 1–23. *A,* Inscription of a single normal QRS complex (0.08 sec.). *B,* Sequential instantaneous vectors generated during this single QRS cycle. *C,* QRS loop results when we connect the arrows which were drawn as if they arose from the same point of origin. *D,* Mean QRS vector which is the vectorial sum of all the instantaneous vectors within a single QRS cycle.

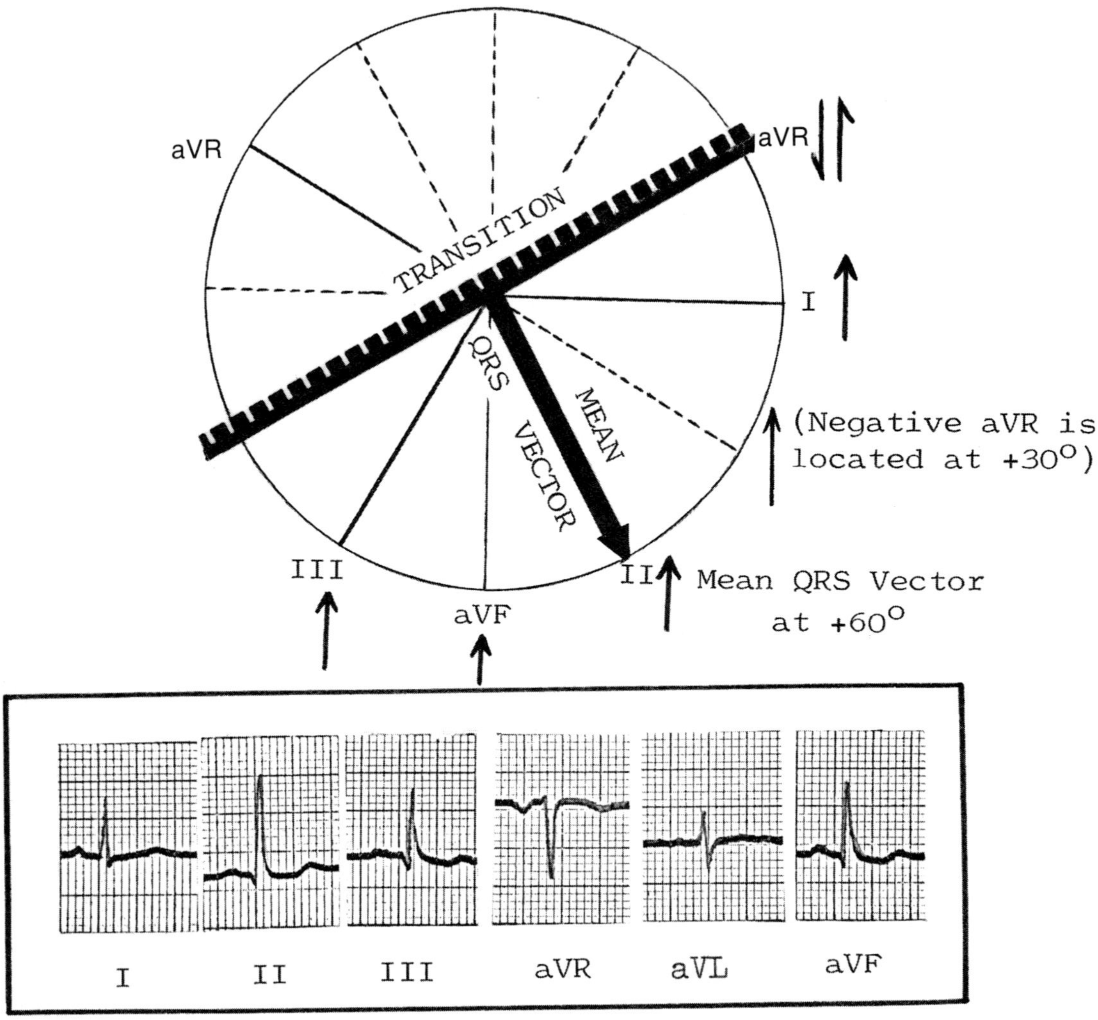

FIGURE 1–24. Determination of the transitional zone and mean QRS vector. See text.

Determination of the Mean QRS Vector in the Frontal Plane

The mean QRS vector is a major determinant of the normality or abnormality of the electrocardiogram. In the following series of electrocardiograms we will determine the mean QRS vector in the *frontal plane.** Prior to starting, this would be a good place to review the Einthoven triangle, the positive, negative and transitional zones of the leads and the "lineup" of the leads around the circle (Figs. 1–8 and 1–10 to 1–12).

**Leads I, II, III, aVR, aVL and aVF* represent electrical activity in the *frontal plane.* The boundaries of the frontal plane are illustrated in Figure 1–54.

In Figure 1–24 let us examine the electrocardiogram as to the positivity and negativity of each QRS complex. In lead I the QRS is positive and is so indicated on the circle next to lead I at 0°. Lead II is also positive, as is lead III. *Negative* aVR is also positive. When lining up the leads remember that *negative* aVR is at +30°; lead aVR must then be inverted before being placed on the circle. Lead aVL is neither predominantly positive nor predominantly negative; it is a transitional lead. Lead aVF is positive. The transition is through lead aVL. The *mean QRS vector* is at right angles to the transitional zone on the positive side. In this electrocardiogram the *transitional zone* is at −30° and the *mean QRS vector* is at 60°.

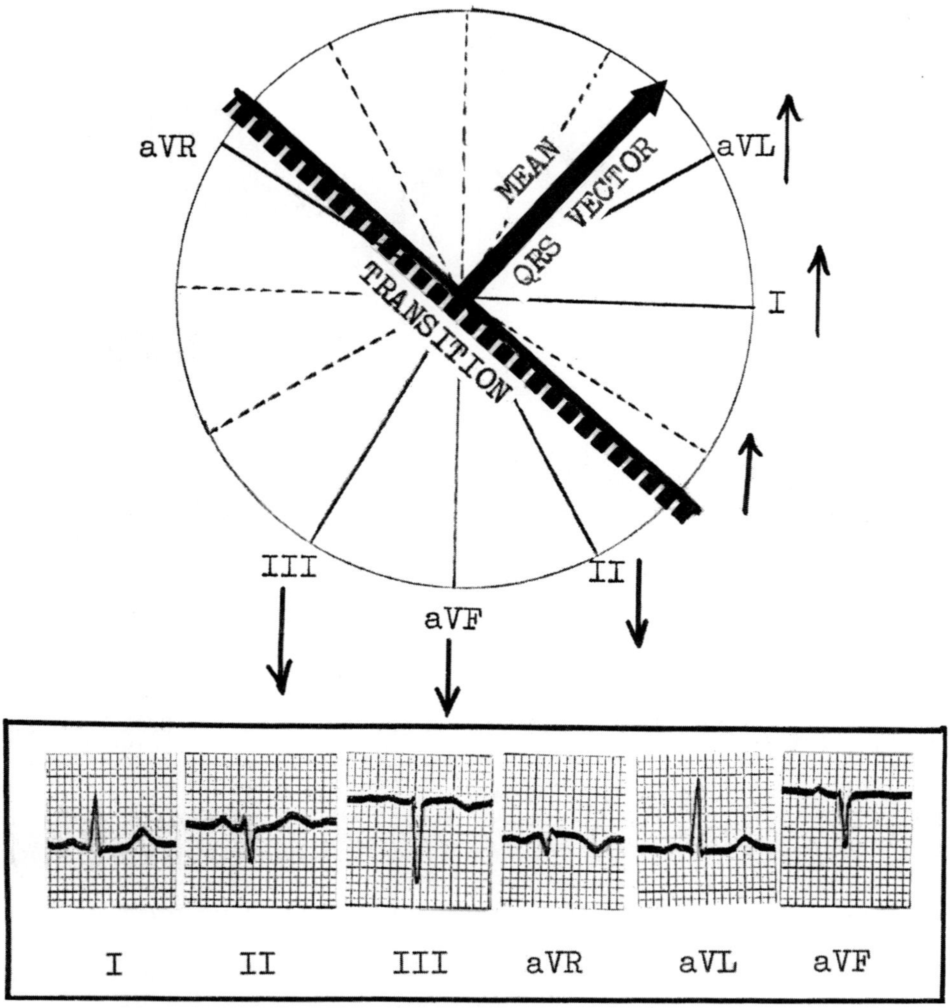

FIGURE 1–25. Mean QRS vector beyond −30°.

In Figure 1–25 lead I is positive, II and III are negative, while *negative* aVR and aVL are positive. Lead aVF is negative. The transitional zone is somewhere between 30° and 60°, with the mean QRS vector at right angles to the transition, on the positive side, beyond −30°. All the positive QRS complexes are in the positive half of the circle and all the negative QRS complexes are in the negative half of the circle. The positive half is the upper part of the circle, hence the mean QRS vector is within this half.

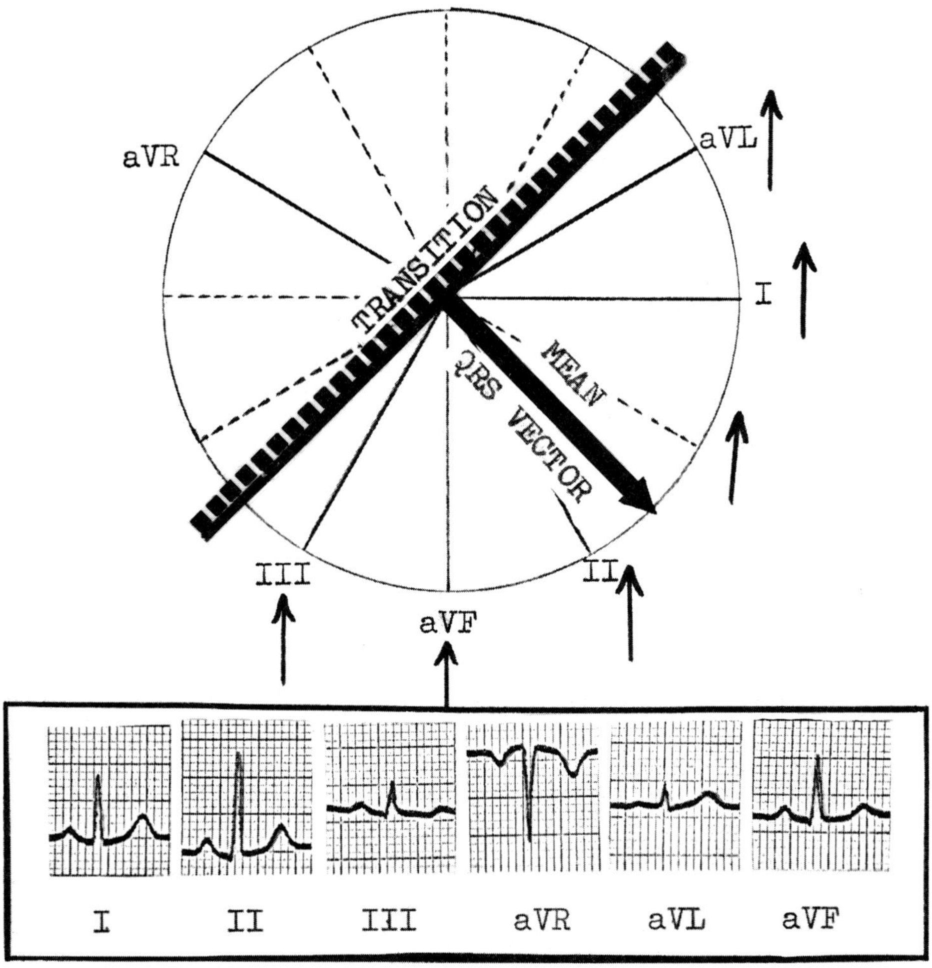

FIGURE 1–26. Mean QRS vector at 45°.

In Figure 1–26 all the QRS complexes are positive. The transitional zone must then bypass all six leads so that all the leads fall within the positive half of the circle. The mean QRS vector, at right angles to the transition, on the positive side, is approximately 45°.

The use of the positivity and negativity of the QRS complexes is a good approximation. The exact measurement of the area under each deflection would not be practical in a clinical setting.

REVIEW

To determine the mean QRS vector in the frontal plane the following should be done sequentially.

1. Line up all six leads on the circle from −30° to +120°. Lead aVR must be inverted at +30°.
2. Draw the transition, dividing the circle into positive and negative halves.
3. The mean QRS vector is at right angles to the transition on the positive side.

The mean QRS vector was studied in three electrocardiograms (Figs. 1–24 to 1–26) and the steps used in this determination were outlined. The following electrocardiograms (Figs. 1–27 to 1–35) are presented for your evaluation. The six leads are seen both in the conventional sequence and also around the circle. Determine the transitional zone and mean QRS vector from the electrocardiogram at the bottom of each figure, then check with the circle above. Do not forget to invert lead aVR since we are dealing with negative aVR at +30°.

PRACTICE ELECTROCARDIOGRAMS FOR THE DETERMINATION OF MEAN QRS VECTOR IN THE FRONTAL PLANE

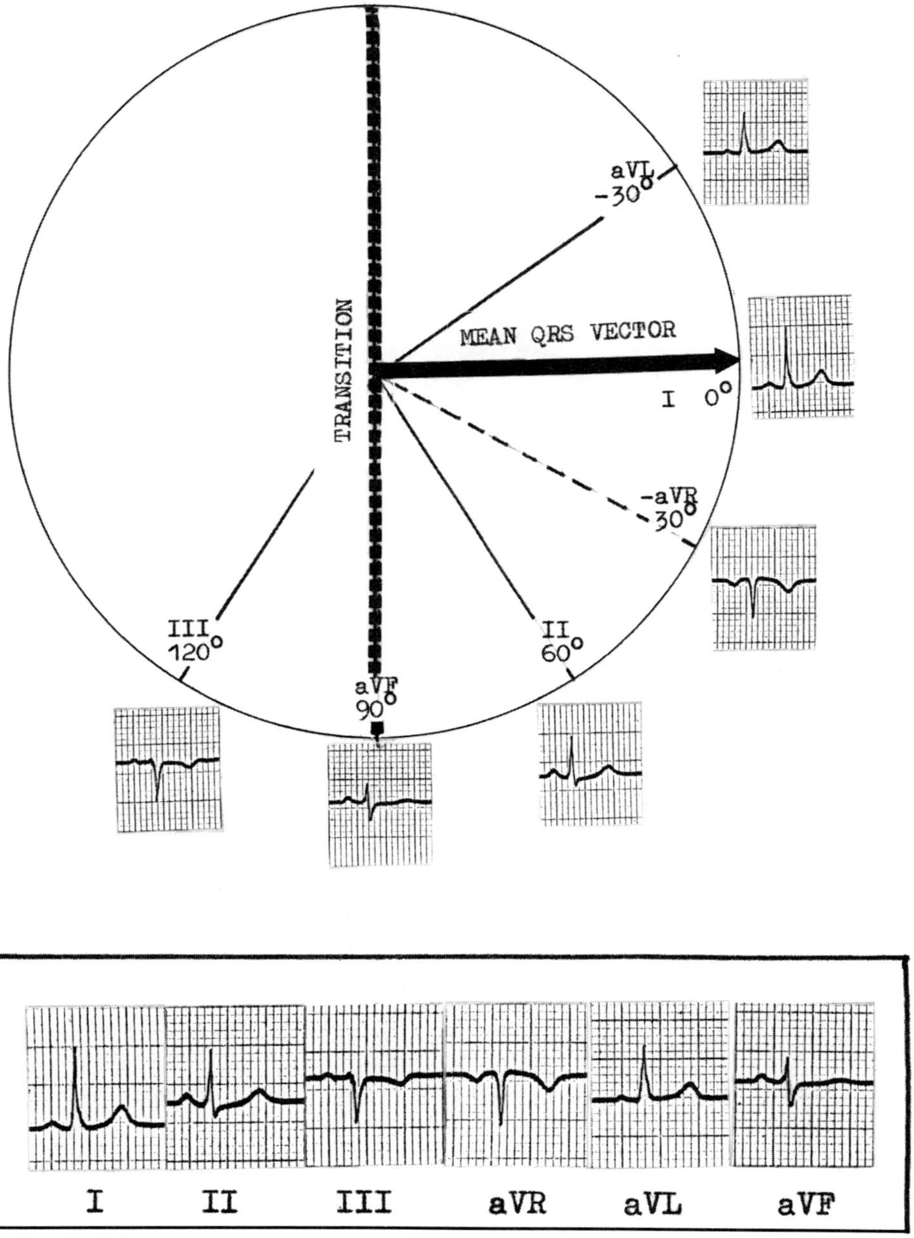

FIGURE 1–27. Leads aVL, I, −aVR and II are positive and lead III is negative. Lead aVF is transitional. We draw the transition at aVF, and the mean QRS vector is perpendicular to the transition, on the positive side (lead I at 0°).

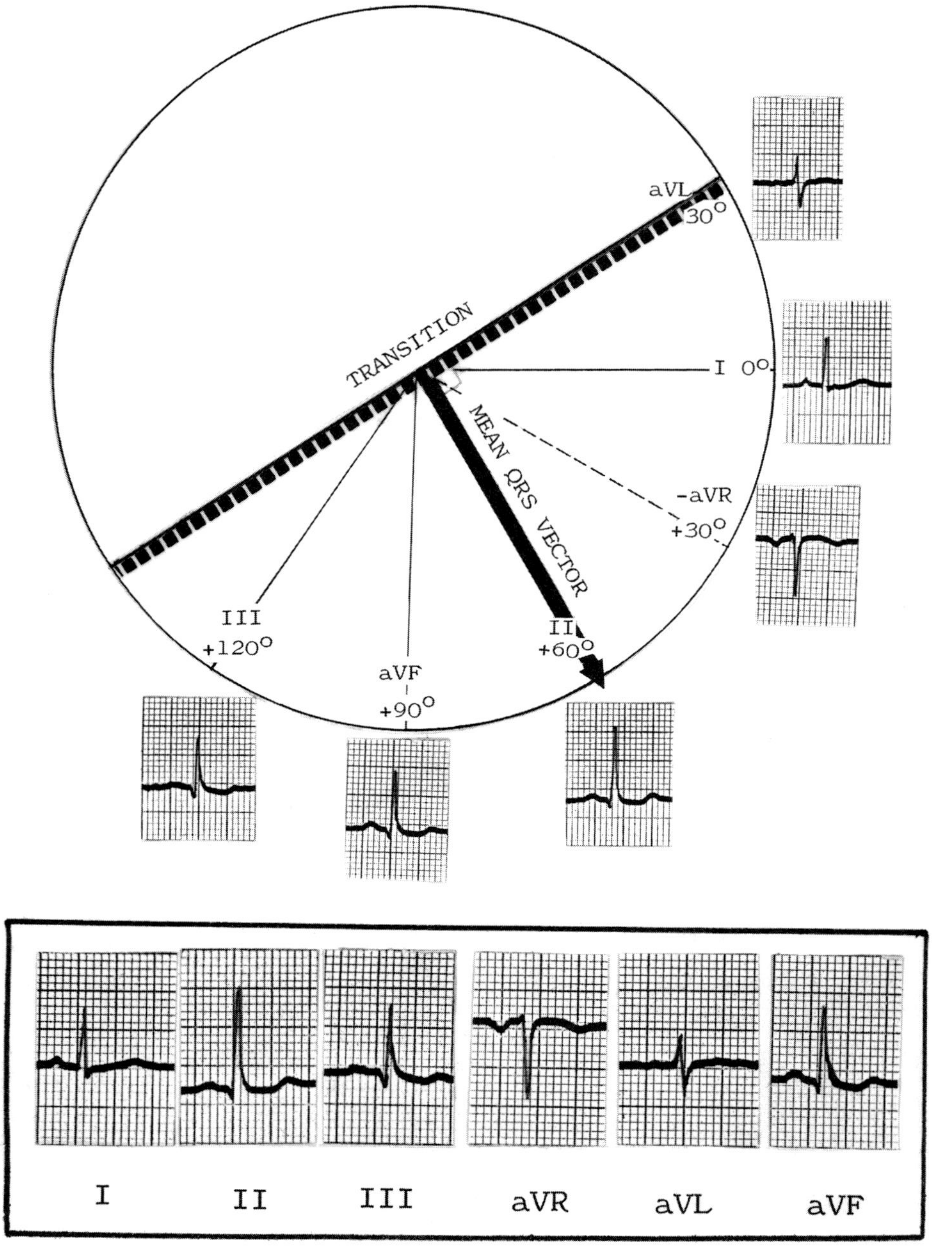

FIGURE 1-28. Leads I, II, III, negative aVR and aVF are positive. Lead aVL is transitional. We therefore draw the transition through the axis of aVL. The mean QRS vector is perpendicular to this transition, towards the positive (lead II at 60°).

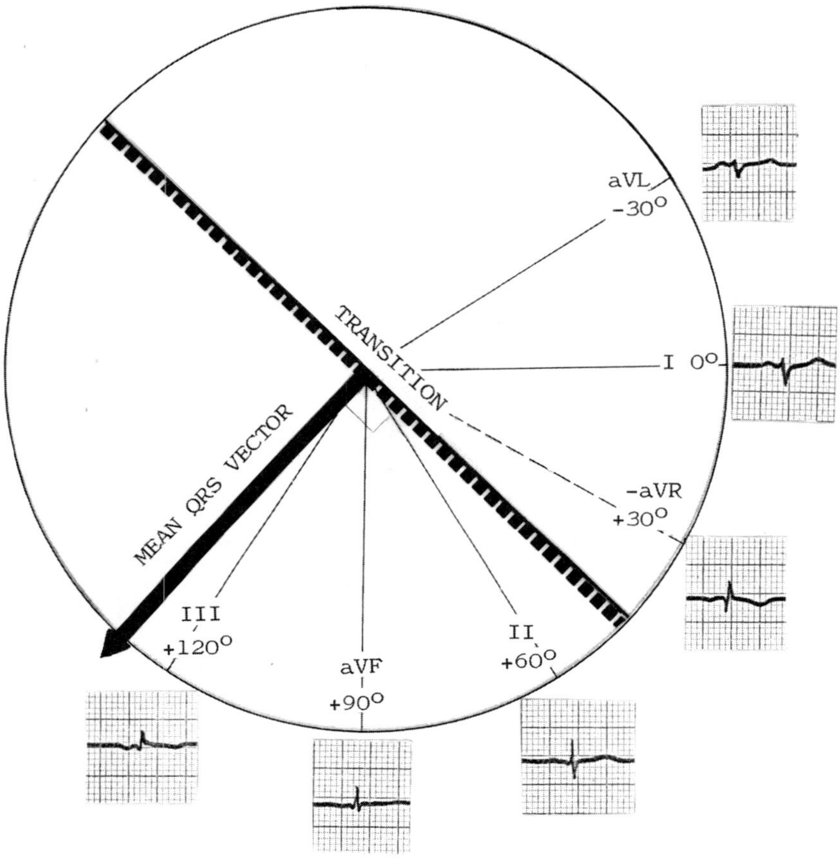

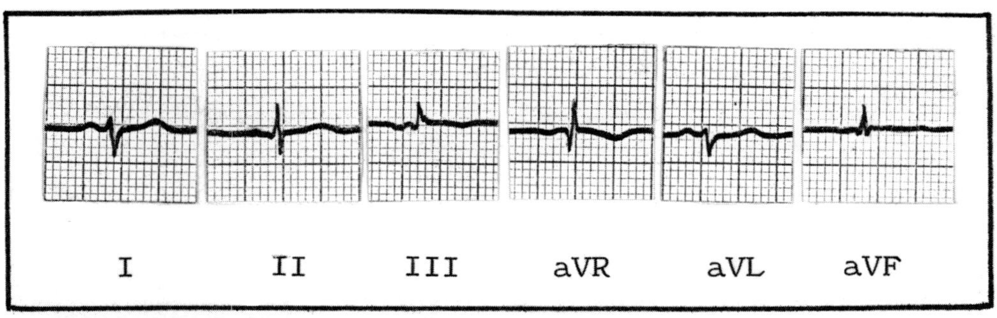

FIGURE 1–29. Leads I and aVL are negative, while leads III and aVF are positive. Lead II is slightly more positive, while negative aVR is slightly more negative. The transition, therefore, falls between leads −aVR and II, with the mean QRS vector beyond lead III (beyond 120°).

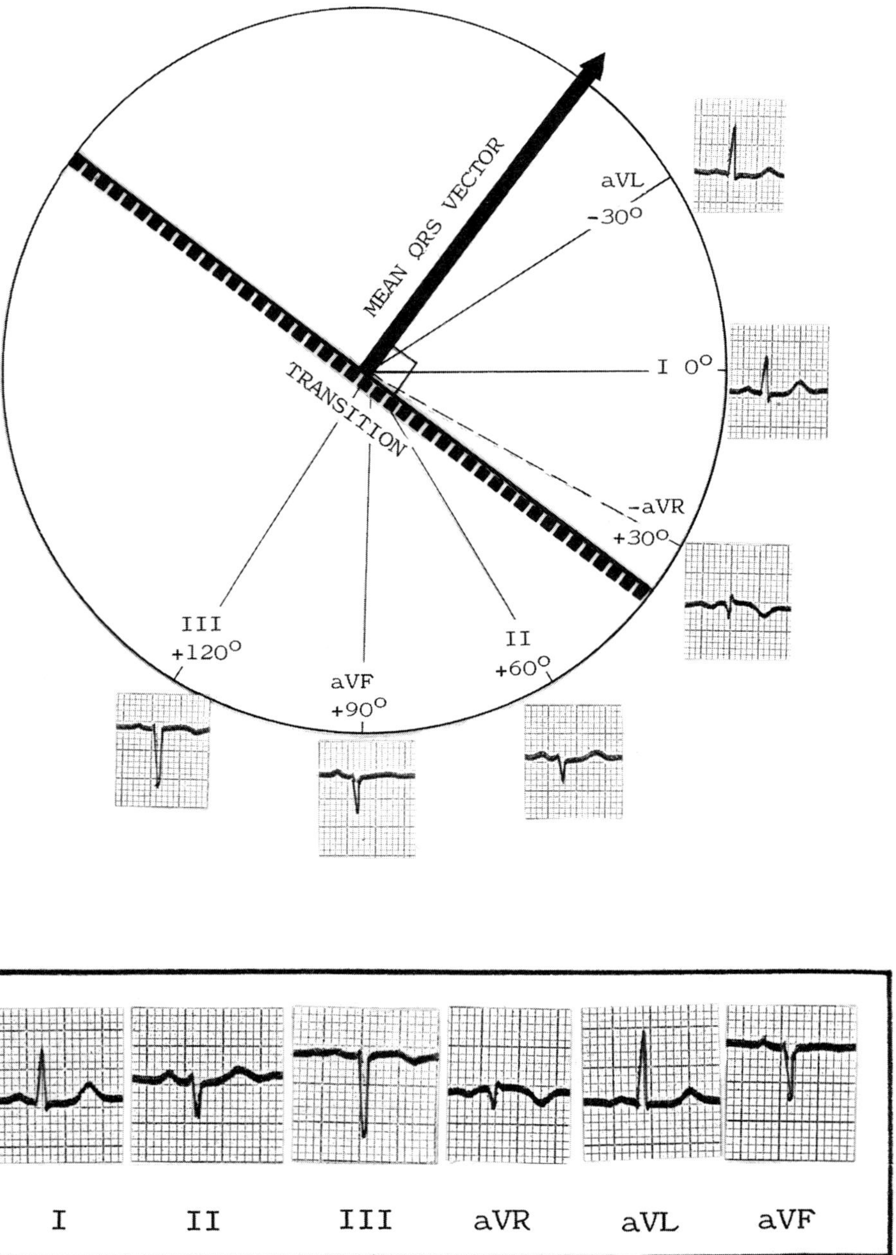

FIGURE 1–30. Leads aVL, I and −aVR are positive and leads II, aVF and III are negative. The transition is between leads −aVR and II, with the mean QRS vector beyond −30°.

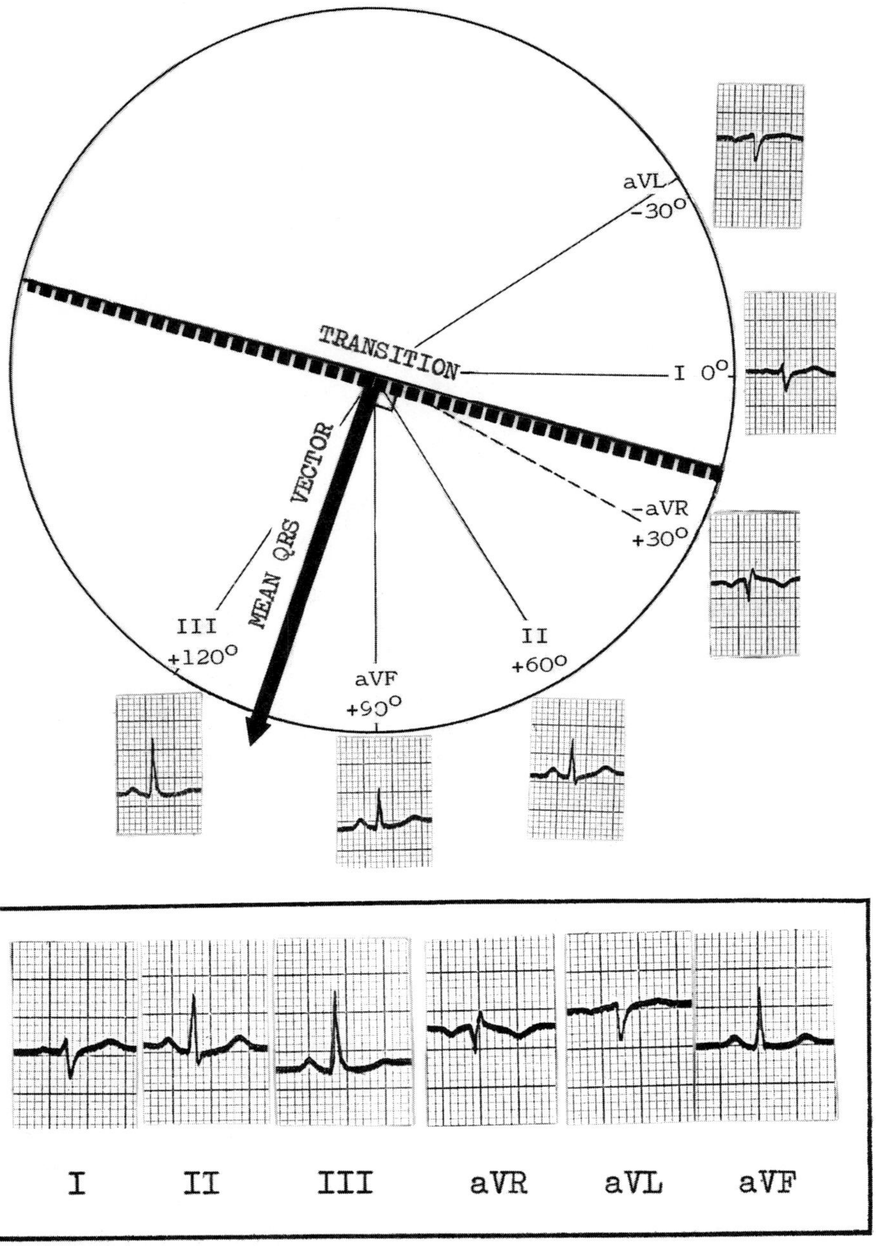

FIGURE 1–31. Leads aVL and I are negative and leads −aVR, II, aVF and III are positive. The transition is between leads I and −aVR and the mean QRS vector is between leads aVF and III (between +90° and +120°).

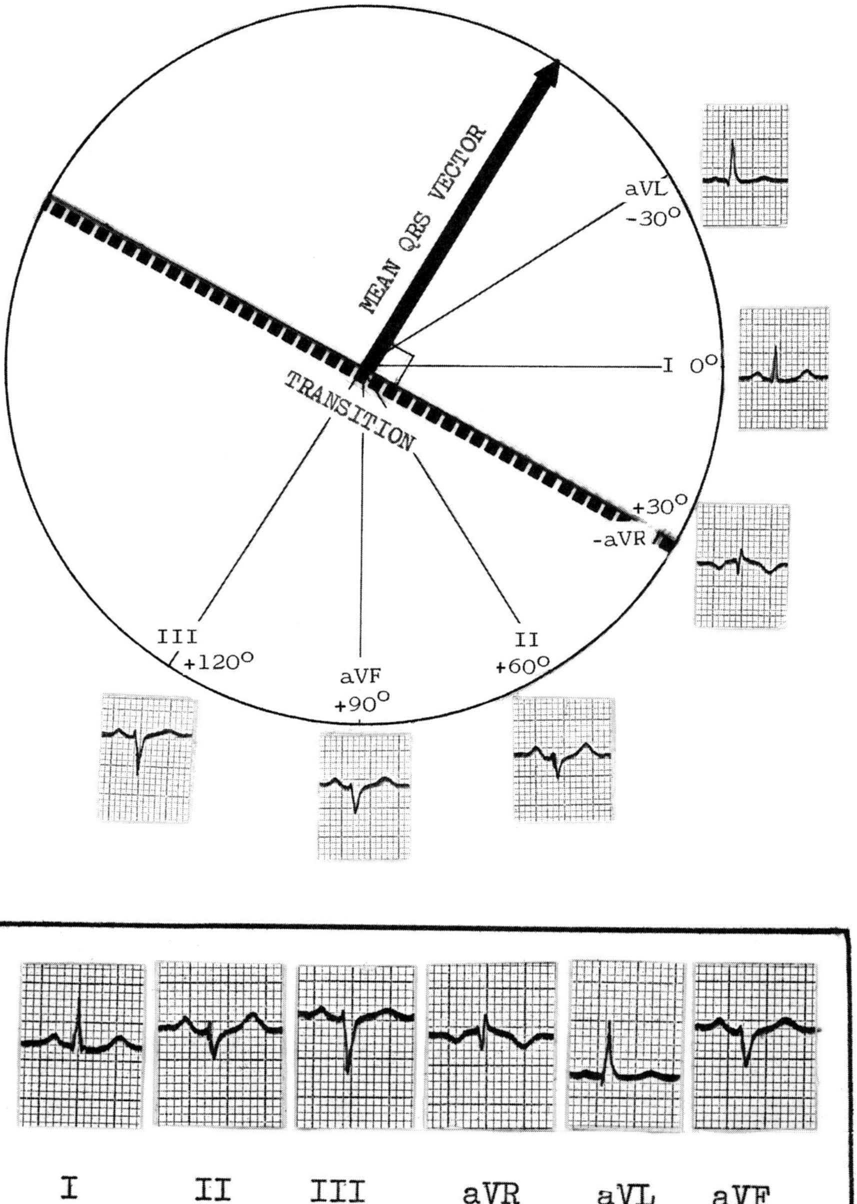

FIGURE 1–32. Leads aVL and I are positive, while leads II, aVF and III are negative. The transition is at lead aVR. The mean QRS vector, perpendicular to the transition toward the positive, is beyond −30° (at −60°).

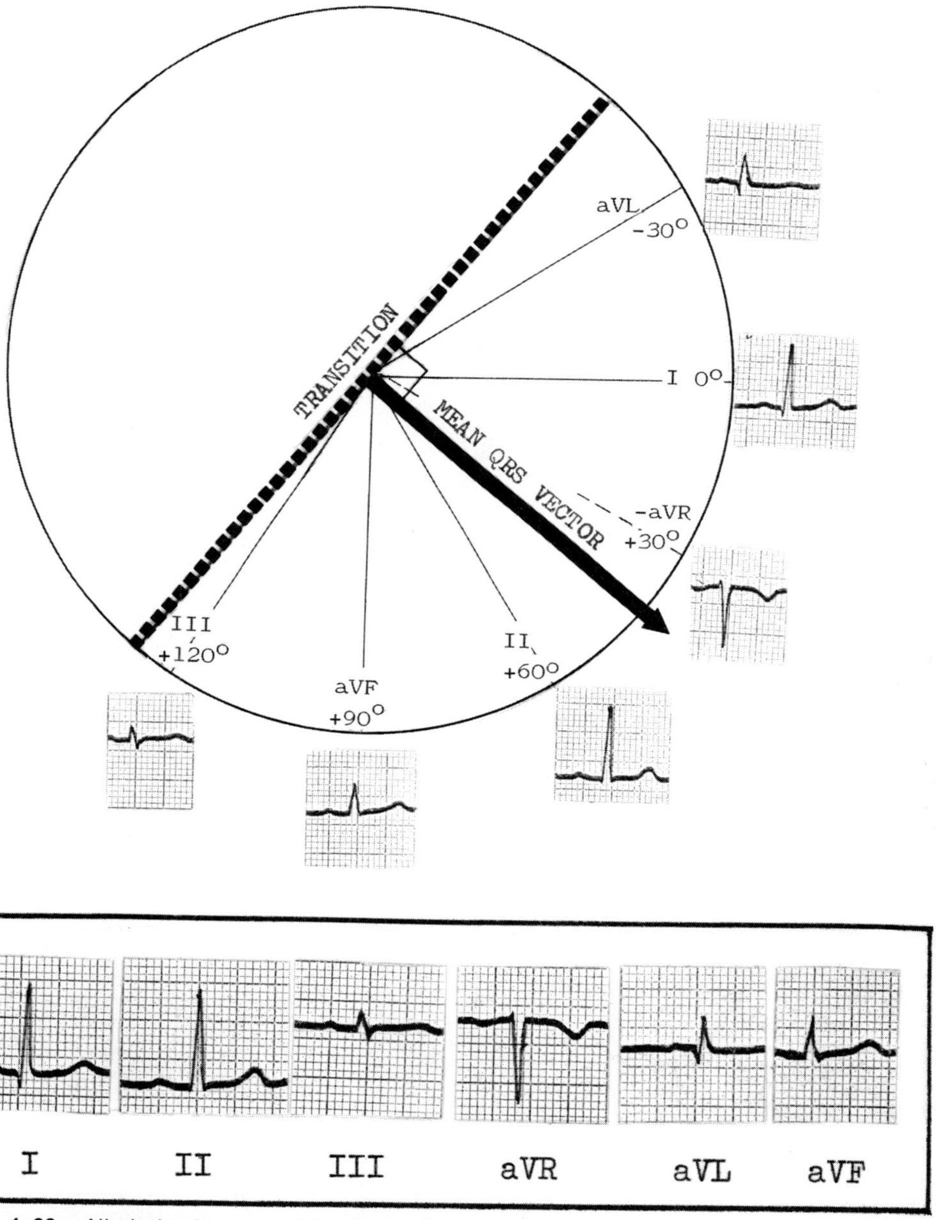

FIGURE 1–33. All six leads are positive (remember to invert aVR). The transition, therefore, bypasses all the leads, and the mean QRS vector falls between +30° and +60°.

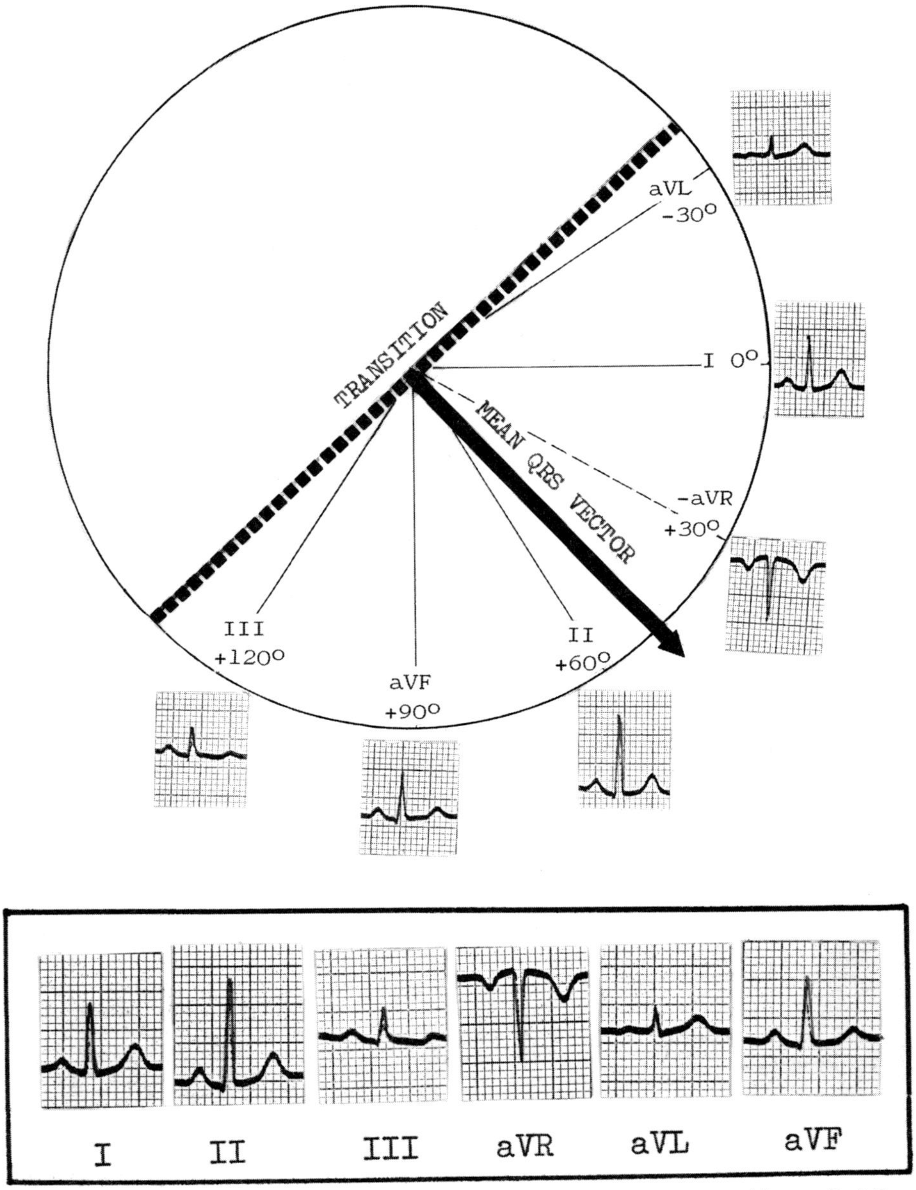

FIGURE 1–34. This figure is similar to Figure 1–33. All the leads are positive so that the transition bypasses all the leads. The mean QRS vector is between +30° and +60°.

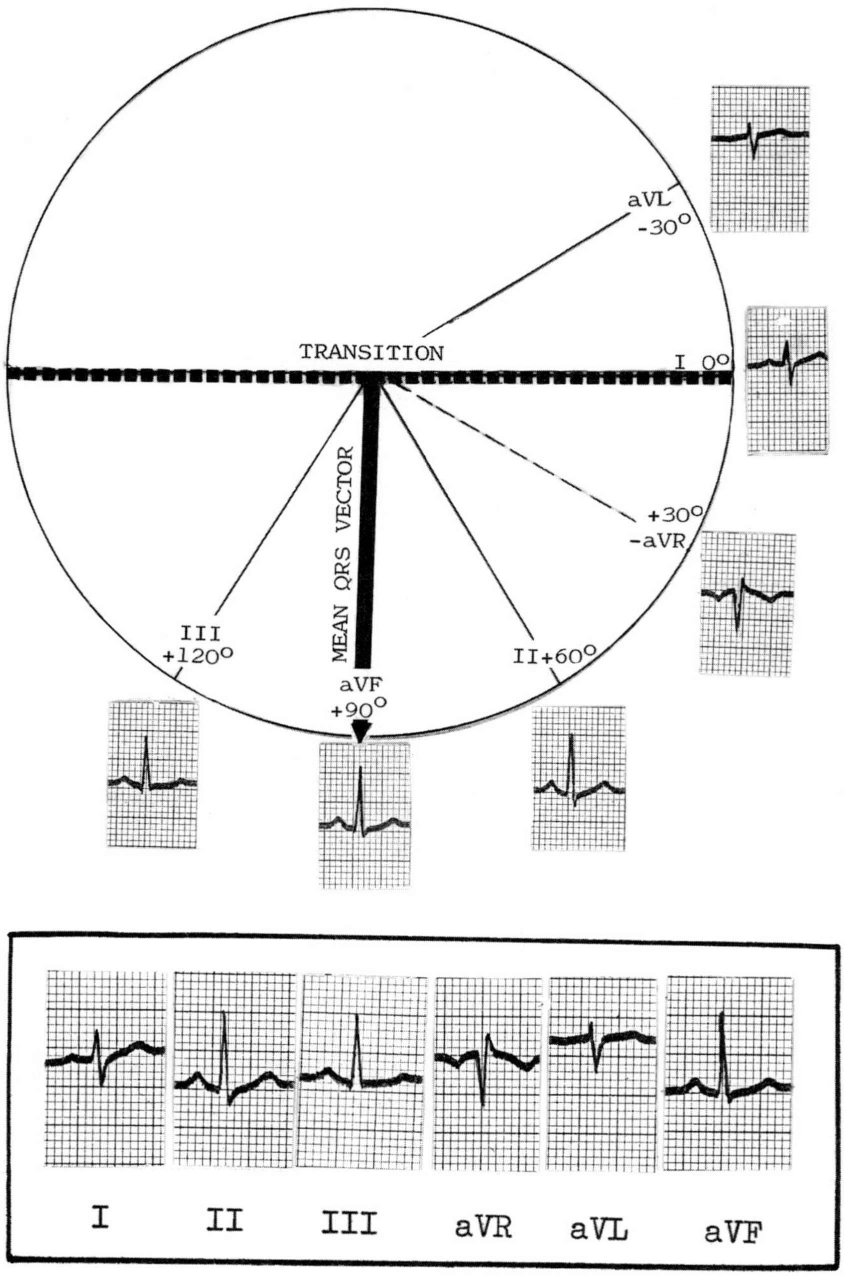

FIGURE 1–35. The transition is at 0° (Lead I). Lead aVL is negative; leads –aVR, II, aVF and III are positive. The mean QRS vector is, therefore, perpendicular to lead I at 90° (lead aVF).

In the normal adult (Fig. 1–36), the mean QRS vector is usually between 0° and 90°. That is, the mean QRS vector is normally between leads I and aVF. There is a shaded area between −30° and 0° and between +90° and +105°. Many cardiologists feel that a mean QRS vector falling within these shaded areas is still within the limits of normal. Beyond −30° is *abnormal left axis deviation (LAD)* and beyond +105° is *abnormal right axis deviation (RAD)*. Study Figure 1–36 well and then review Figures 1–24 to 1–35 and determine which mean QRS vectors are normal and which are abnormal. As you can see by Figure 1–36 there is a wide range of normality. As a general rule the mean QRS vector is more rightward in early life and more leftward with increasing age. Some of the pathological entities responsible for abnormal mean QRS vectors will be discussed later on.

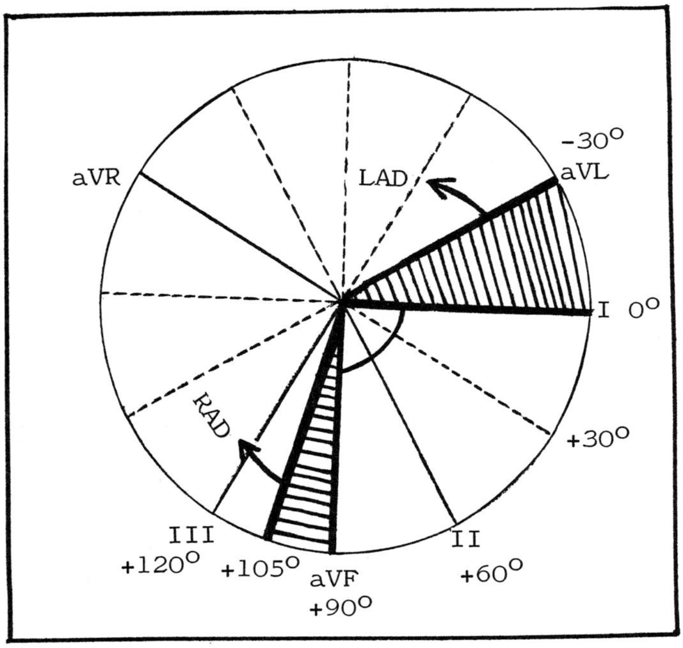

FIGURE 1–36. Normal and abnormal ranges for the mean QRS vector. LAD, Left axis deviation; RAD, right axis deviation.

The Mean T Vector in the Frontal Plane

The mean T vector is determined in the same manner as the mean QRS vector.

In Figure 1–37 the T waves are positive in leads aVL, I, −aVR, II, transitional in aVF and negative in III. The transition for the T wave is along lead aVF. The mean T vector is perpendicular to the transition on the positive side, at 0° (large arrow).

After you have calculated the mean T vector in Figure 1–37 determine the mean T vector in Figures 1–38 to 1–42.

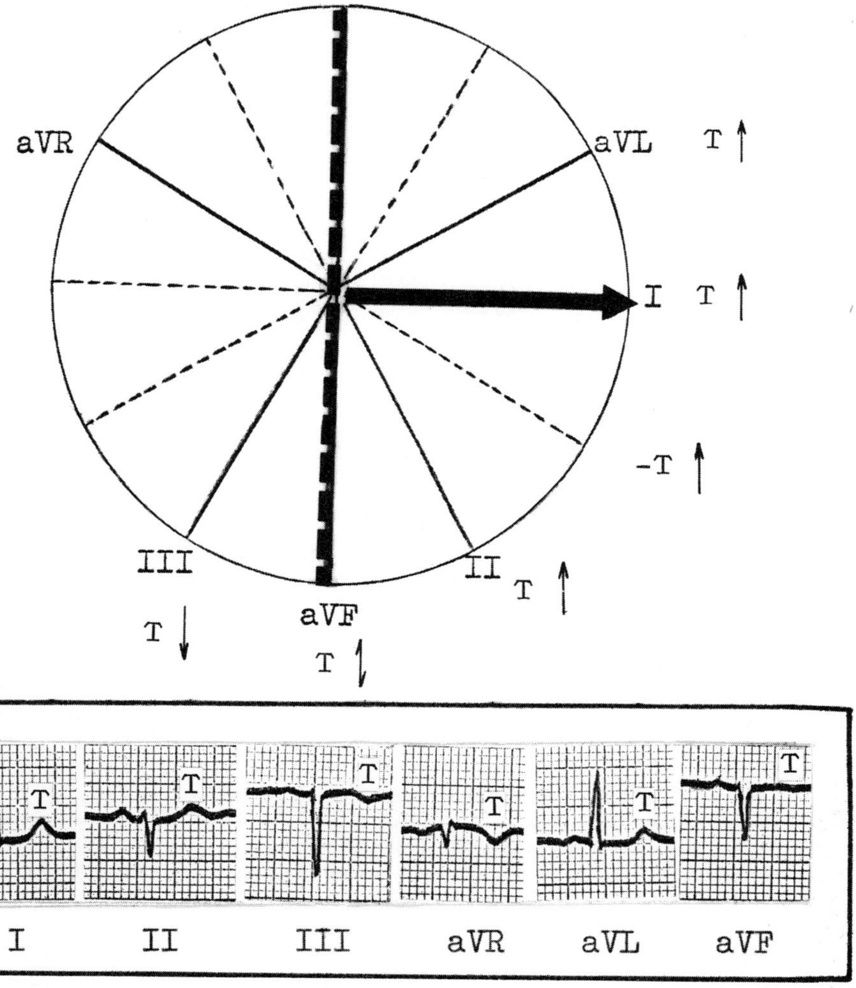

FIGURE 1–37. Mean T vector at 0°.

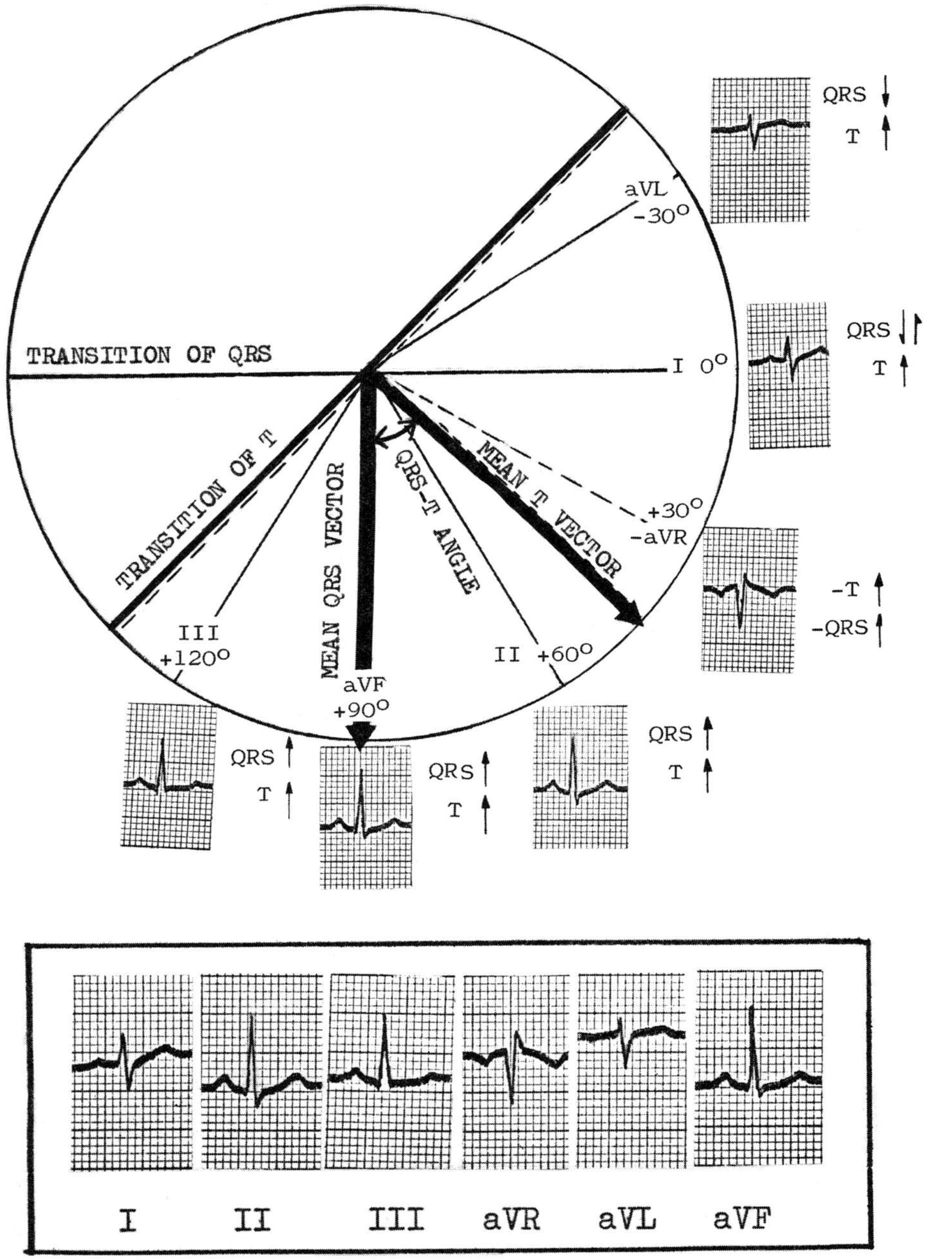

FIGURE 1-38. All the T waves are positive; remember to invert lead aVR. The transition, therefore, bypasses all the leads, and the mean T vector falls between +30° and +60°. Note the angle of 45° between the mean QRS vector and mean T vector. The QRS–T angle is usually 45° or less in the normal and rarely exceeds 60°.

Then return to Figures 1–38 to 1–42 and determine the QRS–T angle. The significance of the QRS–T angle will now be explained.

The QRS–T Angle

The angle formed between the mean QRS vector and the mean T vector is a sensitive method for relating the forces of ventricular depolarization with the forces of ventricular repolarization. In the normal adult the QRS–T angle is rarely wider than 60° and is often less than 45°. This most important relationship is illustrated in Figures 1–38 to 1–42.

Not only the *width* of the QRS–T angle but also the *orientation* of the mean T

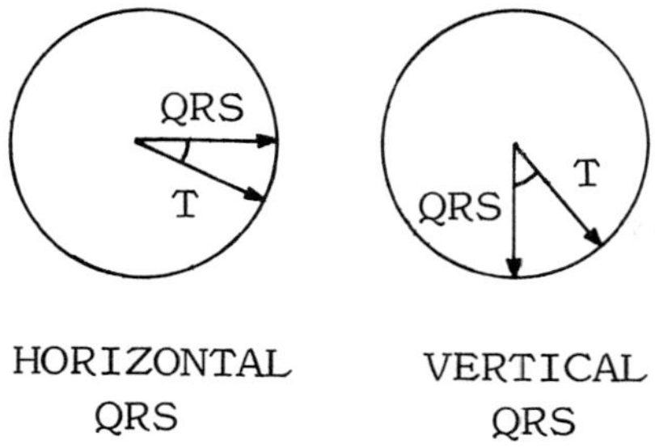

vector in relation to the mean QRS vector are important. If the mean QRS vector is horizontal, the mean T vector is to the right of the mean QRS vector. If the mean QRS vector is vertical, the mean T vector is to the left of the mean QRS vector. If this relationship does not hold, the QRS–T angle may be abnormal although its width is within 60°.

In Figures 1–38 to 1–42 determine the:

1. Mean QRS vector. Normal or abnormal?
2. Mean T vector.
3. QRS–T angle. Normal or abnormal?

Cassette Side 3

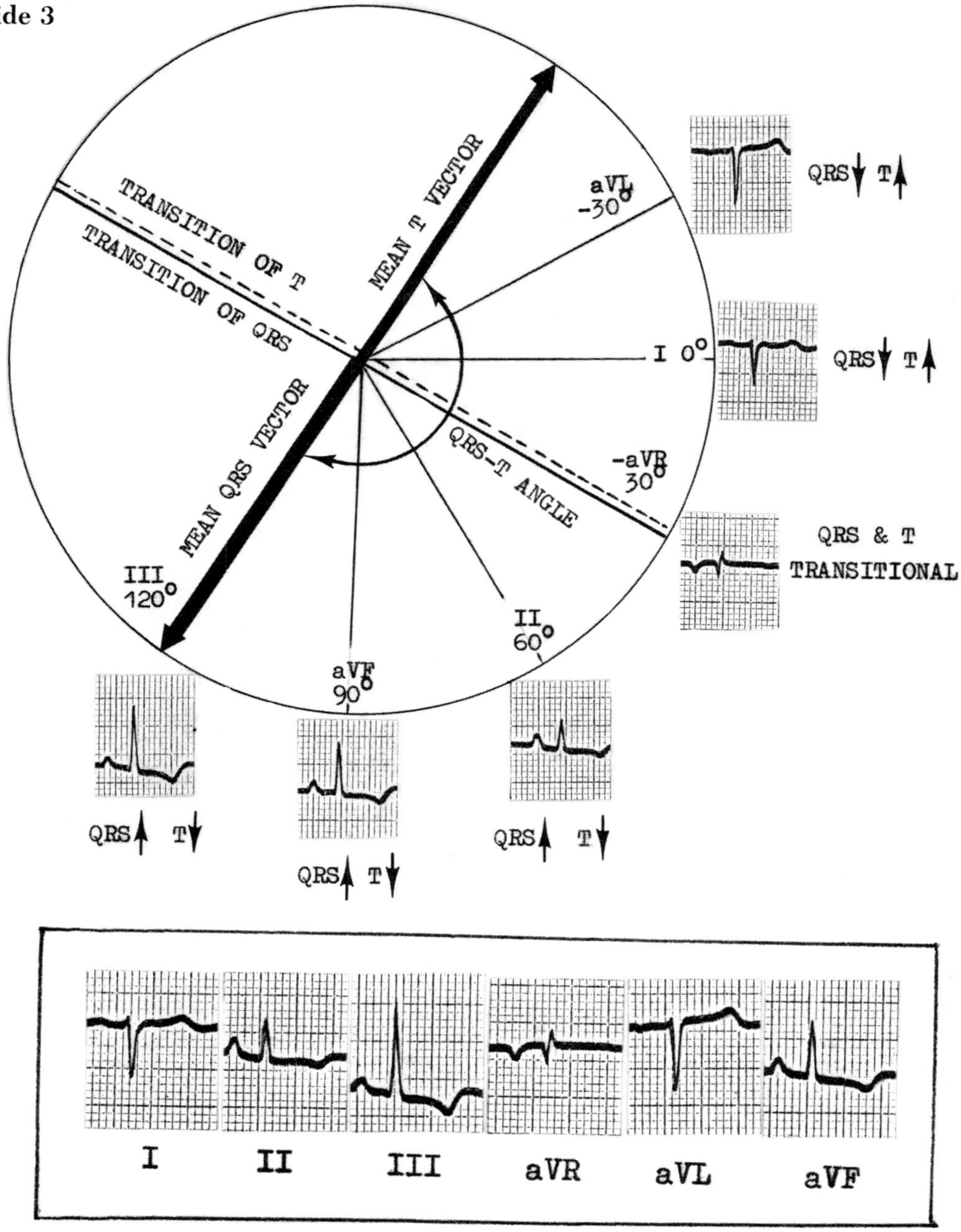

FIGURE 1–39. The transitional zone for both the QRS and T wave is at lead aVR. In all other leads the QRS deflections are opposite the T deflections, an orientation resulting in a very wide QRS–T angle (180°).

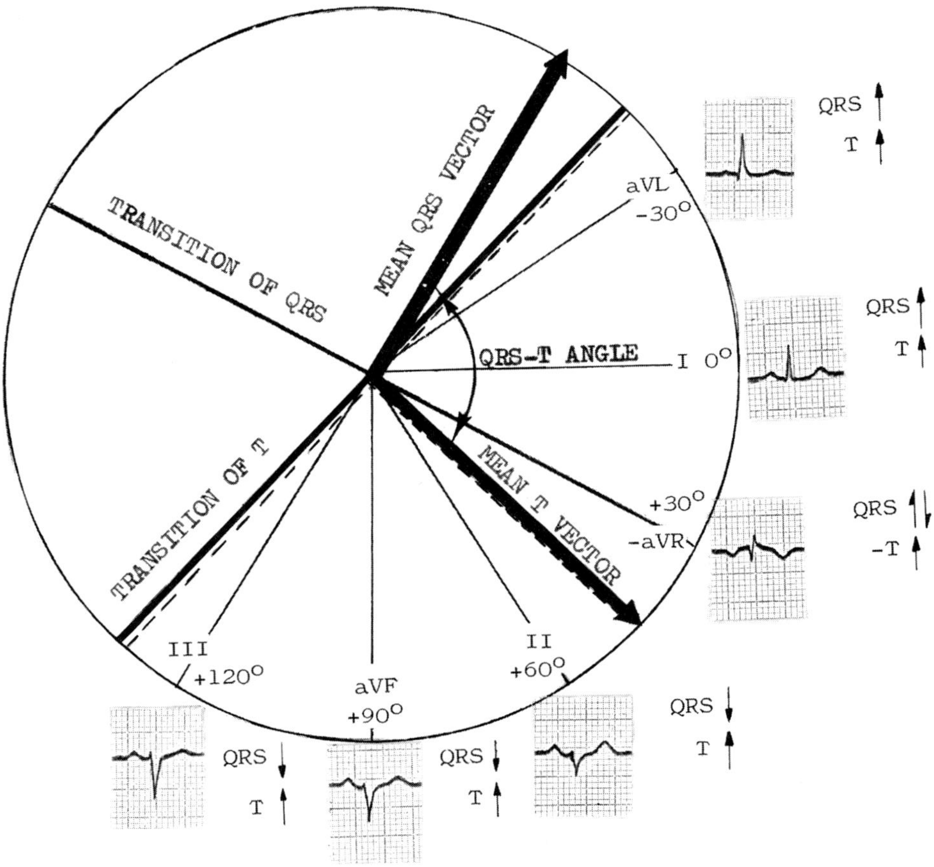

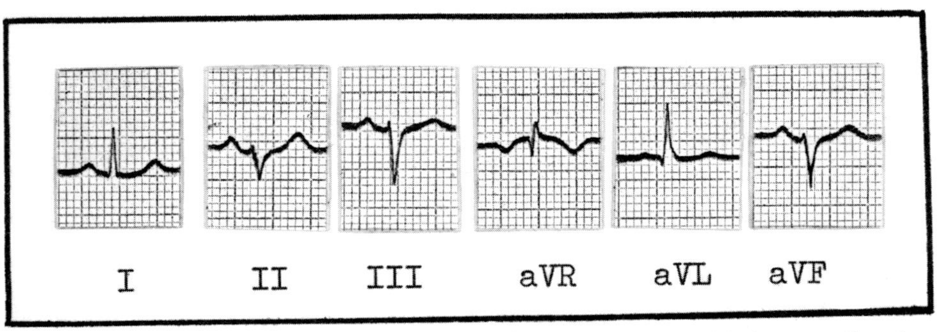

FIGURE 1–40. Once again we find that all the T waves are positive, with the mean T vector at 45°. Due to the marked *left axis deviation (LAD)* of the QRS (−60°), a wide angle is noted between the mean QRS vector and the mean T vector (105°).

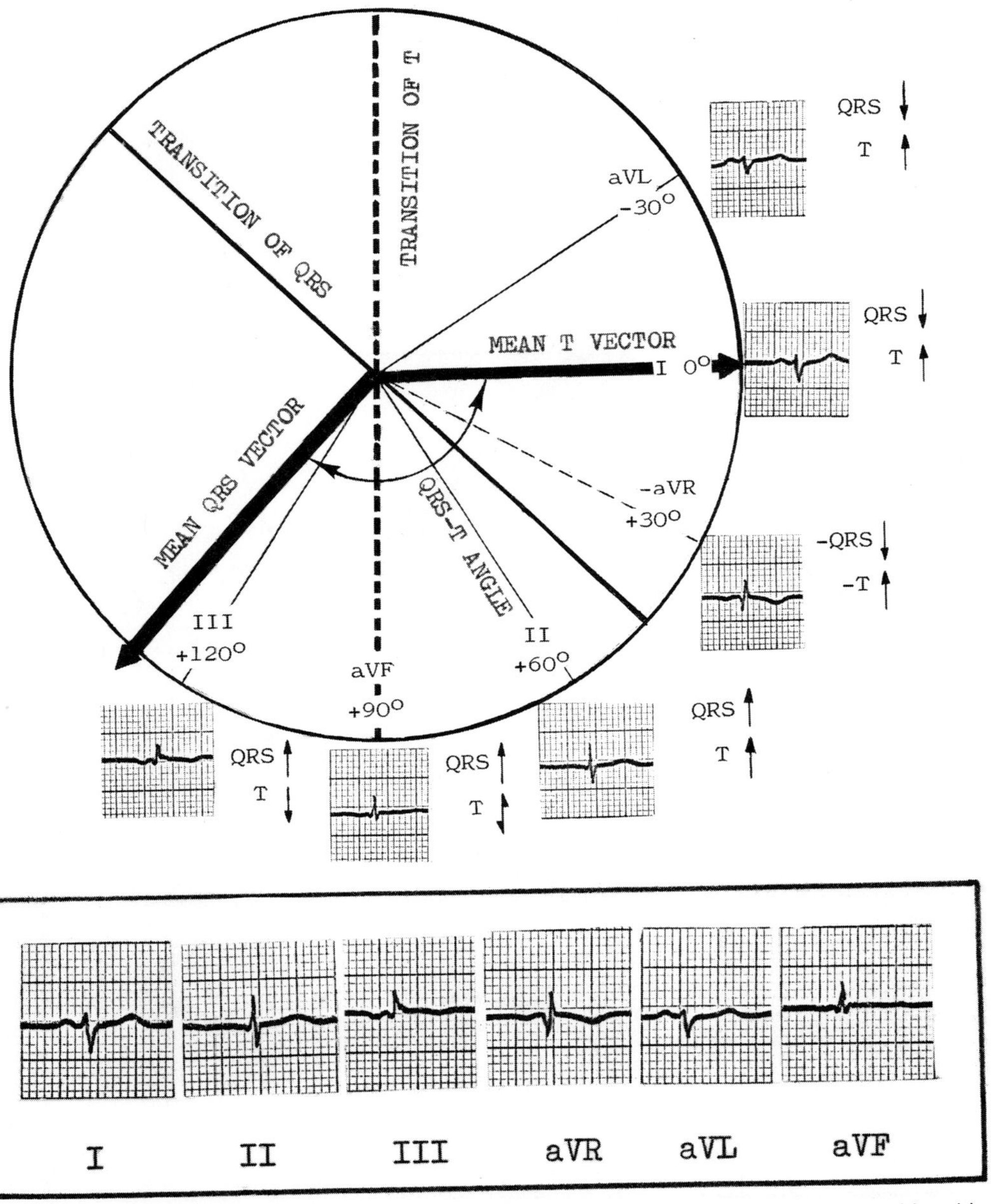

FIGURE 1–41. The T waves in leads aVL, I, −aVR and II are positive. The T wave is transitional in lead aVF and negative in lead III. With the transition at aVF, the mean T vector is at 0°. Note the abnormally wide QRS–T angle.

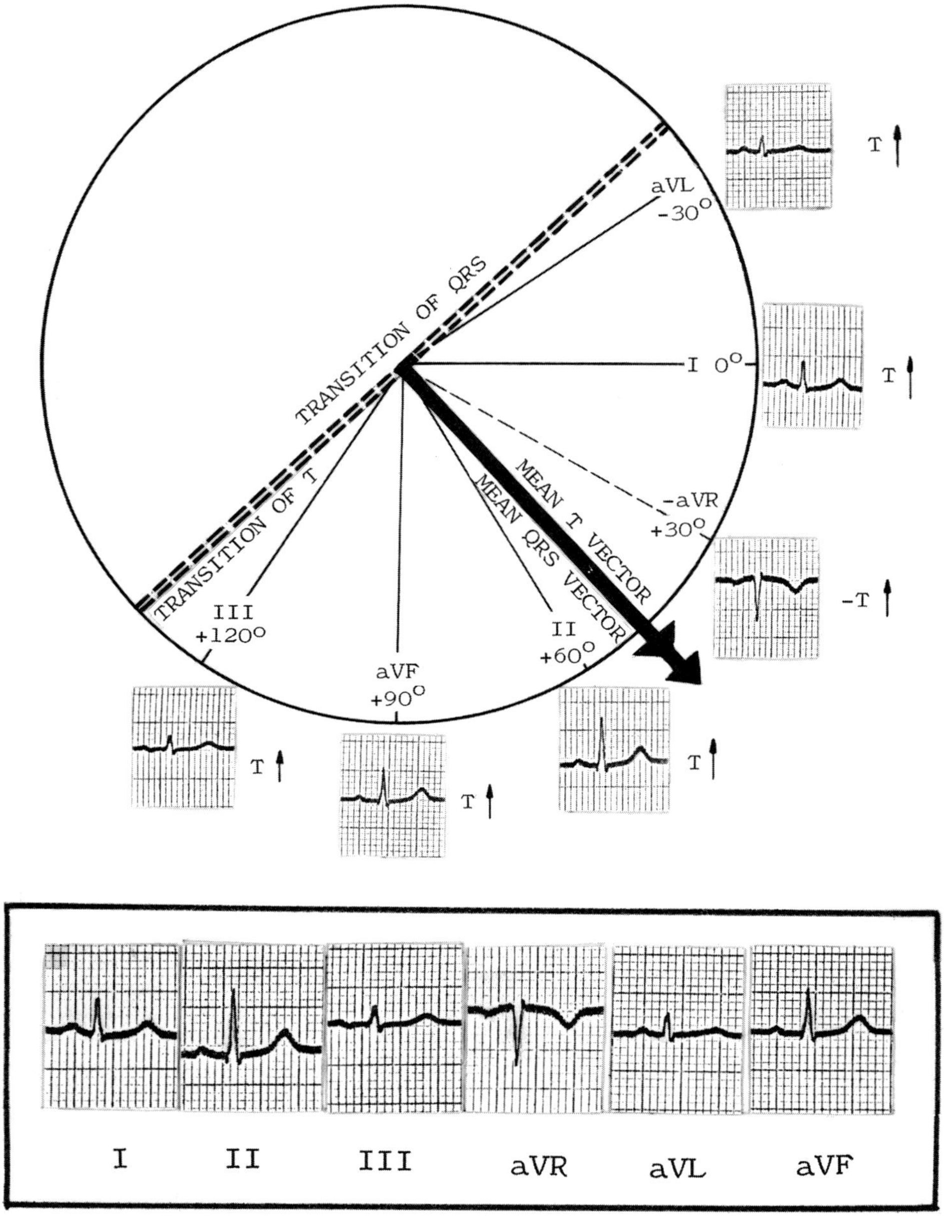

FIGURE 1–42. All the QRS complexes are positive, as are all the T waves. The mean QRS vector and mean T vector are superimposed, thereby forming a very narrow, if any, angle between them.

The Mean P Vector

To find the mean P vector, use the same approach as for the mean QRS and T vectors. The transitional zone is first calculated, then the mean P vector. In Figure 1–43 note that the P waves are upright (positive) in leads I, II and III. The transition, therefore, bypasses these three leads; the mean P vector is perpendicular to the transition and is found along the axis of lead II at 60°. The range for the mean P vector is usually rather narrow in the normal electrocardiogram. The outer limits of normal are between 0° and +90°, usually between +15° and +75°, as indicated by the arc between the arrows outside the circle in Figure 1–43.

Because of this narrow range of normality, pay very close attention to the positivity and negativity of the P waves. A P wave which is negative in lead II, but positive in lead I, is a leftward P (Fig. 1–44) and one which is negative in lead I is a rightward P (Fig. 1–45).

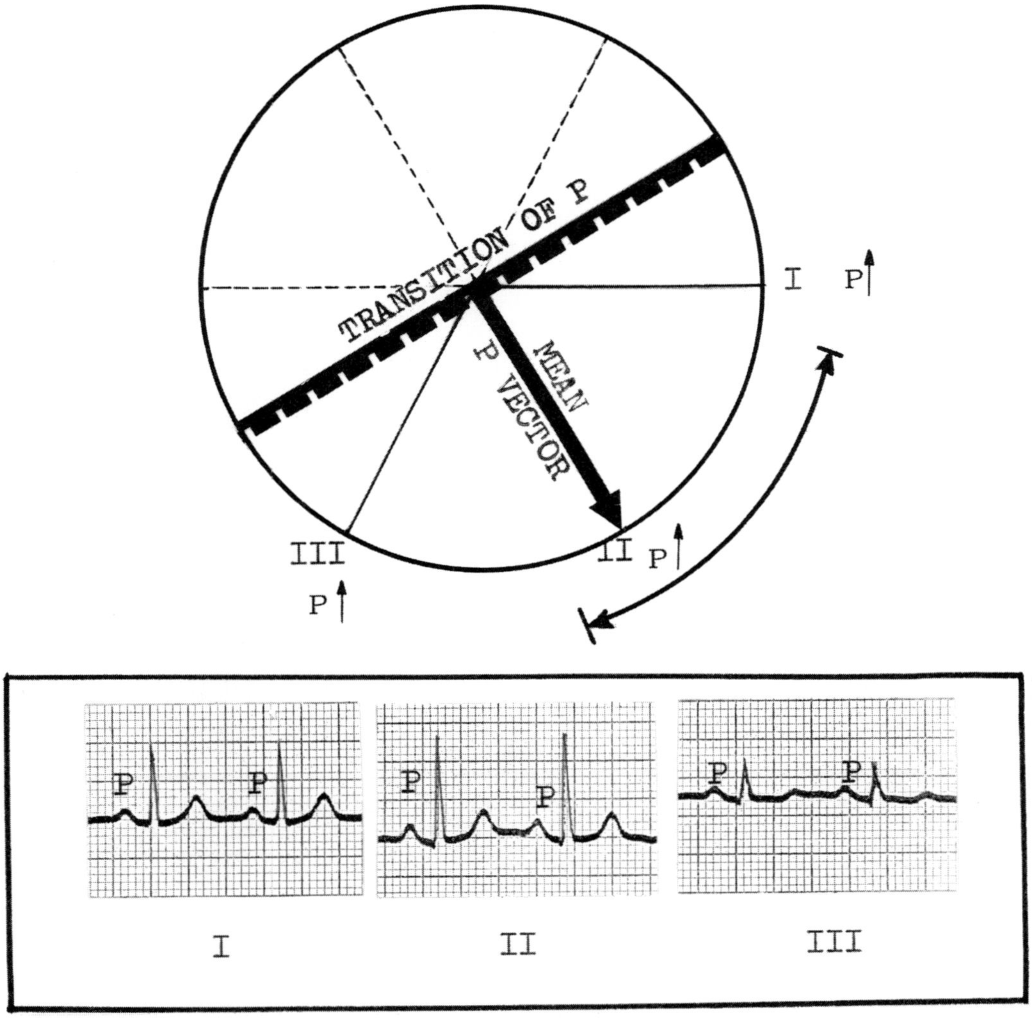

FIGURE 1–43. The mean P vector at 60°.

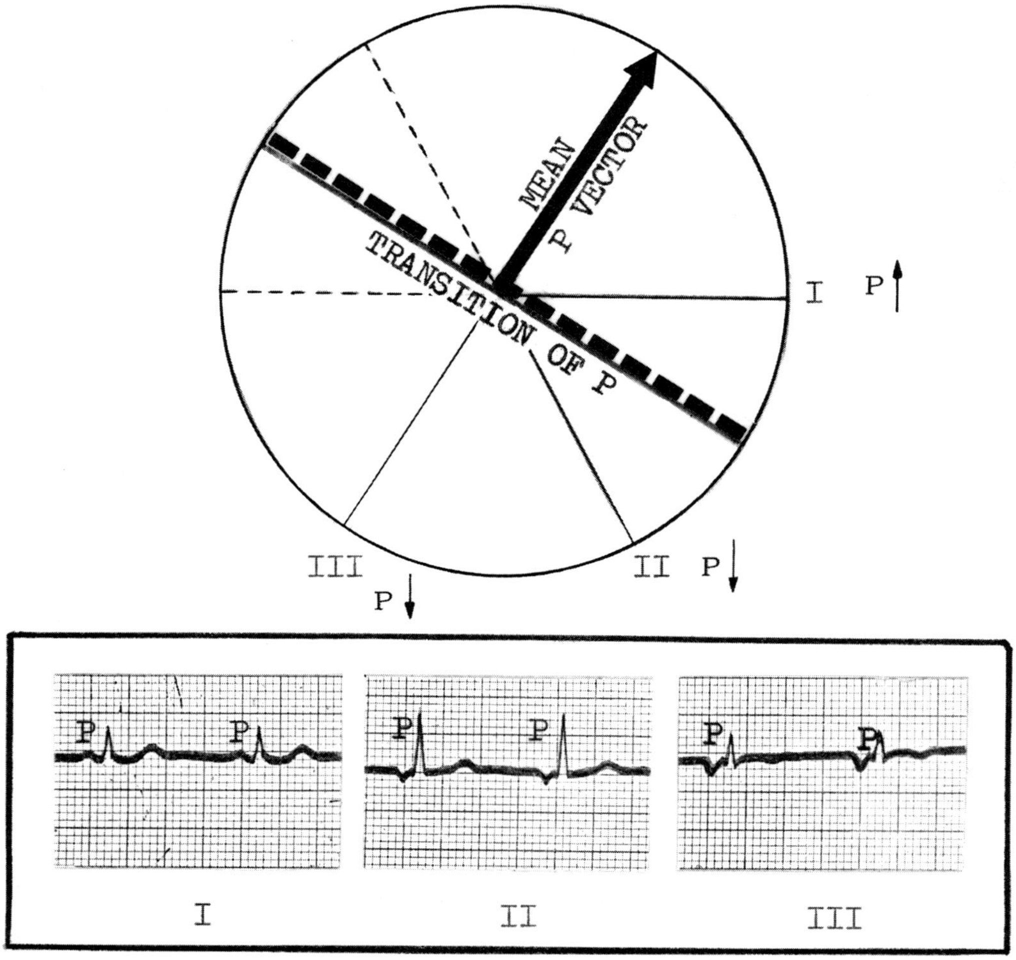

FIGURE 1–44. The P wave is positive in lead I but negative in leads II and III. The transition is, therefore, between leads I and II, resulting in an abnormal *left axis deviation* of the mean P vector. The origin of the impulse is not from the SA node but from some other focus; it is from an *ectopic* focus, representing an abnormal sequence of atrial depolarization.

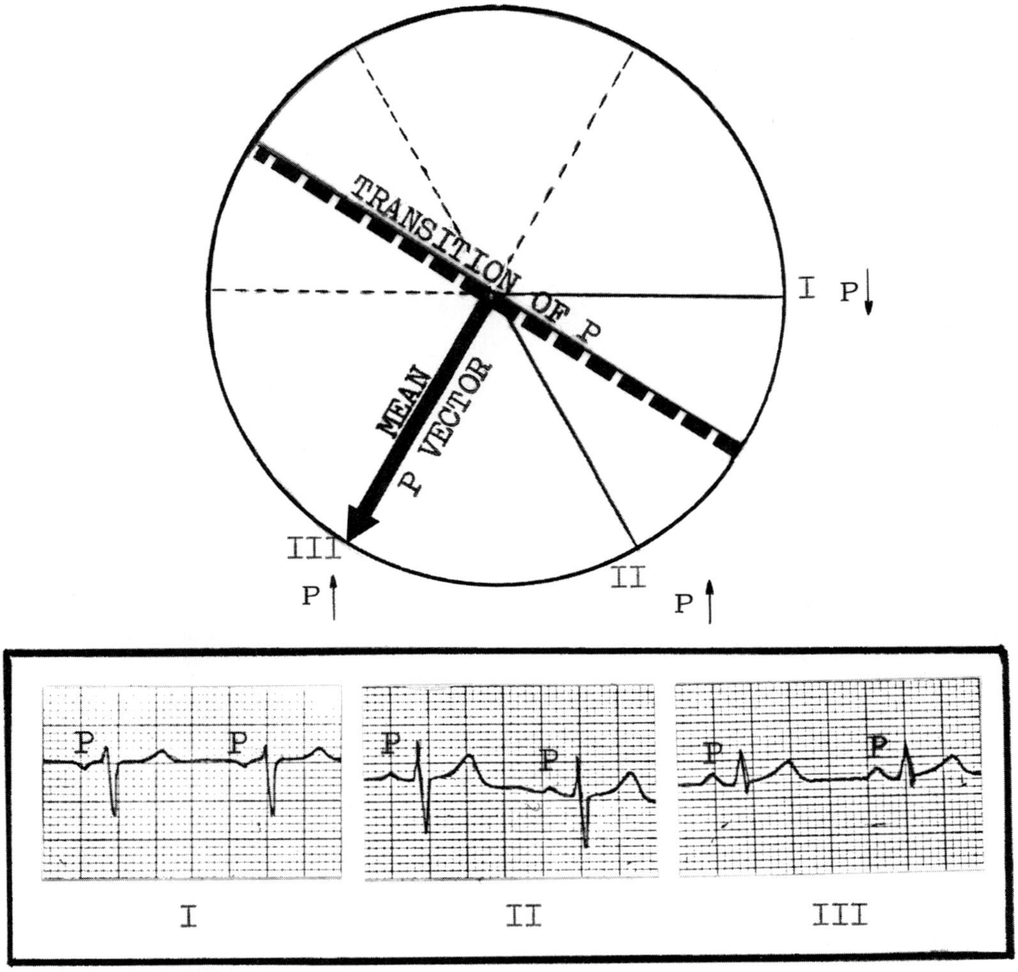

FIGURE 1–45. The P wave is negative in lead I but positive in leads II and III. The transition is, therefore, between leads I and II; the mean P vector is deviated abnormally to the right. This electrocardiogram is from a patient with known dextrocardia. This is an exception to the general rule, for, in the patient with dextrocardia, the P wave is inscribed as a negative wave in lead I even though the origin of the impulse may be in the *SA node.* It is only that the heart is not in the usual location (the heart is on the right side rather than the left).

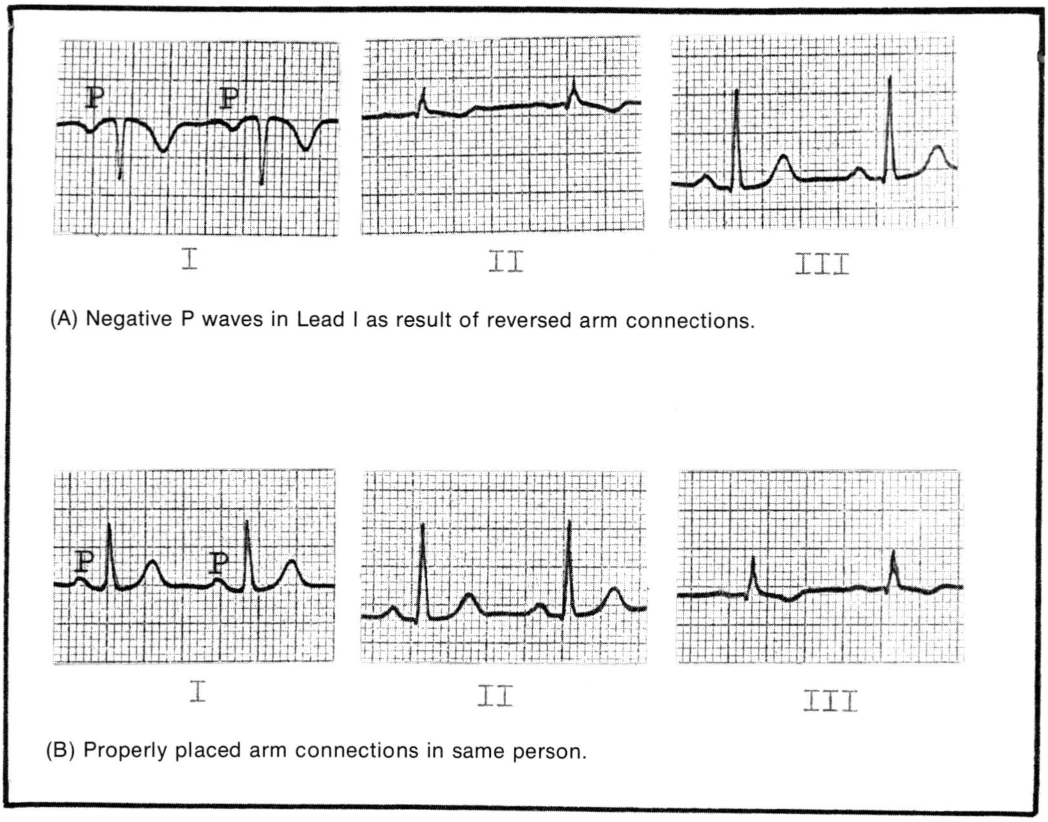

FIGURE 1–46. *A,* Another cause of a negative P wave in lead I is the misplacement of the electrodes (right arm electrode on the left arm and left arm electrode on the right arm). In fact, this misplacement is the most common cause of a negative P wave in lead I; this is a favorite examination question. Dextrocardia is far rarer as a cause of the negative P wave in lead I. Note that in this electrocardiogram (Fig. 1–46*A*), as well as in the previous one (Fig. 1–45), both the P wave and the QRS complex in lead I are predominantly negative. Always recheck the arm connections when encountering this situation. *B,* Properly placed connections on same person.

DETERMINATION OF HEART RATE FROM THE ELECTROCARDIOGRAM

Figure 1–47 illustrates the time and amplitude markings on electrocardiographic paper. The large and small boxes are used to determine the height and duration of all the inscriptions on the electrocardiogram. Each small box is 0.04 sec. in duration and 1 mm. in height. Each large box is 0.2 sec. in duration and 5 mm. in height. The normal standardization on the electrocardiogram of 1 millivolt (mv.) results in a deflection of 2 large boxes (10 mm). This standardization will be used on all electrocardiograms in this course. For printing purposes some electrocardiograms have been enlarged for clarity and others reduced in size.

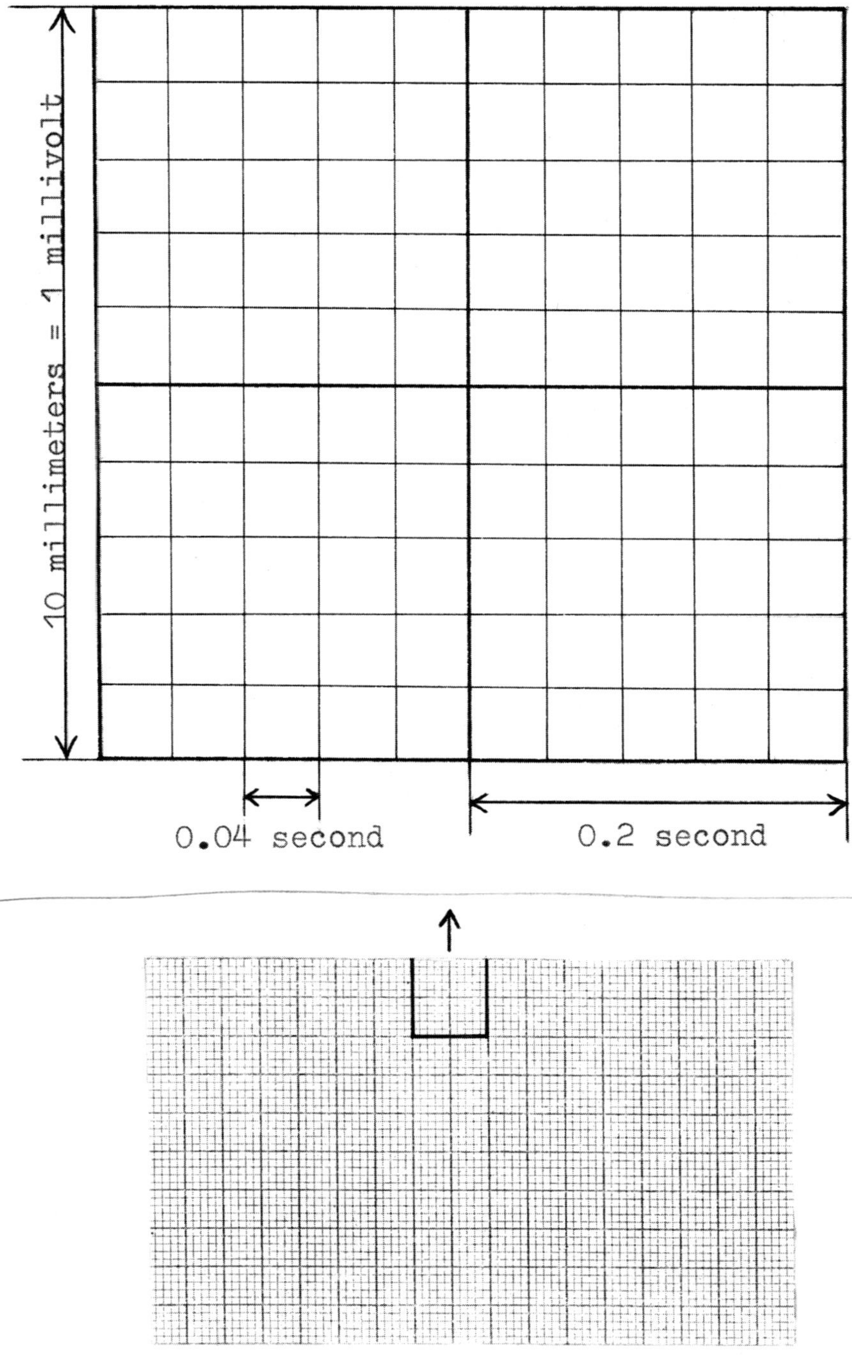

FIGURE 1–47. Time and amplitude markings on electrocardiographic paper.

The usual electrocardiographic speed is 25 mm. per second (five large boxes per second). At this speed, when the rate is 300 per minute, the interval is one large box (0.2 sec.) between two complexes. When the heart rate is 150 per minute, the interval is two large boxes (0.4 sec.) between two complexes. Figure 1–48 illustrates this relationship and three heart rate determinations are presented.

Interval (between two complexes)	*Rate*
1 large box	300 beats per minute
2 large boxes	150 (300/2)
3 large boxes	100 (300/3)
4 large boxes	75 (300/4)
5 large boxes	60 (300/5)
6 large boxes	50 (300/6)

In a perfectly regular rhythm all you need are two complexes and the number of large boxes between them. When the rhythm is irregular you may have to count numerous complexes to arrive at the proper average.

The normal heart rate: 60–100 beats per minute
Above 100 beats/min.: tachycardia (rapid heart)
Below 60 beats/min.: bradycardia (slow heart)

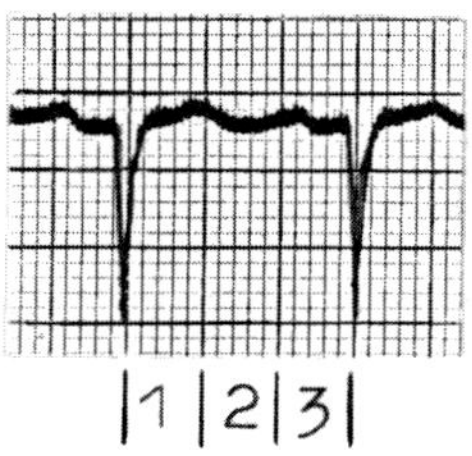

3 boxes between 2 QRS complexes: heart rate = 100 beats per minute (300/3 = 100)

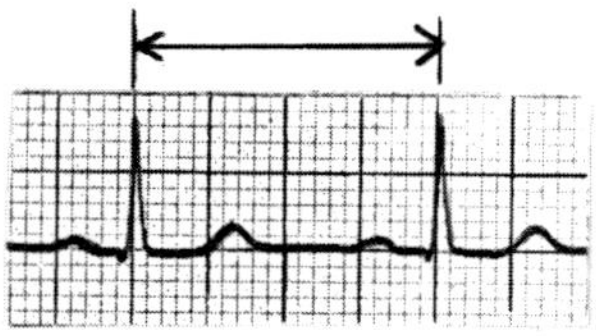

4 boxes between 2 QRS complexes: heart rate = 75 beats per minute (300/4 = 75)

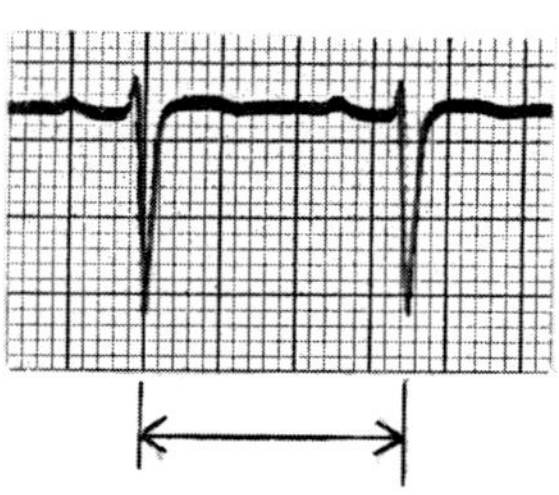

Heart rate = 86 beats per minute (300/3.5 = 86)

FIGURE 1–48. Determination of heart rate from the electrocardiogram.

Sinus Rhythm

In order to describe the rhythm of the heart as *sinus rhythm* (the impulse originating in the sinoatrial node), which is the normal rhythm of the heart, the following conditions must be met:

1. The mean P vector must be normal (see Fig. 1–43).
2. Each P wave must be followed by a QRS complex and each QRS complex must be preceded by a P wave. Abnormalities of this relationship will be studied later in the course.
3. The P–R interval (from the beginning of the P wave to the beginning of the QRS complex) is rarely greater than 0.2 sec. (one large box) in duration in the normal. The normal range is 0.12 to 0.2 sec., and it is constant from beat to beat.
4. The rate is constant between 60 and 100 beats per minute.

The next series of electrocardiograms (Figs. 1–49 to 1–53) contain at least one abnormality or technical error, which can easily be spotted by applying the information acquired so far.

Analyze each electrocardiogram using the following steps:

1. Leads I + III = lead II. Leads aVR + aVL + aVF = 0.
2. Calculate the mean P vector.
3. Calculate the mean QRS vector.
4. Calculate the mean T vector and determine the QRS–T angle.

The abnormality or technical error is described in the legend to each electrocardiogram. Evaluate the electrocardiogram first and then check your work by consulting the legend.

PRACTICE ELECTROCARDIOGRAMS USING INFORMATION LEARNED SO FAR

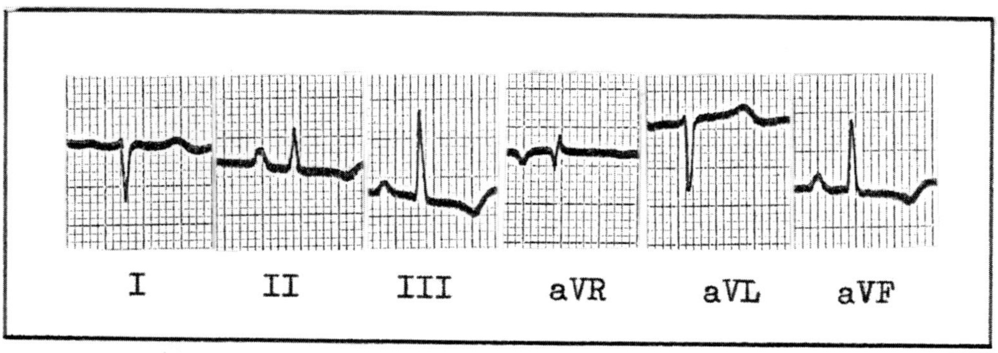

FIGURE 1–49. a. Abnormal right axis deviation (RAD). b. Abnormally wide QRS–T angle.

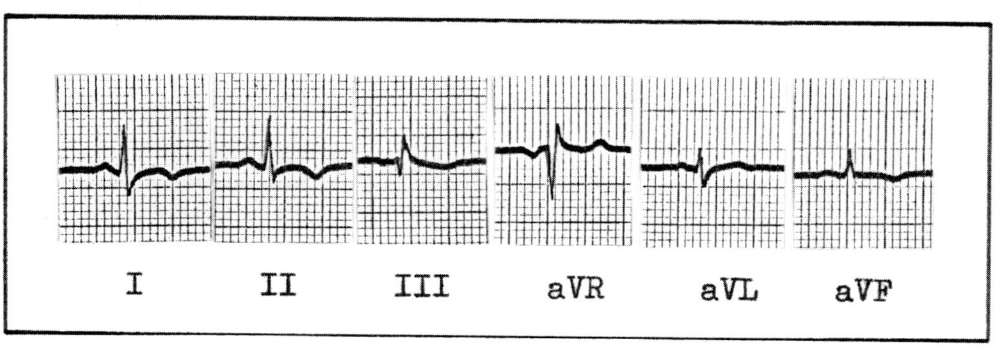

FIGURE 1–50. Abnormally wide QRS–T angle.

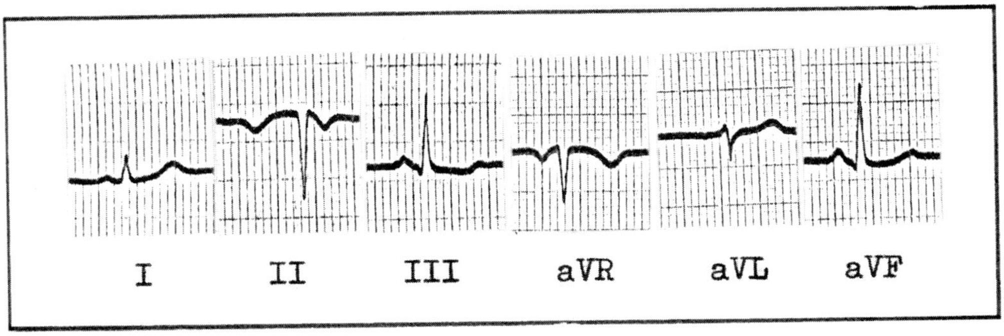

FIGURE 1–51. Lead II has been mounted upside down. Even if you did not recognize this on sight, you would soon see that leads I + III do not add up to lead II.

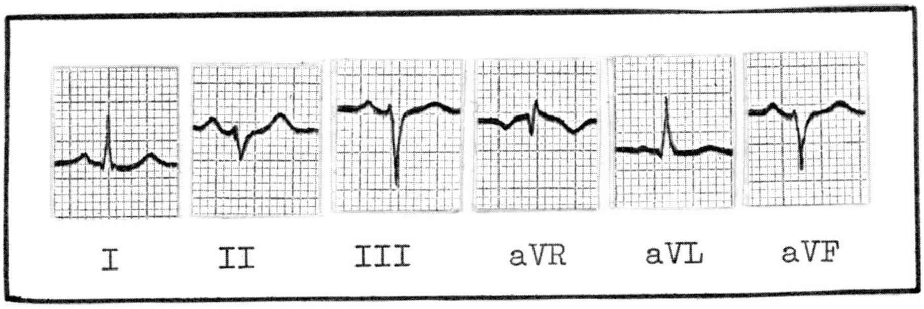

FIGURE 1–52. a. Abnormal left axis deviation (LAD). b. Abnormally wide QRS–T angle.

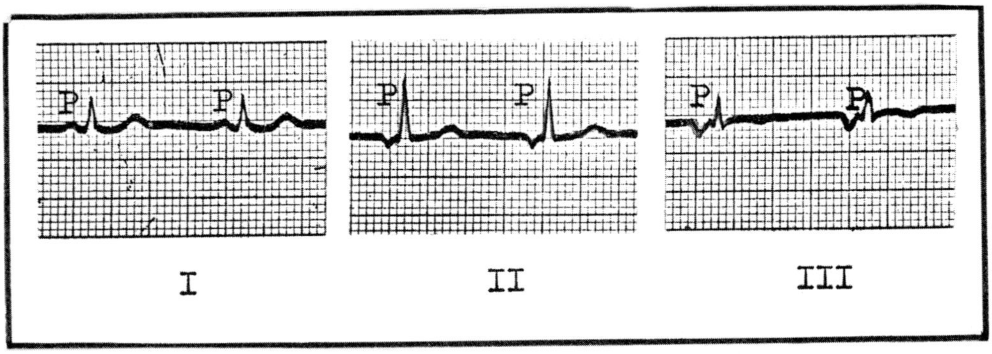

FIGURE 1–53. The mean P vector is abnormal. The site of origin of the impulse is *not* in the S–A node; this is an *ectopic atrial pacemaker.*

The six electrocardiographic leads studied heretofore—I, II, III, aVR, aVL and aVF—are leads in the *frontal* plane. The boundaries of the frontal plane are superior, inferior, right and left (Fig. 1–54).

SUPERIOR

RIGHT

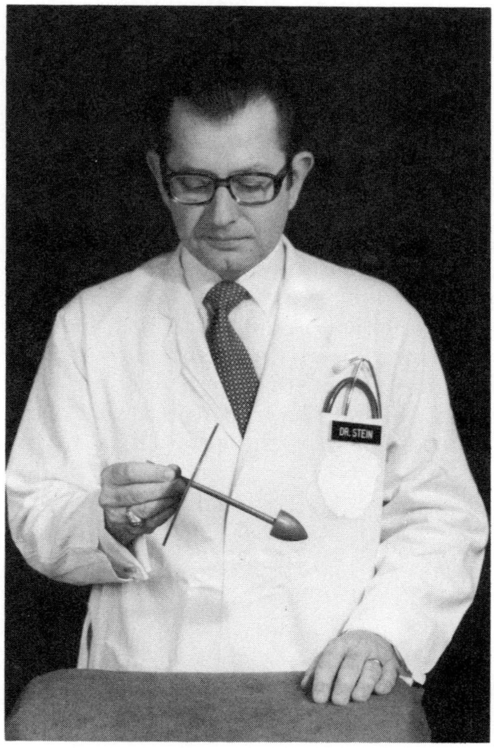

LEFT

INFERIOR

FIGURE 1–54. Boundaries of the *frontal* plane.

When the mean QRS, T and P vectors were indicated by an arrow, only *two* dimensions in space could be described. This is seen in Figure 1–55.

A. The arrow points to the *left* and *inferior*.
B. The arrow points to the *left* and *superior*.
C. The arrow points to the *right* and *inferior*.
D. The arrow points to the *right* and *superior*.

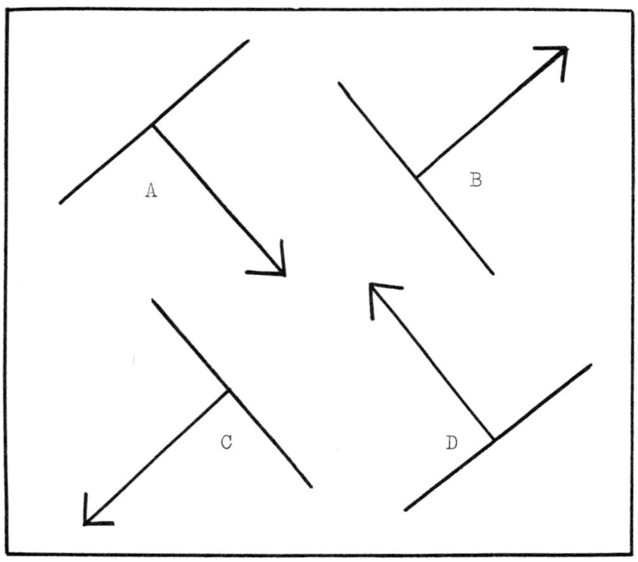

FIGURE 1–55. Describe each arrow in two dimensions.

THE HORIZONTAL PLANE

In order to provide the third dimension in space to describe the cardiac vectors, the *horizontal* plane must be added. The boundaries of the horizontal plane are anterior, posterior, right and left (Fig. 1–56).

Einthoven had no difficulty with the *frontal* plane. There was very little difference in the deflection recorded whether the electrode was placed on the finger, wrist or elbow, or on the toe, ankle or knee of the arm or leg. The frontal plane has convenient projections from the body in the form of arms and legs. It was found that as long as the electrode is at least 15 cm. distant from the heart, moving the electrode still further away records little change on the electrocardiogram. As the electrode is brought very close to the heart—for example, to 3 cm.—a small change in position will result in major changes in the deflections recorded on the electrocardiogram. In the frontal plane, the extremities permit the placement of the electrodes at least 15 cm. from the heart. However, there are no anterior-posterior projections from the chest and from the back to take us 15 cm. from the heart in the horizontal plane. Any position on the chest for recording the horizontal vector is within this critical distance. Einthoven, therefore, in the early days of electrocardiography, abandoned attempts to measure this anterior-posterior vector. It was years later, after many trials, that the chest, or precordial, leads were established and placed in the positions shown in Figure 1–57*A* as V_1 to V_6. Still later, measurements of the cardiac vectors in the horizontal plane were shown to be possible.

POSTERIOR

RIGHT

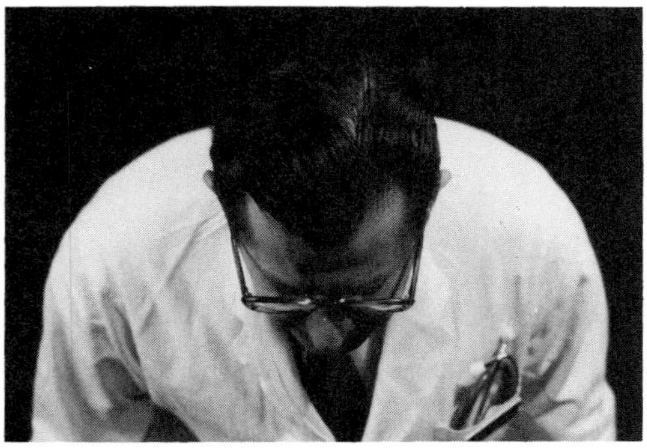

LEFT

ANTERIOR

FIGURE 1–56. Boundaries of the *horizontal* plane.

Although the six precordial leads do not lie in the same horizontal plane (Fig. 1–57*A*), an approximation of the horizontal projection of a QRS loop is illustrated in Figure 1–57*B*. With the addition of the horizontal plane (precordial leads), you will soon be ready to determine the mean spatial vectors in three dimensions.

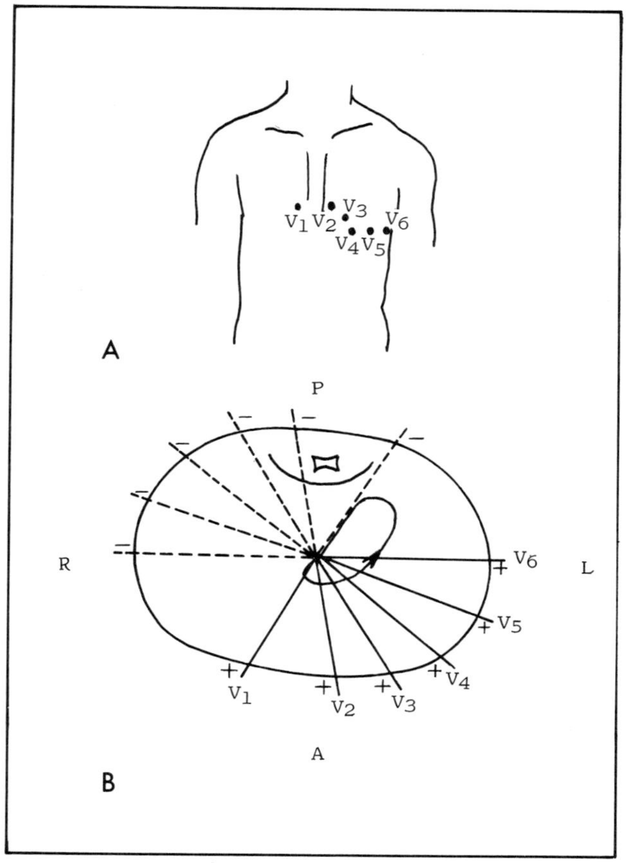

FIGURE 1–57. *A,* Positions of the precordial electrodes. *Electrode positions* are as follows:
- V_1 Fourth intercostal space to the right of the sternum
- V_2 Fourth intercostal space to the left of the sternum
- V_3 Midway between V_2 and V_4
- V_4 Fifth intercostal space—midclavicular line
- V_5 Anterior axillary line—horizontal level of V_4
- V_6 Midaxillary line—horizontal level of V_4

B, QRS loop in the horizontal plane.

While studying the QRS complex in the frontal plane, we were accustomed to drawing a *line* representing the transitional zone, and another line with an arrow perpendicular to it representing the mean QRS vector. We were working with lines since we were limited to only two possible dimensions. An example of this is seen in Figure 1–58. The two-dimensional description of this arrow representing the mean QRS vector is *left* and *inferior.*

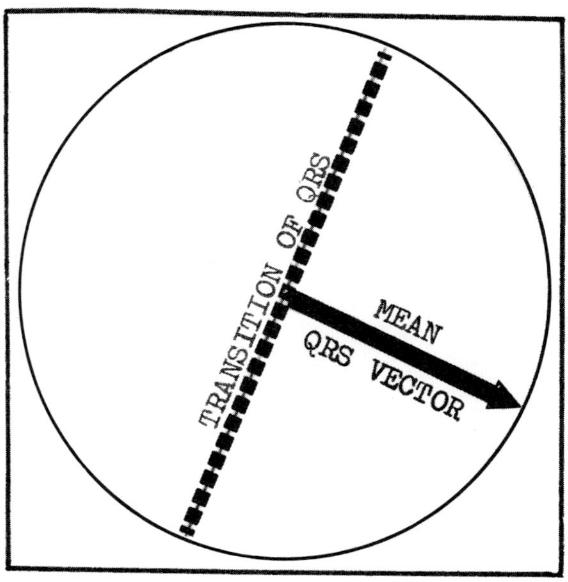

FIGURE 1–58. Mean QRS vector—left and inferior.

We had not really been looking at a transitional *line,* but at a *disk* dividing the body into positive and negative areas. The circumference of this disk viewed on end appeared to be a line (Fig. 1–59A). In a three-dimensional view, as seen in Figure 1–59*B*, the disk and arrow are tilted slightly posteriorly to show that we are not actually looking at a line, but at a disk.

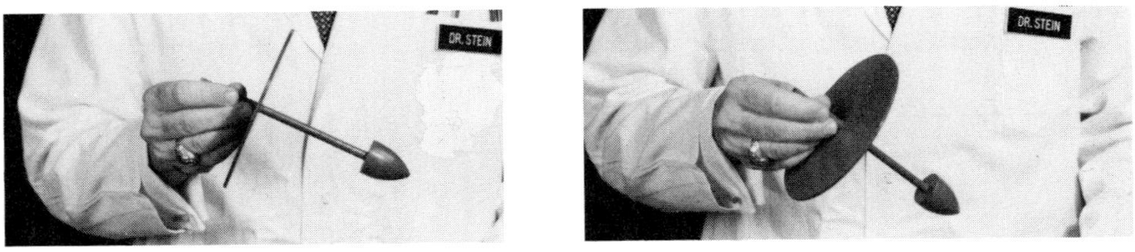

A B

FIGURE 1–59. *A,* In two dimensions, the disk is seen as a line with an arrow. *B,* In three dimensions, the full disk is seen with the posterior tilt of the arrow.

The vector model, seen in Figure 1–60, may be used to better visualize the cardiac vector in three dimensions. The lines, in Figure 1–60*A*, representing the *frontal* plane, are leads I, II and III. The precordial leads, in Figure 1–60*B*, representing the *horizontal* plane are leads V_1 to V_6. The zero on the frontal plane and the zero on the horizontal plane line up, and they line up with the center point of the disk. *We can rotate the disk only through this zero point,* which limits the motion of the disk. We cannot move this disk up and down as we do with a piston. Although inaccuracies are present, since the body is not a cylinder nor a circle, this method facilitates the understanding of the general vectorial concept in three dimensions.

Other possible sources of error should be noted. For example, the precordial leads (Fig. 1–57A) are arbitrarily placed in certain fixed positions on the chest, without regard to the "lie" of the heart. Also, there are wide variations in sizes and shapes of chests among patients.

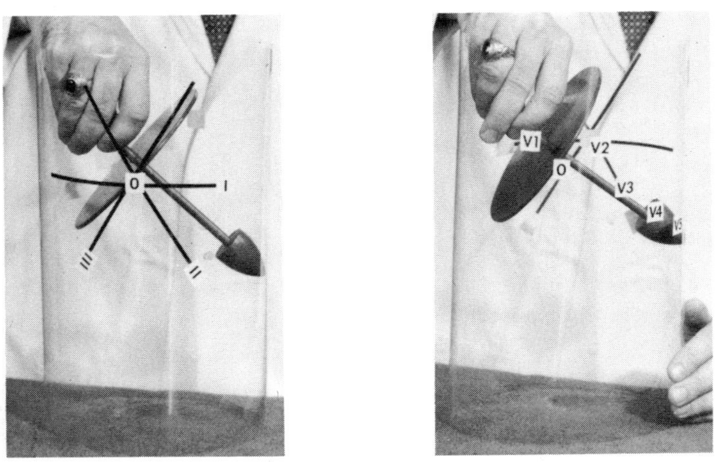

A B

FIGURE 1–60. Vector model, with frontal (*A*) and horizontal (*B*) leads.

STEPWISE DETERMINATION OF MEAN SPATIAL QRS VECTOR (THREE DIMENSIONS)

Determine the mean QRS vector in the frontal plane using leads I, II, III, aVR, aVL and aVF. After plotting the transitional zone and mean QRS vector, check your work with Figure 1–62. The horizontal plane will then be analyzed. Figures 1–62 to 1–65 all relate to Figure 1–61.

On inspection of the electrocardiogram, we see that all six leads are positive, remembering to invert lead aVR. The transitional zone bypasses all of the leads and the mean QRS vector falls between leads II and aVR, to the *left* and *inferior* in the frontal plane.

The disk and arrow (Fig. 1–63), held to the left and inferior, does not actually appear as a disk and arrow, but rather as a line and an arrow. The area facing the arrow is positive and the area away from the arrow, on the other side of the transition, is negative.

Using our vector model in Figure 1–64*A* we see leads I, II and III, and the vector is to the *left* and *inferior*. In Figure 1–64*B*, on the other side of the model, we have a representation of the horizontal plane. *If there were no anterior-posterior rotation,* if the vector were simply to the *left* and *inferior*, V_1 would be *negative* (V_1 is the only precordial lead on the negative side of the disk. The arrow side of the disk is the positive side.) Leads V_2, V_3, V_4, V_5 and V_6 would all be positive.

To review, for emphasis (Fig. 1–64*A*), if the vector were only to the *left* and *inferior*, V_1 (Fig. 1–64*B*) would be negative since it faces away from the arrow side of the disk. On the other hand, leads V_2 to V_6 would all be positive since they

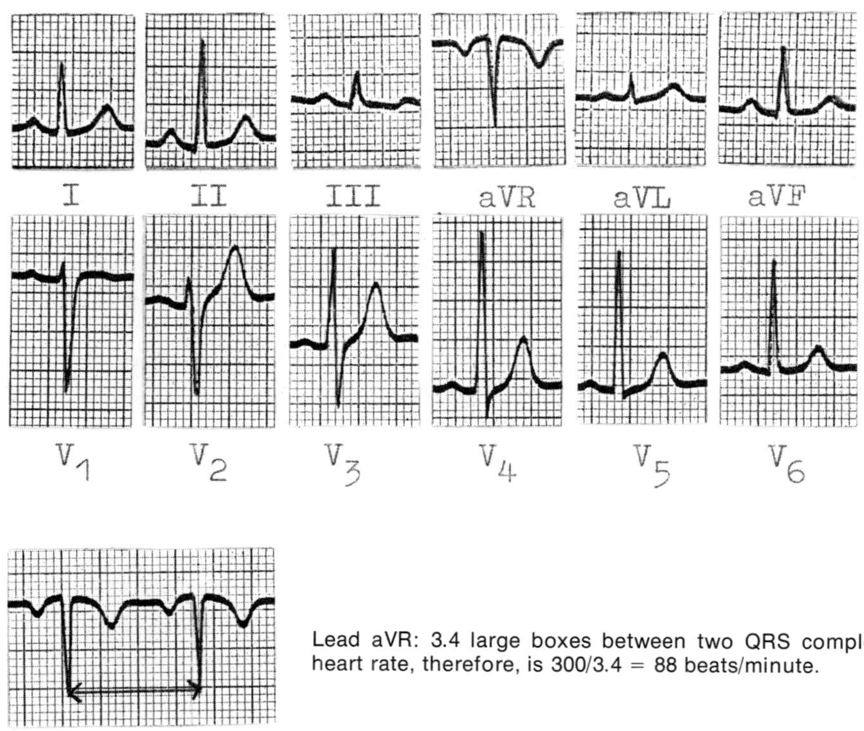

Lead aVR: 3.4 large boxes between two QRS complexes; heart rate, therefore, is 300/3.4 = 88 beats/minute.

FIGURE 1–61. Refer to Figures 1–62 and 1–65 to help visualize the mean QRS vector in three dimensions.

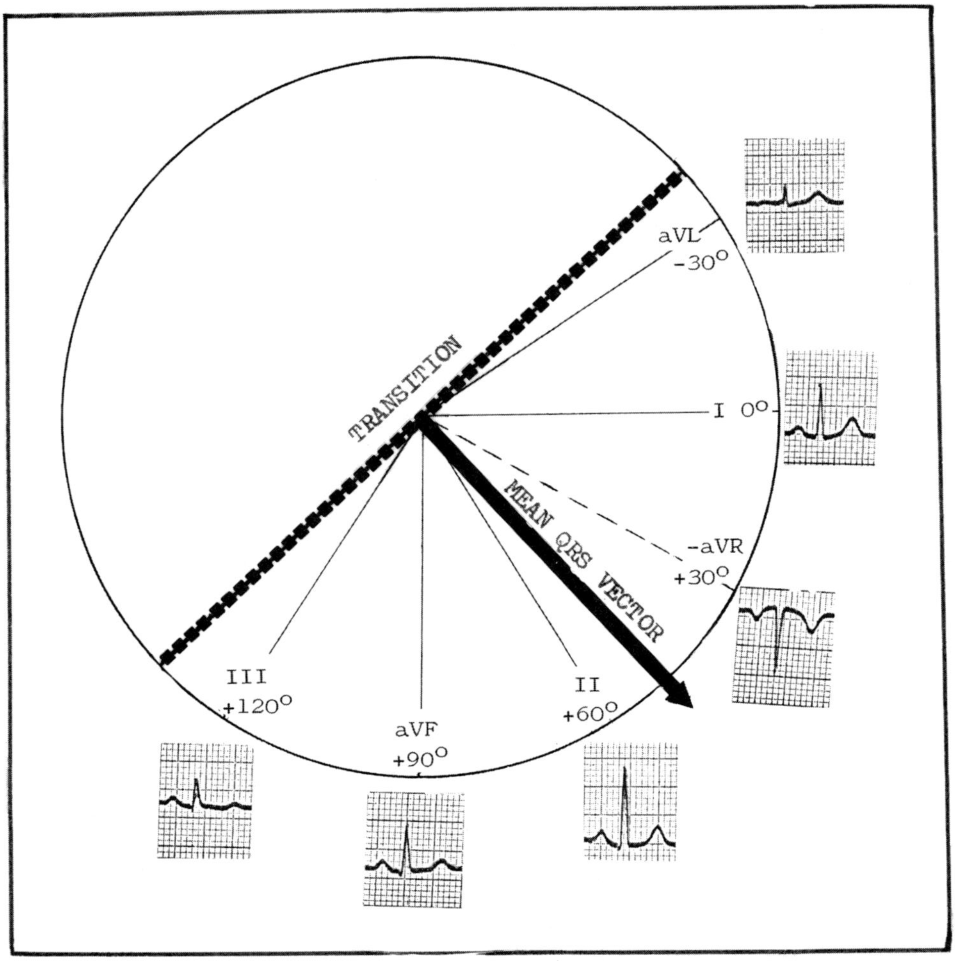

FIGURE 1–62. Mean QRS vector in frontal plane, to left and inferior.

all face the arrow side of the disk.

Is this the case in Figure 1–61? No.

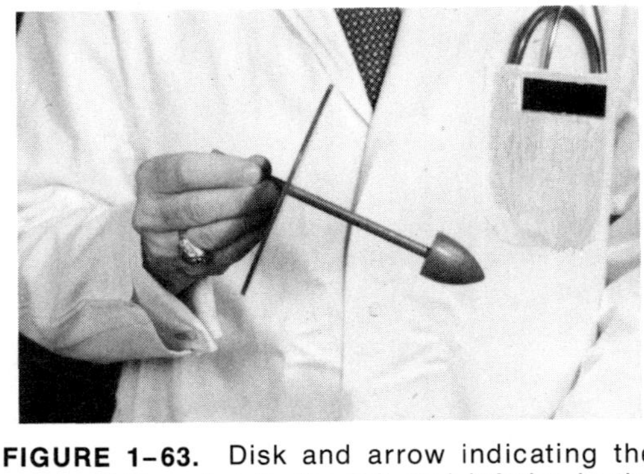

FIGURE 1–63. Disk and arrow indicating the mean QRS vector to the left and inferior in the frontal plane.

On looking again at Figure 1–61 notice that *not only* V_1 *but also* V_2 *is negative.* Leads V_3, V_4, V_5 and V_6 are *positive.* The transition in the horizontal plane is between V_2 and V_3. How do we make our model reflect the electrocardiographic inscription? Note again that the fixed point on this model is the 0, which is aligned with the center of the disk. The disk and arrow cannot be moved up or down, but must be rotated anteriorly or posteriorly. We must tilt the disk so that the arrow faces *posteriorly* (Fig. 1–65). In this position both leads V_1 and V_2 face the negative side of the disk, away from the arrow. Leads V_3, V_4, V_5 and V_6 are positive.

The mean QRS vector, as seen from

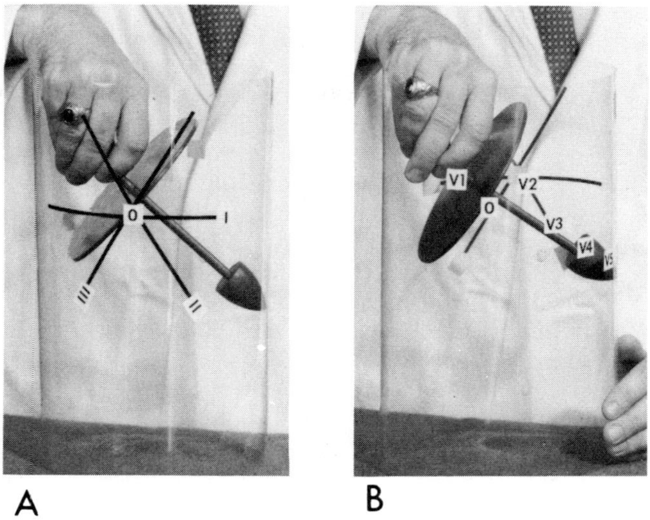

FIGURE 1–64. Vector model, with frontal (*A*) and horizontal (*B*) leads. See text.

Figure 1–61, described in three dimensions, is to the *left, inferior* and *posterior.* This describes the mean spatial QRS vector of the normal adult (Fig. 1–65).

To summarize, whether the mean QRS vector is *left and inferior, left and superior, right and inferior* or *right and superior* is determined from the frontal plane leads, I, II, III, aVR, aVL and aVF. Whether the mean QRS vector is *anterior* or *posterior* must be determined from the *horizontal plane leads* V_1 to V_6.

The vector approach, despite the inaccuracies pointed out earlier, affords us a unifying concept in our understanding of the electrocardiogram. By visualizing the distribution of electrical potential in a three-dimensional way, a single picture, as seen in Figure 1–65, actually indicates what we may find on the twelve lead electrocardiogram.

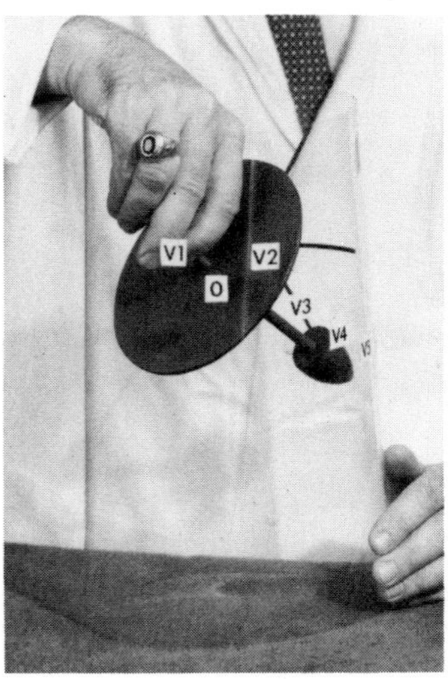

FIGURE 1–65. The mean QRS vector, in three dimensions, is to the left, inferior and posterior.

Cassette Side 4

Analyze Figure 1–66 following the steps used in Figure 1–61. After you have determined the mean QRS vector in three dimensions, check your work with Figures 1–67 and 1–68.

Analyzing the electrocardiogram (Fig. 1–66), we see that once again all six leads are positive, remembering to invert lead aVR. The transitional zone bypasses all of the leads, the mean QRS vector falls between leads II and −aVR. This is diagrammed in Figure 1–67, as you have seen many, many times before. The mean QRS vector, in the frontal plane, is to the left and inferior.

With the mean QRS vector to the left and inferior in the frontal plane (Fig. 1–68*A*), we now turn our attention to the precordial leads for its orientation in the horizontal plane (Fig. 1–68*B*). Leads V_1, V_2 and V_3 are negative, and V_4, V_5 and V_6 are positive. The transition in the precordial leads falls between V_3 and V_4. In the previous electrocardiogram (Fig. 1–61) the transition was between V_2 and V_3, but here it is between V_3 and V_4. We must, therefore, rotate our disk so that the arrow faces more and more posteriorly. Here, too, the mean QRS vector is to the left, inferior and posterior; it is more posterior, however, than in Figure 1–61.

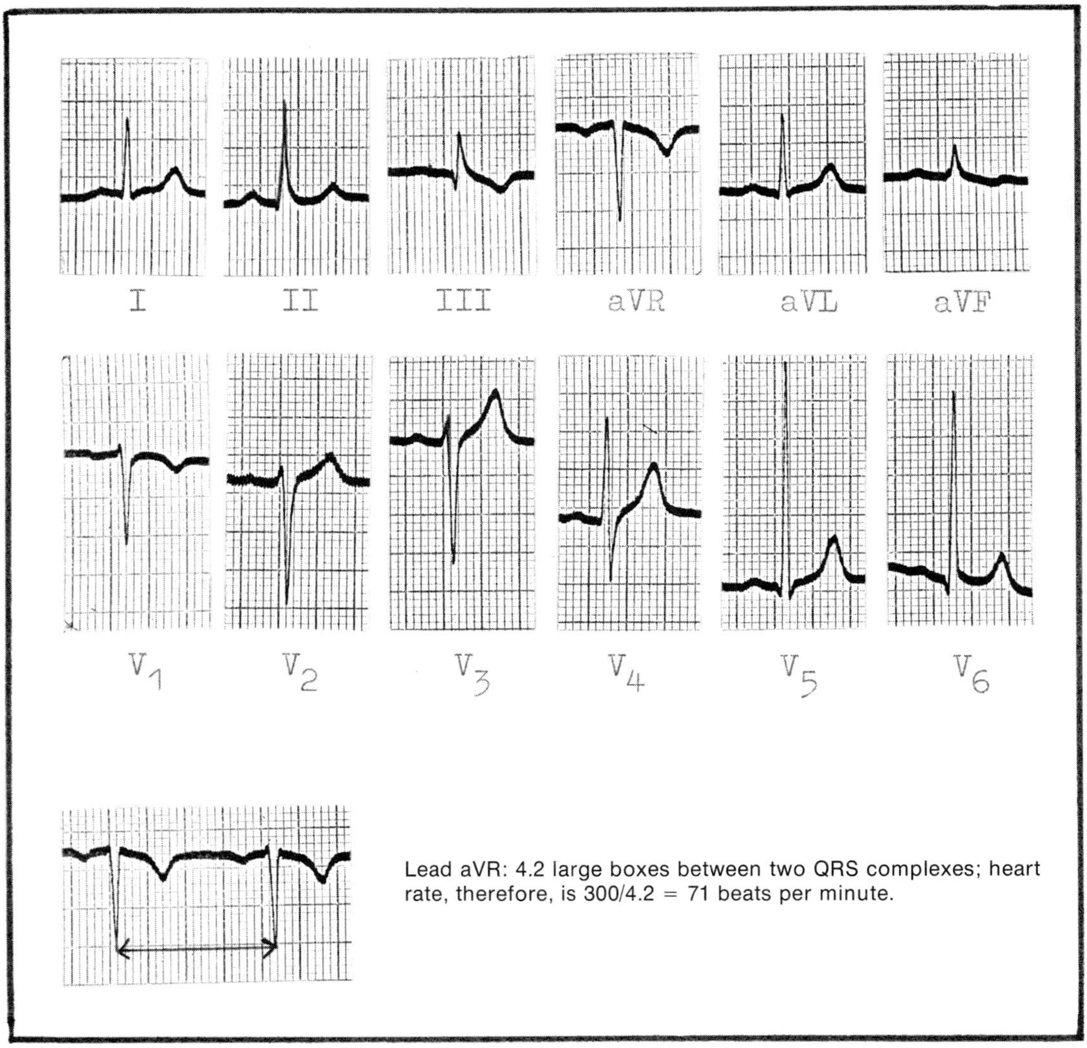

FIGURE 1–66. Refer to Figures 1–67 and 1–68 for visualization of the mean QRS vector in three dimensions.

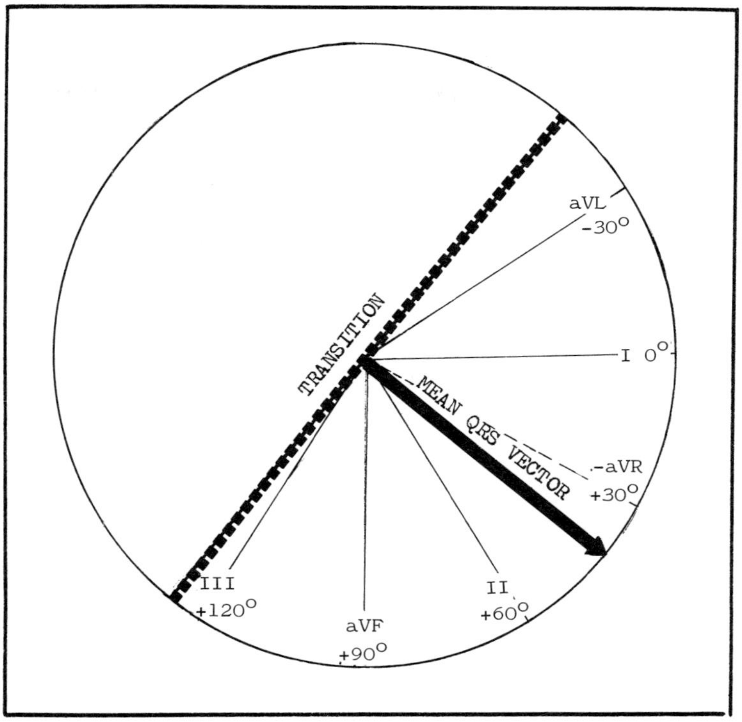

FIGURE 1-67. Mean QRS vector in frontal plane, to left and inferior.

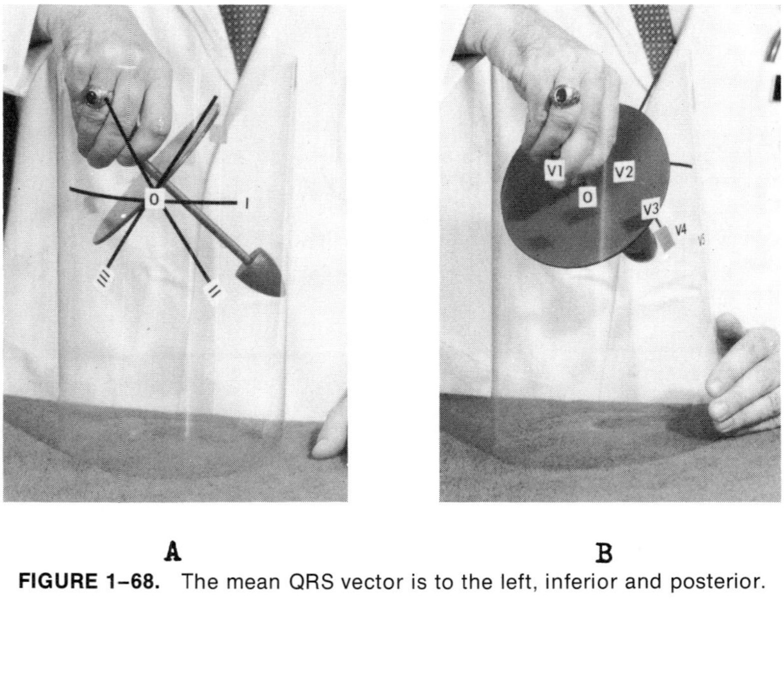

FIGURE 1-68. The mean QRS vector is to the left, inferior and posterior.

In Figure 1–69 the transition is at lead I and the mean QRS vector is at 90°. The mean QRS vector in this frontal plane is neither to the left nor to the right. The arrow is pointing directly inferiorly (Fig. 1–70). This frontal plane mean QRS vector is also illustrated on our vector model in Figure 1–71.

If the mean QRS vector were directly inferior—neither anterior nor posterior (Fig. 1–72*A*)—leads V_1 and V_2 would both be negative and leads V_3 to V_6 would all be positive. The electrocardiogram (Fig. 1–69), however, shows the transition to be between V_3 and V_4. In order to make V_3 negative on the vector model we must tilt the arrow posteriorly. The mean QRS vector is, therefore, inferior and posterior (Fig. 1–72*B*).

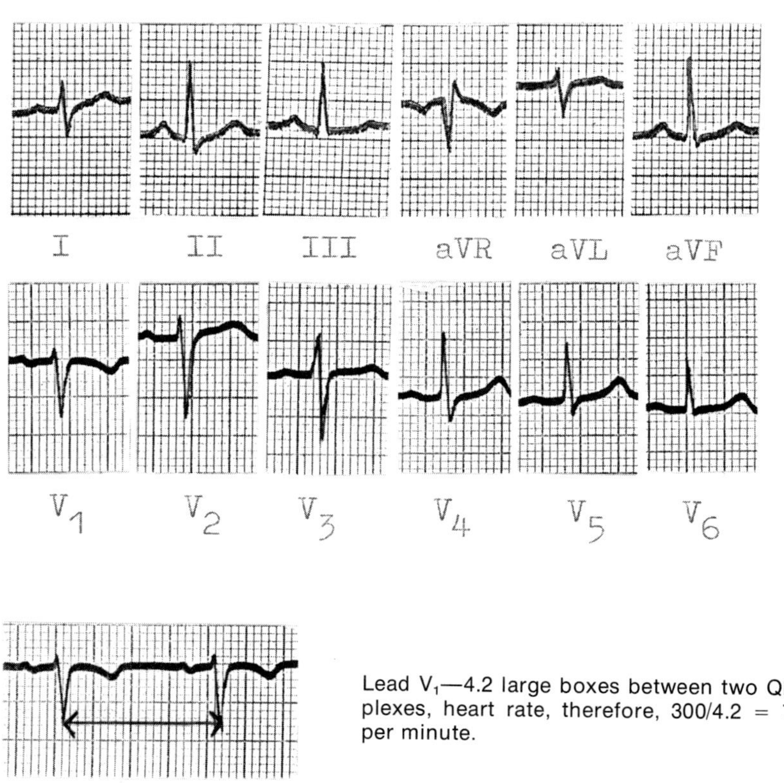

Lead V_1—4.2 large boxes between two QRS complexes, heart rate, therefore, 300/4.2 = 71 beats per minute.

FIGURE 1–69. Refer to Figures 1–70 to 1–72 to help you describe the mean spatial QRS vector.

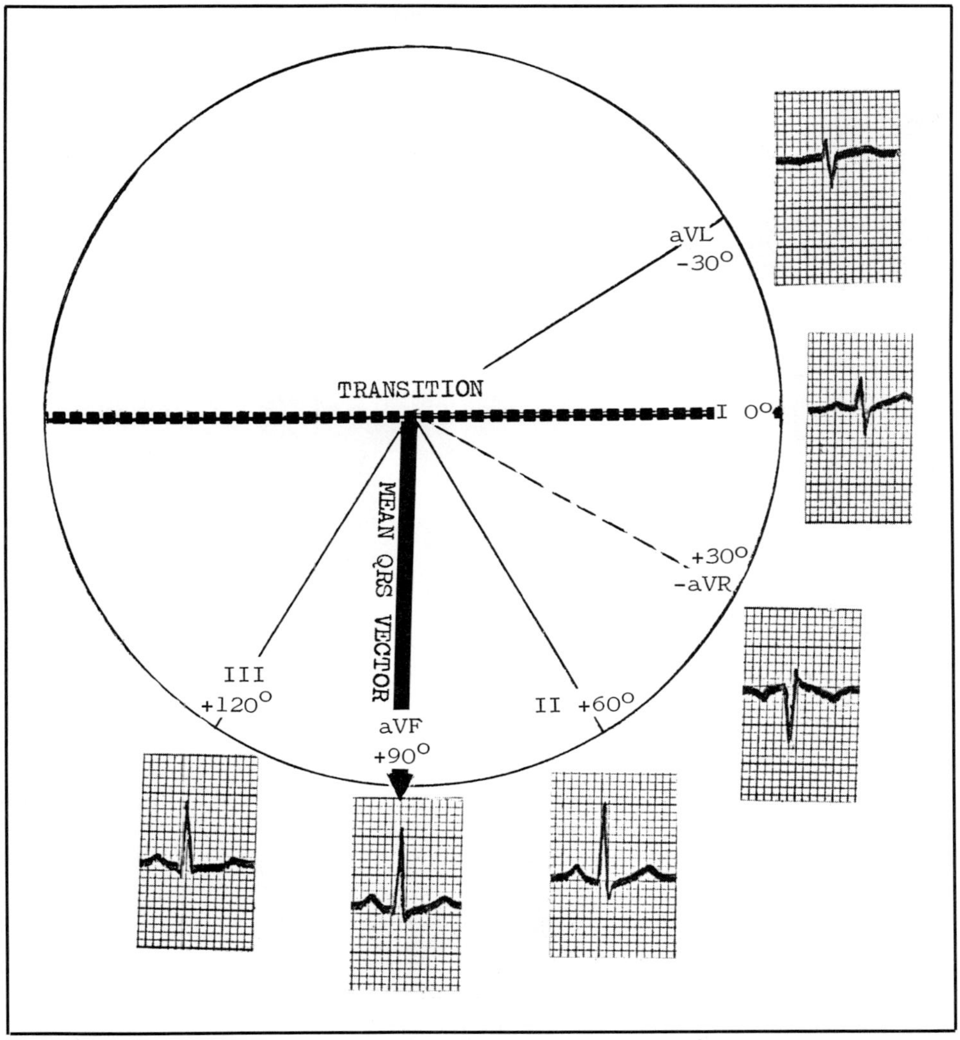

FIGURE 1–70. Mean QRS vector *inferior,* at 90°, in the frontal plane.

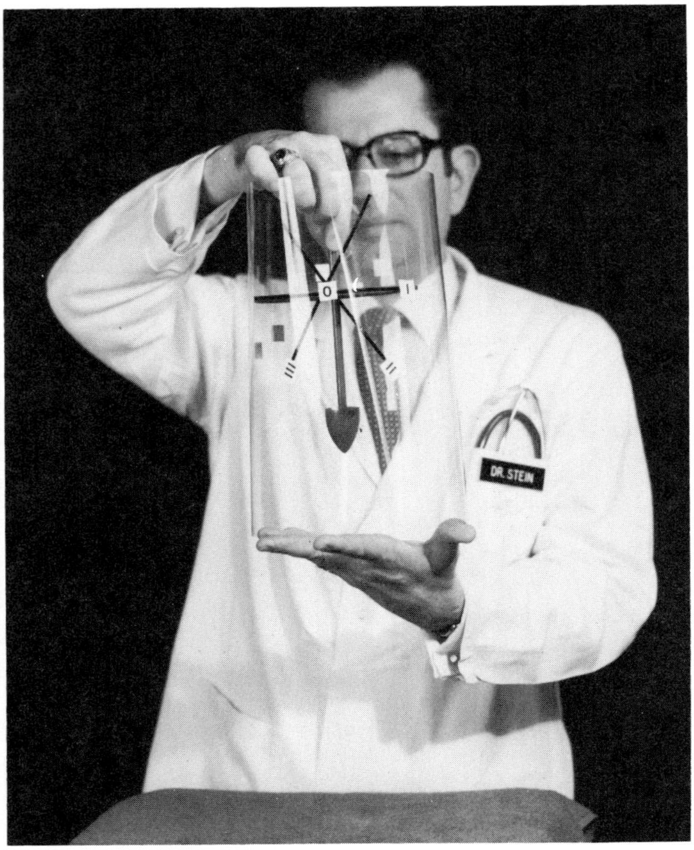

FIGURE 1-71. Mean QRS vector inferior, at 90°, in the frontal plane.

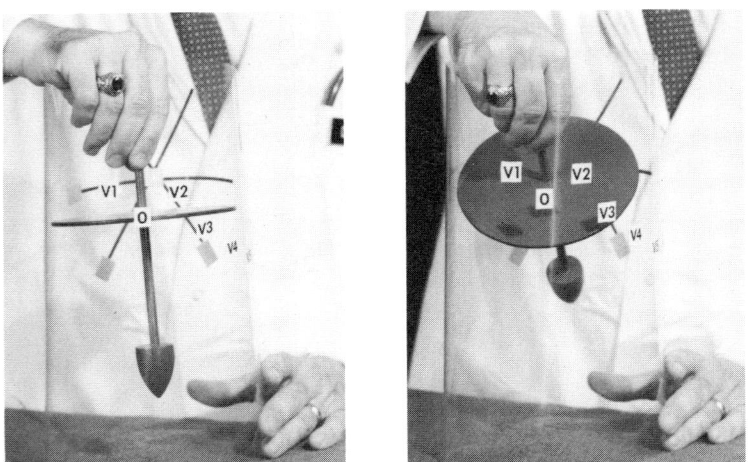

A B

FIGURE 1-72. Vector model for illustration of the mean QRS vector. See text.

Figure 1–73 is from a patient with chronic lung disease and cor pulmonale with enlargement of the right atrium and right ventricle. These entities will be studied in Chapter 2. For the present, evaluate the mean QRS vector as in previous examples.

In the frontal plane, the transition is at lead aVL, with the positive area in the upper part of the circle (Fig. 1–74). The mean QRS vector is to the *right* and *superior*.

The mean QRS vector, on our vector model (Fig. 1–75*A*), is again seen to be to the right and superior, with leads I, II and III all negative, all facing away from the arrow side of the disk. If the mean QRS vector were merely to the right and superior, lead V_1 would be positive and V_2 to V_6 would fall on the negative side of the disk (Fig. 1–75*B*). The electrocardiogram (Fig. 1–73), however, reveals that the transition is between leads V_2 and V_3. We must tilt the disk so that the arrow points anteriorly (Fig. 1–75*C*) and the mean spatial QRS vector is to the *right, superior* and *anterior*.

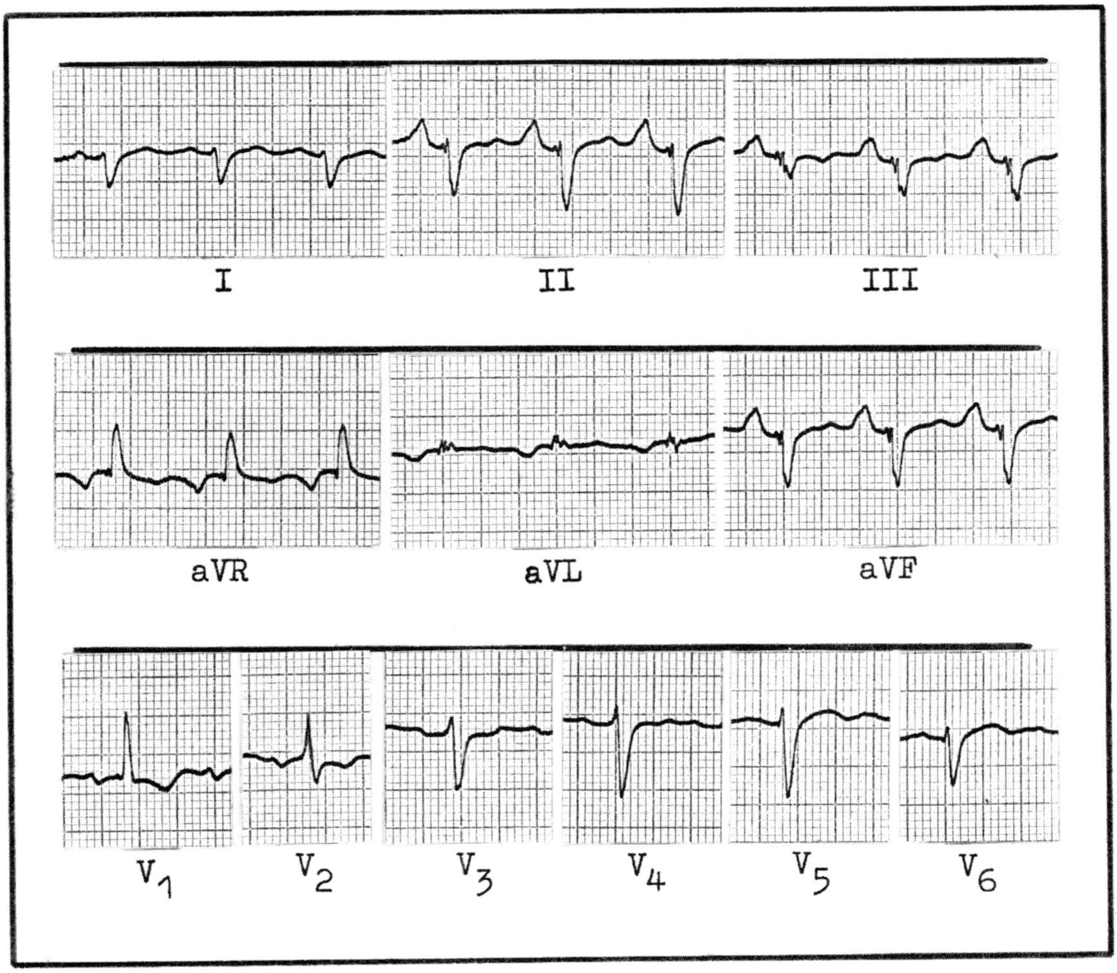

FIGURE 1–73. Calculate the mean spatial QRS vector. Refer to Figures 1–74 and 1–75.

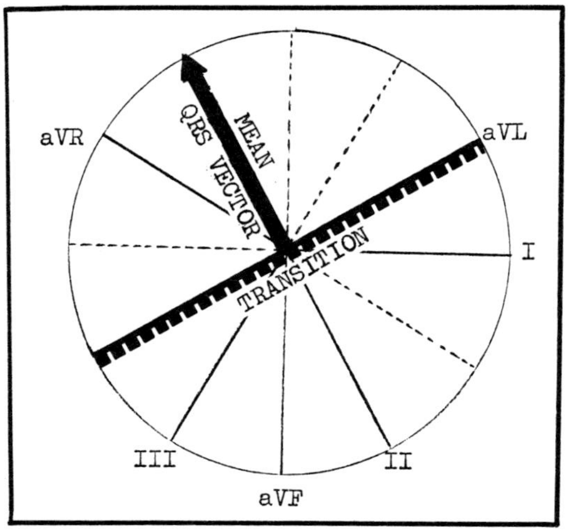

FIGURE 1–74. The mean QRS vector in the frontal plane is to the right and superior.

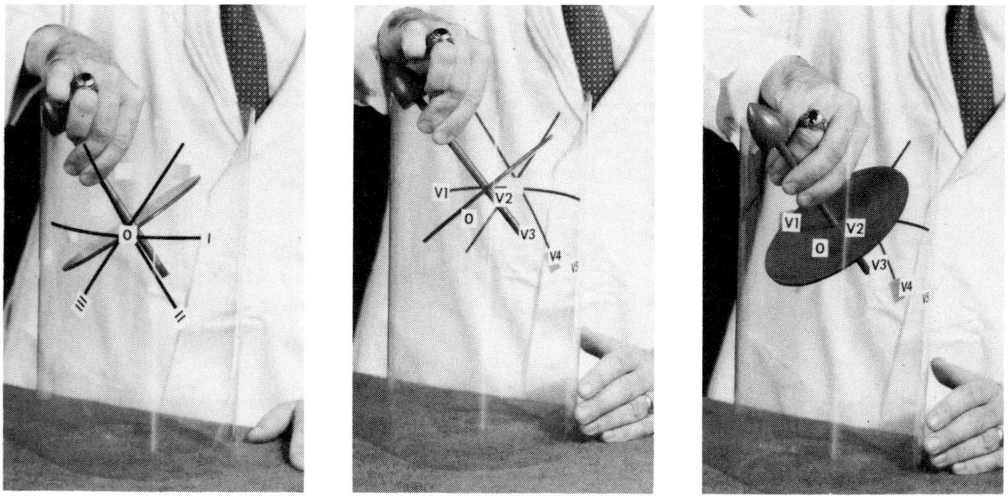

A B C

FIGURE 1–75. Vector model for illustration of mean spatial QRS vector.

Using the steps outlined for the mean QRS vector, the mean T vector may be studied in the horizontal plane. This is important for the determination of the horizontal QRS–T angle, which rarely exceeds 60° in the normal adult.

The S–T segment, representing the early phase of the ventricular repolarization process, is very important in clinical medicine, and will be discussed again in later chapters. The S–T segment is usually isoelectric—neither elevated nor depressed—(the same as the baseline for the electrocardiogram). An S–T segment which is not isoelectric, however, does not automatically indicate abnormality. When a mean S–T vector is measurable it is usually parallel to the mean T vector (the S–T segment follows the T wave in direction). This is commonly seen in the presence of large T waves and will be covered in a later chapter.

Another measurement of importance is the *Q–T interval* (review Fig. 1–22), from the beginning of the QRS complex to the end of the T wave. This interval is related to the heart rate. The mean Q–T intervals for various heart rates are as follows:

Heart Rate (beats per minute)	*Q–T Interval* (sec.)
40	0.46
60	0.39
80	0.35
100	0.31
120	0.29
140	0.26
160	0.25

So far we have discussed the development of the Einthoven triangle, the triaxial system and the hexaxial system including leads I, II, III, aVR, aVL and aVF. These six leads were assigned degrees around the circle from lead aVL at −30° to III at +120°. The summations, leads I + III = II and aVR + aVL + aVF = 0, were studied, as were depolarization, repolarization and the conduction system of the heart, and electrocardiographic waves, intervals and segments. Heart rate and sinus rhythm were discussed. The spatial vector concept was emphasized in the study of the QRS, T and P, as well as the special relationship between the QRS and T, known as the QRS–T angle. The Q–T interval was found to be related to heart rate. Items such as size of QRS complexes and P waves, although important, have not been discussed, since they will be studied in future chapters.

Based on information in this chapter, electrocardiograms will be analyzed as to: rhythm, rate, P–R interval, mean QRS vector, QRS interval, mean T vector, QRS–T angle, S–T segment and Q–T interval.

Following is Table 1–2 which will serve as a general review of this chapter and as a key for the stepwise analysis of electrocardiograms. "Rules of thumb" are also included.

TABLE 1–2. REVIEW AND STEPWISE ANALYSIS OF ELECTROCARDIOGRAMS INCLUDING "RULES OF THUMB" (BASED ON INFORMATION IN CHAPTER 1)

The aim of all the many hours of study has been to emphasize a few, but very basic, concepts to facilitate an understanding of the electrocardiogram. You should, at this point, review all of the material; an additional hour now will save many in the future. Much of what has been covered may be summarized in a few simple steps. Several "rules of thumb" are also included here. As with any summary in which vast amounts of material are condensed into basic rules, you may find some exceptions, but, in general, they work quite well. Any electrocardiograms not strictly fitting the criteria summarized below should be analyzed more carefully; the electrocardiogram may still be within the outer limits of normal.

1. **Leads I + III = Lead II**
   Leads aVR + aVL + aVF = 0
   These are electrical truths and hold for all inscriptions on the electrocardiogram. If these do not add up, recheck the electrocardiogram—for example, for mismounting. Remember it is the *area* which adds up; the height and depth of the complexes may be used as good approximations.
2. **Calculate the mean P vector** to see if it falls within the narrow limits of normal. In order to describe the rhythm of the heart as *sinus rhythm* (the impulse originating in the sinoatrial node), which is the normal rhythm of the heart, the following conditions must be met.
   a. The mean P vector must be normal.
   b. Each P wave must be followed by a QRS complex and each QRS complex must be preceded by a P wave.
   c. The P-R interval (from the beginning of the P wave to the beginning of the QRS complex) is rarely greater than 0.20 sec. (one large box) in duration in the normal.adult. The normal range is 0.12 to 0.20 sec., and constant from beat to beat.
   d. The rate is constant, between 60 and 100 beats per minute. In a regular rhythm divide the number of large boxes (0.20 sec.) between two complexes into 300 to determine the rate per minute.

"Rule of thumb" for normal P vector: The normal P waves must be positive (upright) in leads I and aVF. Leads I and II may be used, as an approximation, if aVF is not given.

3. **Calculate the mean QRS vector.** The QRS complex should be 0.10 sec. (2½ small boxes), or less, in duration.

"Rule of thumb" for normal mean QRS vector in the frontal plane: The QRS deflections must be *positive* in leads I and aVF. Leads I and II may be used, as an approximation, if aVF is not given.
"Rule of thumb" for normal mean QRS vector in the horizontal plane: When the mean QRS vector is normal (leftward and inferior in orientation), leads V_1, V_2 and often V_3 are predominantly negative, reflecting the *posterior* orientation of the vector.

4. **Calculate the mean T vector and determine the QRS–T angle.**

"Rule of thumb" for normal QRS–T angle in the frontal plane: The T waves should follow the QRS complexes, in direction, in leads I and aVF. For example, when the QRS is positive in lead I, the T wave should also be positive. When the QRS is negative, the T wave should also be negative. Leads I and II may be used if aVF is not given. This is, at best, an approximation. The actual calculation is always better than the "rule of thumb."
"Rule of thumb" for normal QRS–T angle in the horizontal plane: The T waves should follow the QRS complexes, in direction, from leads V_3 to V_6, or at least from V_4 to V_6.

In most normal persons the QRS complexes are predominantly positive from leads V_3 or V_4 to V_6. The T waves are predominantly positive from V_2 or V_3 to V_6. A variant of this, in the normal, will be seen later in the course.

5. **Evaluation of the S–T segment.**
   The S–T segment in the normal adult is usually isoelectric (same as baseline for the electrocardiogram), neither elevated nor depressed. An S–T segment which is not isoelectric, however, does not automatically indicate abnormality. When a mean S–T vector is measurable it is usually parallel to the mean T vector (the S–T segment follows the T wave in direction). This is commonly seen in the presence of large T waves and will be studied in a later chapter.

TABLE 1-2. *(Continued)*

6. **Q–T interval.**

Heart Rate (beats per minute)	*Q–T Interval* (sec.)
40	0.46
60	0.39
80	0.35
100	0.31
120	0.29
140	0.26
160	0.25

Note: "Rules of thumb" are given as an aid; they must never be a substitute for a thorough knowledge of the subject.

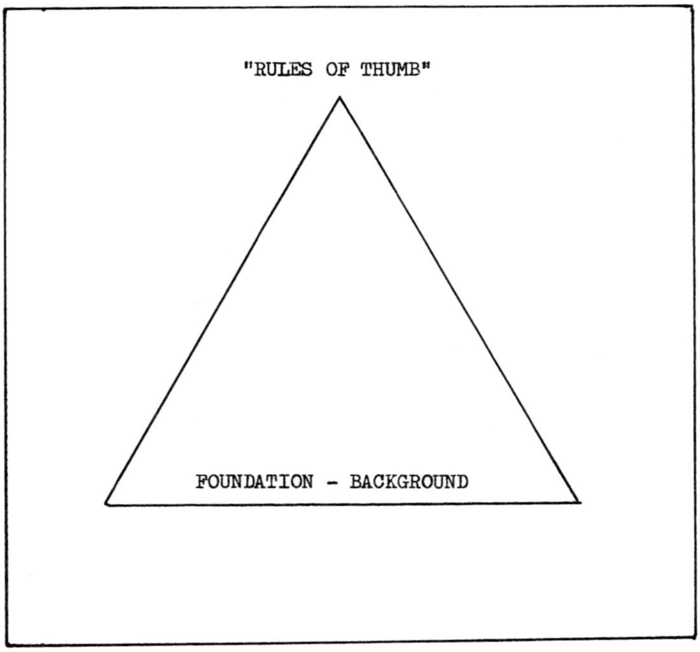

FIGURE 1-76. Whenever "rules of thumb" are given caution must be exercised. "Rules of thumb" must never be used without falling back upon the foundation of knowledge. They are merely the tip of the iceberg, and exceptions will be found. Always be ready to completely analyze any electrocardiogram for which questions arise. Keep reviewing the basis for the "rules."

NORMAL ELECTROCARDIOGRAMS FOR REVIEW AND PRACTICE

Based on the steps outlined in Table 1–2 you will analyze the following series of electrocardiograms. A careful analysis of each of these electrocardiograms will provide a good review of the principles learned in Chapter 1.

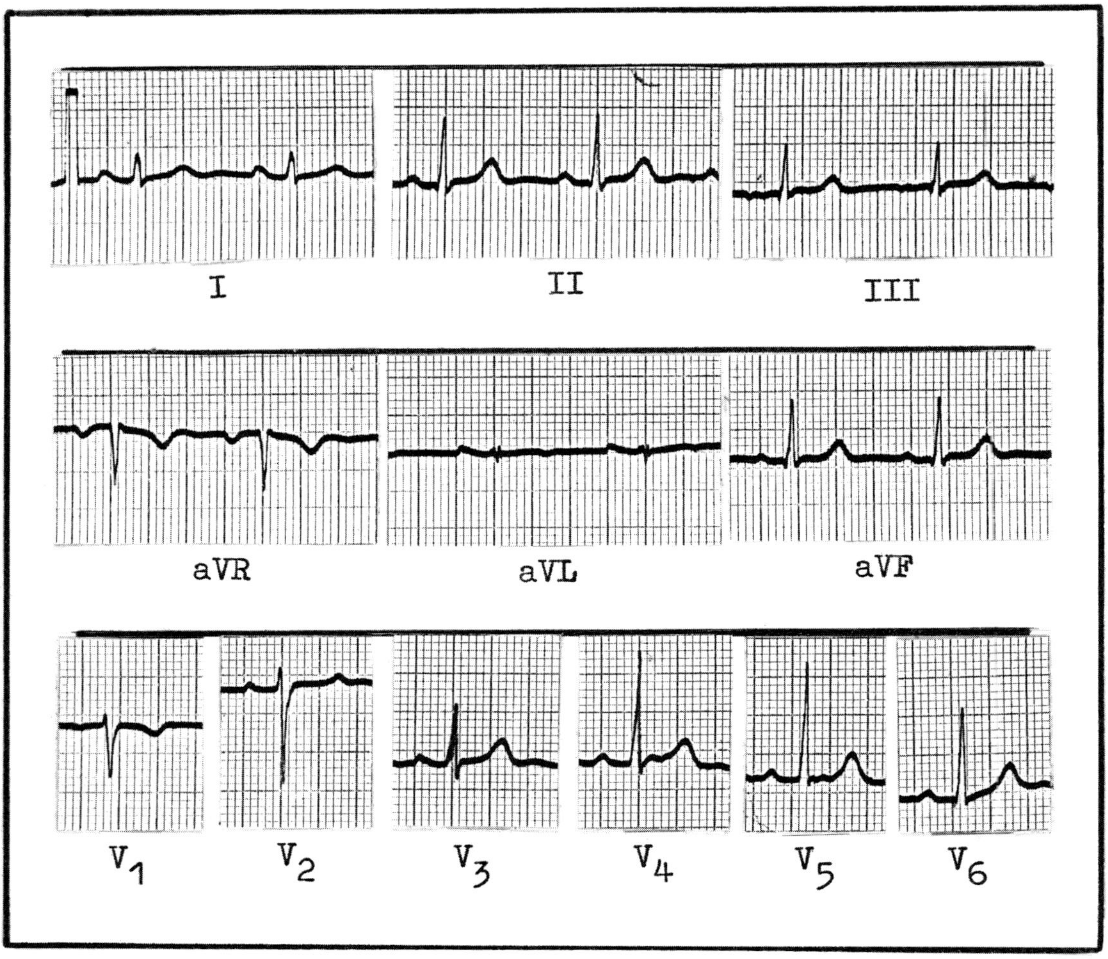

FIGURE 1–77. Normal.

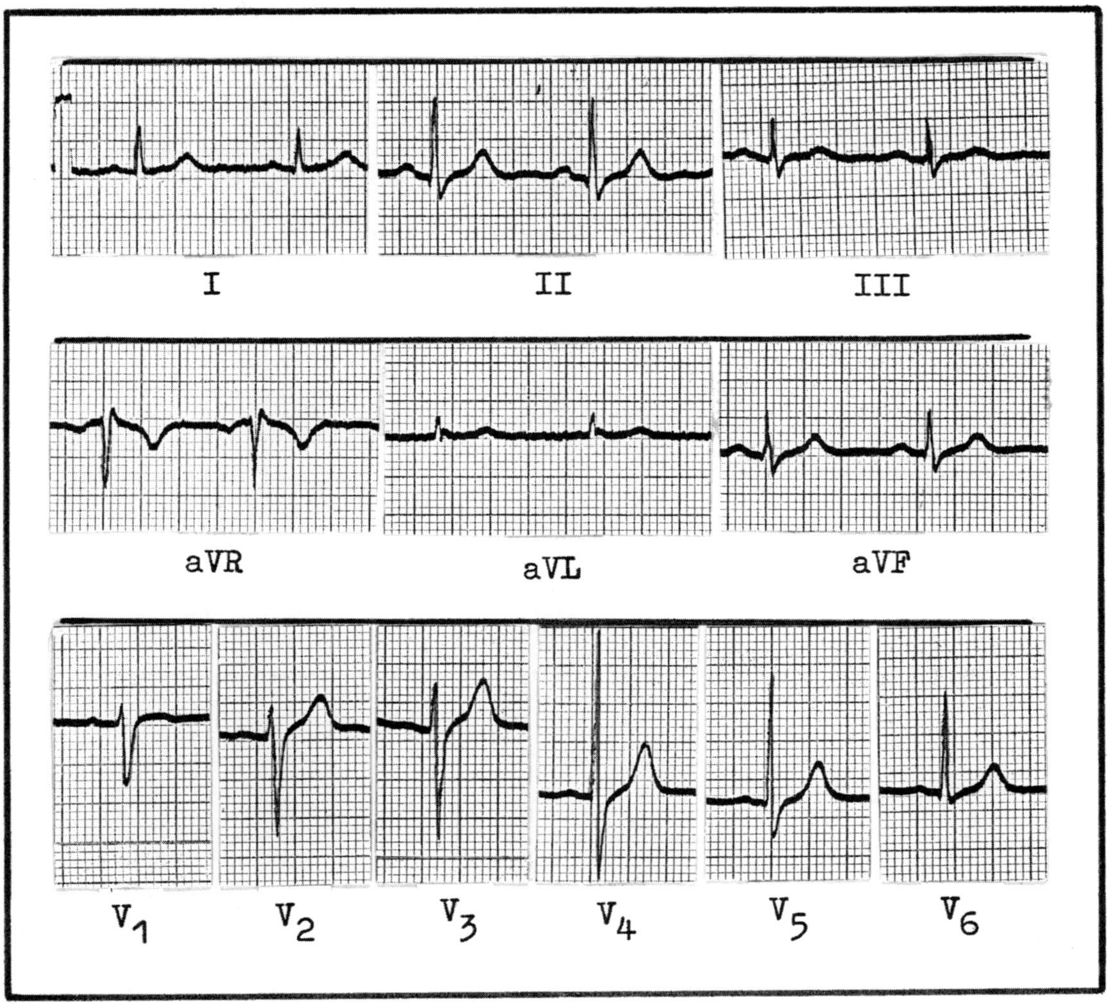

FIGURE 1–78. Normal.

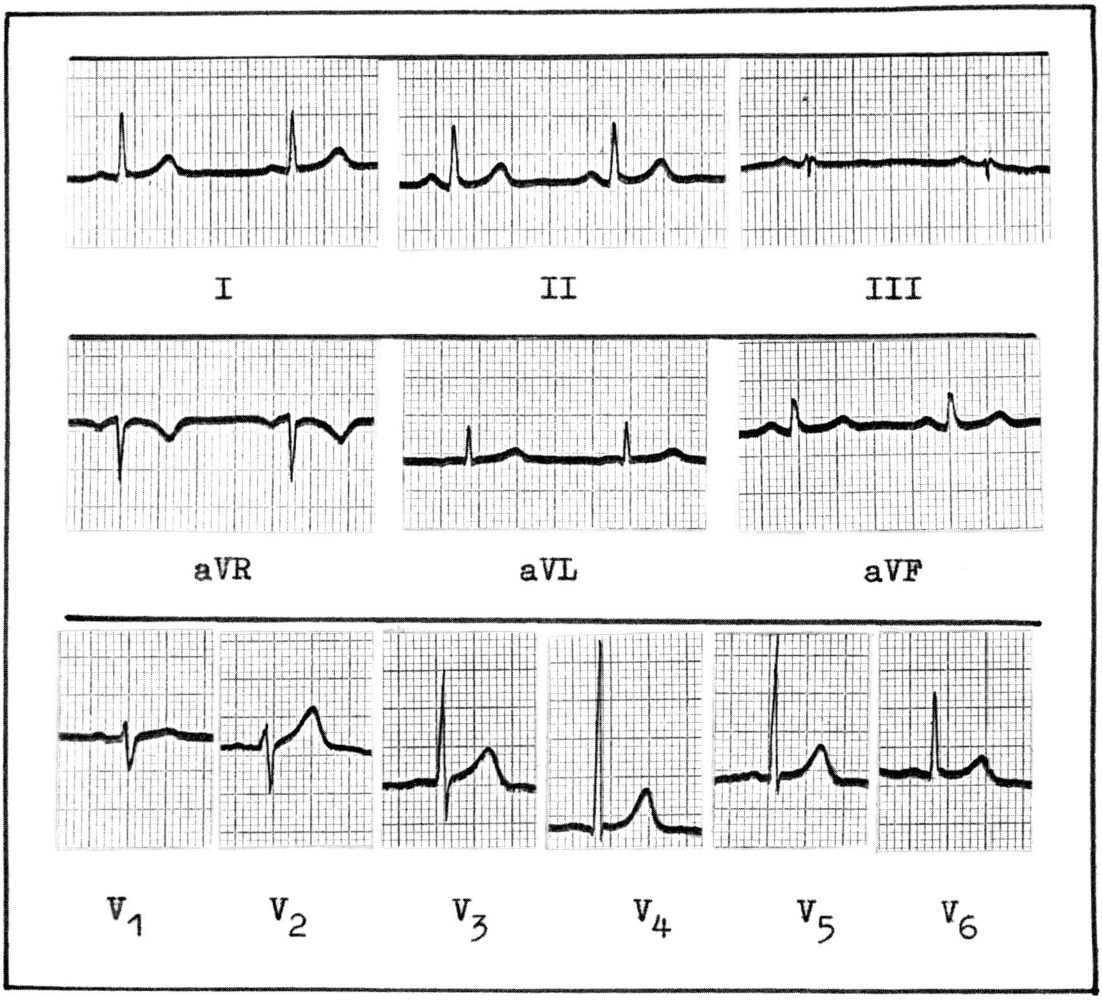

FIGURE 1–79. Normal.

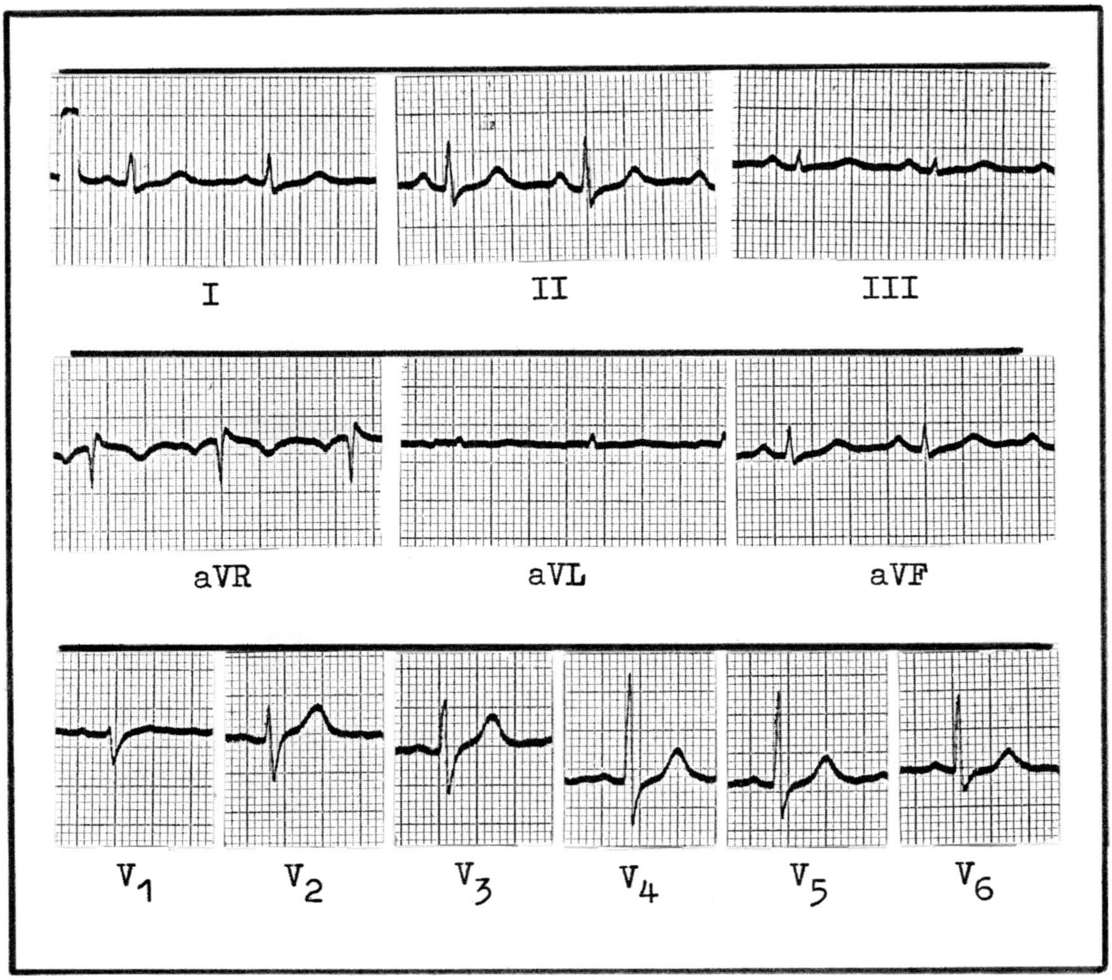

FIGURE 1–80. Normal.

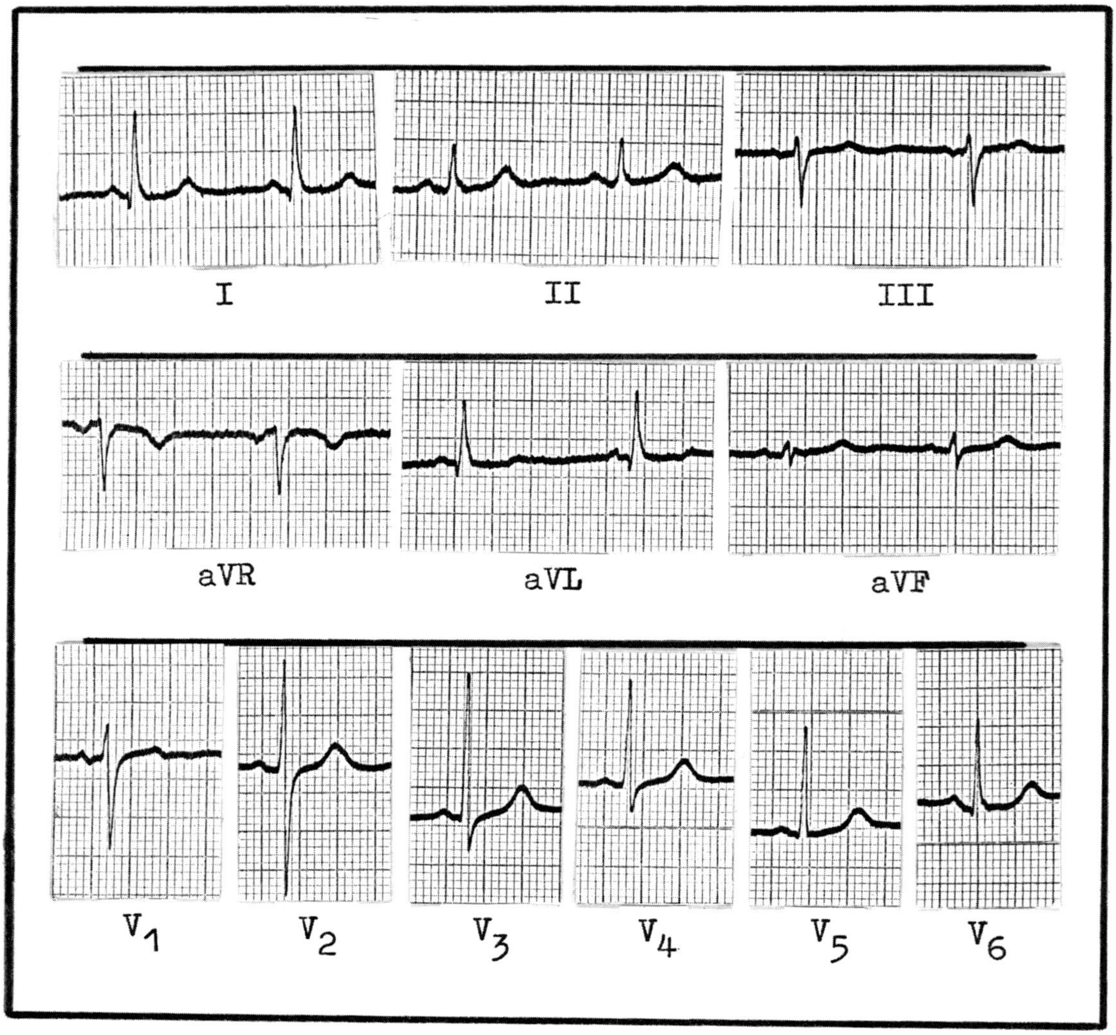

FIGURE 1–81. Normal.

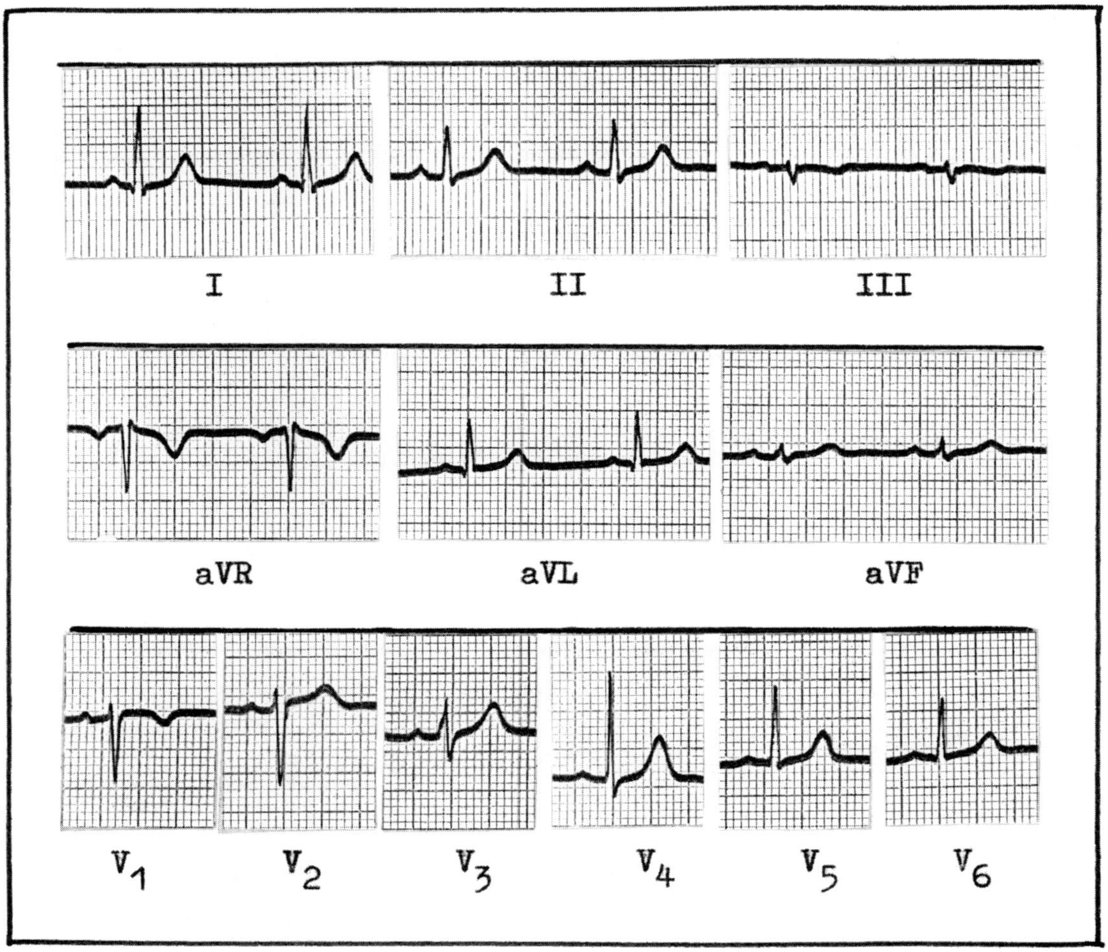

FIGURE 1–82. Normal.

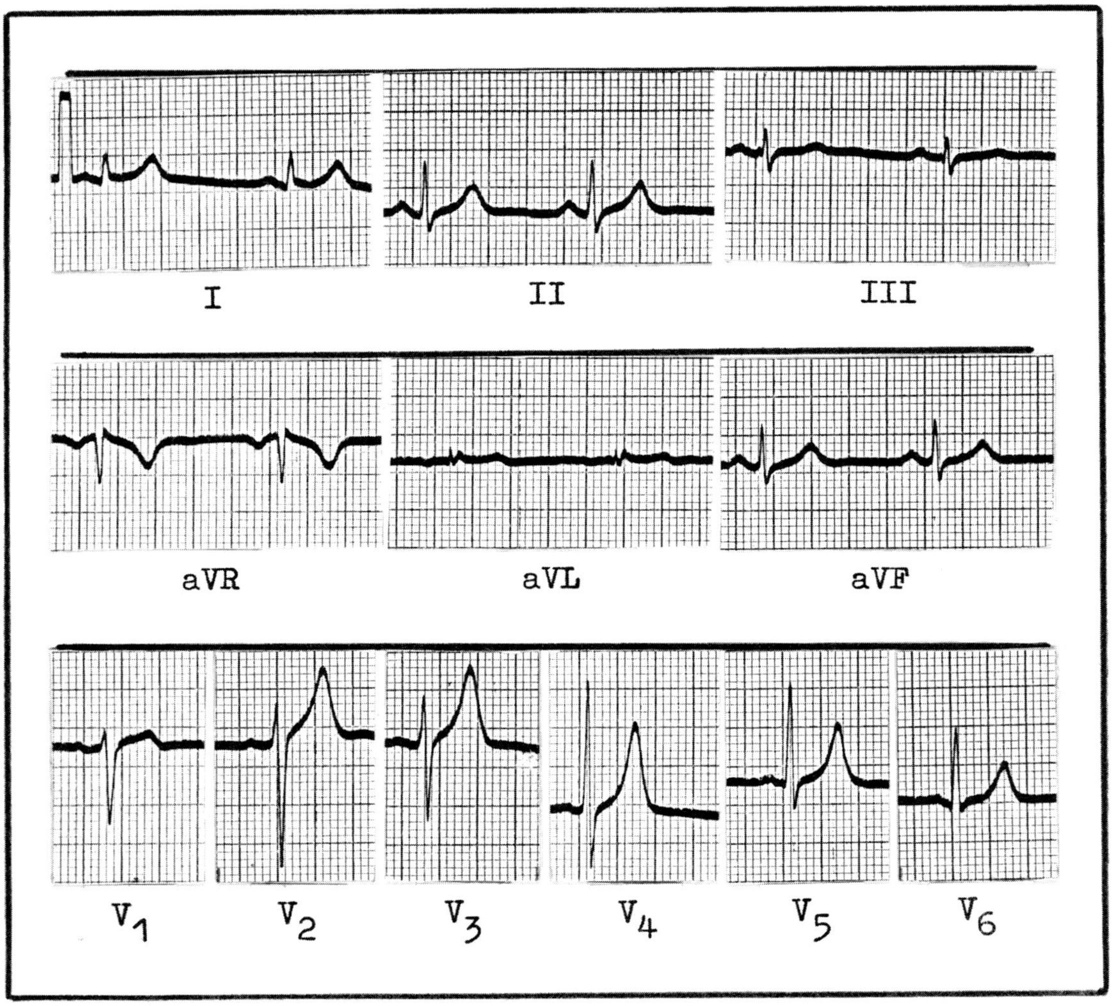

FIGURE 1–83. Normal.

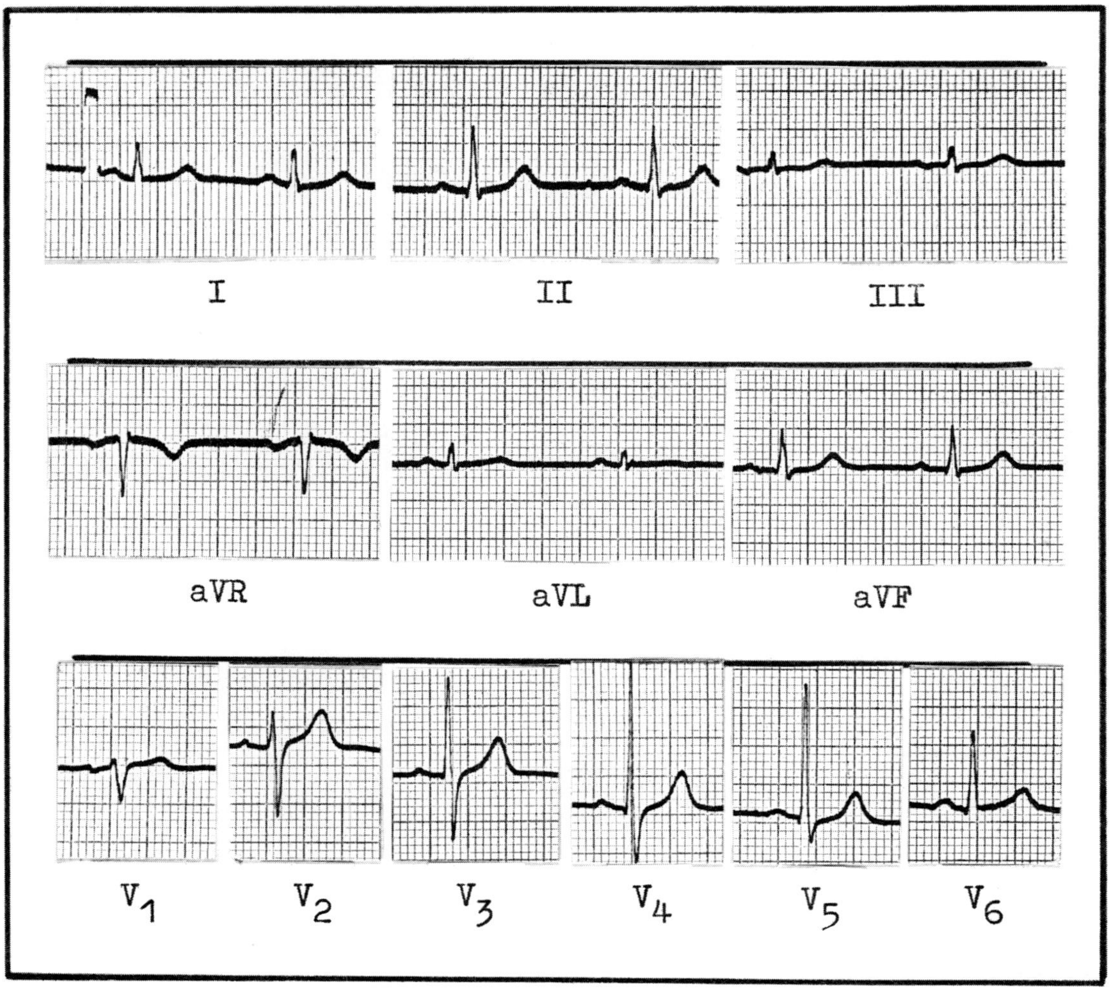

FIGURE 1–84. Normal.

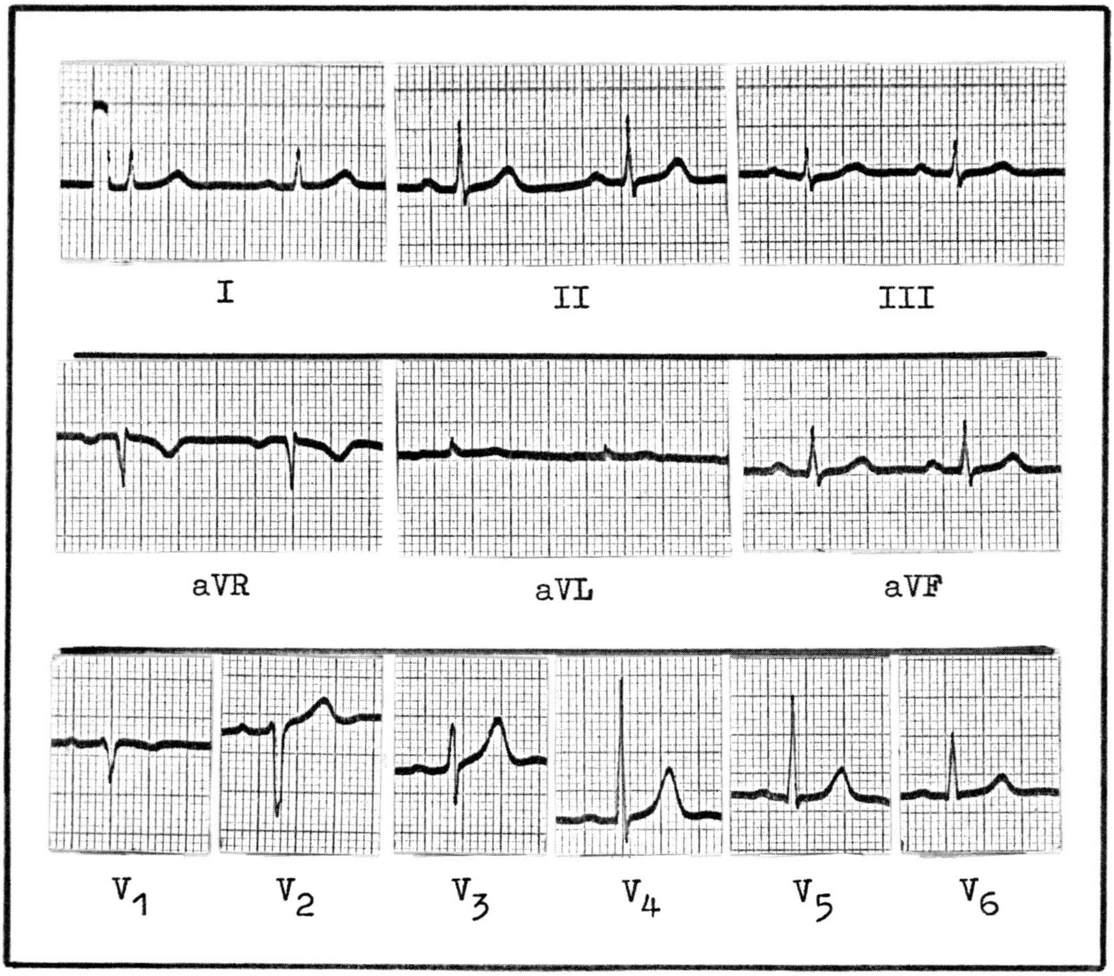

FIGURE 1–85. Normal.

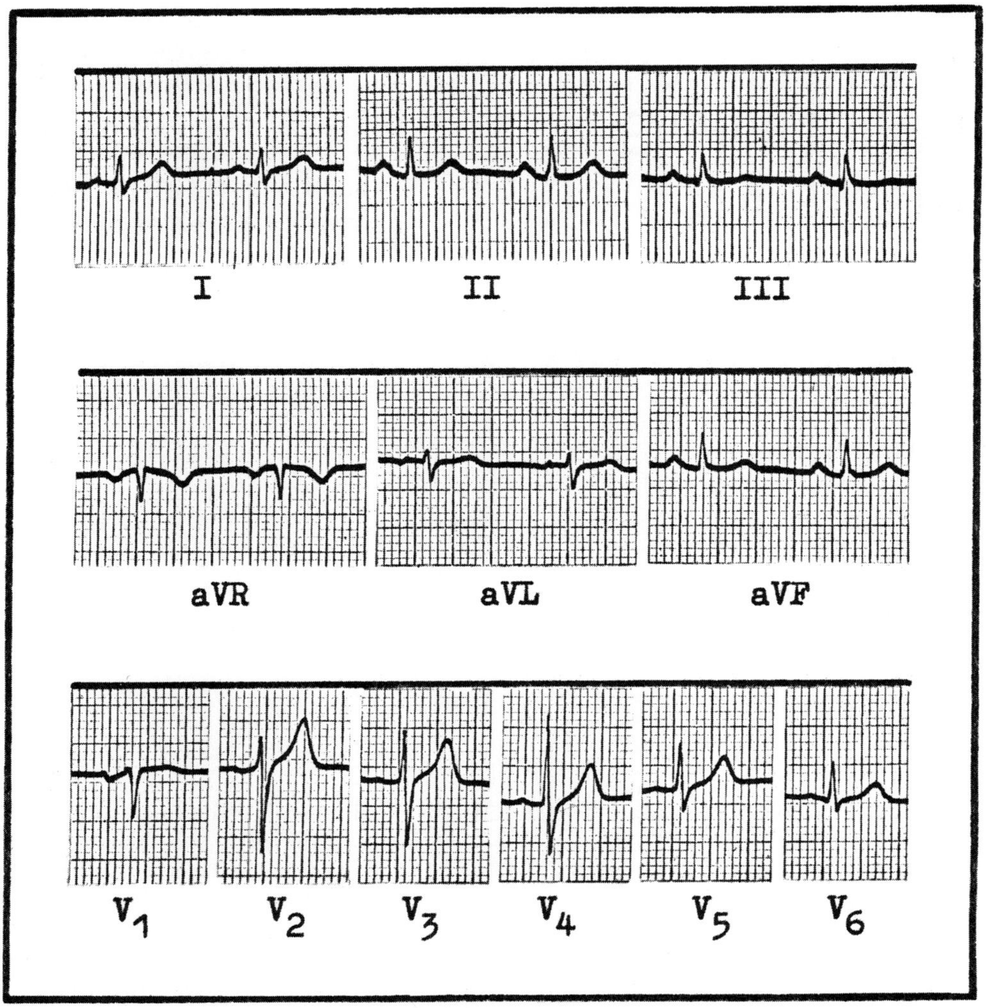

FIGURE 1–86. Normal.

2 RIGHT VENTRICULAR HYPERTROPHY (INCLUDING RIGHT AND LEFT ATRIAL ENLARGEMENT)

Cassette Side 5

RIGHT VENTRICULAR HYPERTROPHY

The diagnosis of right ventricular hypertrophy is frequently difficult to make, electrocardiographically, in the adult. The left ventricle is dominant, and even a very hypertrophied right ventricle may be overshadowed by a normal left ventricle. A normal electrocardiogram does not, therefore, rule out right ventricular hypertrophy. There are, however, certain findings on the electrocardiogram which help us make the diagnosis with reasonable security.

The "presumptive" or indirect evidence of right ventricular hypertrophy has often helped in the absence of direct electrocardiographic evidence. In addition to right atrial enlargement, left atrial enlargement will be discussed, since it may accompany right ventricular hypertrophy (for example, in the presence of mitral stenosis).

The word "hypertrophy" is commonly used. Admittedly, hypertrophy is not the only cause of an enlarged right ventricle and differentiation is often difficult on the electrocardiogram. "Enlargement" is a more inclusive term; both terms are used in this study.

Electrocardiographic diagnosis of right ventricular hypertrophy is made on the basis of:

A. Right axis deviation (of the mean QRS vector).
B. Magnitude of the mean QRS vector.
C. Repolarization abnormalities (abnormalities of the S–T segments and T waves).
D. "Presumptive" evidence.
   a. Right atrial enlargement.
   b. Left atrial enlargement (in presence of mitral stenosis).

A. Right Axis Deviation

In the normal adult, as already learned, the left ventricle is dominant (Fig. 2–1*A*) and the mean spatial QRS vector is usually oriented to the *left, inferiorly* and *posteriorly*. In the newborn (Fig. 2–1*B*) the right ventricle, located anteriorly and to the right of the left ventricle, is dominant and the mean QRS vector, reflecting this dominance, is usually to the *right, inferior* and *anterior*.

The mean QRS vector, which in infancy is to the *right, inferior* and *anterior*, becomes ever more *leftward* and ever more *posterior* throughout life (Fig. 2–2). The left ventricle early becomes, and remains throughout life, the dominant ventricle. Therefore, progression to or persistence of the pattern seen in infancy should cause you to immediately stop and to evaluate the patient for right ventricular hypertrophy. The importance of serial tracings must be stressed, for you may see subtle changes providing the clue to progressive hypertrophy of the right ventricle; this we see so often among our patients with pulmonary disease.

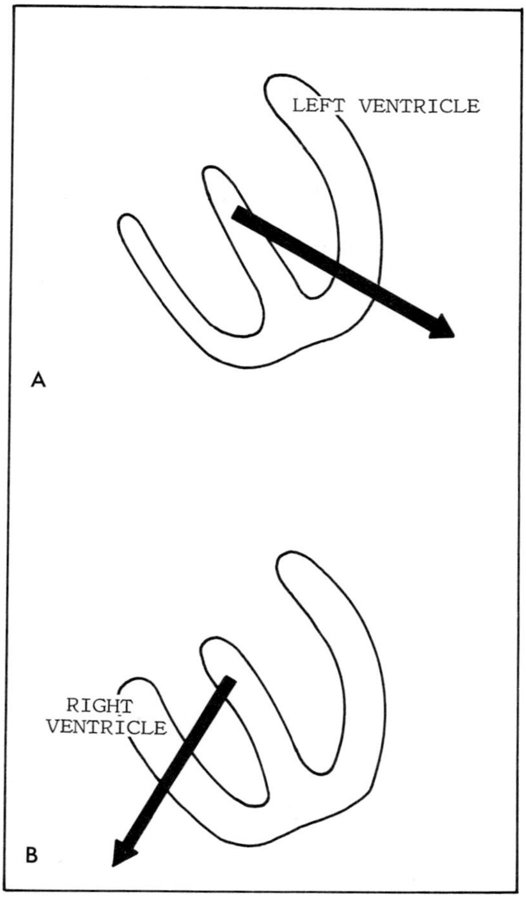

FIGURE 2–1. *A,* In the normal adult the left ventricle is dominant, and the mean QRS vector is usually to the *left, inferior* and *posterior. B,* In early life the right ventricle is dominant and the mean QRS vector is usually to the *right, inferior* and *anterior.*

In Figure 2–3*A* the mean QRS vector is to the *right, inferior* and *anterior*. This is in sharp contrast to the normal (Fig. 2–3*B*). Any time you see the QRS deflections predominantly *negative* in lead I and positive in leads II and III the mean QRS vector is oriented to the *right* and *inferiorly*. Figure 2–4 *A* is a diagram of the mean QRS vector in the frontal plane.

The QRS deflections in lead V_1 are *positive*, and the transition is close to lead V_6. What does this mean? It can easily be understood using the vector model, illustrated in Figure 2–5. The mean spatial QRS vector is not only *inferior* and to the *right*, but also *anterior*.

The two electrocardiographic characteristics of a mean spatial QRS vector oriented to the *right* and *anteriorly* are:

1. QRS deflections in lead I are *negative*.
2. QRS deflections in leads V_1 and V_2 are *positive*.

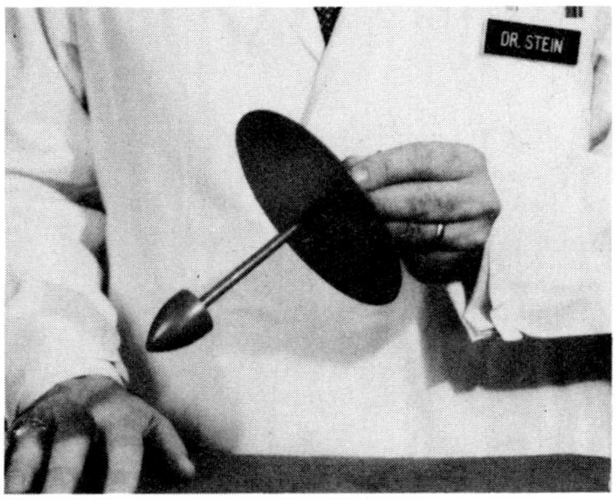

A. Infancy

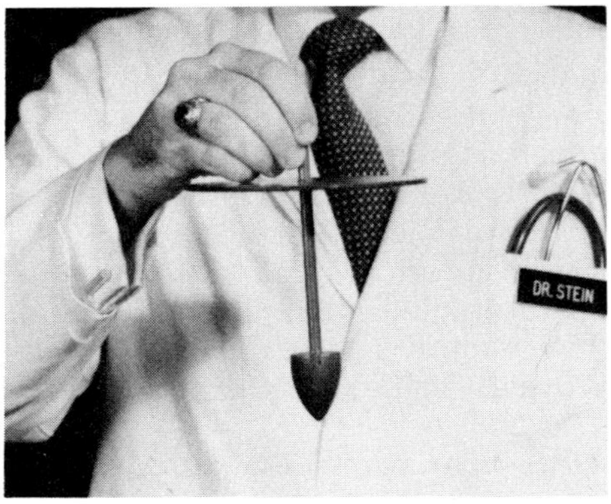

B. Youth

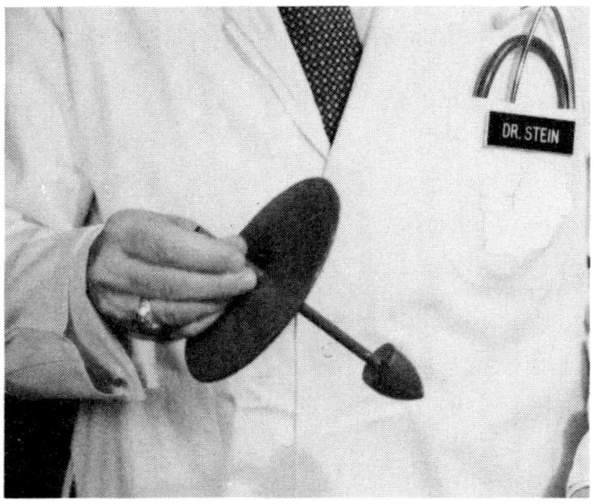

C. Adult

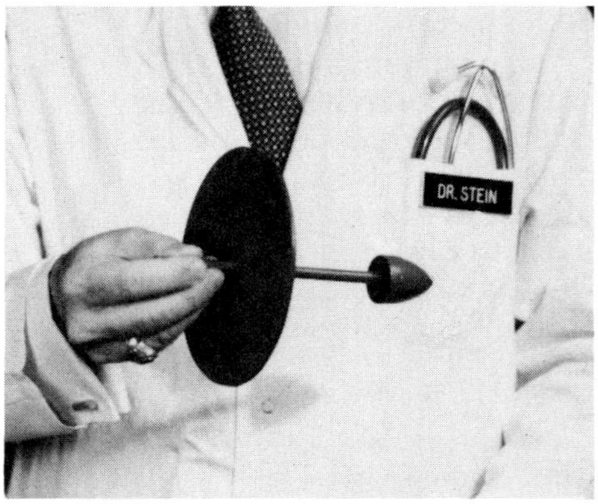

D. Old Age

FIGURE 2–2. Changes in the mean QRS vector from birth to old age.

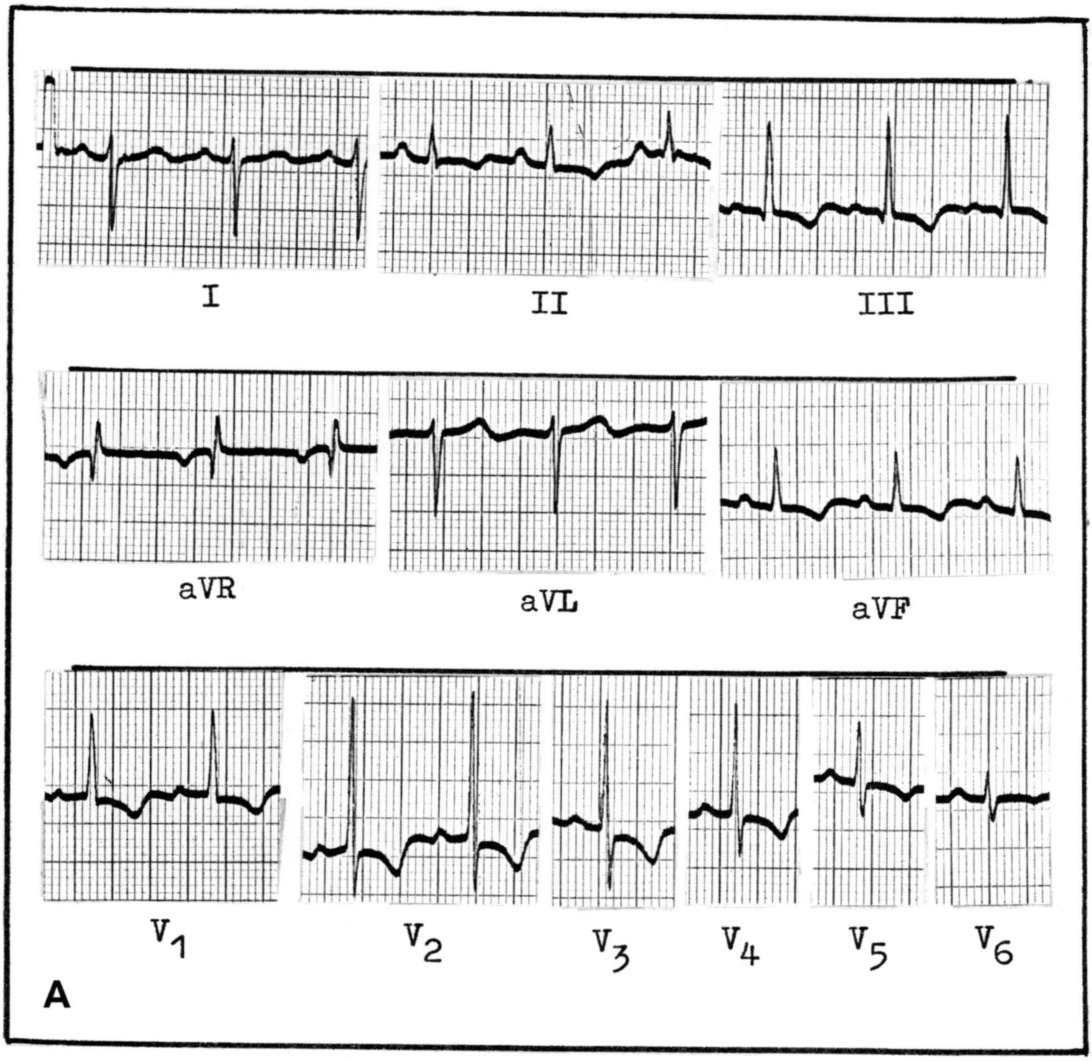

FIGURE 2–3. *A,* Adult with congenital heart disease and right ventricular hypertrophy. The QRS complexes in lead I are almost entirely negative, with positive QRS complexes in leads II and III. The transitional zone falls along the axis of lead aVR, with the mean QRS vector at +120°, clearly in the area of right axis deviation. This is diagrammed in Figure 2–4. Leads V_1 to V_5 are predominantly positive with the transition at V_6. Therefore, the three-dimensional mean QRS vector, in addition to being to the *right* and *inferior,* is also *anterior* (Figure 2–5). From a vectorial point of view, these findings characteristic of the hypertrophied right ventricle, are in such contrast to the normal findings (compare and contrast this electrocardiogram with the normal in Figure 2–3*B*), that they stand out sharply upon inspection of the electrocardiogram.

Illustration continued on following page.

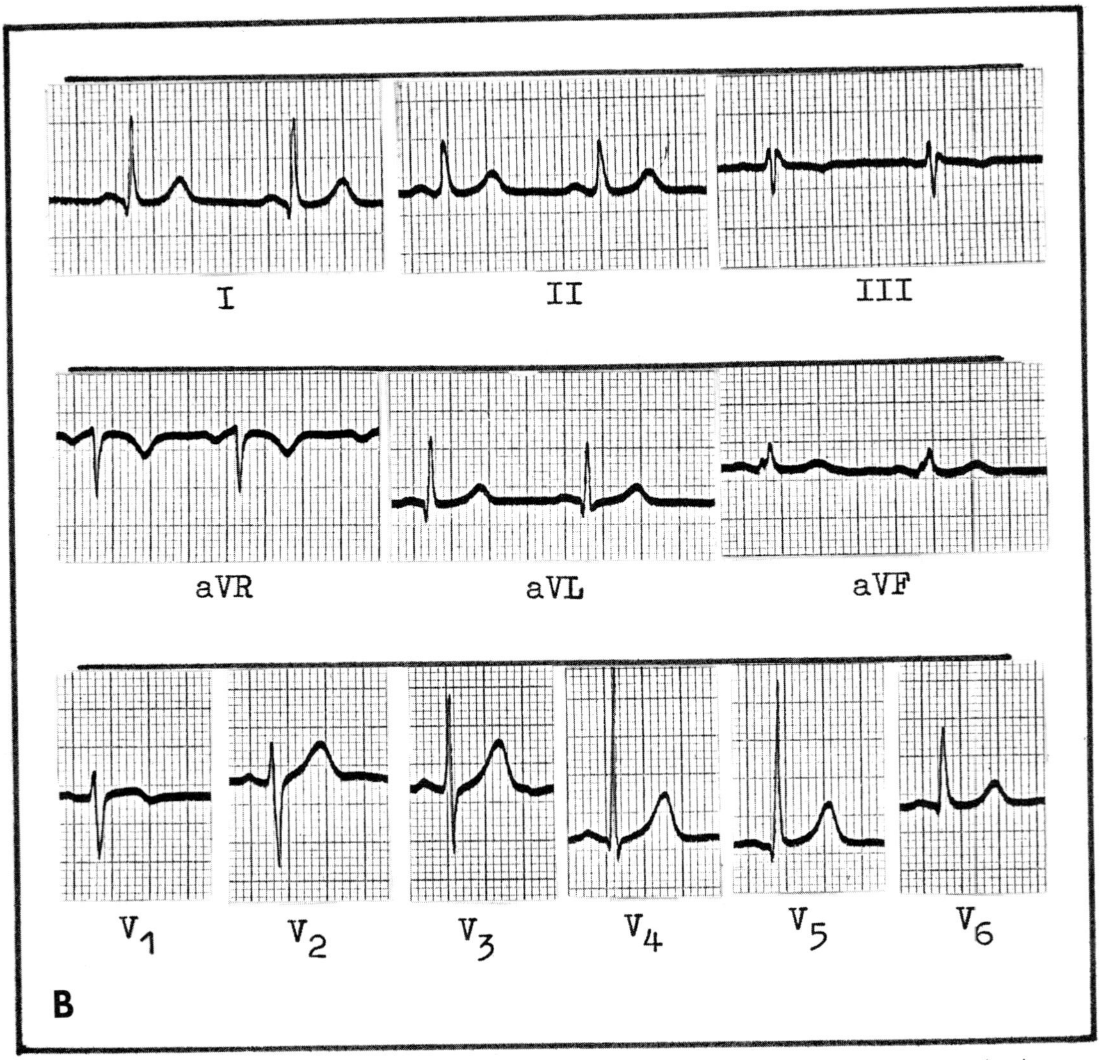

FIGURE 2–3 *Continued.* *B*, Normal electrocardiogram. When studying the abnormal always gc back, compare and contrast with the normal.

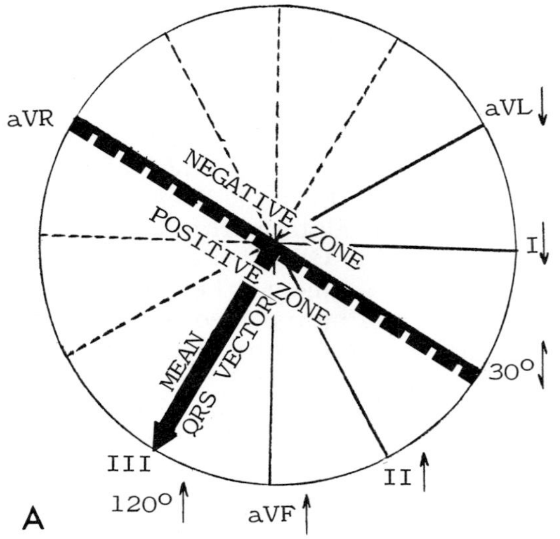

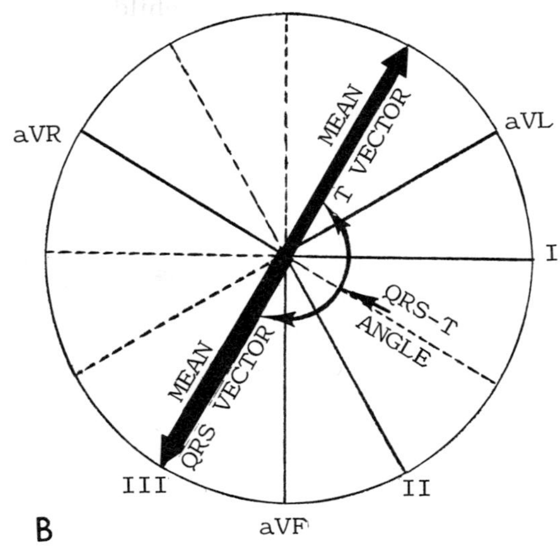

FIGURE 2-4. *A,* The mean QRS vector in Figure 2-3*A* is to the right and inferior at + 120°, in the frontal plane. *B,* In Figure 2-3*A,* in addition to the abnormally oriented QRS vector, the QRS-T angle is also abnormal.

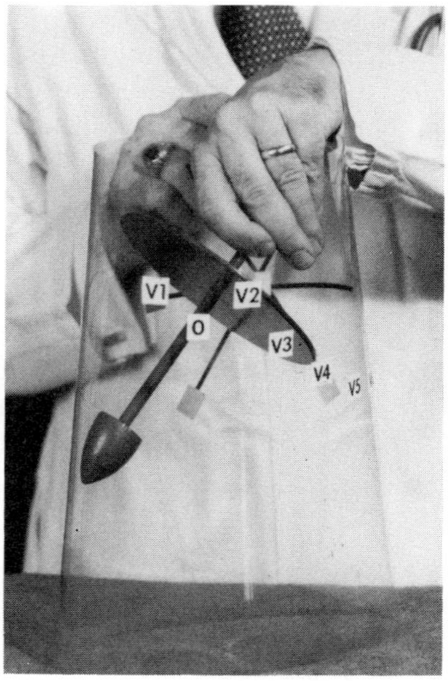

FIGURE 2-5. The addition of the precordial leads permits us to see that the mean QRS vector, in addition to being to the *right* and *inferior,* is also *anterior.* In the face of frank right axis deviation, lead V_1 may be positive without anterior or posterior rotation of the mean QRS vector. However, if V_2 is also positive the mean QRS vector is rotated anteriorly.

B. Magnitude of the Mean Spatial QRS Vector

In the adult with right ventricular hypertrophy the magnitude of the QRS deflections frequently is not increased. In fact, in emphysematous patients, with marked right ventricular hypertrophy, the QRS deflections may actually be small.

Although this course deals principally with adult electrocardiography, examples of congenital heart disease in children are included. The question often arises as to the diagnosis of right ventricular hypertrophy in very young children who *normally* have right ventricular preponderance. Table 2–1 gives one set of suggested criteria. It is in circumstances such as these that the criteria in this table may be helpful. In addition, Figure 2–17, from Nadas and Fyler, gives the R–S ratio in lead V_1 from birth to 13 years. For instance, if at birth the algebraic sum of the R and S waves in lead V_1 is 25 mm., which is well outside the normal range, right ventricular hypertrophy may be strongly suspected.

Most of the adult electrocardiograms do not fit the magnitude criteria in Table 2–1. However, where the R wave is the *main ventricular deflection* in lead V_1, regardless of size, right ventricular hypertrophy enters into the differential diagnosis. Other causes of an R wave (or R′), as the main ventricular deflection in lead V_1, include: true posterior wall myocardial infarction, right bundle branch block (RSR′), and the Wolff-Parkinson-White syndrome. These will be studied later in the course.

C. Repolarization Abnormalities (Abnormalities of the S–T Segments and T Waves)

In Figure 2–3*A* not only is the mean QRS vector abnormally oriented to the right, inferiorly and anteriorly, but the QRS–T angle is also abnormal (Fig. 2–4*B*). Note also the depression of the S–T segments, especially in leads V_2, V_3 and V_4. The wide QRS–T angle has often been referred to as an "ischemia" pattern, and S–T segment abnormalities together with a wide QRS-T angle, in the hypertrophied ventricle, as a "strain" pattern. These terms are unfortunate since they impart a clinical connotation to an electrocardiographic pattern; they will not be used in this course. The term "ventricular repolarization abnormalities," covering both the wide QRS-T angle and the abnormal S–T segment, is better. This same problem will be repeated and reemphasized when left ventricular hypertrophy is studied in Chapter 3.

In order to be able to recognize right ventricular hypertrophy electrocardiographically, we will examine a number of electrocardiograms. In each figure, part *A* represents the hypertrophied right ventricle, and part *B* is the normal for comparison.

In Figure 2–6*A* the QRS complex is predominantly negative in lead I and positive in leads II and III. The mean QRS vector is to the *right* and *inferior* in the frontal plane. In leads V_1 and V_2 the QRS deflections are positive. The mean QRS vector is, therefore, not only to the right and inferior, but also *anterior*. Note the repolarization abnormalities; the QRS–T angle is wide, with S–T segment abnormalities.

None of the deflections is unusually large, but three important findings of right ventricular hypertrophy are present.

1. Right axis deviation (mean QRS vector oriented to the right).
2. The R wave is the main ventricular deflection in lead V_1. See criteria for adult in Table 2–1.
3. Repolarization abnormalities (wide QRS–T angle and S–T segment abnormalities).

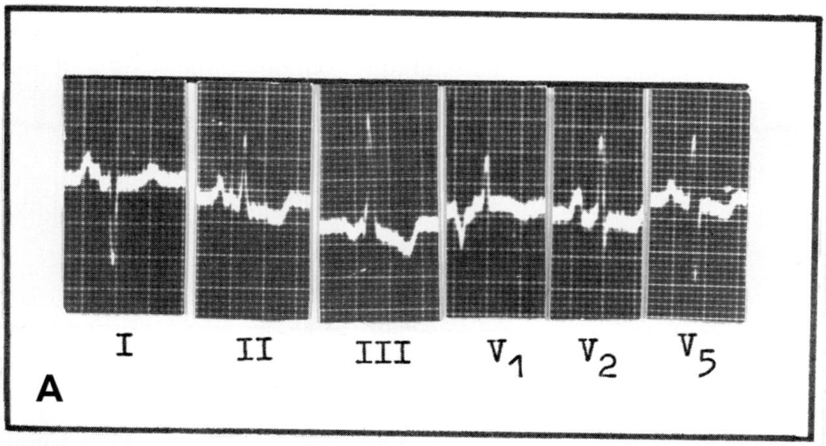

FIGURE 2–6. *A,* Right ventricular hypertrophy in a patient with mitral stenosis. (Electrocardiogram reduced in size.)

Illustration continued on following page.

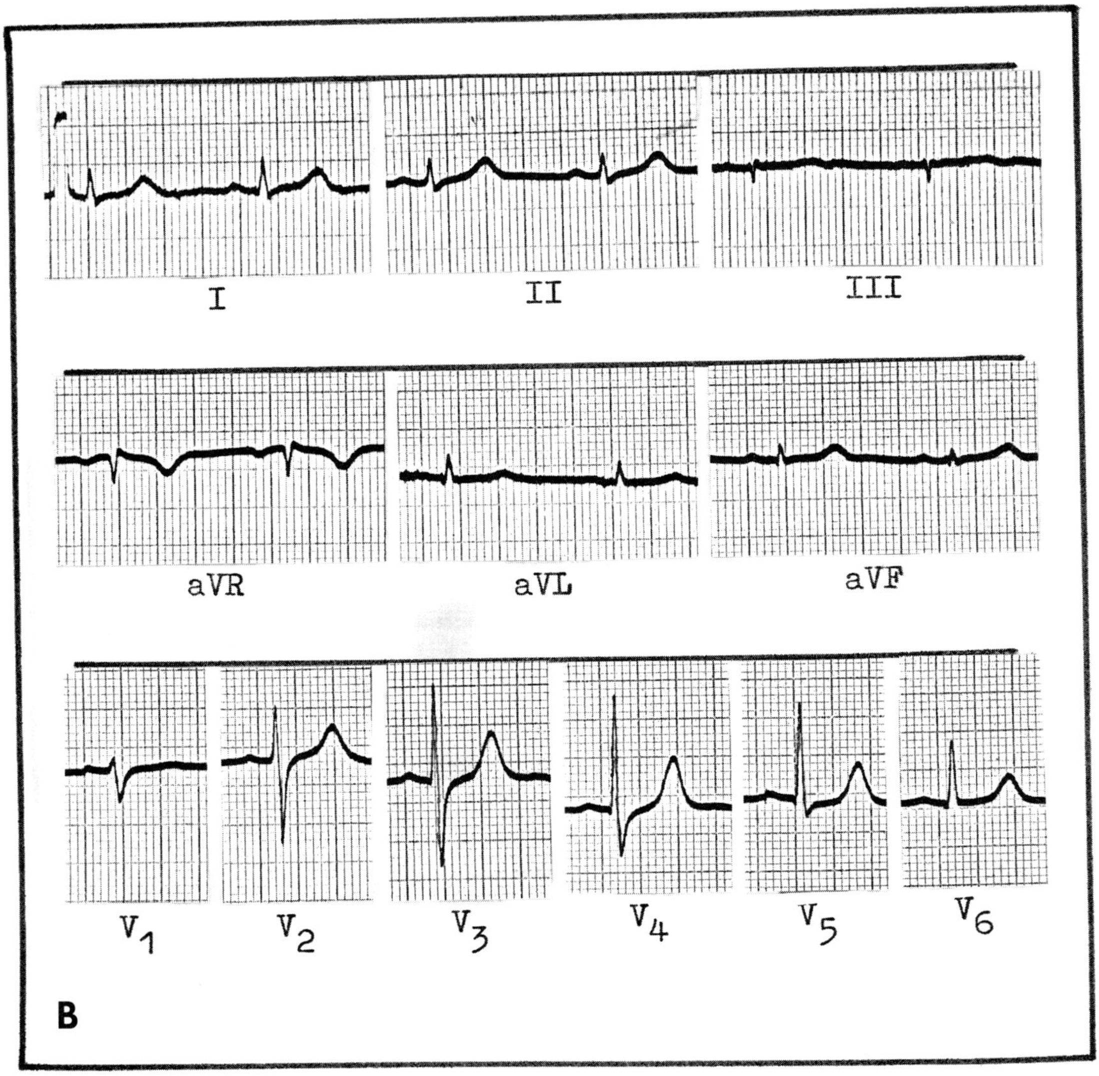

FIGURE 2–6 *Continued.* *B,* Normal electrocardiogram. How do the findings here differ from those in the electrocardiogram in Figure 2–6*A*?

In Figure 2–7*A* the QRS complex in lead I is negative with the transition at aVR. The QRS in lead V_1 is positive and of great magnitude. The mean spatial QRS vector is to the *right*, *inferior* and *anterior*, in contrast to the normal (Fig. 2–7*B*), where the mean QRS vector is to the *left*, *inferior* and *posterior*.

This child, who had congenital heart disease, has an R wave magnitude greater than 25 mm. in lead V_1, which would permit an electrocardiographic diagnosis of right ventricular hypertrophy even at birth (see Fig. 2–17).

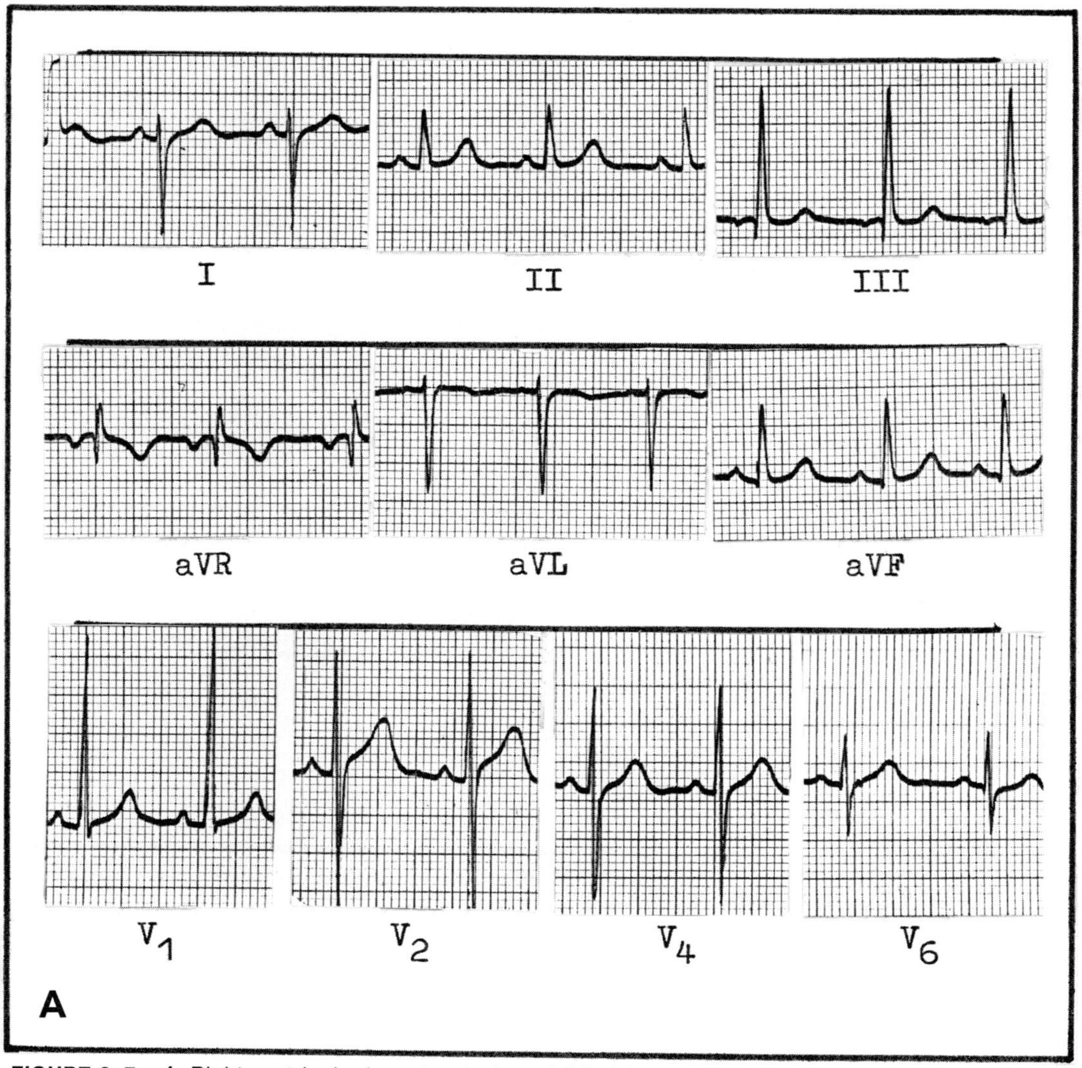

FIGURE 2–7. *A,* Right ventricular hypertrophy in a child with congenital heart disease.

Illustration continued on following page.

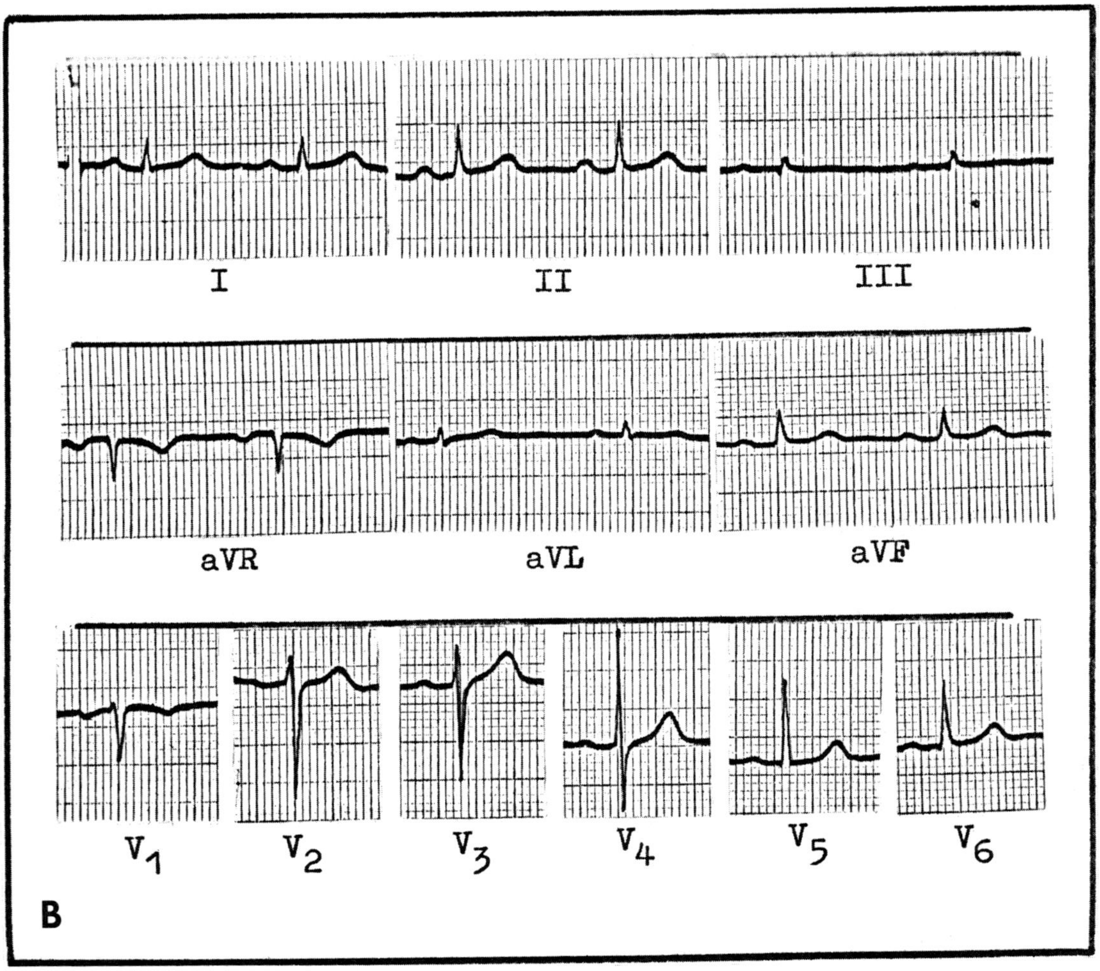

FIGURE 2–7 *Continued.* *B*, Normal electrocardiogram. Compare with the electrocardiogram in Figure 2–7*A*.

In Figure 2–8*A* the QRS complex in lead I is negative, with the transition at aVR, and the QRS in V_1 and V_2 is positive. The mean spatial QRS vector is to the *right, inferior* and *anterior.*

Although the complexes are not large, the important findings of right ventricular hypertrophy in the adult are once again seen:

1. Right axis deviation.
2. The R wave in lead V_1 is the main ventricular deflection.
3. Repolarization abnormalities.

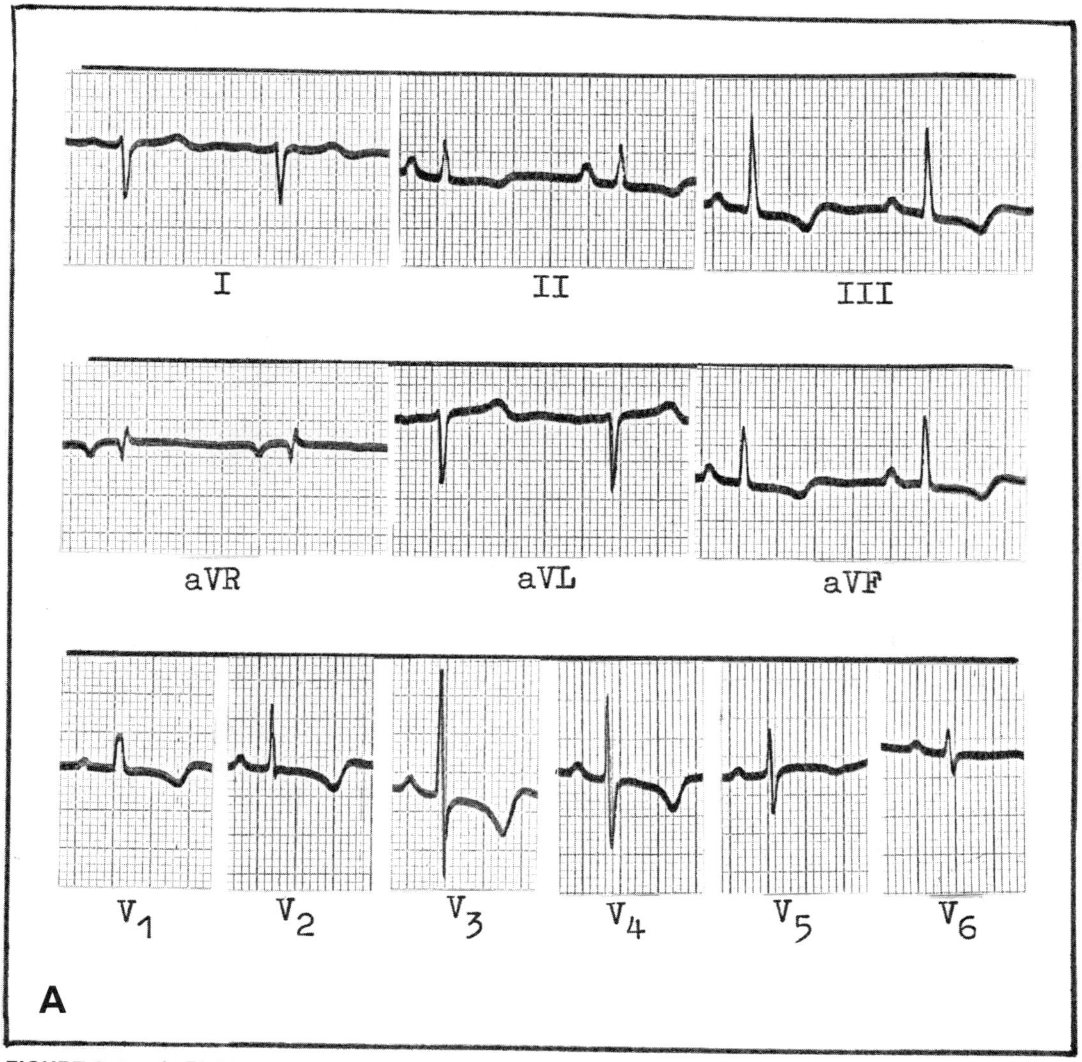

FIGURE 2–8. *A,* Right ventricular hypertrophy in an adult with congenital heart disease.

Illustration continued on following page.

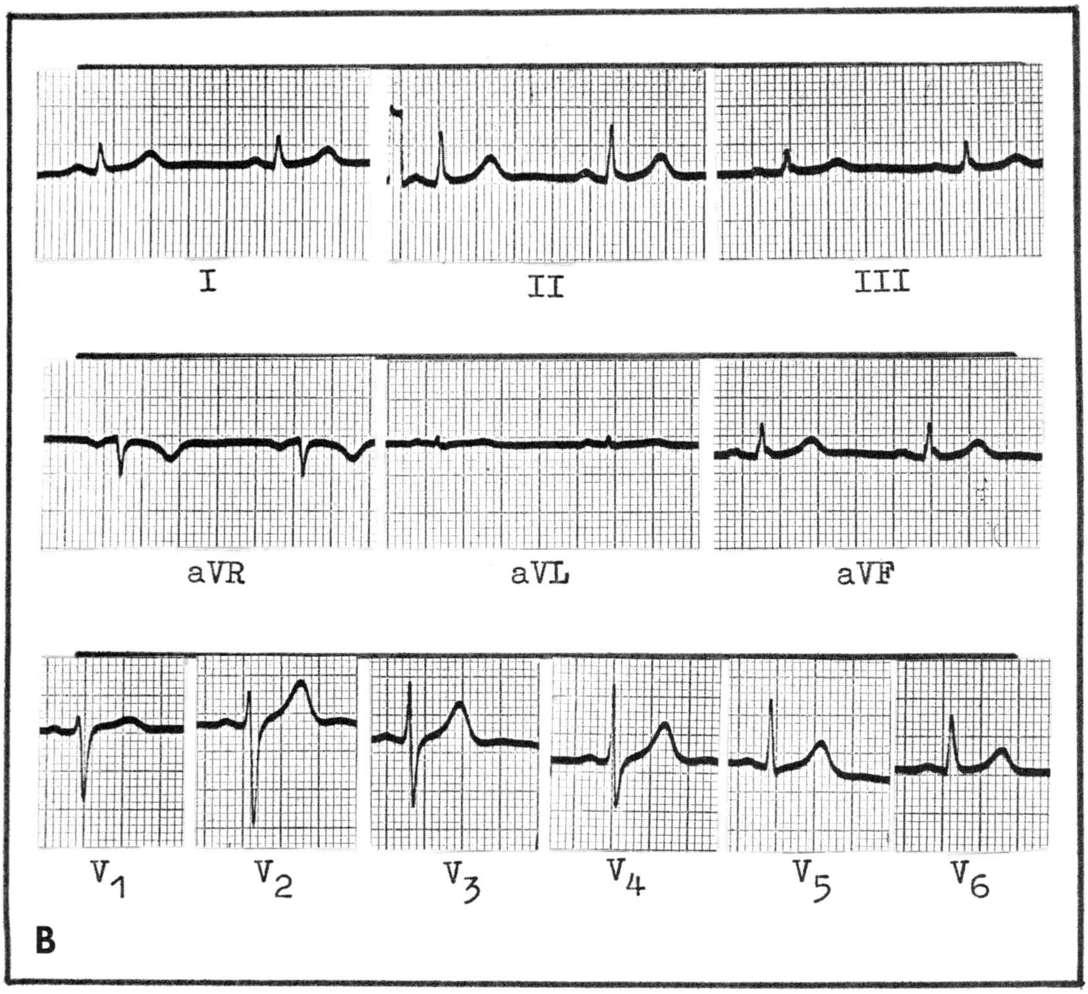

FIGURE 2–8 *Continued.* *B,* Normal electrocardiogram. Compare with electrocardiogram in Figure 2–8*A.*

Figure 2–9A, from a patient with advanced chronic obstructive lung disease with cor pulmonale, was studied once before (Chapter 1, Fig. 1–73); this figure emphasizes the importance of understanding the vectorial forces. In the previous electrocardiograms representing right ventricular hypertrophy in this chapter, lead I was negative while leads II and III were positive. Here we have an electrocardiogram in which leads I, II and III are all negative and the transition is near lead aVL. This is diagrammed in Figure 2–10. In the precordial leads, V_1 and V_2 are predominantly positive and the rest are predominantly negative (review Fig. 1–75 in Chapter 1). The mean spatial QRS vector is to the *right, superior* and *anterior*.

Again the criteria, so far learned, for right ventricular hypertrophy are met:

1. Right axis deviation.
2. The R wave in lead V_1 is the main ventricular deflection.
3. Repolarization abnormalities.

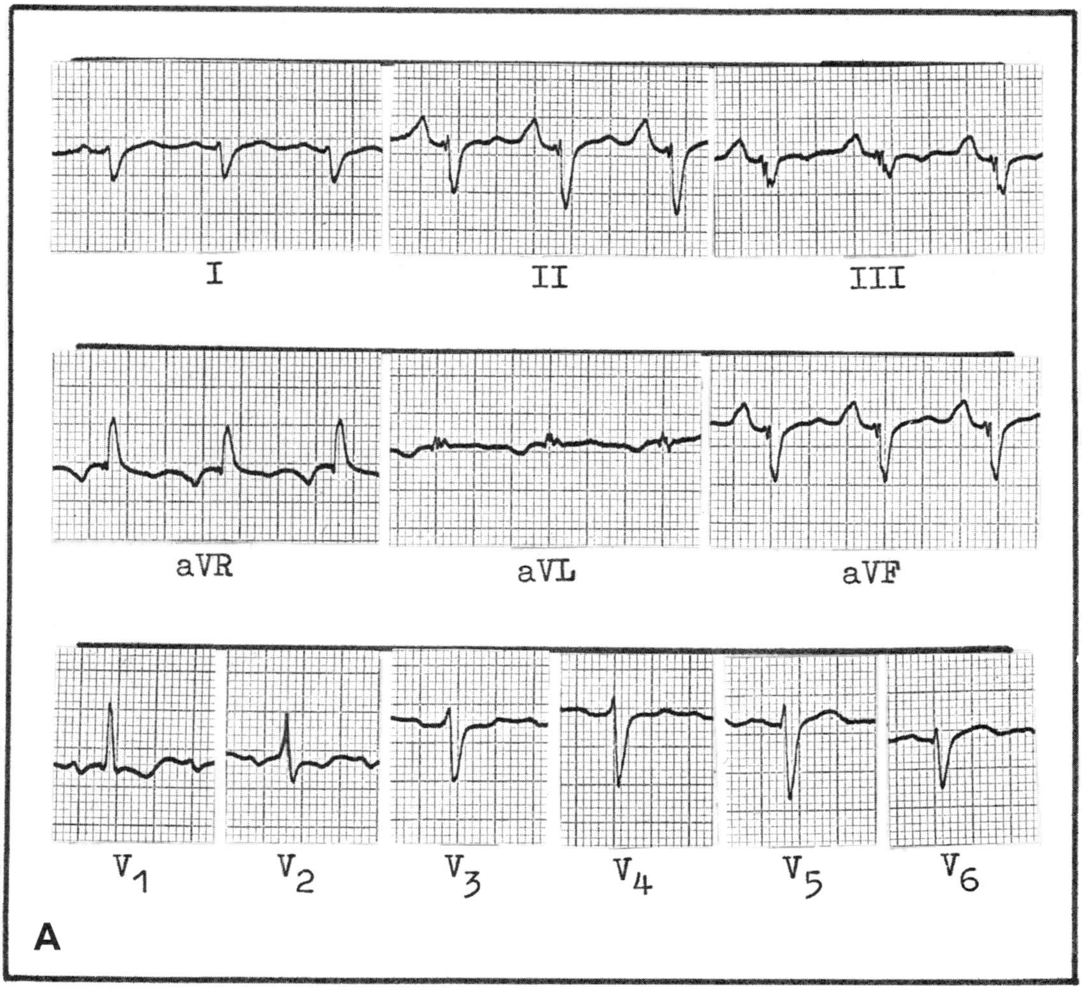

FIGURE 2–9. *A,* How does the mean QRS vector differ in this electrocardiogram, representing right ventricular hypertrophy, from the mean QRS vectors seen in the previous electrocardiograms representing right ventricular hypertrophy in this chapter? This is diagrammed in Figure 2–10.

Illustration continued on following page.

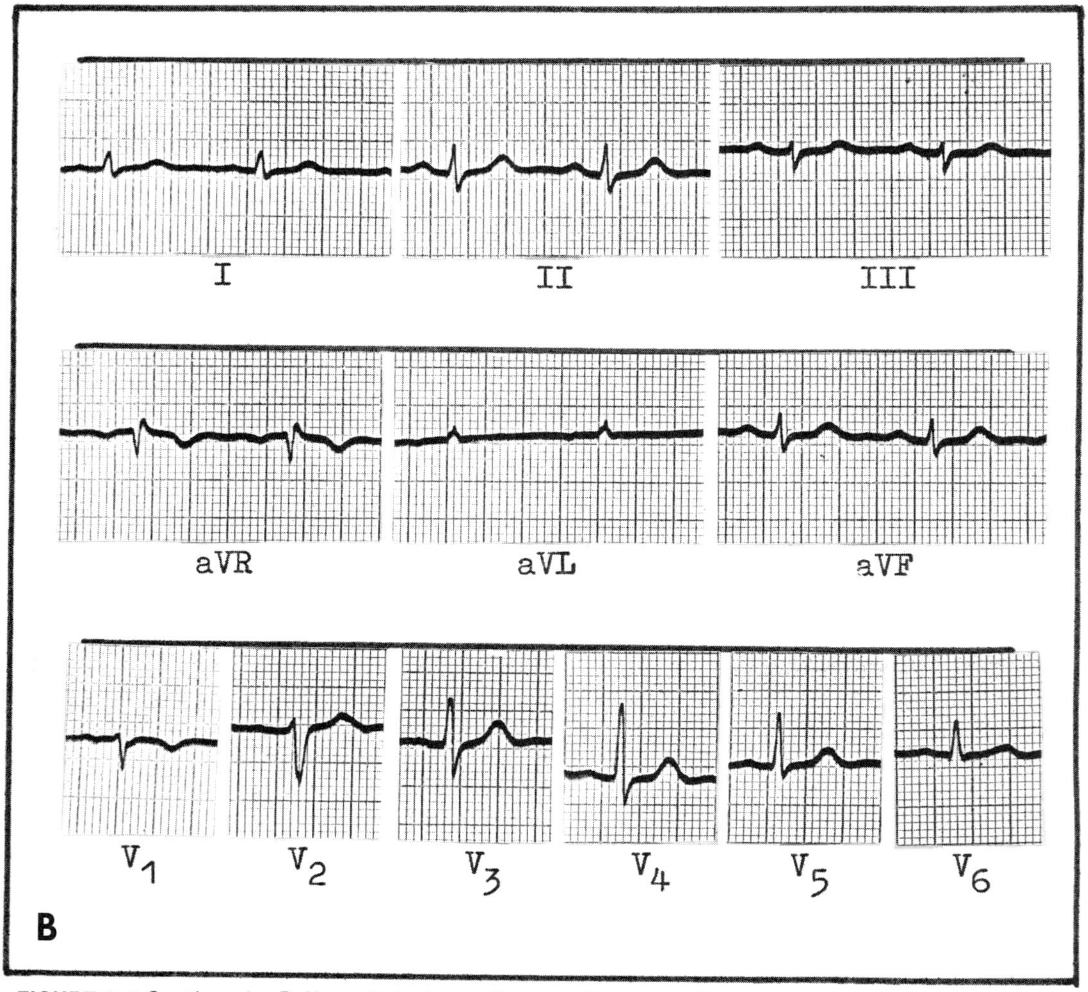

FIGURE 2–9 *Continued.* *B,* Normal electrocardiogram. Compare with electrocardiogram in Figure 2–9*A.*

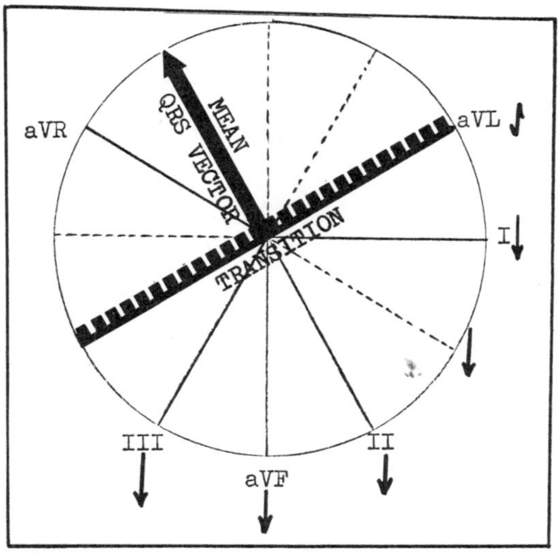

FIGURE 2–10. The mean QRS vector in Figure 2–9*A* is to the *right* and *superior* in the frontal plane.

RIGHT AND LEFT ATRIAL ENLARGEMENT

The hypertrophied right ventricle does not occur in a vacuum. It is often accompanied by the enlargement of the right atrium and at times by enlargement of the left atrium (mitral stenosis). The electrocardiographic manifestations of atrial enlargement will now be studied.

As seen in Chapter 1 (Fig. 1–21), the sinoatrial (S–A) node is the normal pacemaker of the heart. The impulse arises in the S–A node, then spreads across the atria, depolarizing both atria, first the right, then the left, and inscribing the P wave on the electrocardiogram. Both atria are represented in the P wave. The right atrial vector is more rightward and anterior compared to the left atrial vector, which is more leftward and posterior. The early part of the P wave represents the right atrium and the later part of the P wave the left atrium (Fig. 2–11). Enlargement of the right atrium, therefore, results in tall peaked P waves in leads II and III. Since the right atrial vector is oriented *anteriorly*, a tall peaked P wave may be seen in lead V_1. Electrocardiographic manifestations of right atrial enlargement are seen in Figure 2–12. Electrocardiographic manifestations of left atrial enlargement are explained in Figure 2–13. Please note that in the *normal* electrocardiogram the P wave is rarely, if ever, greater than 3 mm. in any lead.

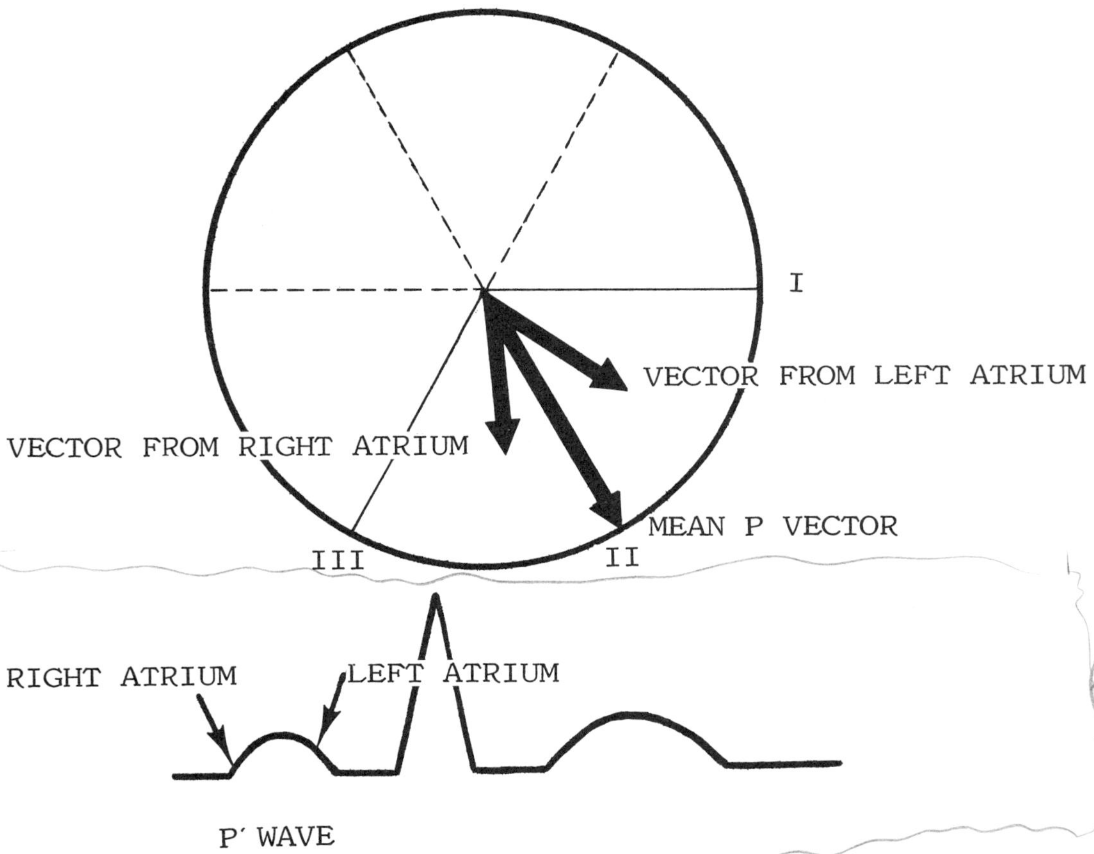

FIGURE 2–11. The mean P vector, representing both atria, is usually in the area of lead II, with the P waves positive in leads I and aVF and often in lead III as well (Fig. 1–43). In the above diagrams are illustrated, in addition to the mean P vector, the right and left atrial vectors. The earlier right atrial vector is more rightward and anteriorly oriented compared with the left atrial vector, which is more leftward and posteriorly oriented.

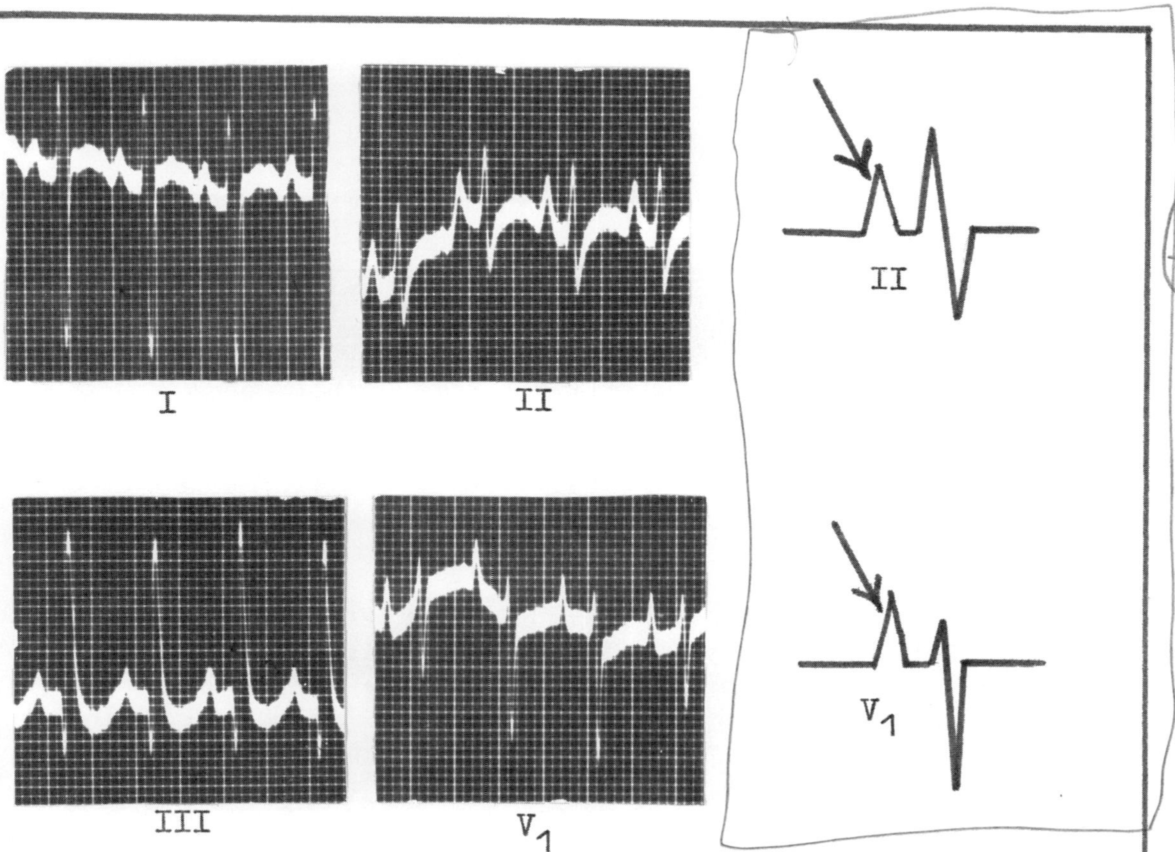

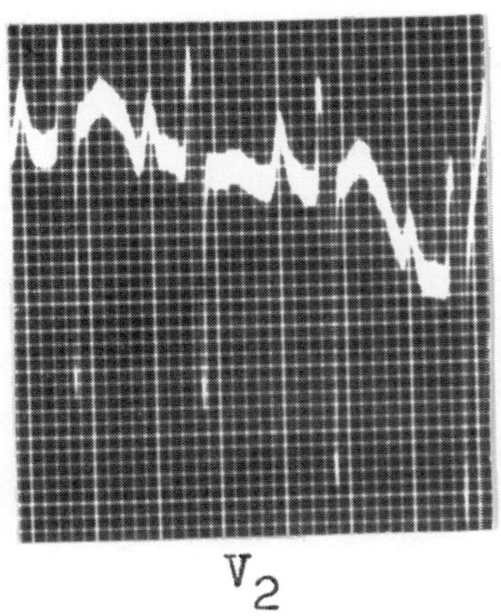

The right atrial vector is earlier, more rightward and anterior compared to the left atrial vector. The right atrial vector faces leads II and III. *Enlargement of the right atrium,* therefore, results in the following electrocardiographic manifestations:

A. Tall, peaked P waves in leads II and III or even in leads I, II and III.

B. Since the right atrial vector is also anterior, the early part of the P wave, or even the entire P wave, may be positive and of great magnitude in lead V_1 or leads V_1 and V_2.

(Electrocardiogram enlarged for clarity.)

FIGURE 2–12. Electrocardiographic manifestations of right atrial enlargement.

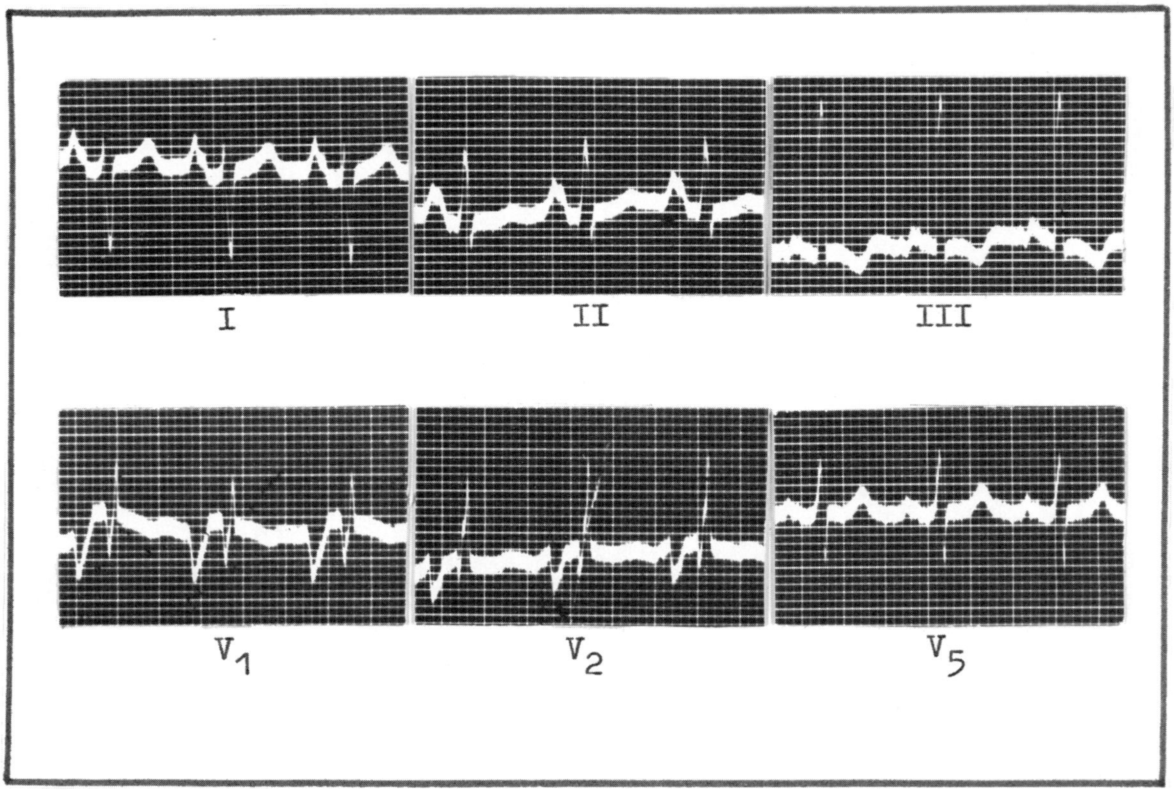

FIGURE 2–13. Electrocardiographic manifestations of left atrial enlargement. Left atrial depolarization starts later than right atrial depolarization. The left atrial vector is more leftward and posterior compared with the right atrial vector, and faces leads I and II. *Enlargement of the left atrium,* therefore, results in the following electrocardiographic manifestations:

a. Broad, notched and sometimes tall P waves in leads I and II or even in leads I, II and III. The notching is due to the fact that the right atrial inscription is seen first, in the early part of the P wave, which is followed by the delayed depolarization of the enlarged left atrium.
b. The vector is posteriorly oriented, so that the latter part, sometimes the entire P wave, may be negative and of great magnitude in lead V_1.

Rarely, if ever, is the P wave deflection in the normal electrocardiogram greater than 3 mm. in any lead. If a P wave of this magnitude is found, atrial enlargement must be considered.

Biatrial enlargement, together with right ventricular enlargement, is not uncommon (mitral stenosis). Although left atrial enlargement is most prominent in this figure, the enlarged right atrium may be represented by the early peaking of the P waves, especially in leads I and II. The initial Q wave, seen here in leads V_1 and V_2, together with the other findings, provides additional evidence of right ventricular hypertrophy.
(Electrocardiogram enlarged for clarity.)

Figure 2–14 is a representation of trichambered cardiac enlargement (right ventricular and right and left atrial enlargement), which may be seen in patients with mitral valve stenosis. We will start at the left atrium. Between the left atrium and the left ventricle is the mitral valve. If the mitral orifice is significantly narrowed (stenotic), the left atrium enlarges, since it cannot empty its contents properly into the left ventricle. As the pressure in the left atrium rises, it is reflected backwards into the pulmonary veins. This increased pressure in the pulmonary circuit is, in turn, reflected backwards into the right ventricle, whose pressure must increase to get blood into the pulmonary circuit. Progressive pressure rise in the right atrium accompanies the increased pressure in the right ventricle. The left ventricle, on the other hand, appears to be protected, since the amount of blood entering it is limited because of the significantly stenotic mitral valve. The left ventricle empties its contents into the aorta, and if there is no significant aortic valve disease the left ventricle may remain relatively normal in size or even smaller than normal.

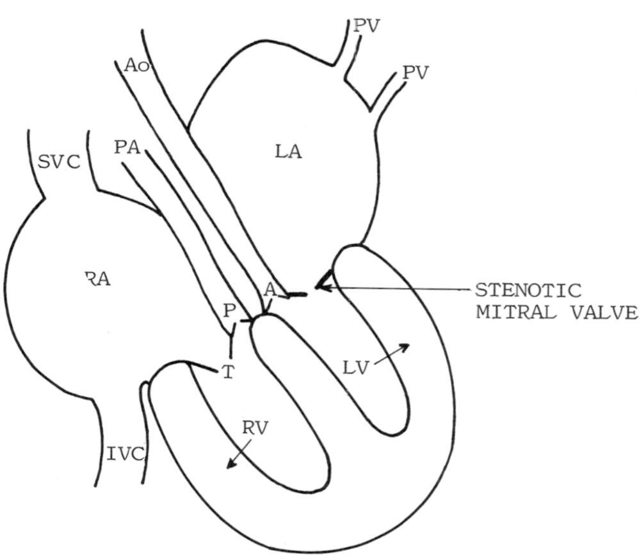

SVC	Superior vena cava
IVC	Inferior vena cava
RA	Enlarged right atrium
LA	Enlarged left atrium
RV	Enlarged right ventricle
LV	Left ventricle
PA	Pulmonary artery
Ao	Aorta
PV	Pulmonary vein
T	Tricuspid valve
P	Pulmonic valve
A	Aortic valve

FIGURE 2–14. The hypertrophied right ventricle is not infrequently accompanied by an enlarged right atrium and an enlarged left atrium (as seen in mitral stenosis).

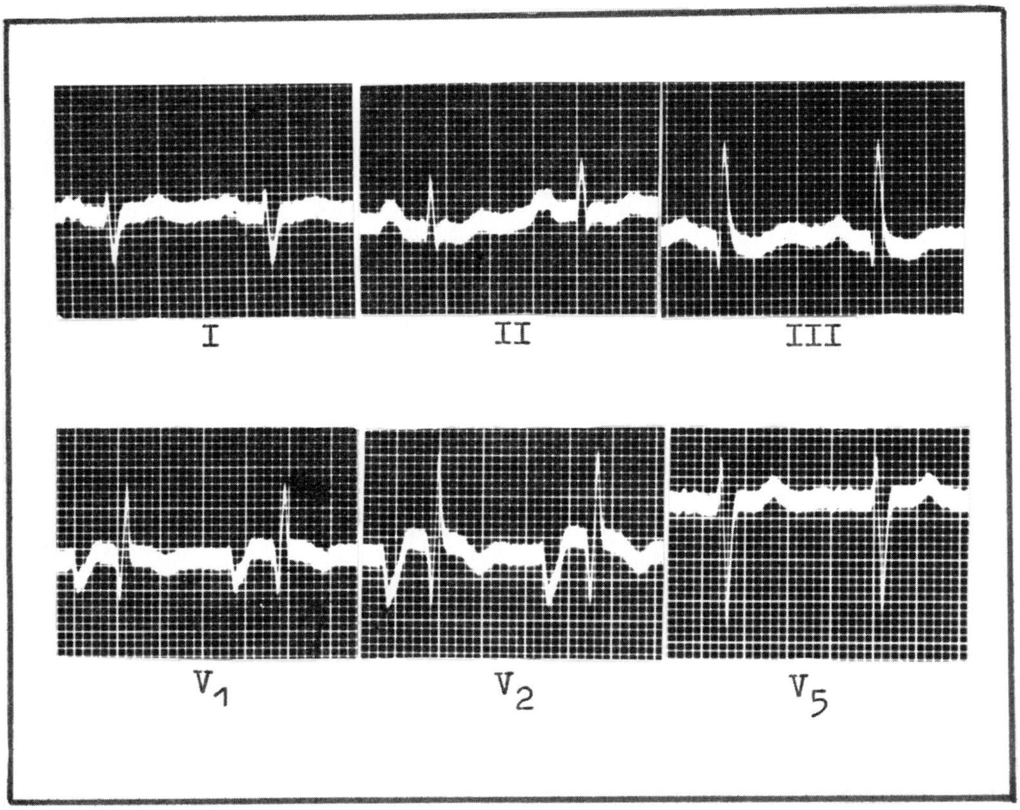

FIGURE 2–15. Adult with mitral stenosis. List all the criteria for (1) right ventricular and (2) left atrial enlargement.
(Electrocardiogram enlarged for clarity.)

Cassette Side 6

D. "Presumptive" Evidence for Right Ventricular Hypertrophy

As mentioned in the introduction to this chapter, and as described in Table 2–1, the diagnosis of right ventricular hypertrophy is frequently difficult to make electrocardiographically in the adult. The left ventricle is dominant, and even a very hypertrophied right ventricle may be overshadowed by a normal left ventricle. A normal electrocardiogram does not, therefore, rule out right ventricular hypertrophy. The "presumptive" or indirect evidence of right ventricular hypertrophy has often helped in the absence of direct electrocardiographic evidence. Presumptive evidence refers to the clearly defined evidence of atrial enlargement in the *absence* of clear-cut evidence of right ventricular enlargement. The assumption is that atrial enlargement, right or left, is not an isolated finding.*

Figure 2–16 is from an elderly patient with severe chronic obstructive pulmonary disease and cor pulmonale. Although right ventricular hypertrophy might be suspected, the criteria are not strictly met. Note, however, the size and configuration of the P waves, especially in lead II, representing the enlarged right atrium and constituting good presumptive evidence for the enlarged right ventricle.

The emphasis in this course continues to be on the concept and not on long lists of memorized data. Table 2–1 is presented as one set of suggested criteria, covering children and adults. Before studying specific data read the introduction to this table carefully.

---

*We have been studying the electrocardiographic manifestations of left atrial enlargement associated with right ventricular enlargement (mitral stenosis). A more common cause, however, of left atrial enlargement is left ventricular enlargement (Chapter 3).

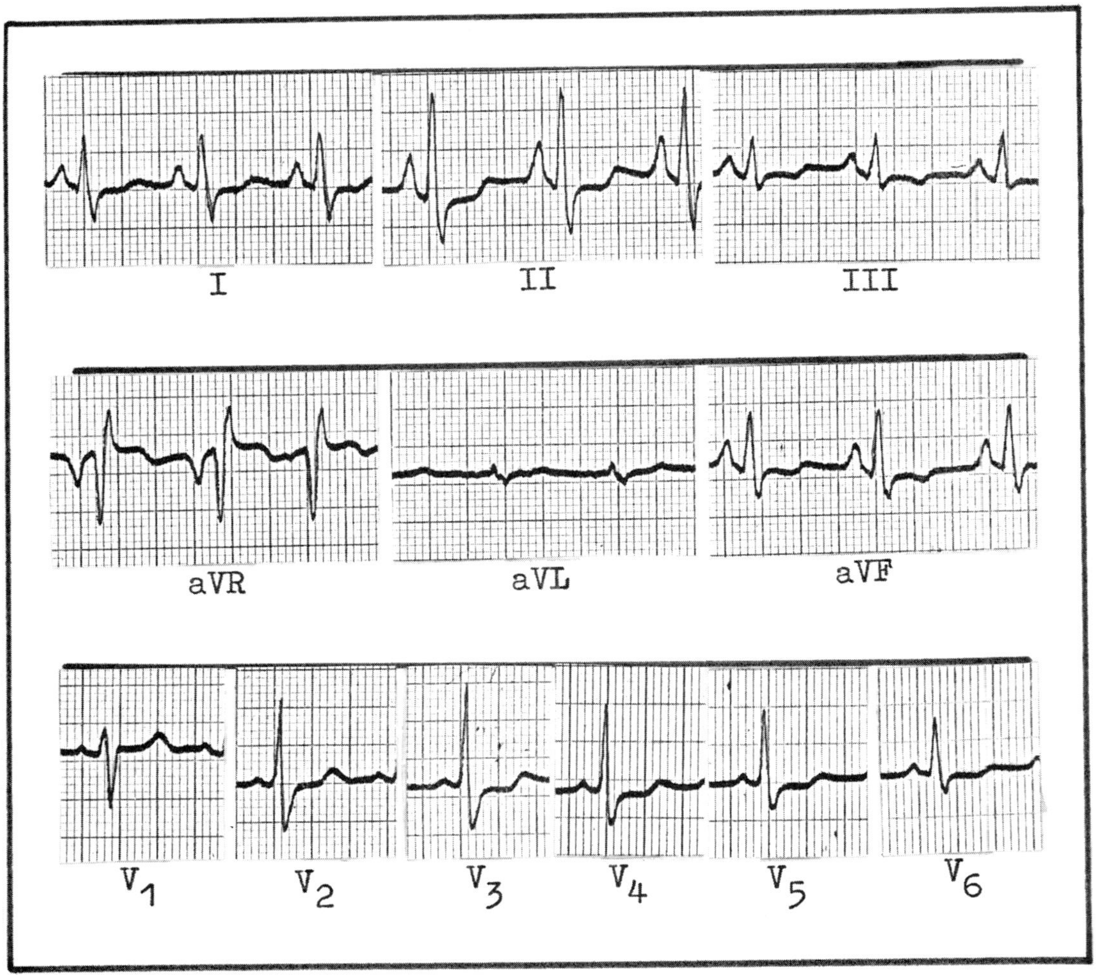

FIGURE 2-16. Elderly patient with chronic obstructive lung disease and cor pulmonale. What is the "presumptive" evidence which makes you suspicious of right ventricular hypertrophy?

TABLE 2–1. RIGHT VENTRICULAR HYPERTROPHY

Once the basic concepts of the vectorial forces of right ventricular and right and left atrial enlargement are understood, the criteria are easily learned. The emphasis in this course has always been on the concept rather than on the "criteria." Do not be a slave to figures; they frequently change in the face of evolving information. The following values are general, especially for infants and children in whom the changes progress rapidly during the first few years.

Right Ventricular Hypertrophy in Children

A. RIGHT AXIS DEVIATION (RAD)
Evaluate carefully since right axis deviation is normal in the very young.

B. MAGNITUDE OF THE MEAN QRS VECTOR
Standard Leads: I, II and III.
At times the mean QRS vector is of great magnitude, so that the S wave in lead I plus the R wave in lead III summate to more than 35 mm.

$$S_I + R_{III} > 35 \text{ mm.}$$

aV Leads: aVR, aVL and aVF.
The great vectorial magnitude described above may result in the S wave in lead aVL plus the R wave in lead aVF summating to more than 35 mm.

$$S_{aVL} + R_{aVF} > 35 \text{ mm.}$$

The R or R′ in lead aVR may be more than 6 mm. in height.

$$R_{aVR} \text{ or } R'_{aVR} > 6 \text{ mm.}$$

The R in lead aVR becomes taller with increased magnitude of the mean QRS vector, especially as the vector becomes more rightward (toward +aVR).
Chest Leads: V_1 to V_6.
Algebraic sum of R and S waves in lead V_1 more than 15 mm. in height (Fig. 2–17). At birth a tall R wave in lead V_1 may still be normal. An R wave in lead V_1 greater than 15 mm., however, may represent an abnormally enlarged right ventricle even in the newborn.

C. REPOLARIZATION ABNORMALITIES (WIDE QRS–T ANGLE AND S–T SEGMENT ABNORMALITIES)
The term "strain" is commonly used, but it is an unfortunate one since it imparts a clinical connotation to electrocardiographic deflections. What is meant is that there is a wide angle between the mean QRS vector and the mean T vector, together with abnormalities of the S–T segments. These repolarization abnormalities are frequently found in ventricular hypertrophy.

Right Ventricular Hypertrophy in Adults

In addition to the above:
If the R wave is the main ventricular deflection in lead V_1, regardless of its size, the possibility of right ventricular enlargement must be considered. This finding alone does not always point to the enlarged right ventricle. In your differential diagnosis should be:

a. True posterior wall myocardial infarction.
b. Right bundle branch block (RSR′).

Table continued on following page.

TABLE 2–1. RIGHT VENTRICULAR HYPERTROPHY *(Continued)*

c. Preexcitation (Wolff-Parkinson-White) syndrome.
These will be studied later.

D. PRESUMPTIVE EVIDENCE OF RIGHT VENTRICULAR HYPERTROPHY
Presumptive evidence refers to the clearly defined evidence of atrial enlargement in the *absence* of clear-cut evidence of right ventricular enlargement. Review the criteria for right and left atrial enlargement as explained in Figures 2–12 and 2–13, and remember that a more common cause of left atrial enlargement is left ventricular enlargement. In the adult the normal right ventricular wall is only one third as thick as the left ventricular wall. Even a 100 per cent increase in the thickness of the right ventricle will not cause it to be as thick as the predominant left ventricle. As a result, even marked hypertrophy of the right ventricle may not be manifest on the clinical electrocardiogram. On the other hand, clear evidence of right atrial enlargement, in the absence of tricuspid valve stenosis, is good presumptive evidence of right ventricular enlargement.

This is a "summary of a summary" and should be used only after you have mastered the basic concepts.

Right Ventricular Hypertrophy

IN CHILDREN

A. RAD

B. Magnitude criteria

Standard leads:

$S_I + R_{III} > 35$ mm.

aV leads:

$S_{aVL} + R_{aVF} > 35$ mm.

R_{aVR} or $R'_{aVR} > 6$ mm.

Chest leads:

$R - S_{V_1} > 15$ mm. at birth (Fig. 2–17)

C. Repolarization abnormalities

IN ADULTS (in addition to above)

R_{V_1} is main ventricular deflection. Differential diagnosis:

a. True posterior wall myocardial infarction.
b. Right bundle branch block (RSR′).
c. Preexcitation (Wolff-Parkinson-White) syndrome.

D. Presumptive evidence

Right Atrial Enlargement

See Figure 2–12 for explanation and illustration of tall, peaked P waves in leads II, III and V_1.

P wave

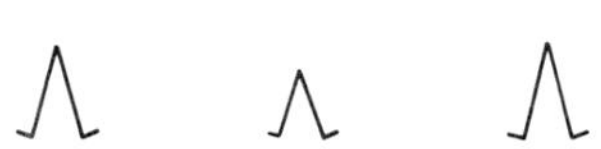

Leads II III V_1

Left Atrial Enlargement

See Figure 2–13 for explanation and illustrations of broad, notched P waves in leads I, II and V_1.

P wave

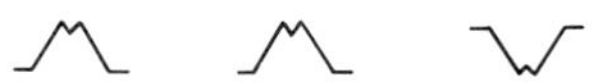

Leads I II V_1

Figure 2–17, from Nadas and Fyler, gives the algebraic sum of the R and S waves in lead V_1 from birth to 13 years. For instance, as seen earlier in this chapter, if at birth the algebraic sum of the R and S waves is 25 mm., which is well outside the normal range, right ventricular hypertrophy is strongly suggested.

Most of the adult electrocardiograms do not fit the criteria in Table 2–1, as previously noted. However, when the R wave in lead V_1 is the main ventricular deflection, regardless of size, right ventricular hypertrophy enters into the differential diagnosis.

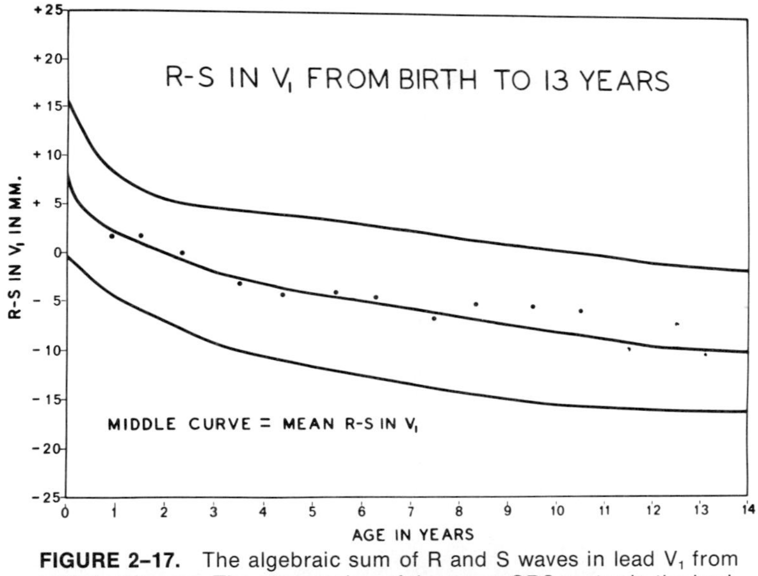

FIGURE 2–17. The algebraic sum of R and S waves in lead V_1 from birth to 13 years. The progression of the mean QRS vector in the horizontal plane, from anterior to posterior is reflected in the R–S ratio in lead V_1. (From A. S. Nadas and D. C. Fyler, Pediatric Cardiology, 3rd ed. Philadelphia, W. B. Saunders Company, 1972. Used by permission.)

REVIEW ELECTROCARDIOGRAMS

You will now examine many electrocardiograms as you ponder the manifestations of right ventricular and right and left atrial enlargement. Review, with each electrocardiogram, the criteria for each of these entities, and compare them with the many normal electrocardiograms you have already seen.

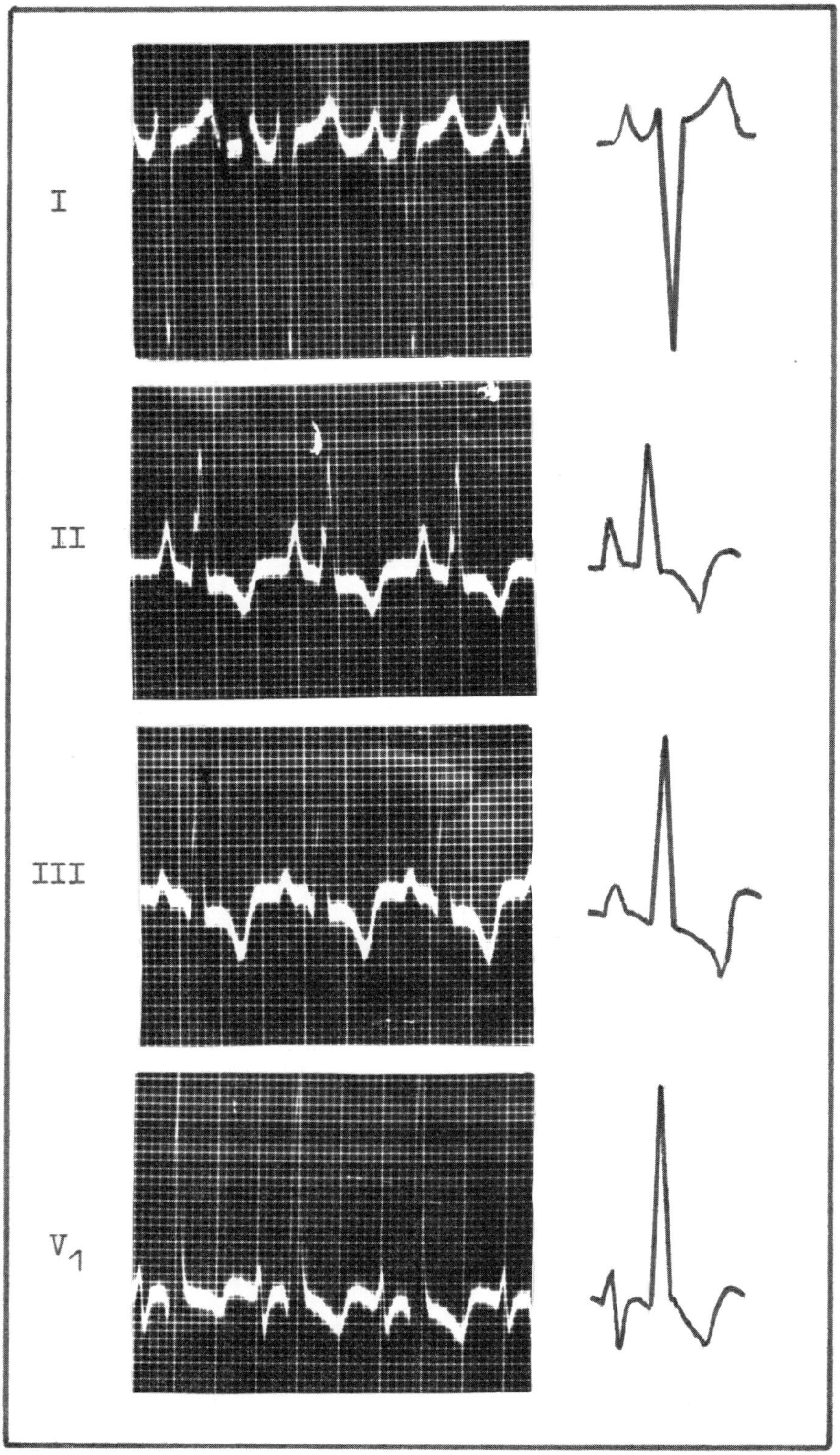

FIGURE 2–18. Right ventricular hypertrophy in a child. Review the criteria as given in Table 2–1.
(Electrocardiogram enlarged for clarity.)

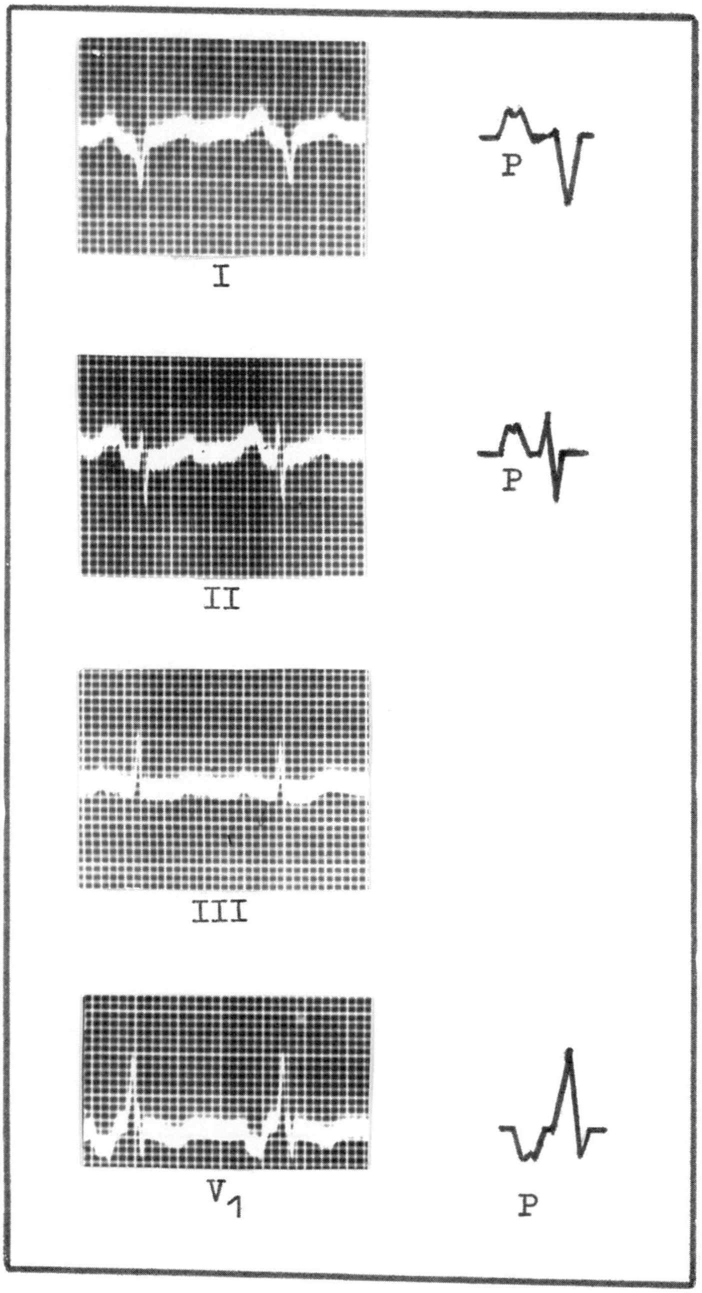

FIGURE 2–19. Adult with mitral stenosis. Describe the characteristics of right ventricular and left atrial enlargement. (Electrocardiogram enlarged for clarity.)

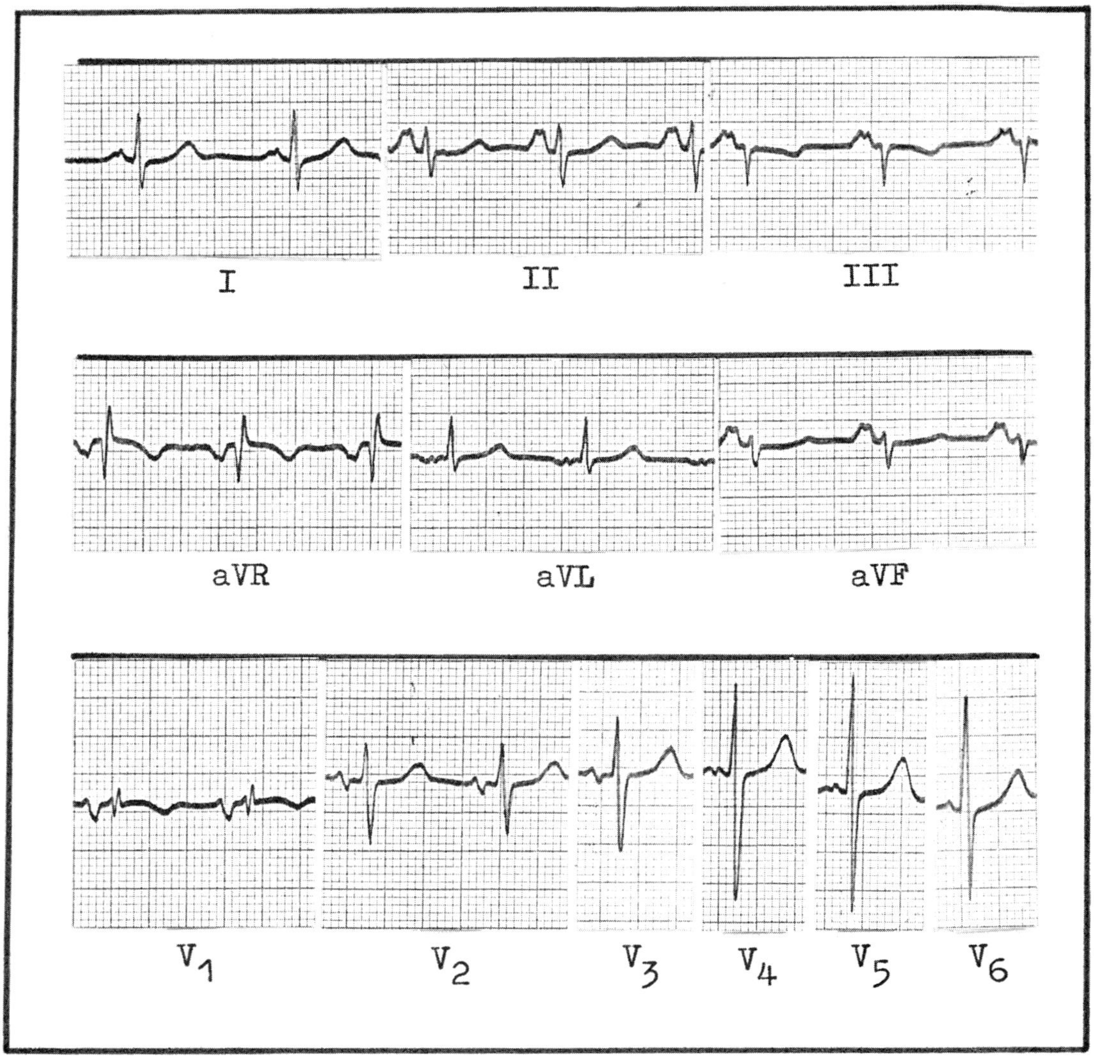

FIGURE 2–20. Review all the electrocardiographic evidence of an enlarged left atrium.

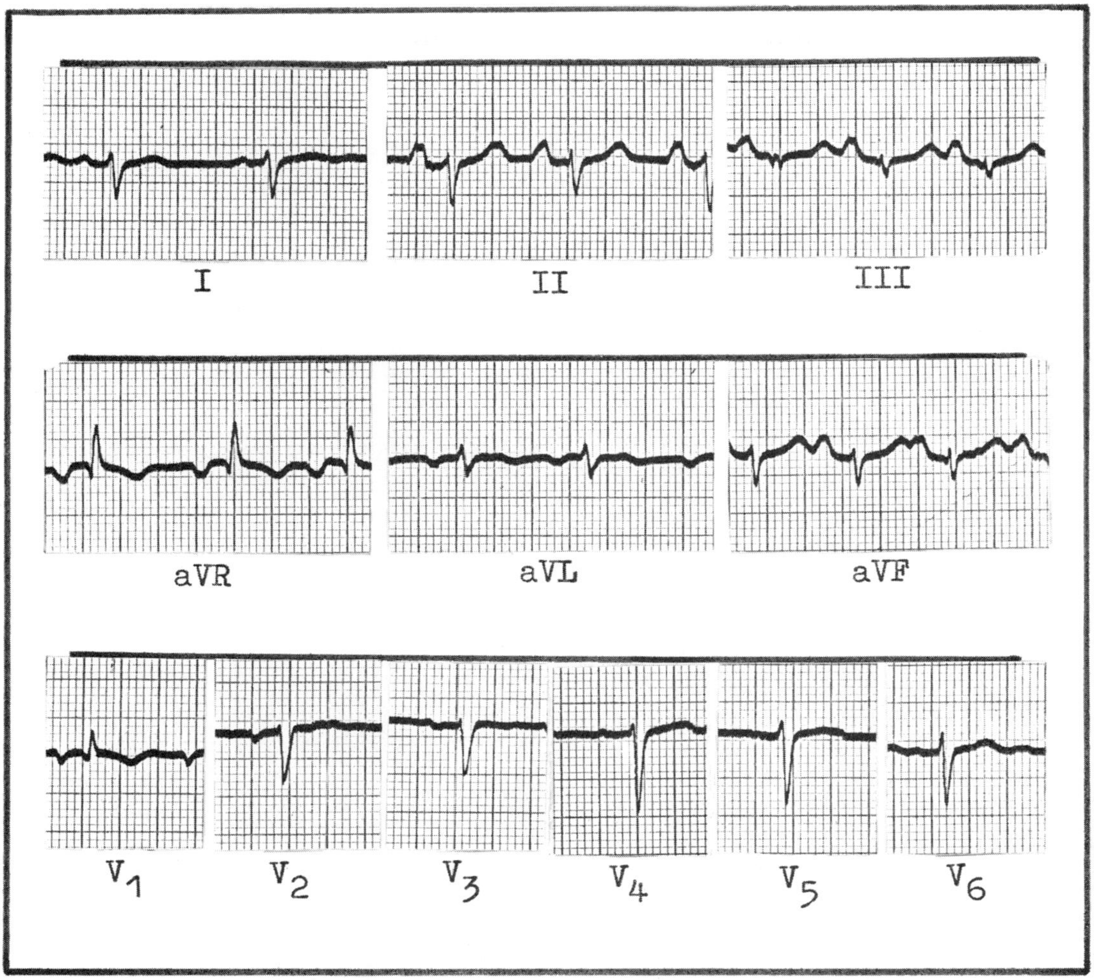

FIGURE 2–21. Right ventricular hypertrophy in a patient with chronic lung disease and cor pulmonale. Note that, although it is small, the R wave is the main ventricular deflection in lead V_1.

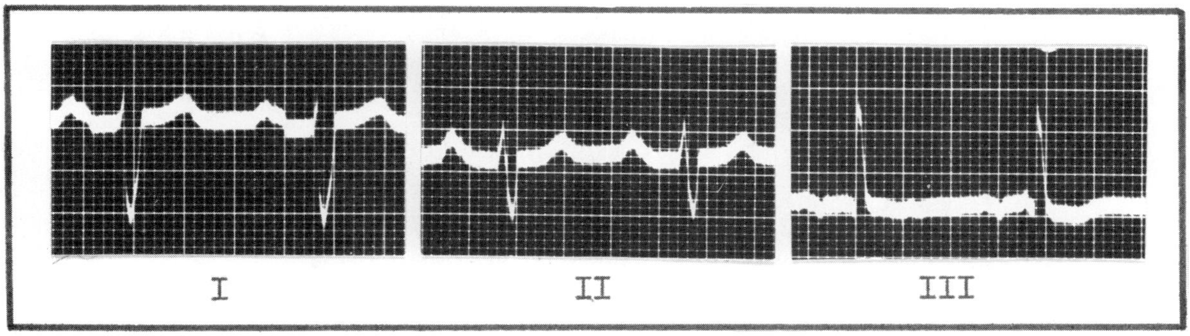

FIGURE 2–22. Right ventricular hypertrophy. Right axis deviation is a common finding in right ventricular hypertrophy. Also evident is the broad, notched P wave, especially in lead I, and the wide QRS–T angle. The distance from the beginning of the P wave to the beginning of the QRS complex is greater than 0.2 sec. (one large box). This is known as first degree atrioventricular block and will be observed again later. This patient had mitral stenosis.
(Electrocardiogram enlarged for clarity.)

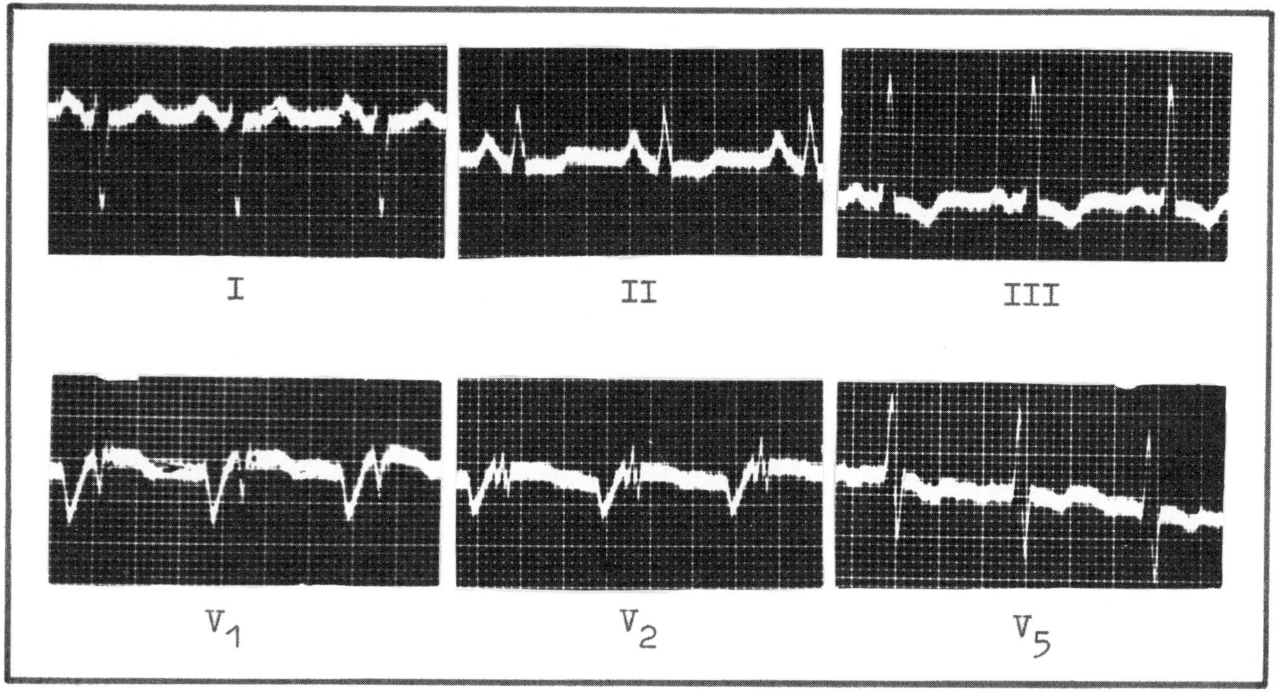

FIGURE 2–23. Right ventricular hypertrophy. Note right axis deviation, broad and notched P waves, especially in lead I, tall P waves in lead II, deep negative P waves in lead V_1 (the P waves are of greater magnitude than the QRS complexes) and a wide QRS–T angle.

Although we have clear evidence of right ventricular enlargement, the QRS vector in the horizontal plane is posterior, as seen from the negative QRS complexes in lead V_1. One does not need all the criteria in each and every case to make the diagnosis. This patient had mitral stenosis with right ventricular and biatrial enlargement. (Electrocardiogram enlarged for clarity.)

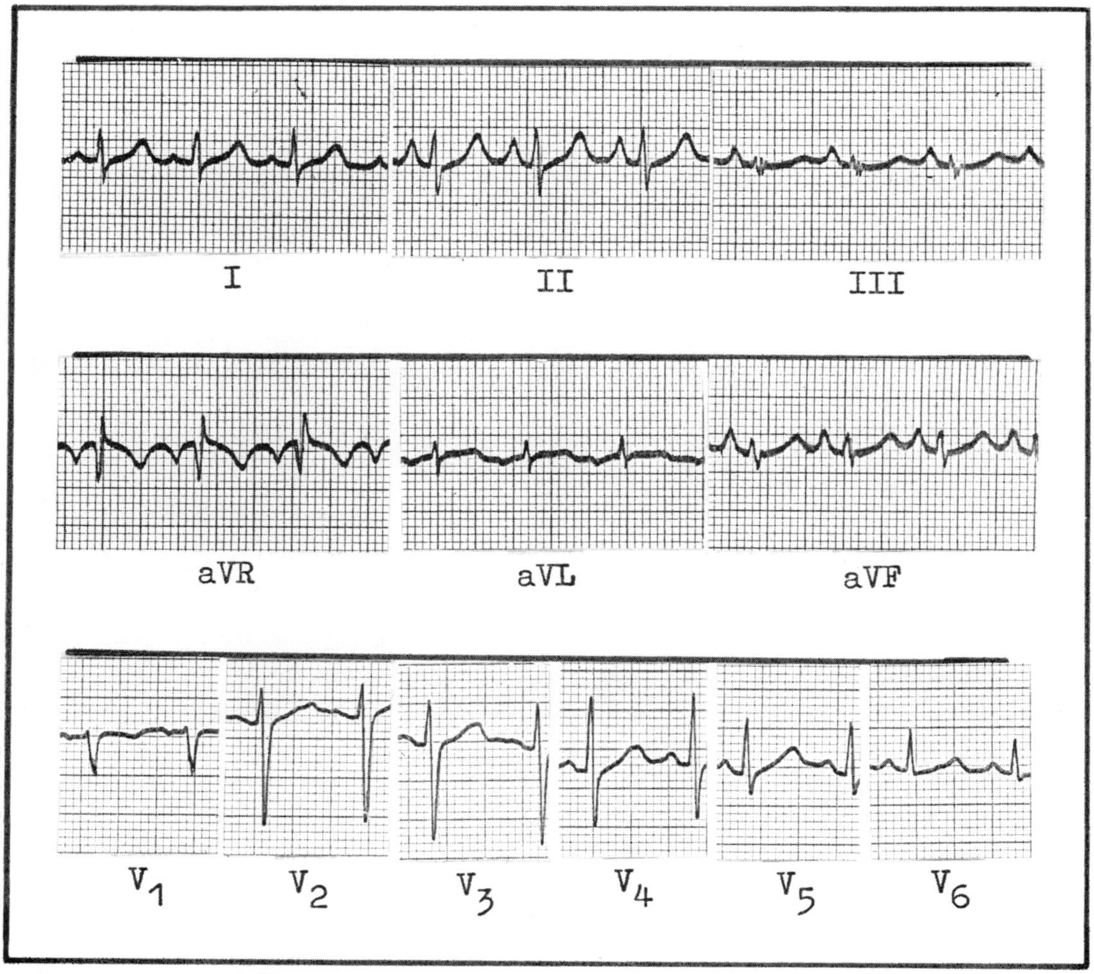

FIGURE 2–24. What evidence can you assemble to support the diagnosis of right ventricular hypertrophy? Up to this point your diagnosis would be based on "presumptive" evidence. In a later chapter (Chapter 6) you will study the "$S_1S_2S_3$ syndrome," which includes right ventricular hypertrophy in the differential diagnosis.

Figure 2–25 emphasizes a concept of great importance, the contribution of serial electrocardiograms in following a patient. In Figure 2–25*A* the QRS complex is predominantly positive in leads I, II and III; the mean QRS vector is within normal limits. The very tall peaked P waves in lead II and, to a lesser degree, in leads I and III, represent right atrial enlargement in this elderly patient and constitute good presumptive evidence of right ventricular enlargement.

A year and a half later we no longer had to look for "presumptive" evidence because the QRS deflections in lead I in Figure 2–25*B* had become predominantly negative; the mean QRS vector had shifted rightward. The importance of serial electrocardiograms in patient follow-up will be stressed again and again.

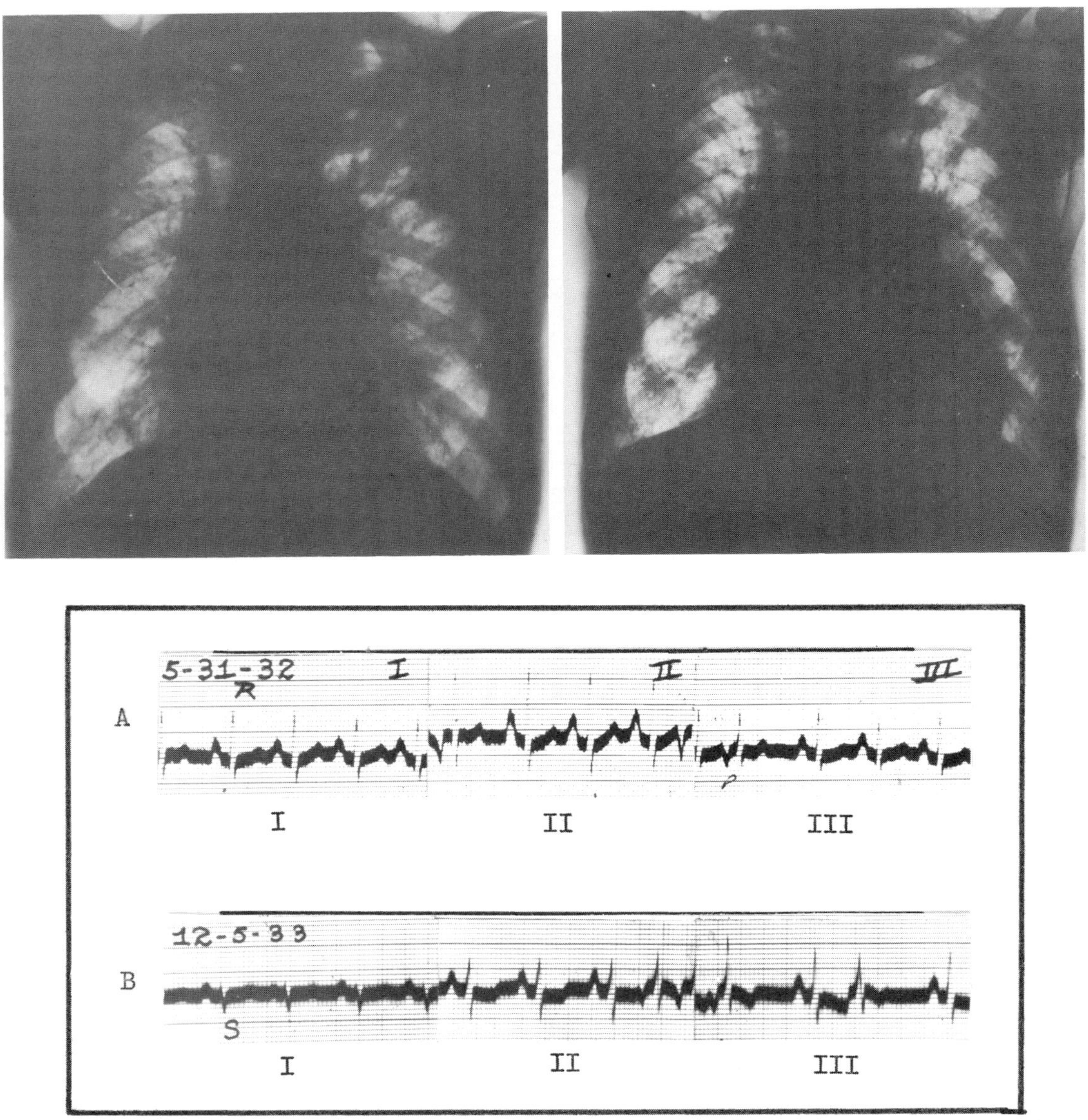

FIGURE 2–25. Enlargement of the right ventricle (progressive). What changes have occurred in the interim between the two electrocardiograms?
(Electrocardiogram reduced in size.)

In Figure 2–26*A* the mean QRS vector is within normal limits. Several months later, as seen in Figure 2–26*B*, the QRS deflections in lead I had become predominantly negative; the mean QRS vector had shifted rightward with the progression of this man's pulmonary disease and cor pulmonale.

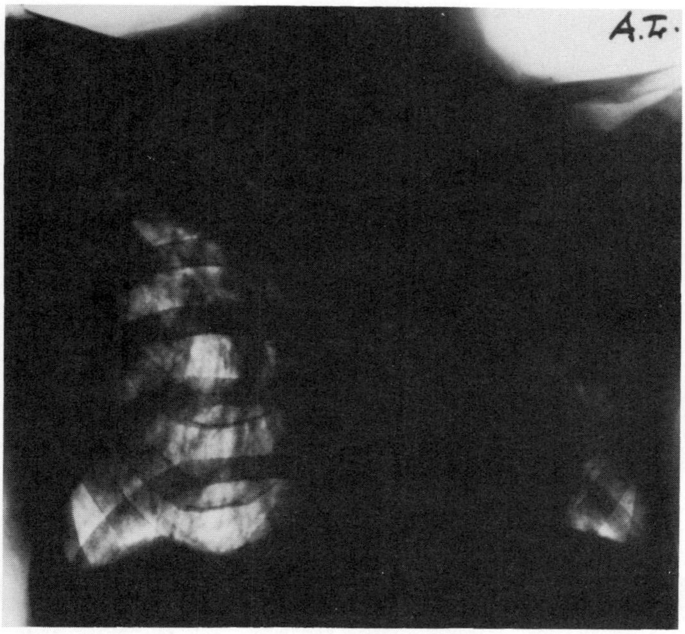

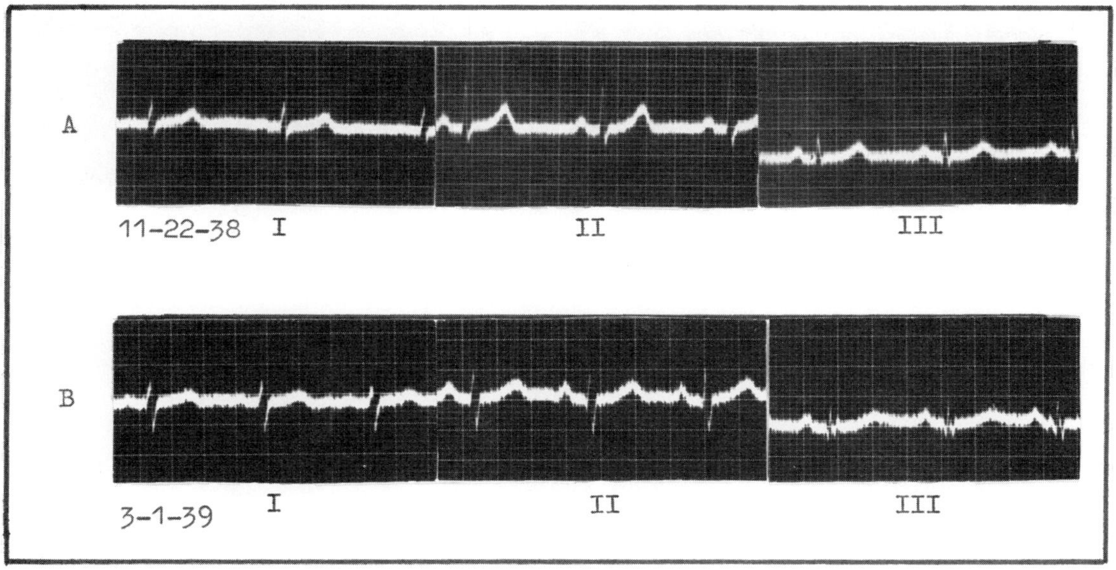

FIGURE 2–26. Axis shift from normal to right with progression of pulmonary disease and cor pulmonale. (Electrocardiogram reduced in size.)

In Figure 2–27*B* not only has the mean QRS vector shifted rightward but the P waves have also become more prominent, especially in lead II, with progression of the disease.

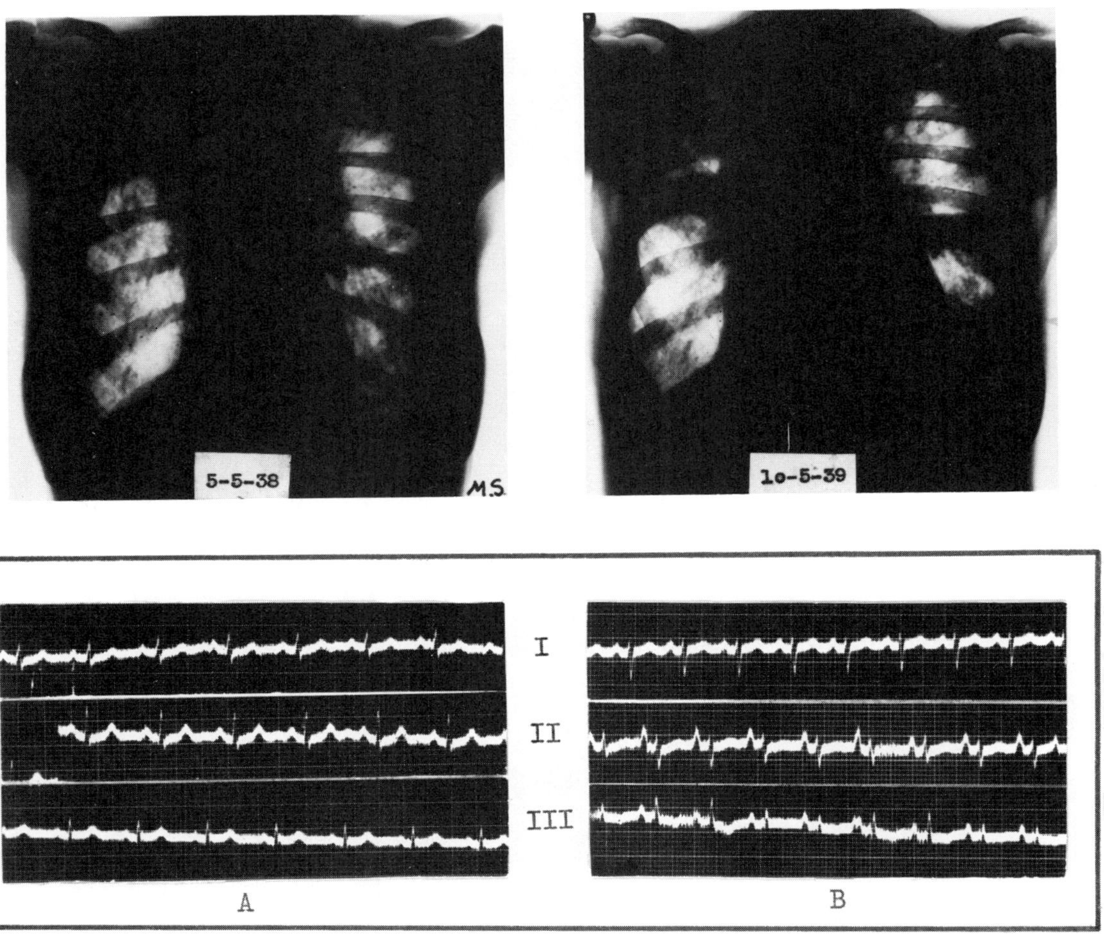

FIGURE 2–27. Note the rightward shift of the mean QRS vector in *B.* What P wave changes are noted? Another example of the importance of serial electrocardiograms in patient follow-up.
(Electrocardiogram reduced in size.)

Figure 2–28*A* represents the "stable" pattern in a patient with long-standing chronic obstructive lung disease. During a clinic visit this patient stated that he felt well and just wanted renewal of his medication. An astute house officer detected slightly increased shortness of breath and ordered an electrocardiogram as part of the evaluation. Figure 2–28*B*, showing a rightward shift of the mean QRS vector, was taken at that time. The patient was immediately hospitalized and treated.

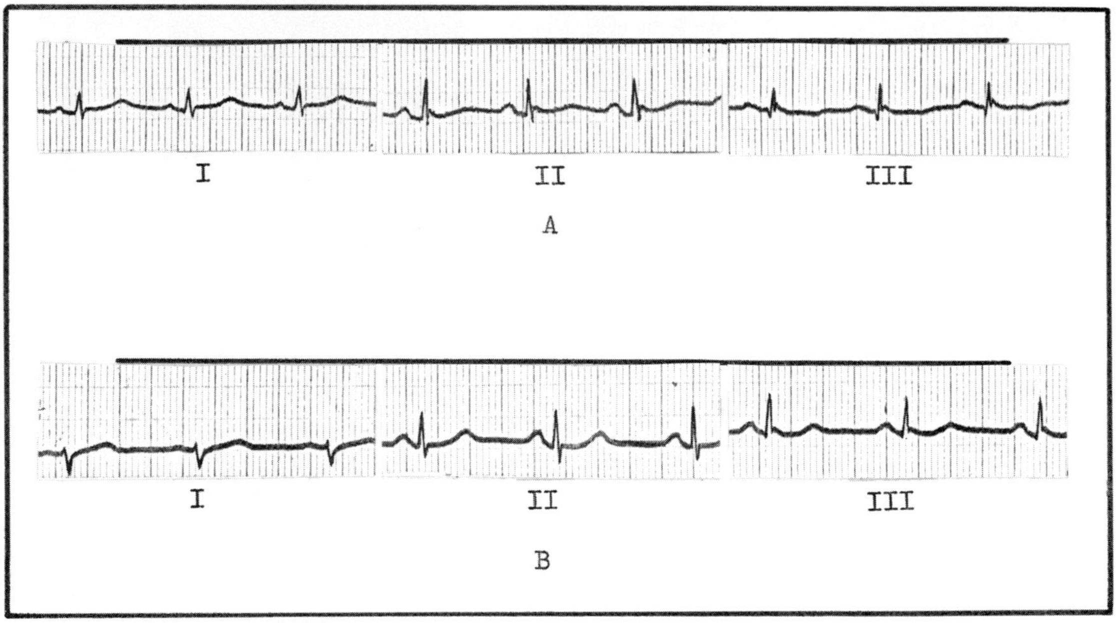

FIGURE 2–28. A mean QRS vector shift to the right confirmed clinical findings (see text). (Electrocardiogram reduced in size.)

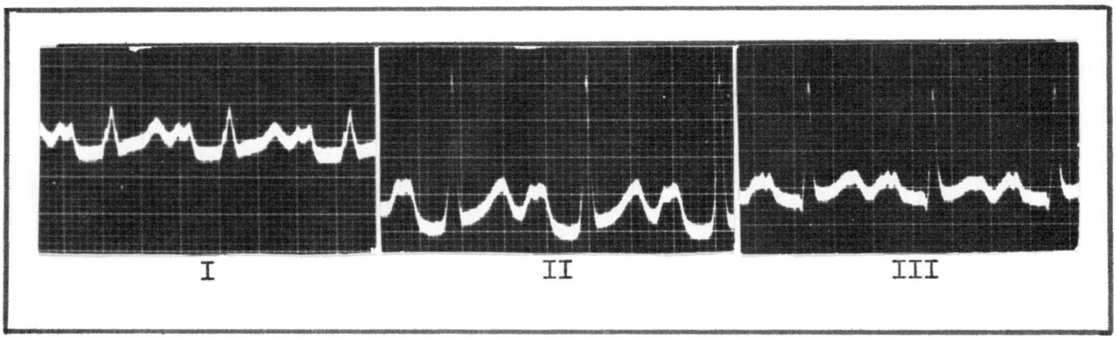

FIGURE 2–29. This electrocardiogram will be studied again in a later chapter. For the present, note the following:

1. Size of P waves.
2. Configuration of P waves.
3. Duration of P–R interval.
4. Depression of P–R segment (atrial repolarization).

Diagnosis?

(Electrocardiogram enlarged for clarity.)

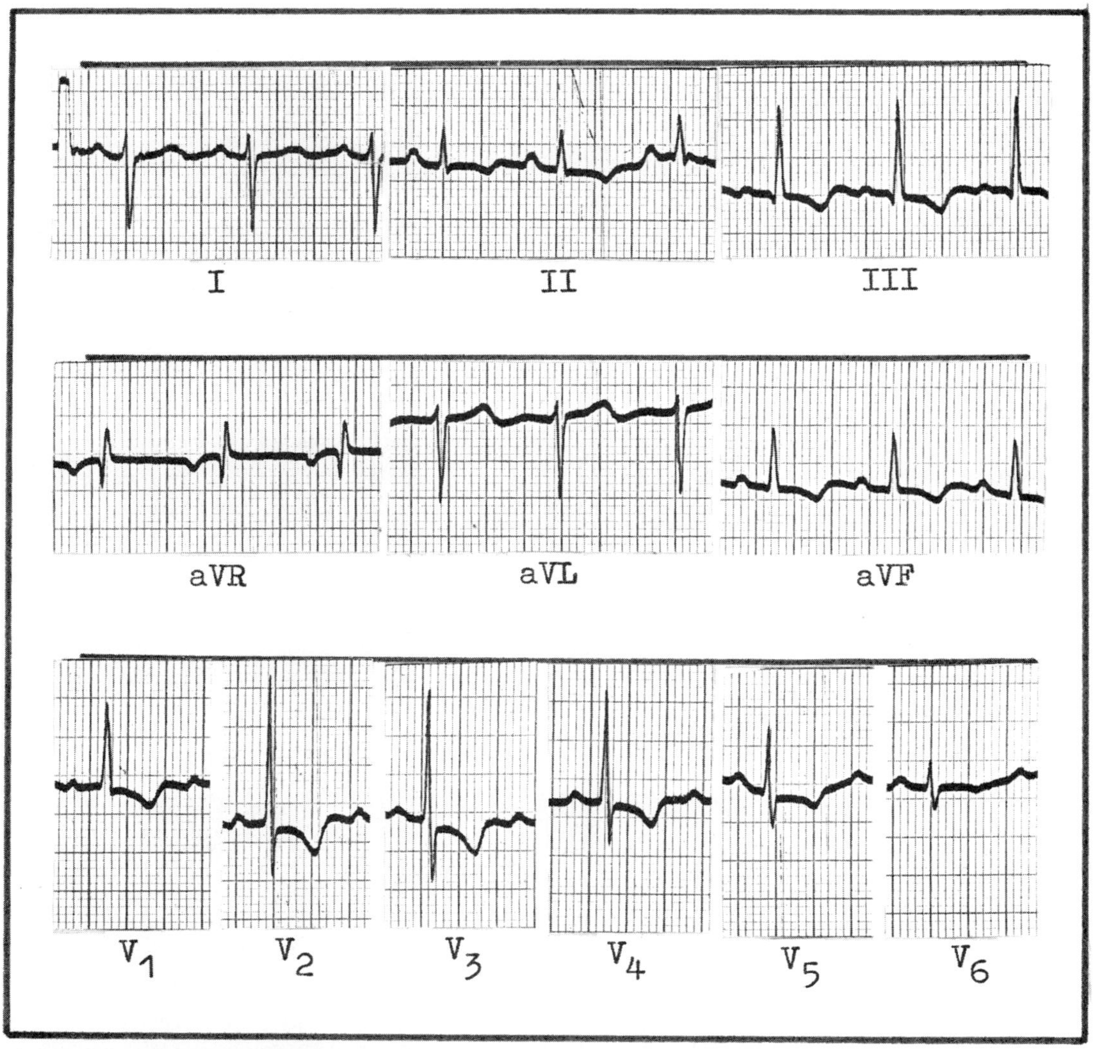

FIGURE 2–30. Right ventricular hypertrophy. Figures 2–30 to 2–35 are labeled "right ventricular hypertrophy." Analyze each using all the criteria learned for right ventricular hypertrophy.

A. Right axis deviation.

B. Magnitude of the mean QRS vector (remember RV_1 as the main ventricular deflection in the adult).

C. Repolarization abnormalities.

D. "Presumptive" evidence. Pay attention to evidence of atrial enlargement.

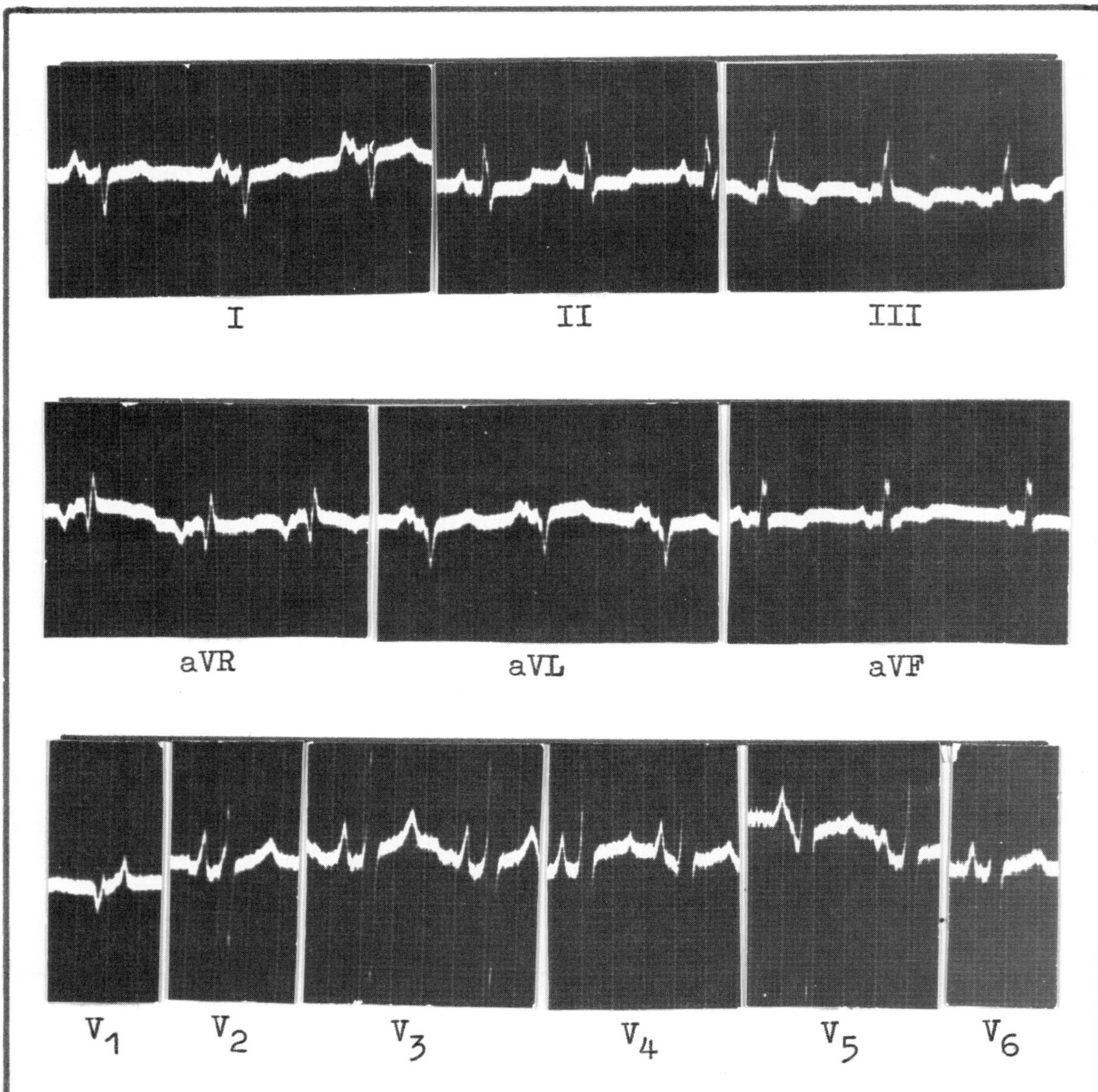

FIGURE 2–31. Right ventricular hypertrophy. (Electrocardiogram reduced in size.)

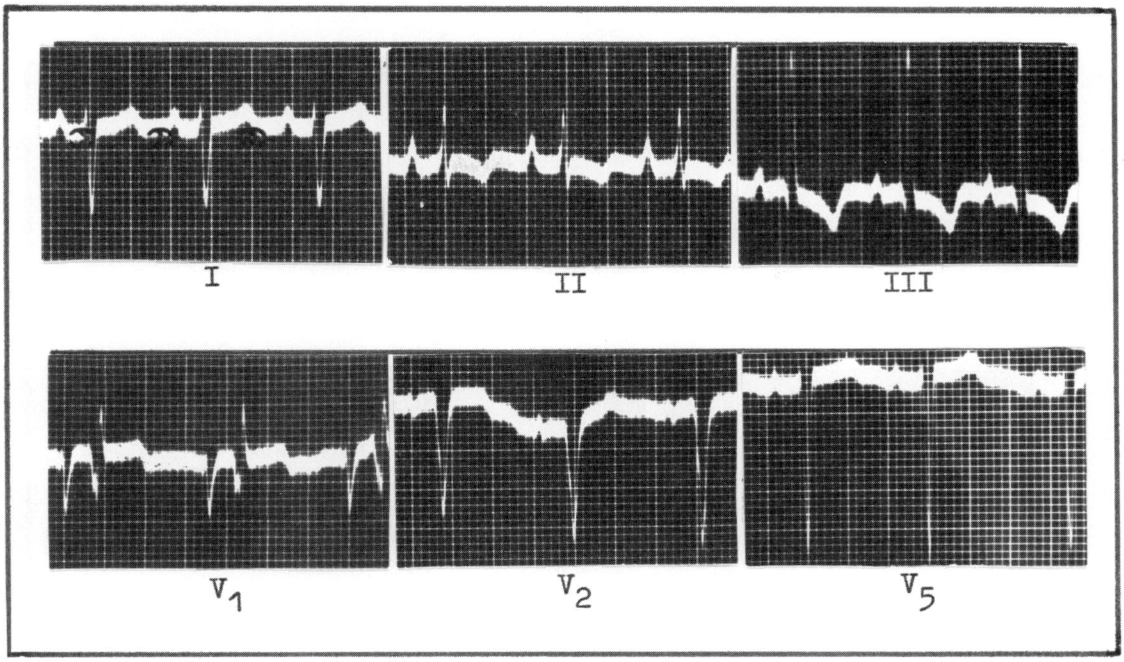

FIGURE 2–32. Right ventricular hypertrophy. (Electrocardiogram enlarged for clarity.)

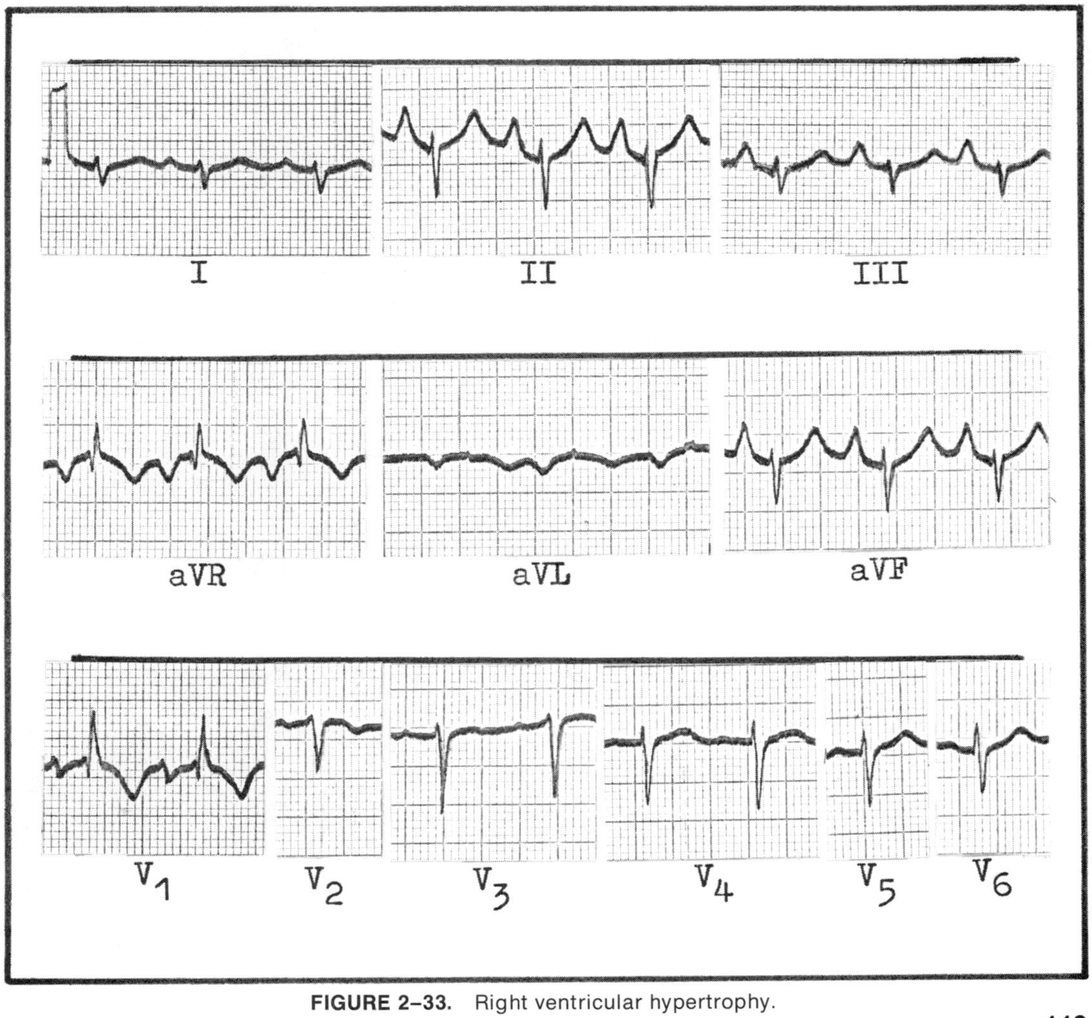

FIGURE 2–33. Right ventricular hypertrophy.

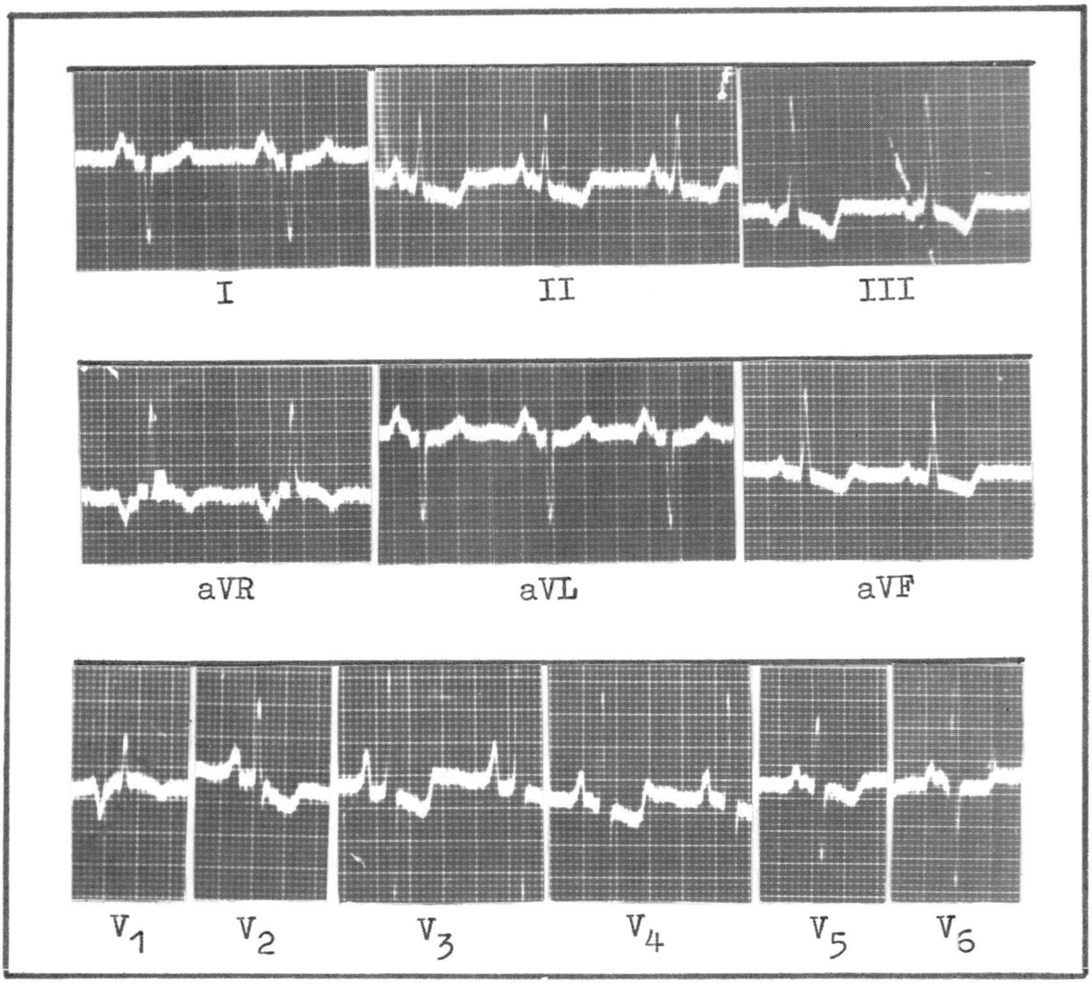

FIGURE 2–34. Right ventricular hypertrophy. (Electrocardiogram reduced in size.)

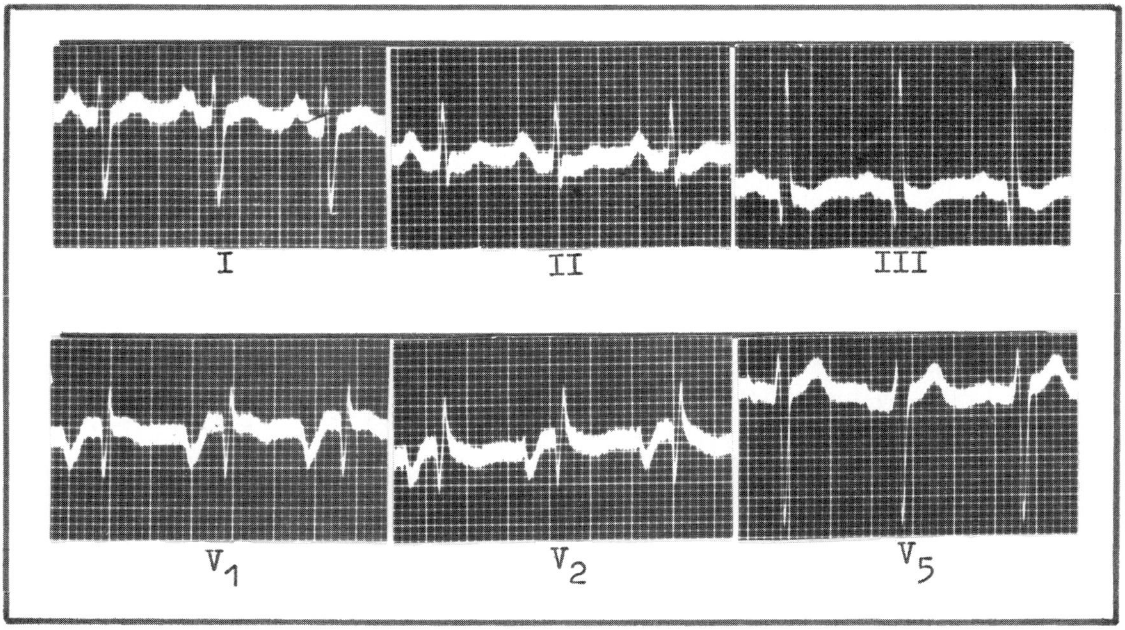

FIGURE 2–35. Right ventricular hypertrophy. (Electrocardiogram enlarged for clarity.)

3 LEFT VENTRICULAR HYPERTROPHY

Cassette Side 7

LEFT VENTRICULAR HYPERTROPHY

The following factors will be considered in the determination of left ventricular hypertrophy.

A. Increase in magnitude of the mean QRS vector.

B. Repolarization abnormalities (abnormalities of the S–T segments and T waves).

C. Left axis deviation.

A. Increase in Magnitude of the Mean QRS Vector

In discussing left ventricular hypertrophy we should remember that the *normal left ventricle*, having a wall several times as thick as the normal right ventricle, is the dominant ventricle. Therefore, the normal mean QRS vector, reflecting this dominance, is to the *left*, *inferior* and *posterior*. This was emphasized in the study of the normal electrocardiogram and in the "rules of thumb" (Chapter 1).

In contrast to right ventricular hypertrophy (Chapter 2), left ventricular hypertrophy is often accompanied by an *accentuation of the normal vector*. This is diagrammed in Figure 3–1. The pointers at the top of the figure represent the mean QRS vector of left ventricular hypertrophy and the normal mean QRS vector. Often associated with the increase in magnitude of the mean QRS vector are repolarization abnormalities.

B. Ventricular Repolarization Abnormalities (Abnormalities of the S–T Segments and T Waves)

Figure 3–1*B* shows the *wide angle* between the mean QRS vector and mean S–T and T vectors. The wide QRS–T angle has been referred to as an "ischemia" pattern and S–T segment abnormalities together with a wide QRS–T angle, in

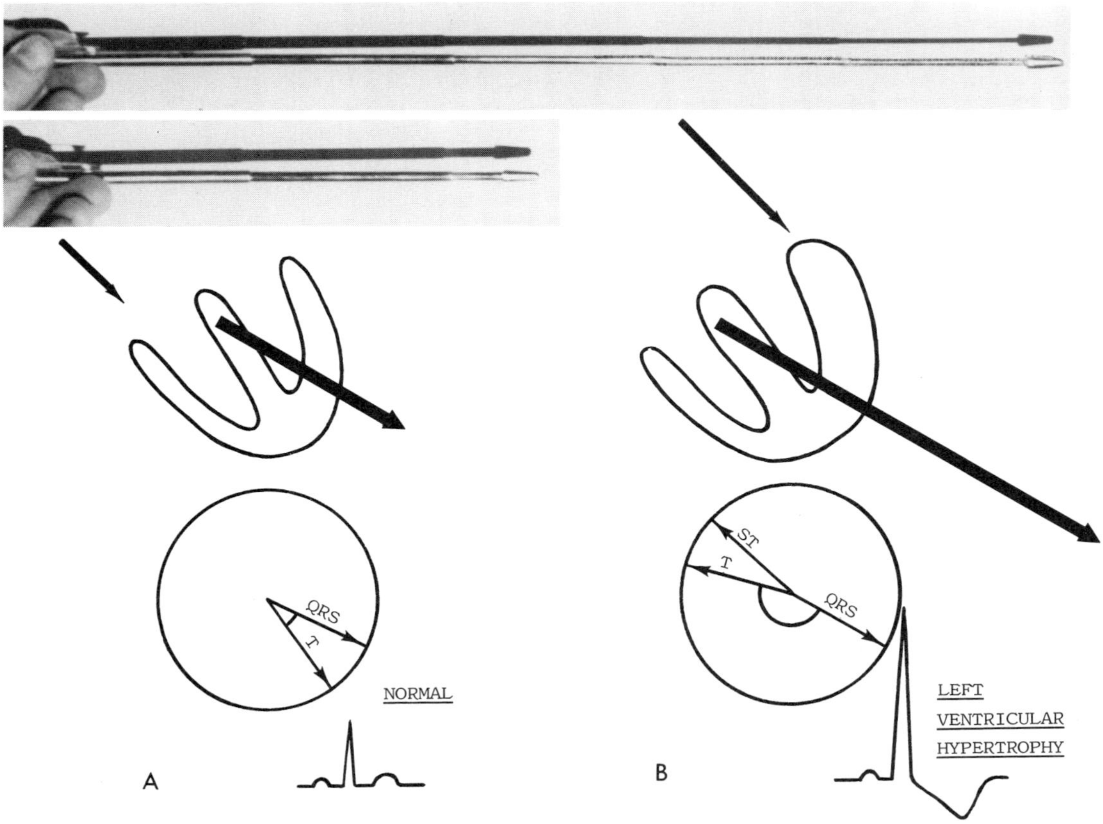

FIGURE 3–1. Normal left ventricle (*A*) and hypertrophied left ventricle (*B*). The normally oriented mean QRS vector is increased in magnitude in left ventricular hypertrophy. The pointers, at the top of the figure, represent the mean QRS vector of left ventricular hypertrophy and the normal mean QRS vector. Accompanying the hypertrophy of the left ventricle are repolarization abnormalities resulting in a wide angle between the mean QRS vector and the mean S–T and T vectors.

the hypertrophied ventricle, as a "strain" pattern. These terms are unfortunate as they impart a clinical connotation to an electrocardiographic pattern; they will not be used in this course. Think of the feeling of a patient who is told that he has left ventricular "strain." Immediately visualized is a heart that is weak and struggling; the opposite may actually be true. The heart may not be near failure and may not necessarily be straining. The previously asymptomatic patient may leave the physician's office with symptoms. The term "ventricular repolarization abnormalities" covering both the wide QRS–T angle and the abnormal S–T segment, is a better term. Occasionally "left ventricular strain" has been listed as the number one criterion for left ventricular hypertrophy. Our findings, however, agree with Grant's that there should be QRS evidence of hypertrophy *(Increase in Magnitude of the Mean QRS Vector)* before even making the diagnosis of "left ventricular strain," for other conditions may produce S–T and T vector abnormalities similar to it.

Before delving into specific values for the hypertrophied left ventricle, compare Figure 3–2*A* with Figure 3–2*B* for (*A*) magnitude of the mean QRS vector and (*B*) ventricular repolarization abnormalities.

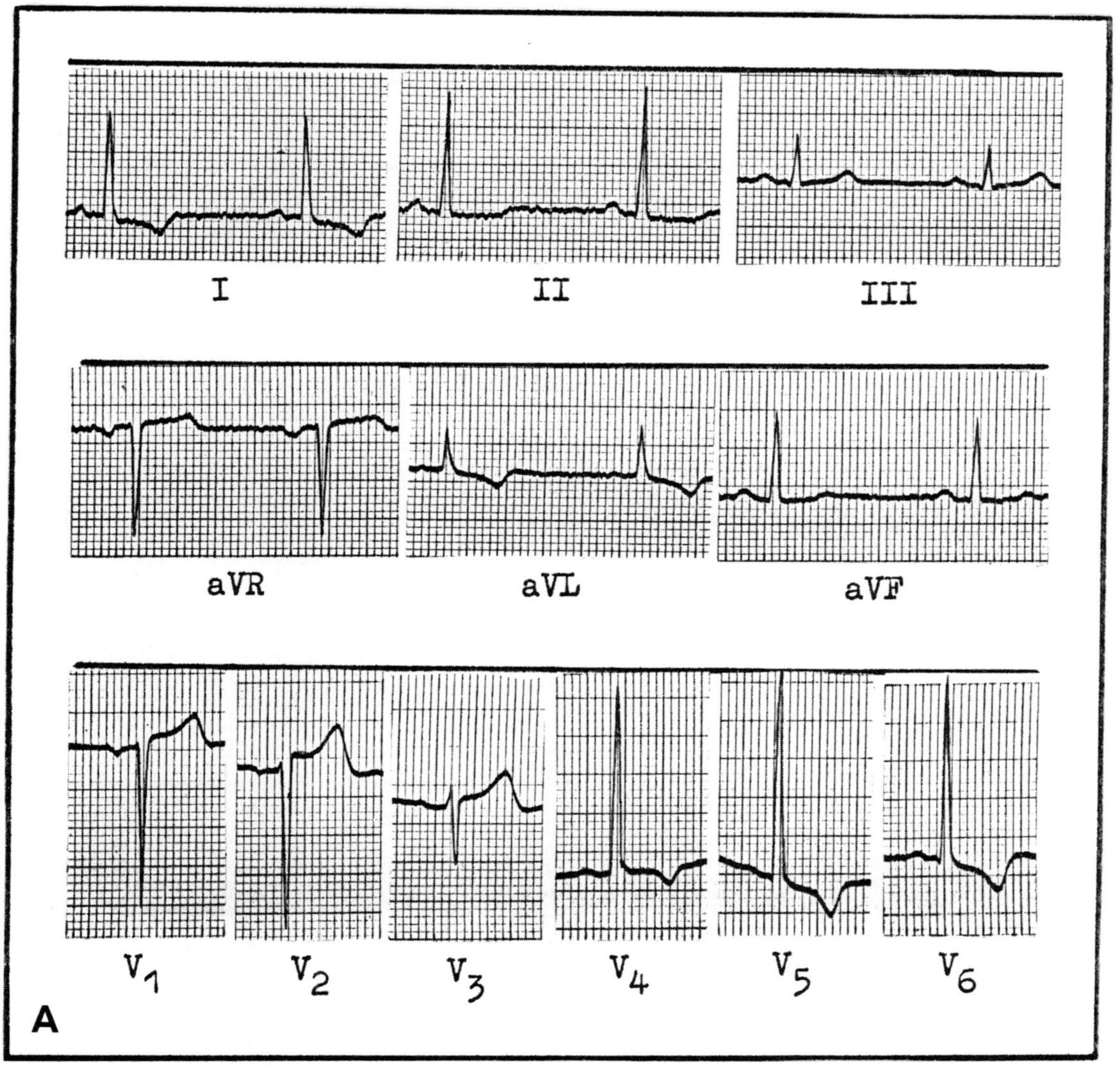

FIGURE 3-2. *A,* Left ventricular hypertrophy. Compare the size of the deflections with those in Figure 3-2*B*, especially in leads V_1, V_2, V_4, V_5 and V_6. The mean QRS vector in each electrocardiogram is to the *left, inferior* and *posterior.*

The QRS–T angle is wide and the S–T segments reveal elevations and depressions. Normally the S–T segment is iso-electric; it is neither elevated nor depressed. See schematic in Figure 3–1. This wide QRS–T angle plus the abnormal S–T segments (repolarization abnormalities of the ventricle) are often referred to as "strain." The term "strain" is unfortunate since it imparts a clinical connotation to an electrocardiographic pattern. The term "repolarization" abnormalities, covering both the wide QRS–T angle and the abnormal S–T segment, is a better term.

The increased magnitude of the mean QRS vector and repolarization abnormalities of the ventricle play an important role in the electrocardiographic diagnosis of hypertrophy of the left ventricle.

Illustration continued on following page.

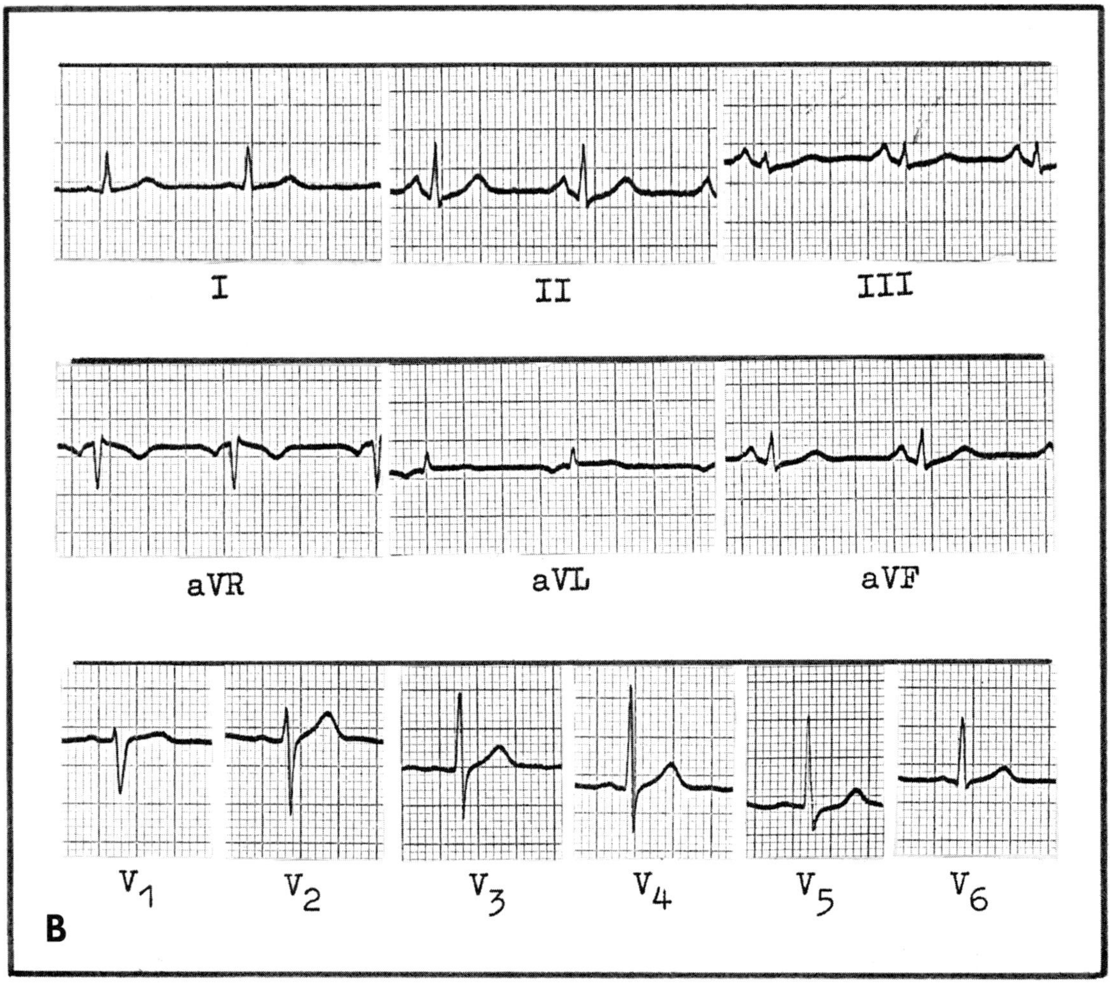

FIGURE 3–2 *Continued.* *B,* Normal. Compare the QRS deflection size, QRS–T angle and S–T segments with those in Figure 3–2*A*.

C. Left Axis Deviation (LAD)

Left axis deviation is defined as a mean QRS vector which is beyond −30° (see Fig. 1–36, page 32). At one time it was thought strongly suggestive of left ventricular hypertrophy. It is now, however, considered to be a conduction disturbance which may or may not accompany left ventricular hypertrophy. That it may be found alone, without any other evidence of left ventricular hypertrophy, is seen in Figure 3–3. Left axis deviation is *not* a major criterion for left ventricular hypertrophy; it is included here because of the frequent association of left axis deviation with left ventricular hypertrophy. This is in contrast to right ventricular hypertrophy, for in right ventricular hypertrophy *right axis deviation* is a *major* electrocardiographic criterion (Chapter 2). Some of the causes of left axis deviation will be studied in a later chapter.

Following the same pattern used in the study of right ventricular hypertrophy, a set of suggested criteria is presented for left ventricular hypertrophy in Table 3–1. Figure 3–4 is then analyzed using these criteria. The expression "suggested criteria" is used since there are numerous sets of criteria in use today, including a "point score" system,* in weighing the diagnosis of left ventricular hypertrophy. The fact that different sets of criteria are used emphasizes that caution must be exercised and that no system is infallible.

*Romheit, D. W., and Estes, E. H., Jr.: A point score system for the ECG diagnosis of left ventricular hypertrophy. Amer. Heart J., 75:752, 1968.

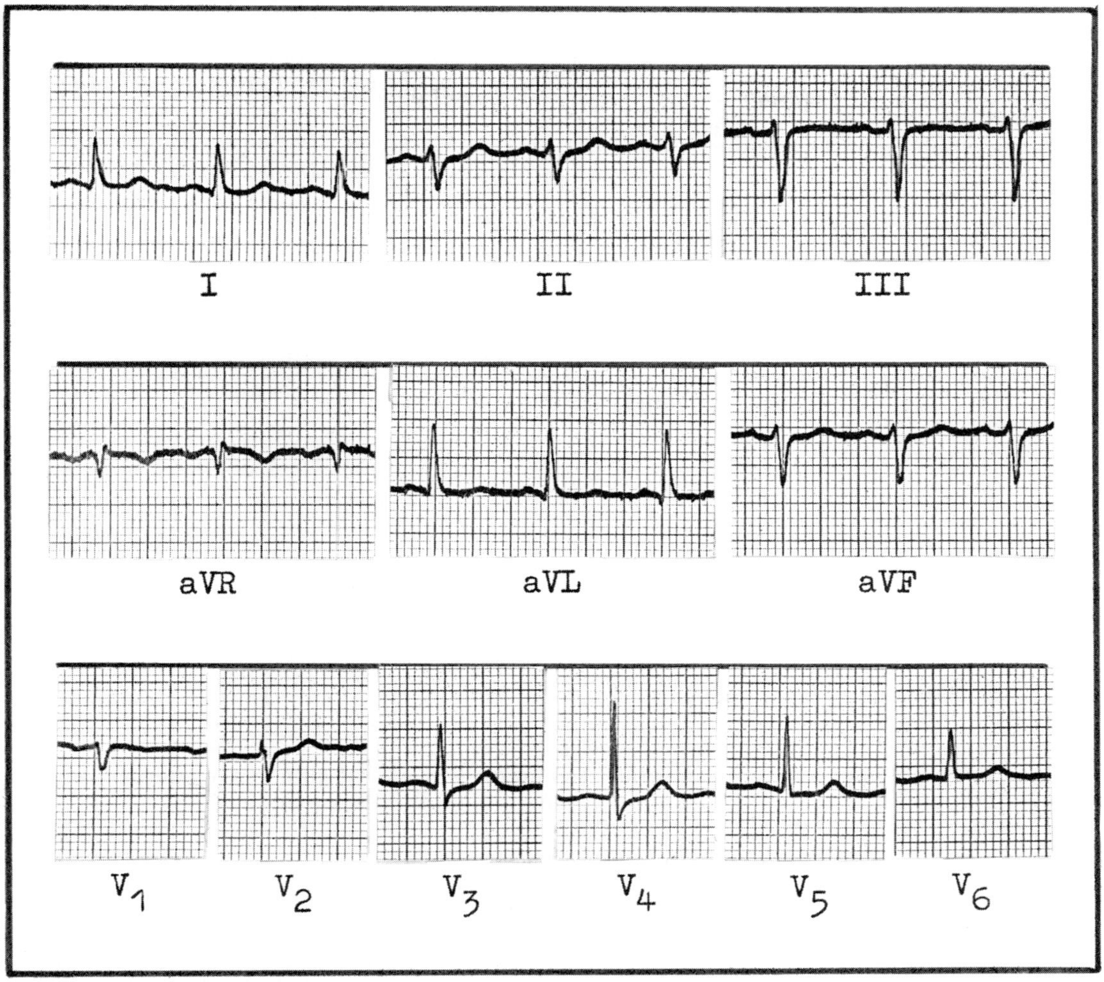

FIGURE 3–3. Left axis deviation (LAD) in a normal sized heart. LAD is not a necessary criterion for the diagnosis of left ventricular hypertrophy. Left ventricular hypertrophy may occur without LAD and LAD may occur without left ventricular hypertrophy. Some of the causes of LAD will be studied later in this course.

For example, in Table 3–1, a statement is made that the magnitude criteria in the chest leads (leads V_1 to V_6) apply to an adult over the age of 30 years, of normal height and weight. This is very important since in the very thin and very young subjects with normal sized hearts, magnitude of the QRS complexes may be well within the range for left ventricular hypertrophy. On the other hand, an obese individual with left ventricular hypertrophy may not have QRS complexes greater than normal amplitude. This again stresses the importance of knowing your patients. Keep in mind that a normal electrocardiogram does not rule out left ventricular hypertrophy.

The mean QRS vector, increased in magnitude, is the prime electrocardiographic evidence of left ventricular hypertrophy. The diagnosis of left ventricular hypertrophy should not be made in the absence of this increased magnitude, and it should not be made on repolarization abnormalities alone; these are nonspecific.

Although a suggested set of criteria is presented in Table 3–1, the emphasis in this course is on concept. Once the basic concept of the vectorial forces of left

TABLE 3–1. LEFT VENTRICULAR HYPERTROPHY

A. Increased Magnitude of the QRS Vector
Mild QRS complex prolongation may occur with increasing left ventricular hypertrophy, e.g., 0.08→0.09→0.10→0.11 second.
Standard Leads: I, II and III.

$R_I + S_{III} > 35$ mm.

aV Leads: aVR, aVL and aVF.

$R_{aVL} + S_{aVF} > 35$ mm.

$R_{aVL} > 12$ mm. (especially in presence of a *normally oriented* mean QRS vector)

Chest Leads: V_1 to V_6 (*mean QRS vector magnitude criteria in an adult over the age of 30 years, of normal height and weight*)

S_{V_1} or $S_{V_2} + R_{V_5}$ or $R_{V_6} > 40$ mm.

S_{V_1} or $S_{V_2} > 30$ mm.

R_{V_5} or $R_{V_6} > 30$ mm. (especially if $R_{V_6} > R_{V_5}$).

B. Repolarization Abnormalities (Wide QRS–T Angle and S–T Segment Abnormalities)
This applies to all leads—standard, aV and chest.

C. Left Axis Deviation (LAD)
This is a conduction disturbance not necessarily associated with the hypertrophied left ventricle. Either may be found independently. It is included here because of the frequent association of LAD with left ventricular hypertrophy.
Once you are thoroughly familiar with these criteria, you will be able to scan electrocardiograms and look for left ventricular hypertrophy in the following order:
A. Increased magnitude of the mean QRS vector.
B. Ventricular repolarization abnormalities.
C. Left axis deviation (LAD).
Note: Clear evidence of *left atrial enlargement* (in absence of mitral stenosis—see Chapter 2) may be the clue that left ventricular hypertrophy is present. Not all of the above criteria are necessary for the electrocardiographic diagnosis of left ventricular hypertrophy. The more the evidence, however, the more secure the diagnosis. The diagnosis should not be made without at least some of the magnitude criteria. Keep in mind that a normal electrocardiogram does not rule out left ventricular hypertrophy.

ventricular hypertrophy is understood, the specific figures are easily understood. The values given should never be taken as absolute truths; they frequently change in the face of evolving information.

To illustrate how tenuous even well recognized criteria may be, just one study will be cited. Several of our hypertensive patients with all the manifestations of left ventricular hypertrophy, especially the "magnitude" criteria, were effectively treated with antihypertensive agents. Some of the group showed either diminution or complete disappearance of the "magnitude" criteria, without real change in the thickness of the left ventricle. Factors such as afterload (resistance to ejection) must, therefore, be given consideration in the electrocardiographic diagnosis of left ventricular hypertrophy. Always remember that the more the available criteria, the more secure the diagnosis.

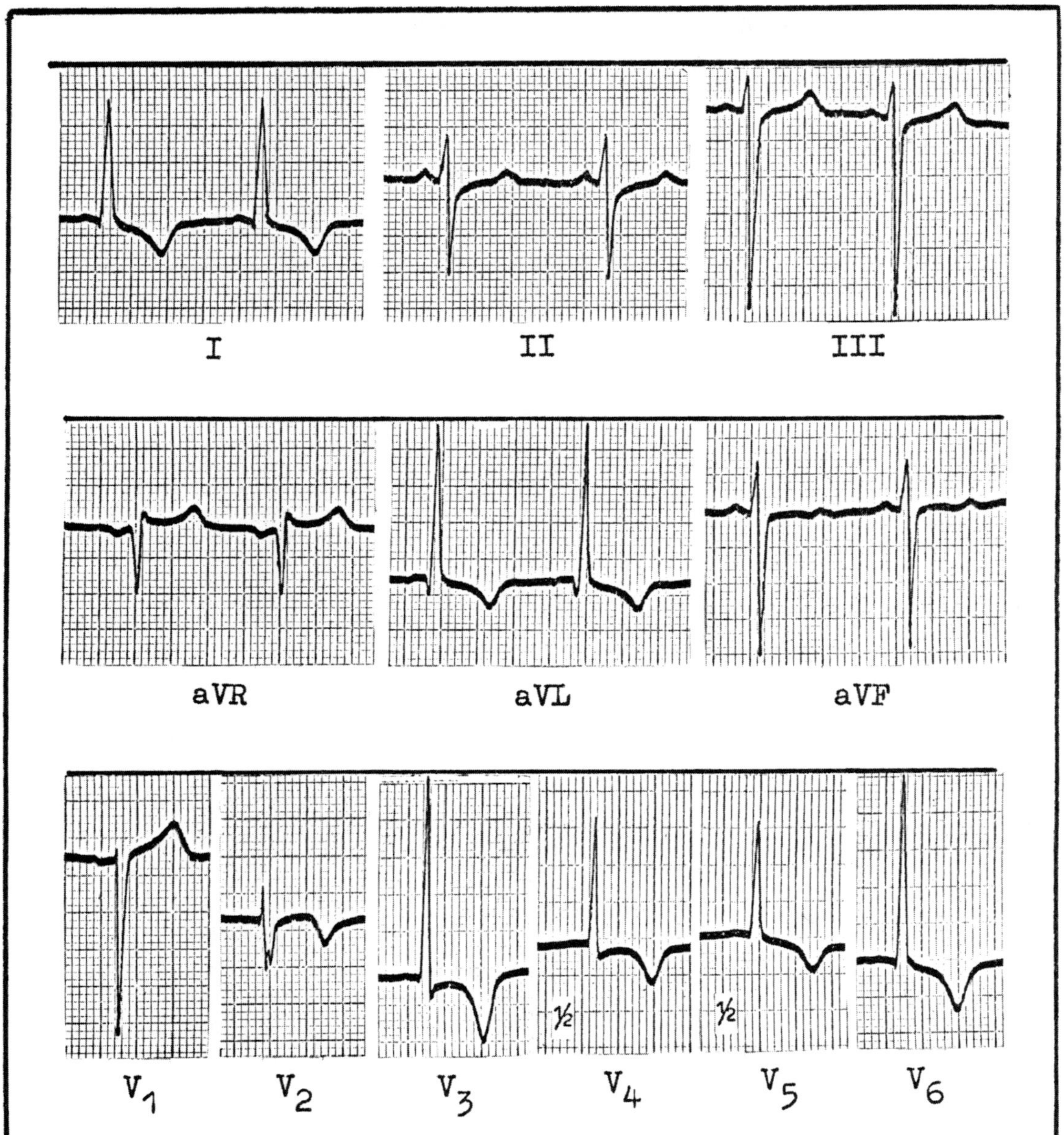

FIGURE 3–4. Left ventricular hypertrophy. The criteria for the electrocardiographic diagnosis of left ventricular hypertrophy were presented in Table 3–1. Let us now analyze this electrocardiogram in the following order:

A. Increased magnitude of the mean QRS vector.
B. Ventricular repolarization abnormalities.
C. Left axis deviation (LAD). As noted, a mean QRS vector beyond −30° is not essential to the diagnosis of left ventricular hypertrophy, *although it is frequently associated with it.* LAD is generally considered a conduction disturbance and will be studied later.

A. Increased magnitude of the mean QRS vector.

Standard leads: I, II and III. The millimeter measurements are approximate.

R wave in lead I = 17 mm.
S wave in lead III = 27 mm.
summate to 44 mm.

Legend continued on following page.

FIGURE 3–4 *Continued.*

aV leads: aVR, aVL and aVF.

R wave in lead aVL = 22 mm.
S wave in lead aVF = 20 mm.
summate to 42 mm.

Chest leads: V_1 to V_6.

S wave in lead V_1 = 24 mm.
R wave in lead V_6 = 25 mm.
summate to 49 mm.

B. The T waves do not follow the QRS complexes in direction. Where the QRS complexes are positive the T waves are generally negative, and vice versa. Therefore, there is a wide QRS–T angle. The S–T segments are not isoelectric and tend to follow the general direction of the T waves, so that we have "repolarization" criteria in addition to "magnitude." Figure 3–1 shows the difference between the normal QRS–T angle and the QRS–T angle and S–T vectors frequently found in the hypertrophied left ventricle.
C. Left axis deviation (LAD) is present (beyond −30°).

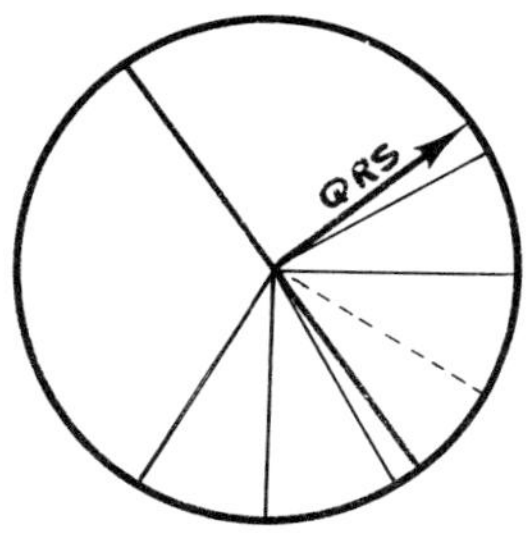

Note that the precordial V_4 and V_5 are one half standard. Remember, therefore, to double the size of these leads in making your "magnitude" calculations.

It must be continually stressed that the electrocardiogram should be viewed as an adjunct to the practice of medicine. It should never be an absolute and must be studied sequentially. It must not at any time be a substitute for a careful history and physical examination.

Figure 3–5*A*, from a patient with known left ventricular hypertrophy, meets the major criteria for left ventricular hypertrophy. Both "magnitude" and "repolarization" criteria are present. A question, however, arises. Since the mean QRS vector is increased in magnitude in the horizontal plane (precordial leads), why do not the frontal plane leads (I, II, III, aVR, aVL and aVF) show this manifestation of increased vectorial magnitude?

It is possible for a three-dimensional vectorial force of increased magnitude to appear normal in one plane (frontal) and large in another plane (horizontal). This is common in left ventricular hypertrophy since the mean QRS vector in the progression of the hypertrophy is often oriented ever more posteriorly. This is explained and illustrated in Figure 3–5*B*; it is seen again in Figure 3–6. It is necessary to examine all the leads, in both planes. The "magnitude" criteria do not necessarily have to be fulfilled in all the leads, but must be fulfilled in some, to show the increased magnitude of the mean QRS vector.

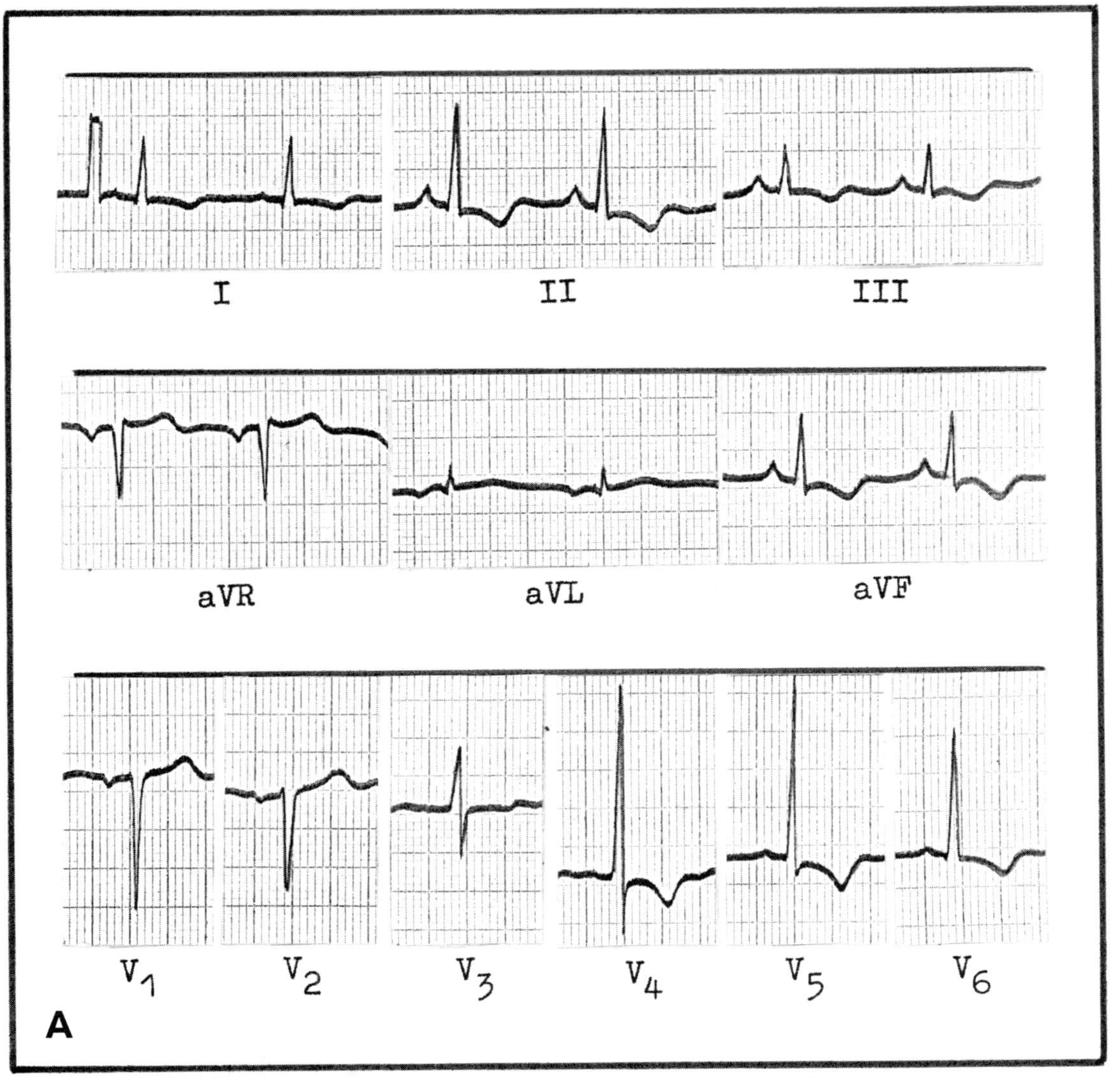

FIGURE 3–5. *A,* Enlarged left ventricle. Analyze, following the steps outlined in Figure 3–4 and Table 3–1.

Illustration continued on following page.

B

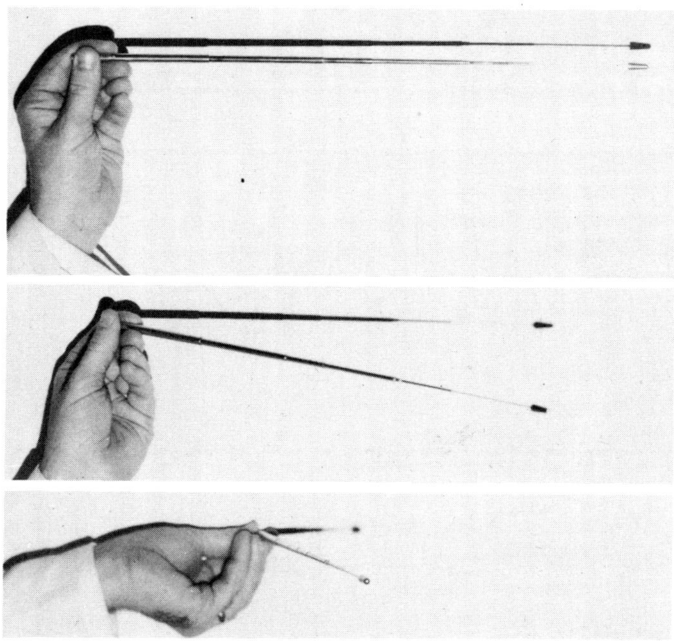

FIGURE 3–5 *Continued.* *B,* Influence of vectorial position on electrocardiographic deflections. You will see many electrocardiograms of the enlarged left ventricle (e.g., Figs. 3–5*A* and 3–6) with markedly enlarged QRS deflections in the horizontal plane (leads V_1 to V_6). The frontal plane (leads I, II, III, aVR, aVL and aVF) QRS deflections, however, are not exceptionally large. How is this possible when all the deflections reflect just one mean QRS vector in space?

The pointers in the upper, middle and lower panels in the above figures are the same size. In the upper panel, you see the pointer in its full length—note the size of the shadow. As the pointer is moved posteriorly, or anteriorly, it appears to be shorter (middle panel). In the lower panel, it appears to be still shorter. When you see the pointer on end, it only *appears* to be short; in reality it may be quite long. So it is with the mean QRS vector. In a markedly posterior (common in the enlarged left ventricle) mean QRS vector, the QRS deflections in the horizontal plane reflect the vector more in its fuller length. The deflections in the frontal plane reflect the vector more on end. The *very same, very large* mean QRS vectorial force may, therefore, seem to be large in some leads and small in others. You must look at all the leads and not jump to conclusions from any given lead.

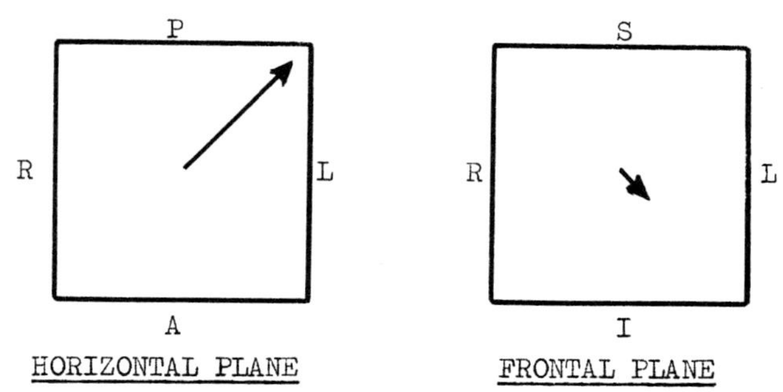

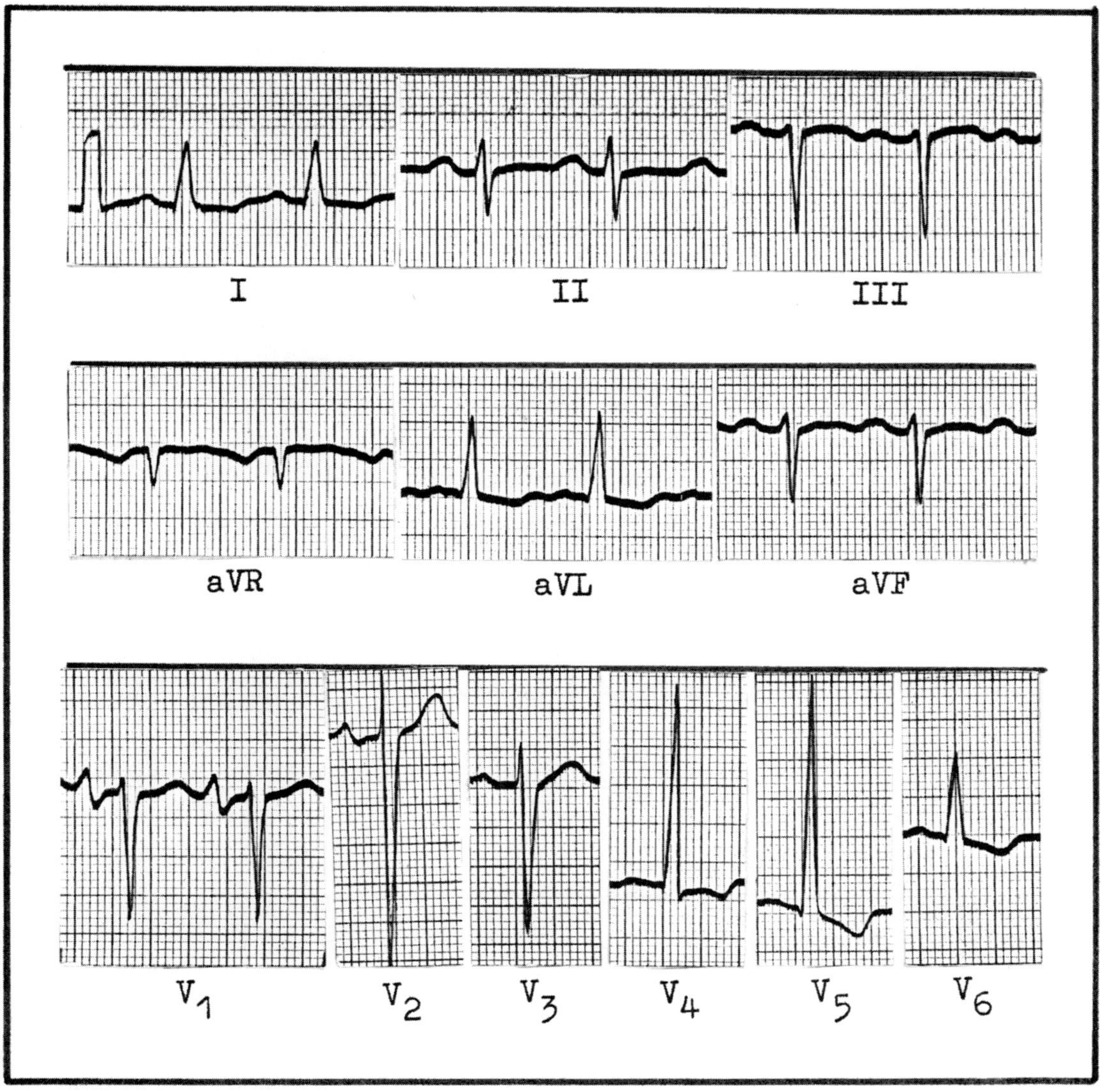

FIGURE 3–6. Left ventricular hypertrophy. Review all the criteria stepwise. Why are the voltage criteria so prominent in the chest leads compared with the standard and aV leads? See explanation in Figure 3–5*B*. Do the P waves help in elaborating the diagnosis? Review the subject of atrial enlargement in Chapter 2.

To this point we have not specifically discussed mean QRS vector magnitude criteria in the normal person. I have already imparted my feelings on the memorization of normal values. However, after covering the "magnitude" criteria for right and left ventricular hypertrophy, you already know the upper limits of the normal mean QRS vector magnitude. What are the lower limits of normal? Is Figure 3–7 a possible example of hypothyroidism or pericardial effusion (among the causes of low amplitude deflections)?

This electrocardiogram is from a normal adult patient. There is much overlap in the normal values, which is why I waited until you had studied the hypertrophy criteria for both ventricles. The lower limits of normal may be stated as follows:

Frontal plane (leads I, II, III, aVR, aVL and aVF) = *5 mm.*
Horizontal plane (leads V_1 to V_6) = *10 mm.*

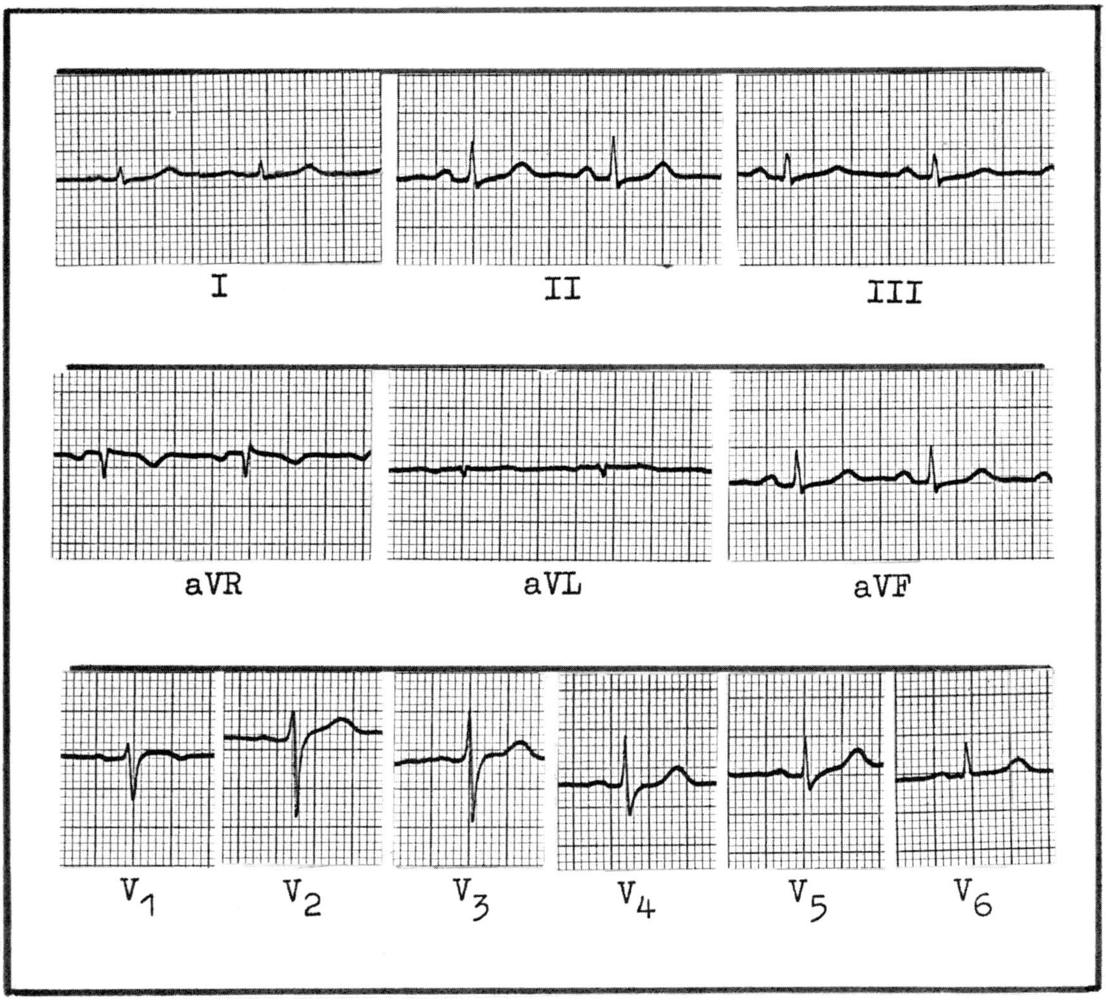

FIGURE 3–7. Normal. See discussion in text on lower limits of normal for mean QRS vector magnitude.

The importance of serial electrocardiograms must again be emphasized. It is vital to know if changes have occurred.

1. Were the deflections taller last year?
2. Is the heart enlarged on physical examination and on x-ray? And yet does it show small deflections on the electrocardiogram?

It is important for physicians to be able to read their own electrocardiograms and interpret them sequentially and in light of the patient's history. The electrocardiogram must never be viewed in isolation from the patient. No better evidence for this is seen than in Figure 3–8*A* and *B*.

Cassette Side 8

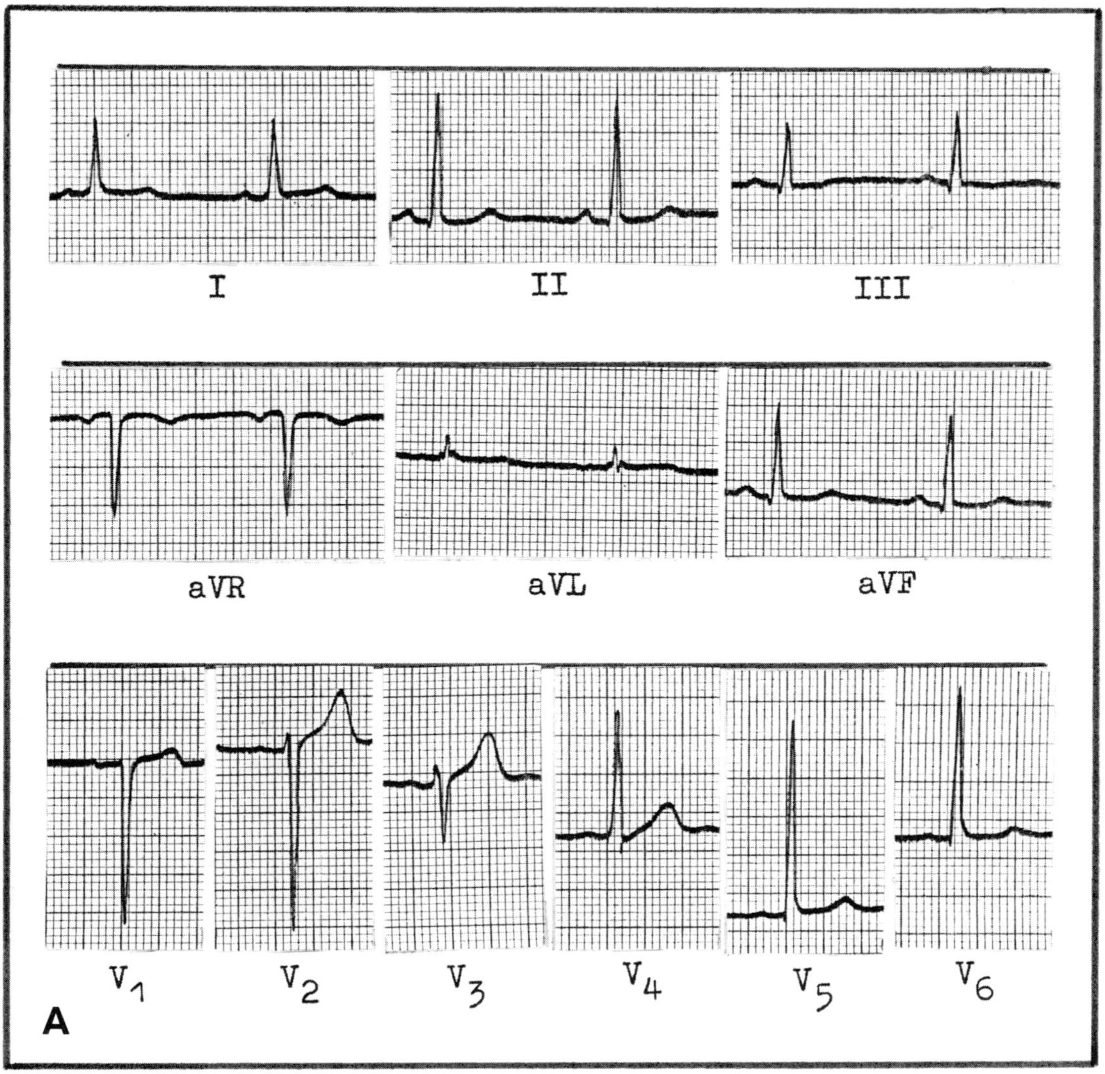

FIGURE 3–8. *A,* Left ventricular hypertrophy. This electrocardiogram and the next (Figure 3–8*B*) belong to the same adult patient. Note similarity in QRS deflection amplitude. Have there been any changes in the repolarization phase (S–T segments and T waves)?

In the interim the patient underwent the repair of a defective aortic value and the insertion of a prosthesis. The patient felt "better" but the electrocardiogram was "worse." Again, emphasis must be placed on

1. Sequential study of the electrocardiogram.
2. Patient history.

The electrocardiogram must never be dissociated from the patient; it must never be read in a vacuum. You do not tell the patient that he is "worse" because his electrocardiogram is "deteriorating."

It may well be that the repolarization abnormalities in Figure 3–8*B* reflect a worsened condition of the myocardium following the surgical procedure. The patient may be feeling better because of the positive *net* effect of heart valve replacement versus continued myocardial deterioration.

Illustration continued on following page.

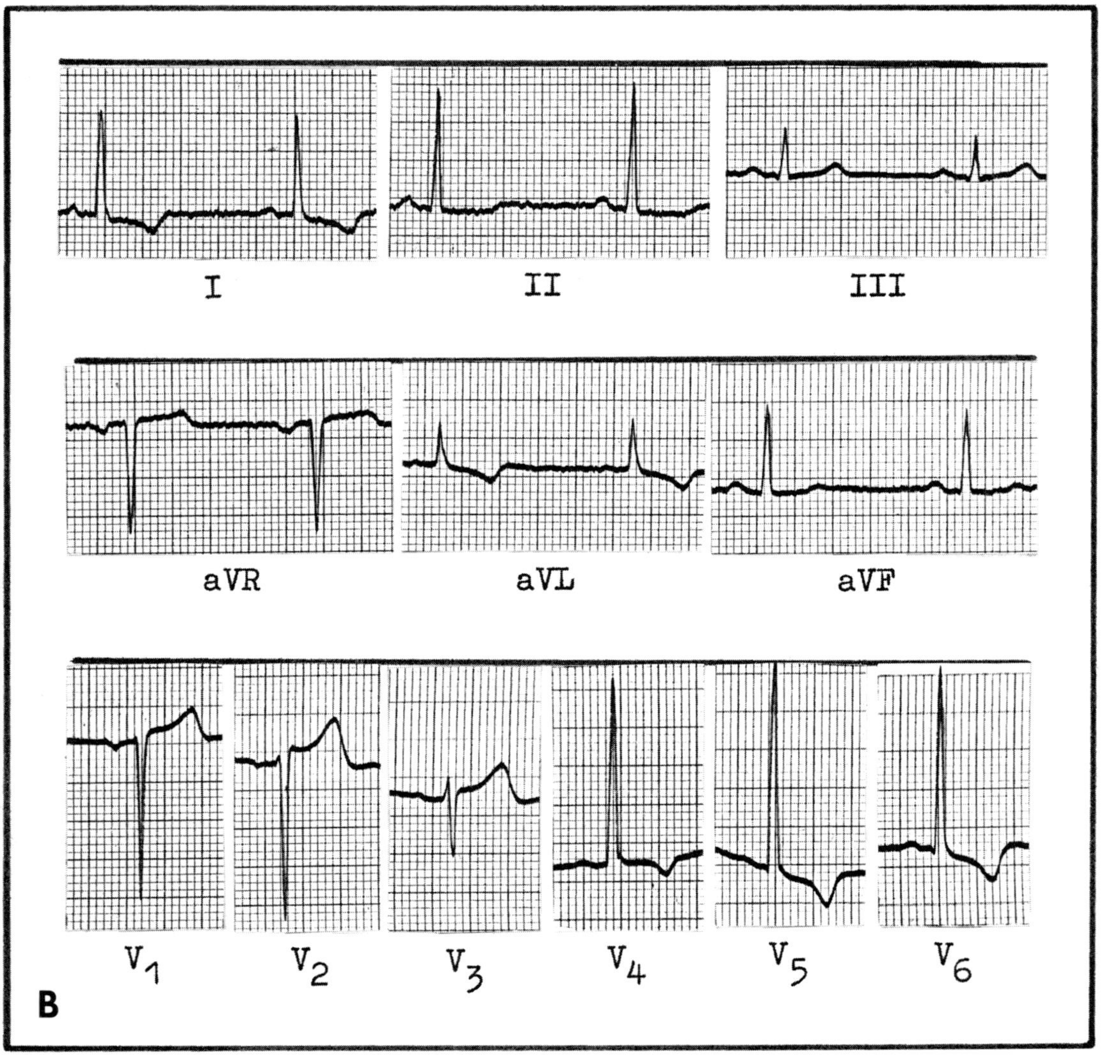

FIGURE 3-8 *Continued.* *B,* Left ventricular hypertrophy. See discussion in legend to Figure 3–8*A*.

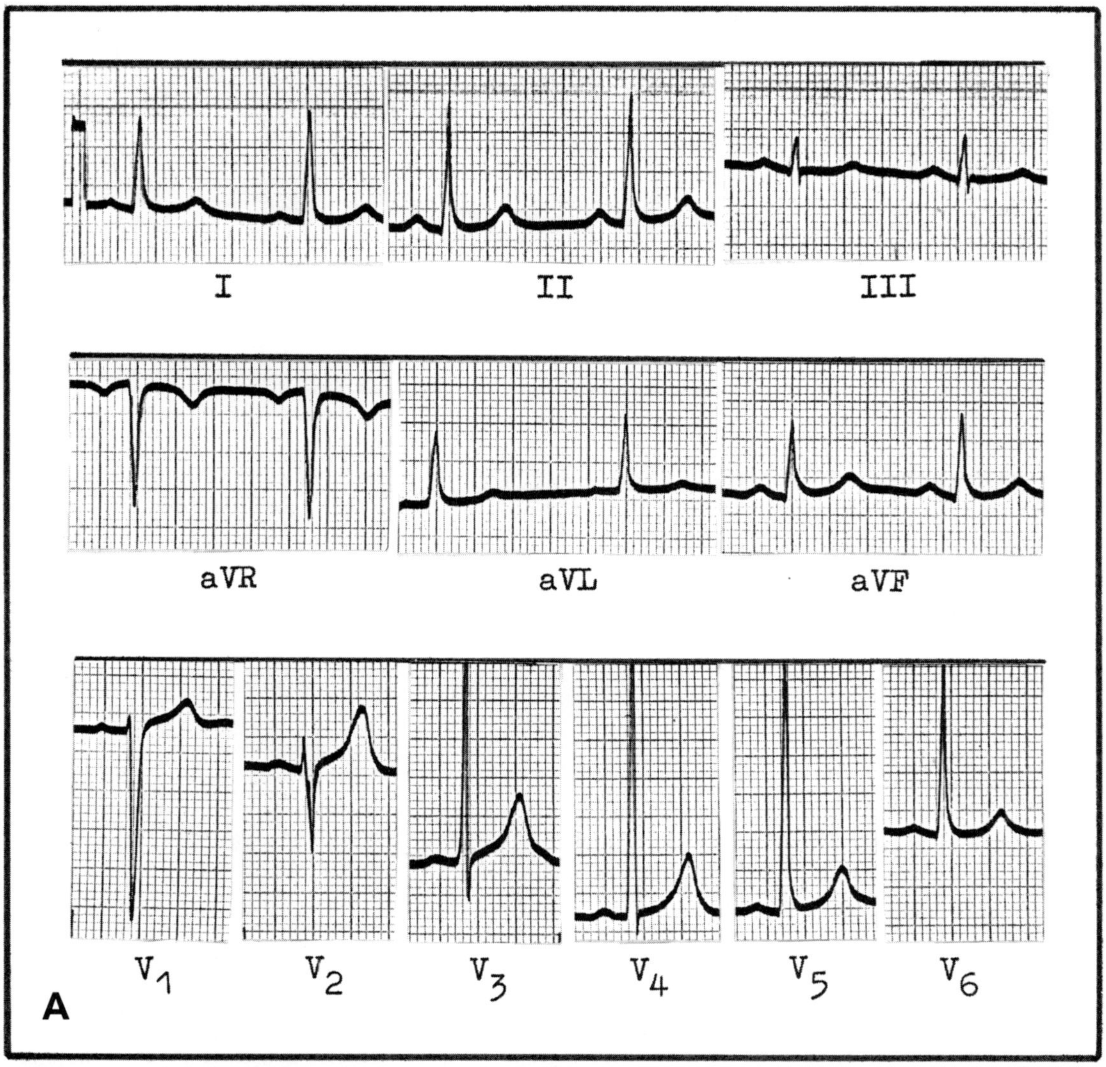

FIGURE 3-9. *A,* Left ventricular hypertrophy. The patient is a young adult with marked hypertension. Do you have the "magnitude" criteria for left ventricular hypertrophy? Do you have the repolarization abnormalities? If the patient were a 16 year old, thin high school student with a small heart on physical examination and on chest X-ray, would you read this electrocardiogram as diagnostic of left ventricular hypertrophy? A mean QRS vector of increased magnitude, in the horizontal plane, without repolarization abnormalities, is not rare among thin and young normal patients. For this reason, when studying the "magnitude" criteria for hypertrophy of the ventricle, it was stated that the patient should be over the age of 30 and of normal height and weight.

Illustration continued on following page.

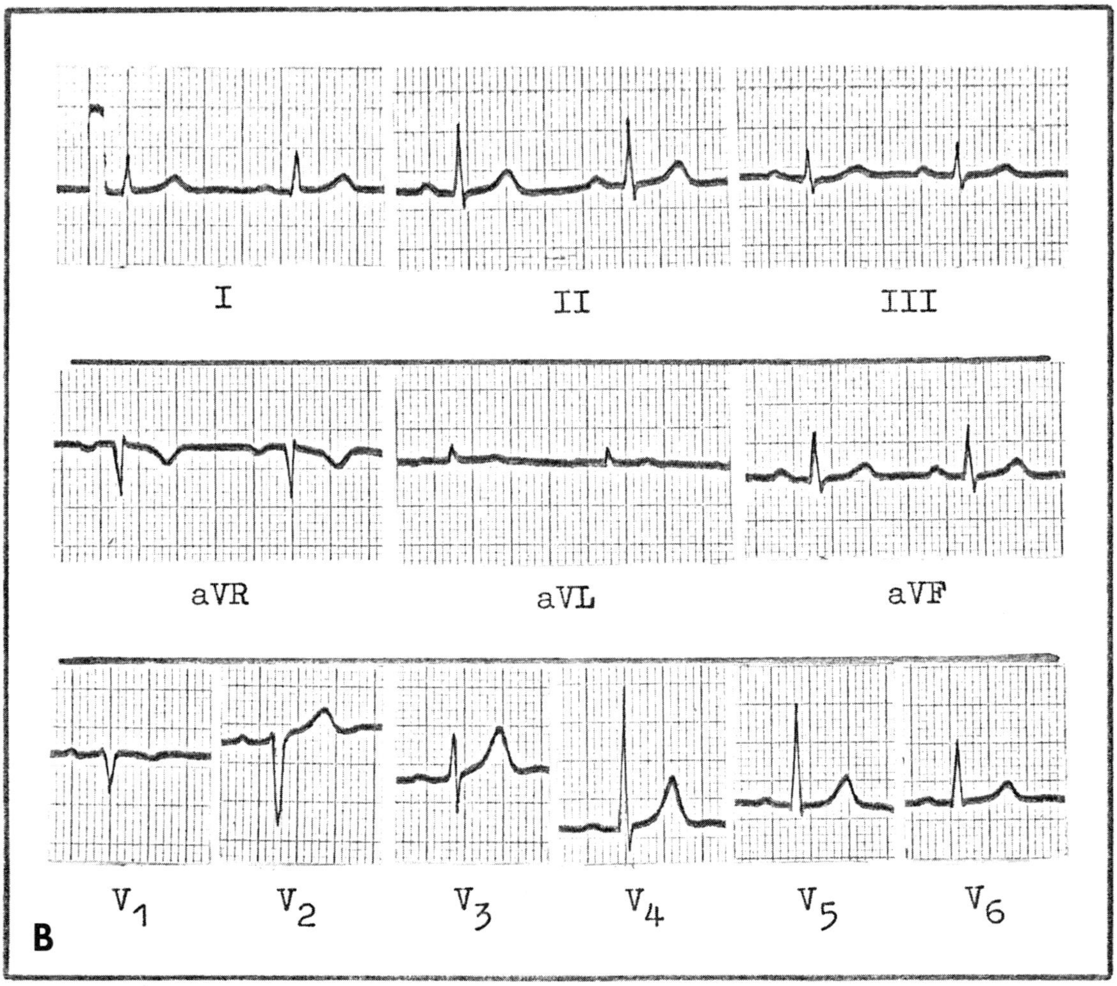

FIGURE 3-9 *Continued.* *B,* Normal. Compare with the hypertrophied left ventricle in Figure 3-9*A.* In the following figures, part *B* will be a normal electrocardiogram to help reinforce the criteria of left ventricular hypertrophy.

REVIEW ELECTROCARDIOGRAMS

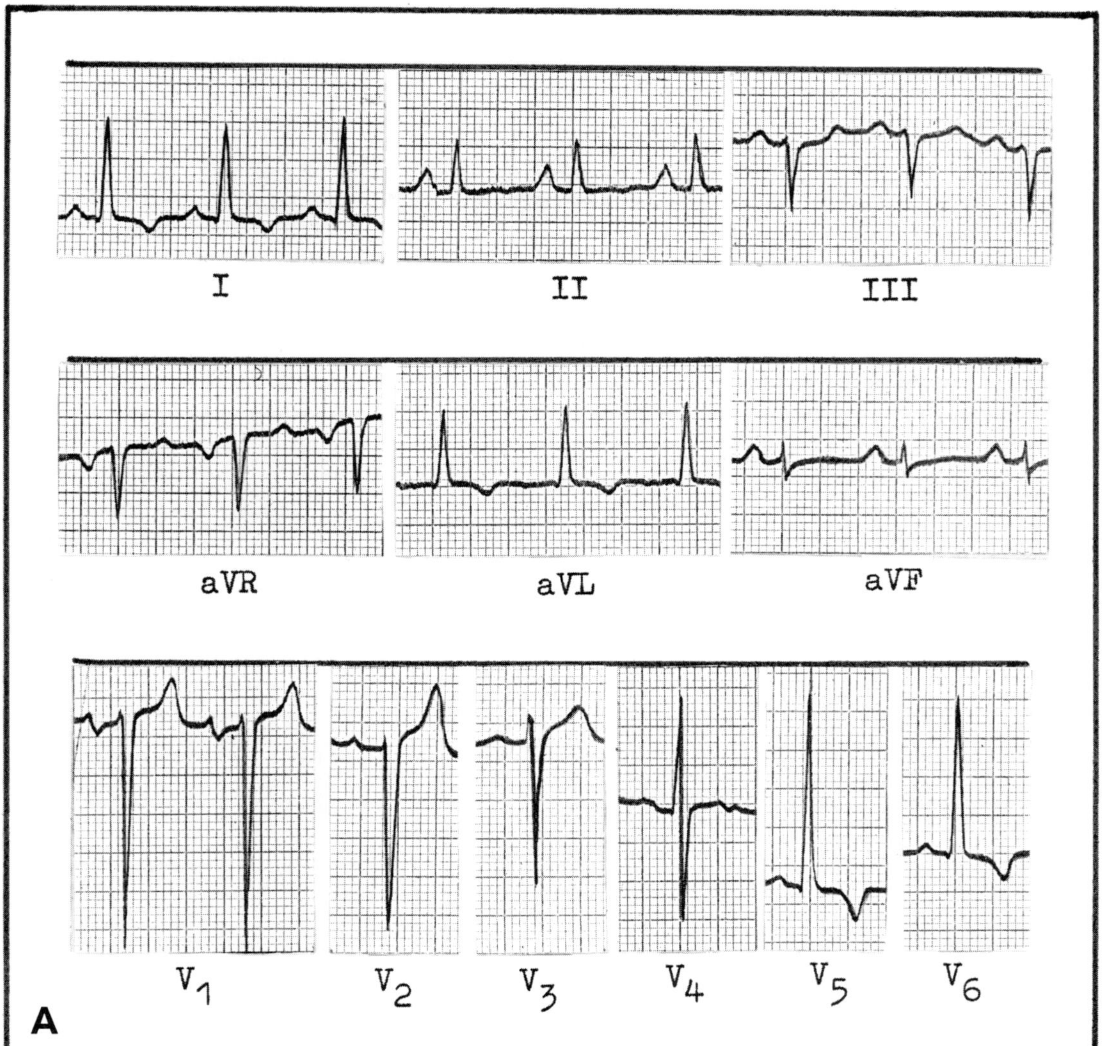

FIGURE 3-10. *A,* Hypertrophied left ventricle in an elderly patient. Review the criteria and the reasons for normal sized QRS complexes in the frontal plane (leads I, II, III, aVR, aVL and aVF) and large QRS complexes in the horizontal plane (leads V_1 to V_6). See explanation in legend to Figure 3-5*B*.

Illustration continued on following page.

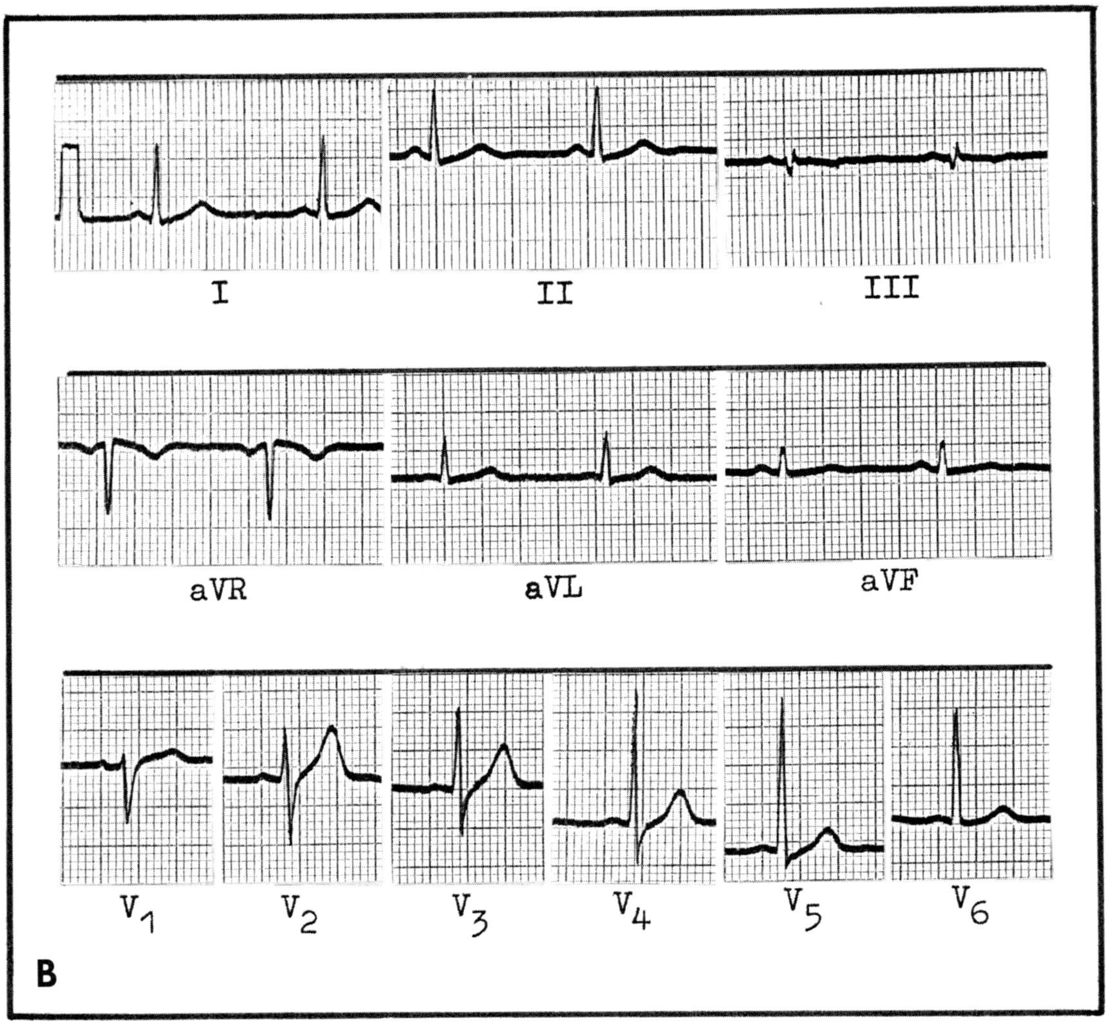

FIGURE 3–10 *Continued.* *B,* Normal. Compare with the hypertrophied left ventricle in Figure 3–10*A.*

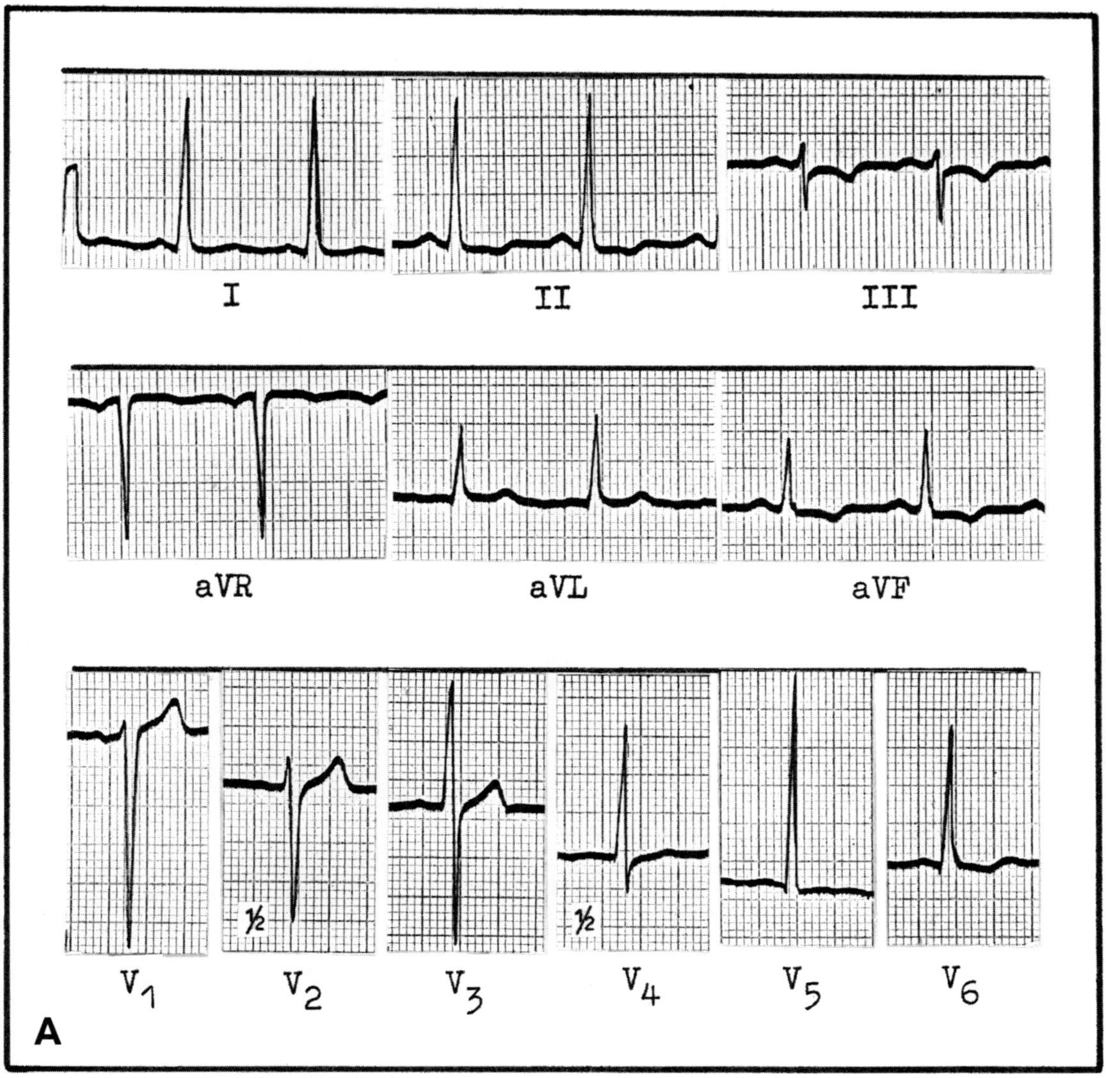

FIGURE 3–11. *A,* Left ventricular hypertrophy in an elderly adult with aortic valve disease. The chest leads V_2 and V_4 are on half standard (remember, therefore, to double the size of these leads in making your "magnitude" calculations).

Illustration continued on following page.

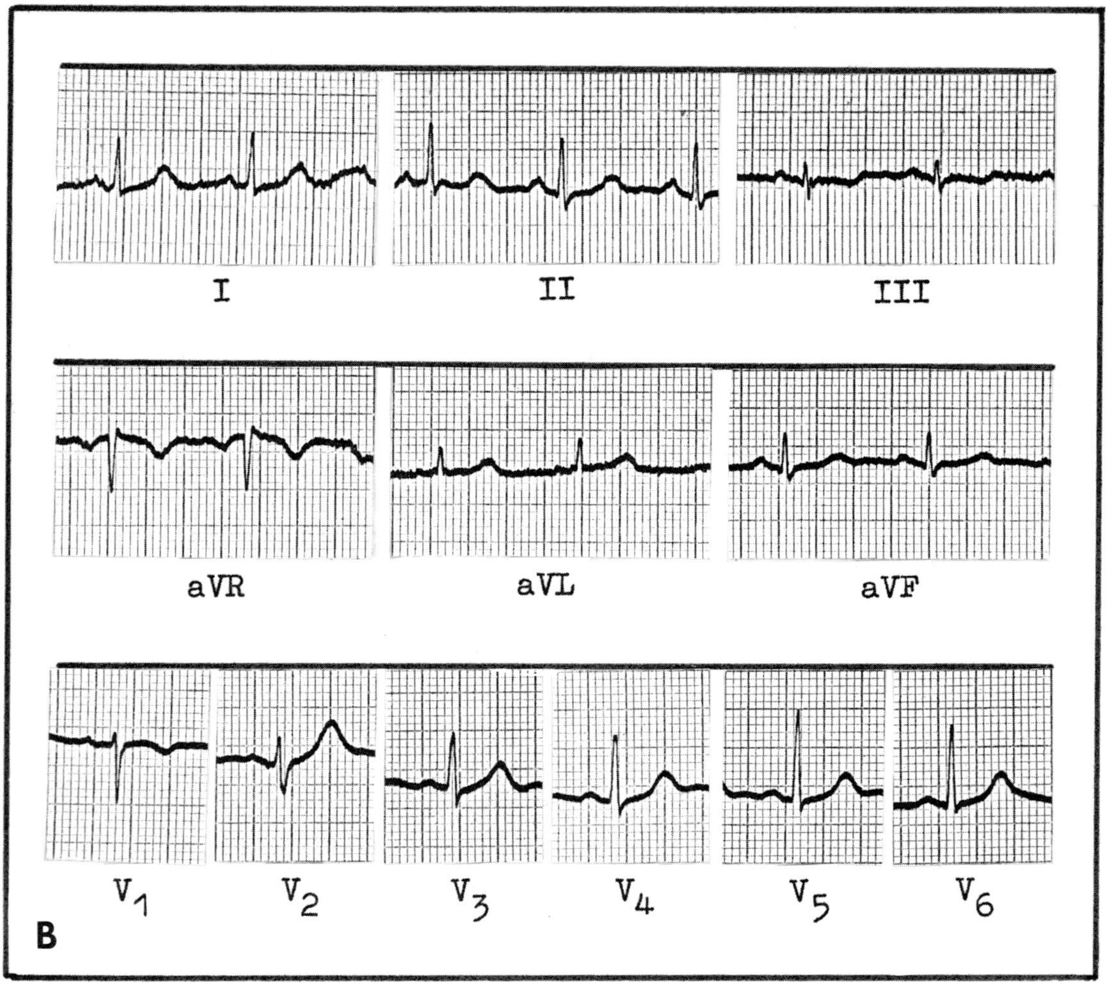

FIGURE 3-11 *Continued.* *B*, Normal. Compare with the hypertrophied left ventricle in Figure 3-11*A*.

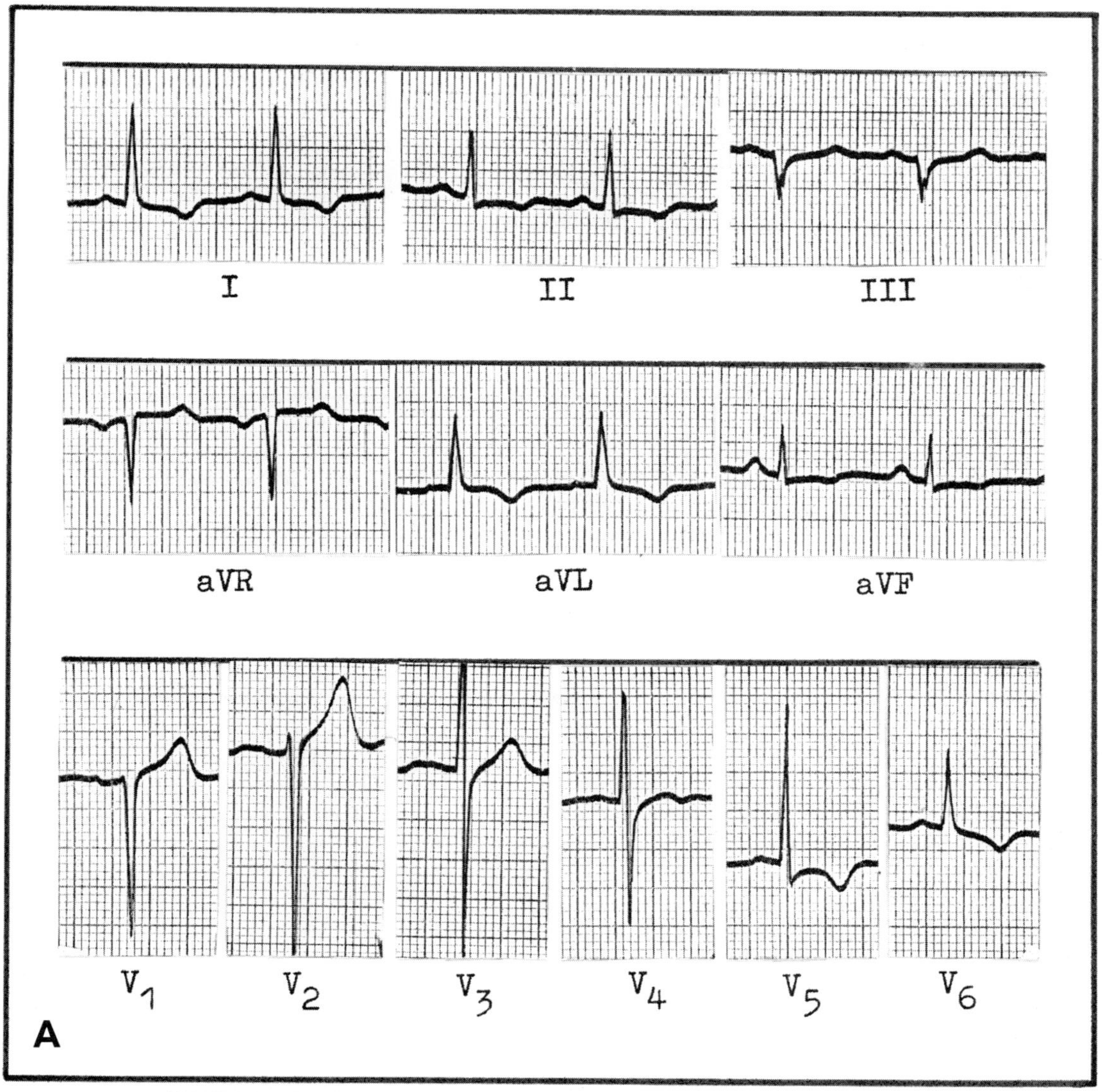

FIGURE 3–12. *A,* Hypertrophied left ventricle in an adult with hypertension.

Illustration continued on following page.

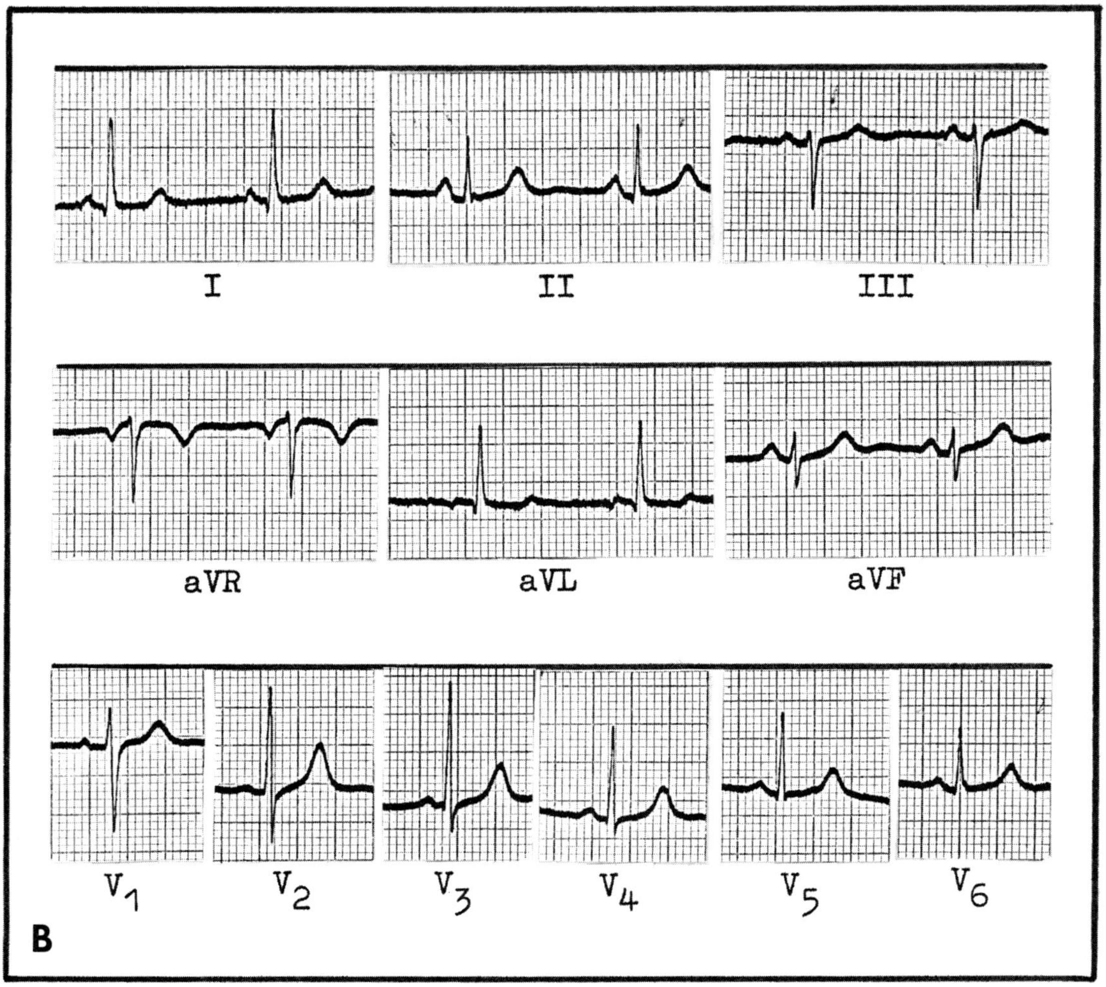

FIGURE 3–12 *Continued.* *B,* Normal. Compare with the hypertrophied left ventricle in Figure 3–12*A.*

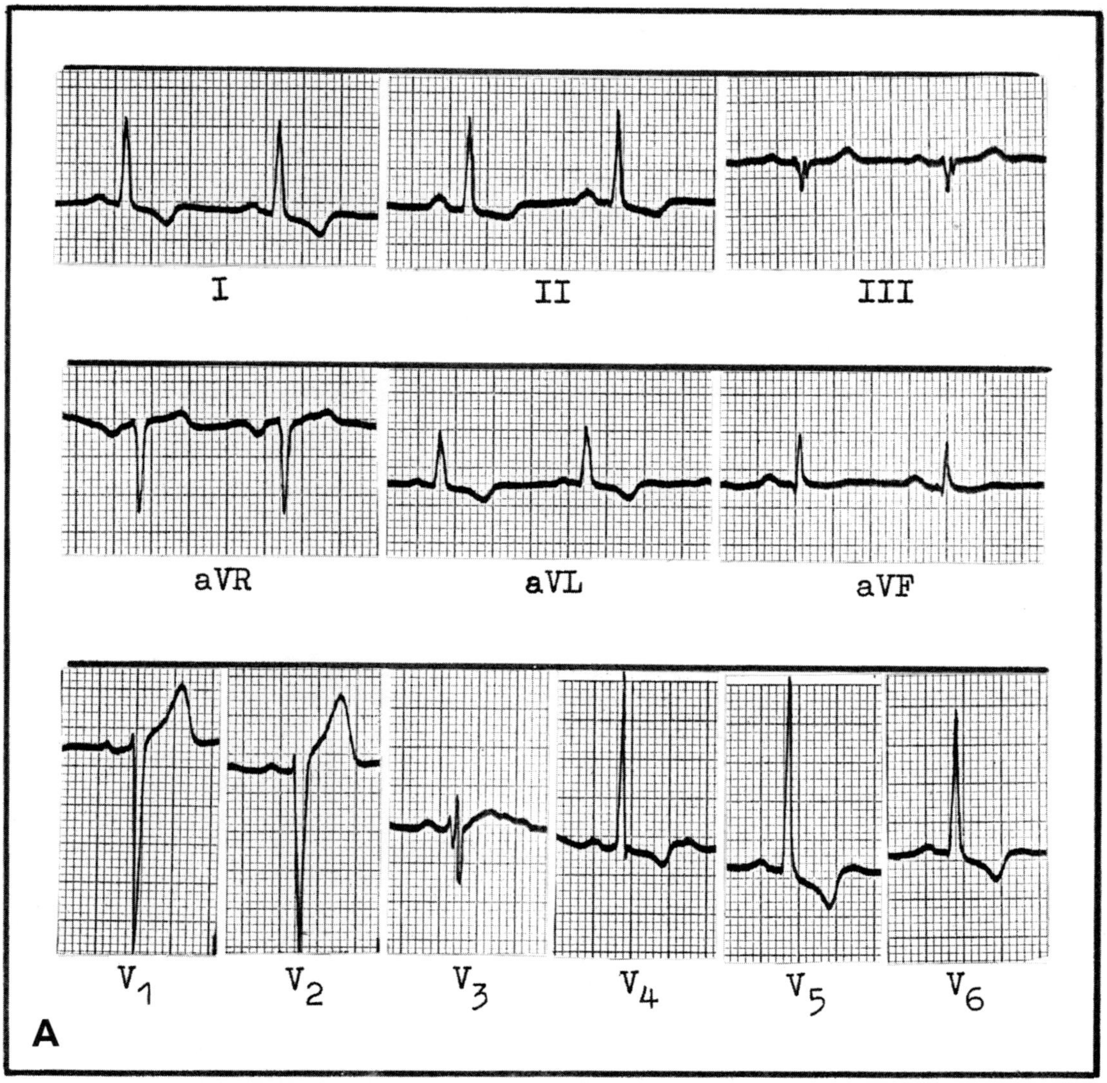

FIGURE 3–13. *A,* Hypertrophied left ventricle in an adult with aortic valve disease.

Illustration continued on following page.

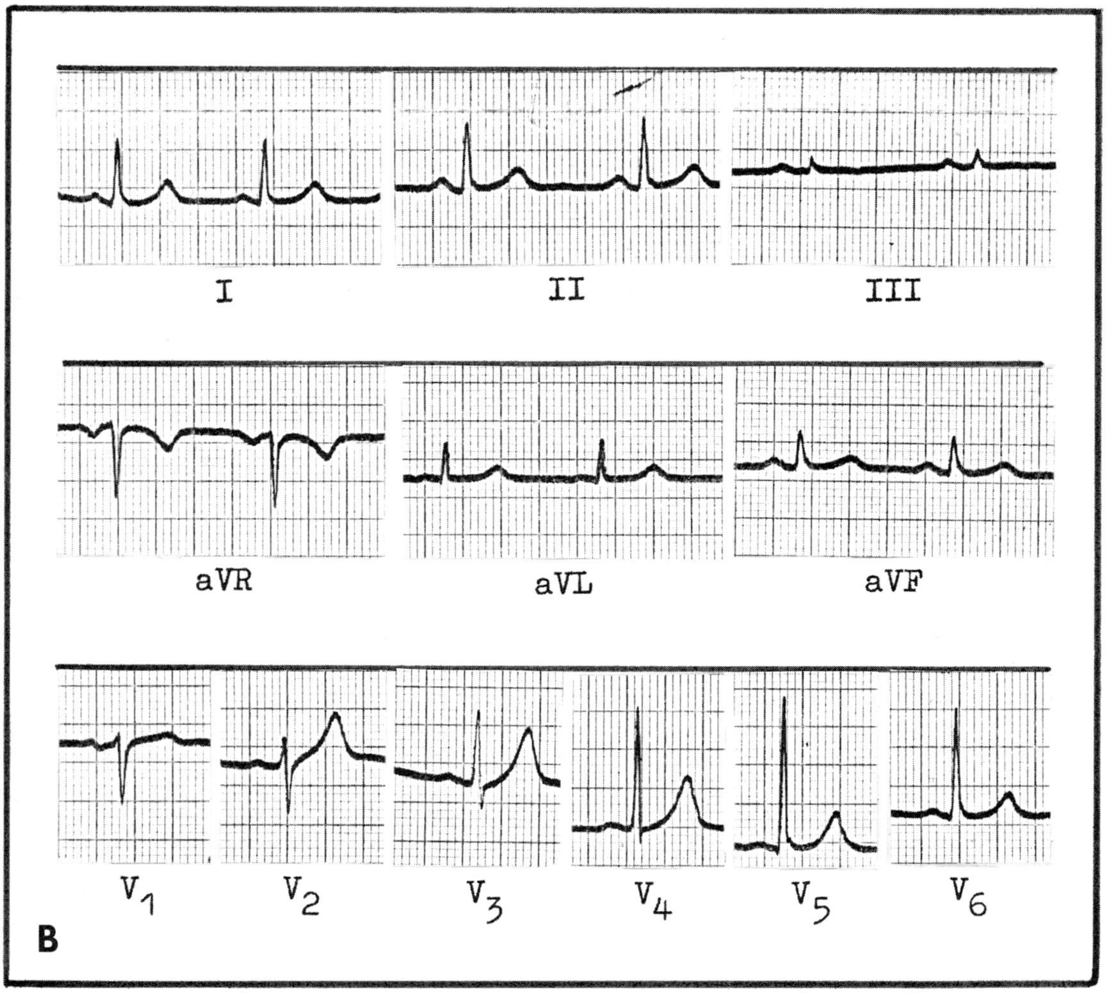

FIGURE 3–13 *Continued.* *B,* Normal. Compare with the hypertrophied left ventricle in Figure 3–13*A*.

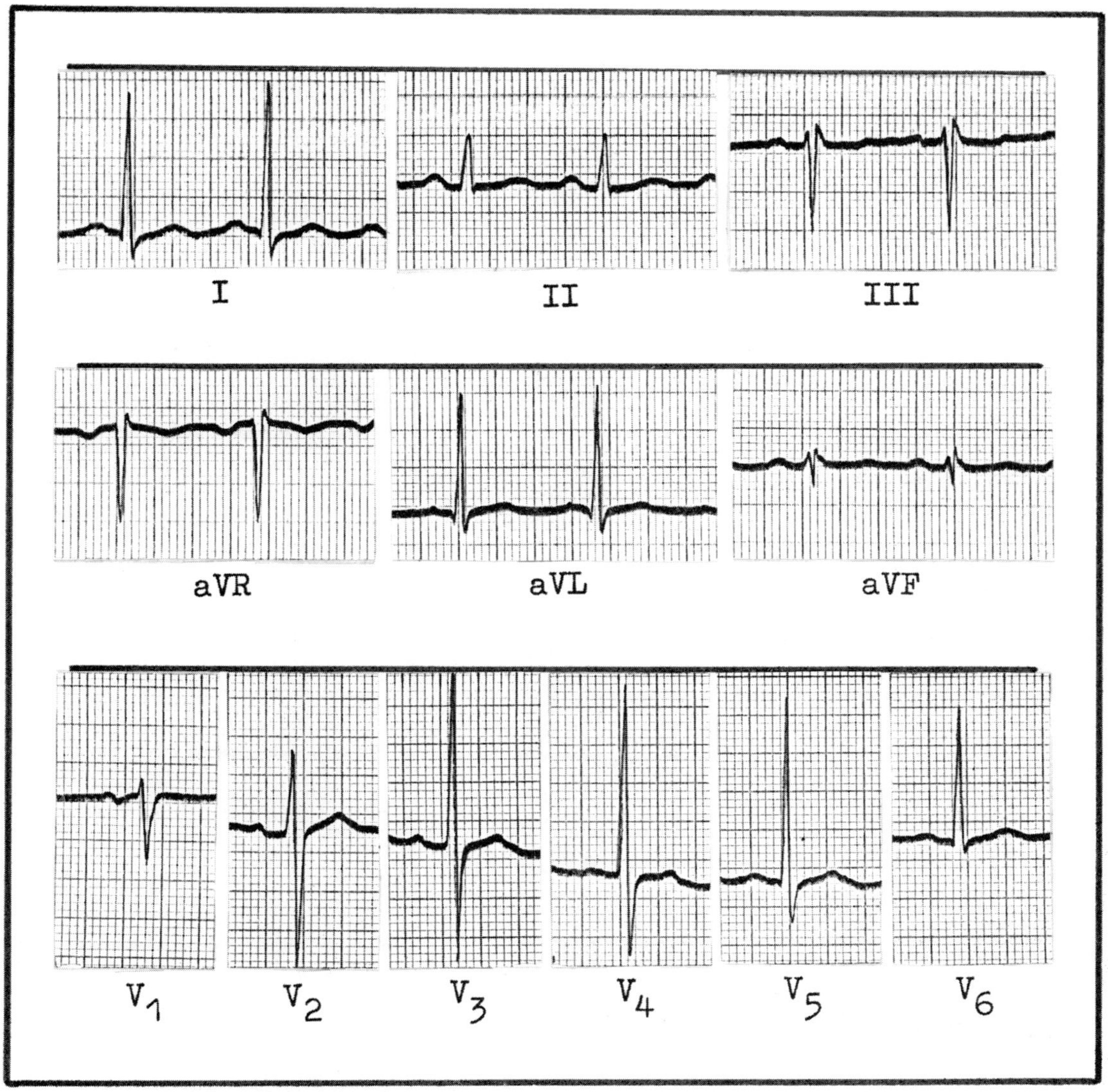

FIGURE 3–14. Left ventricular hypertrophy in an adult with hypertension.

The following electrocardiograms, Figures 3–15 to 3–24, are from adults with known left ventricular hypertrophy. Although there may be other associated abnormalities, the emphasis for the present should be on left ventricular hypertrophy. Review all the criteria for left ventricular hypertrophy with each of these electrocardiograms. Use the following order:

A. Increase in magnitude of the mean QRS vector.
B. Repolarization abnormalities (S–T and T wave abnormalities).
C. Left axis deviation. Review the discussion at the beginning of this chapter.

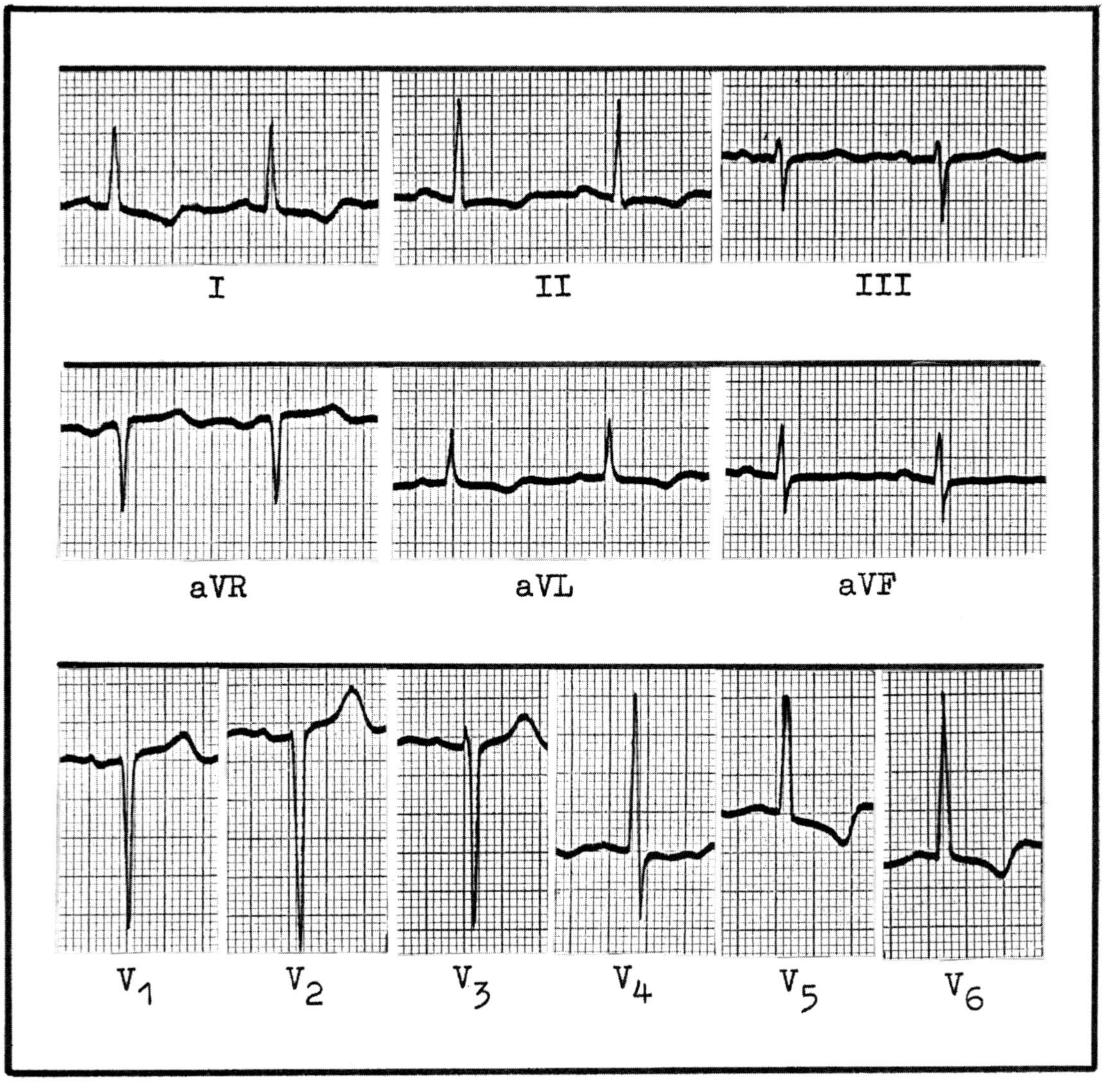

FIGURE 3–15. Left ventricular hypertrophy.

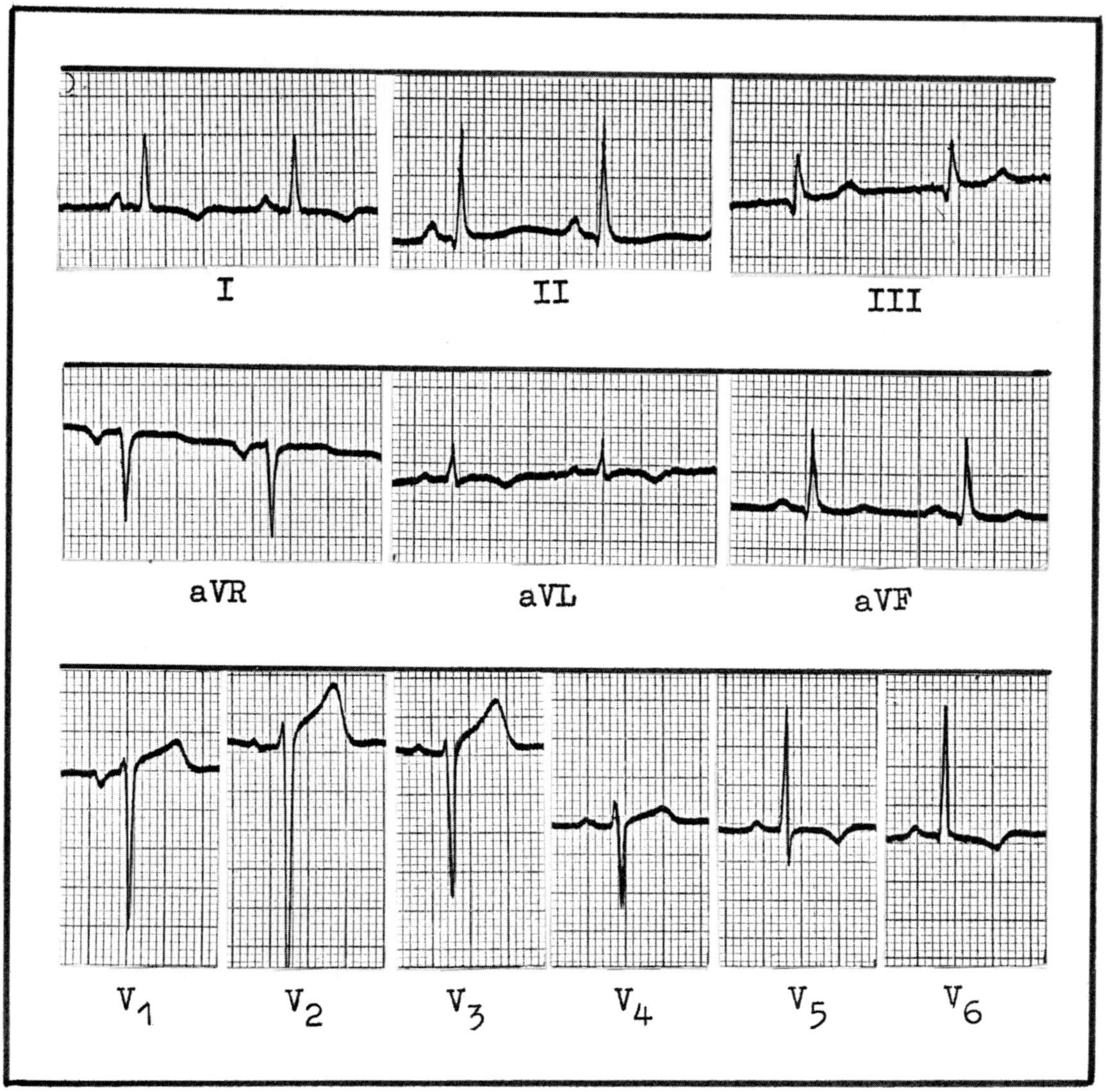

FIGURE 3–16. Left ventricular hypertrophy.

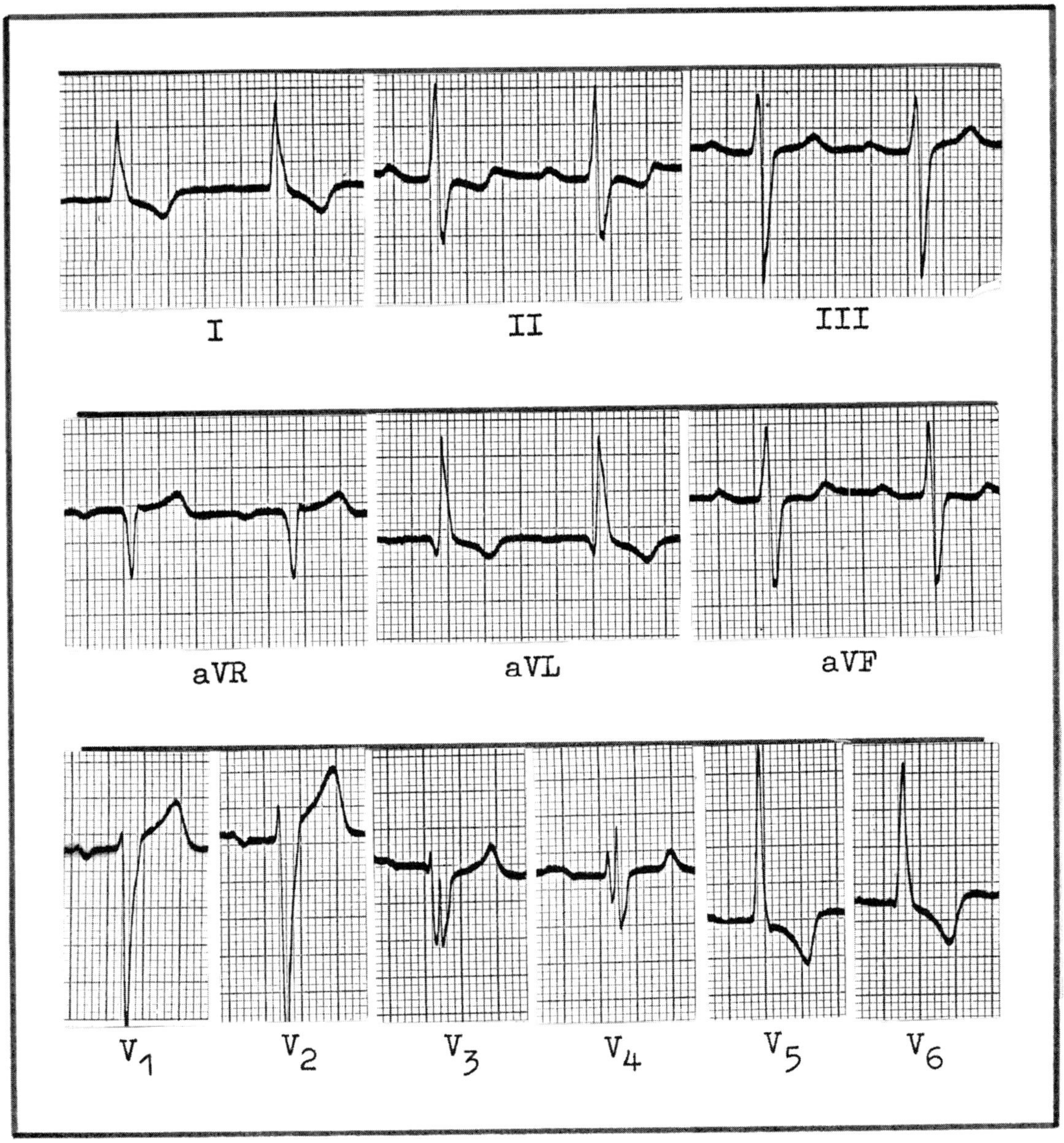

FIGURE 3–17. Left ventricular hypertrophy.

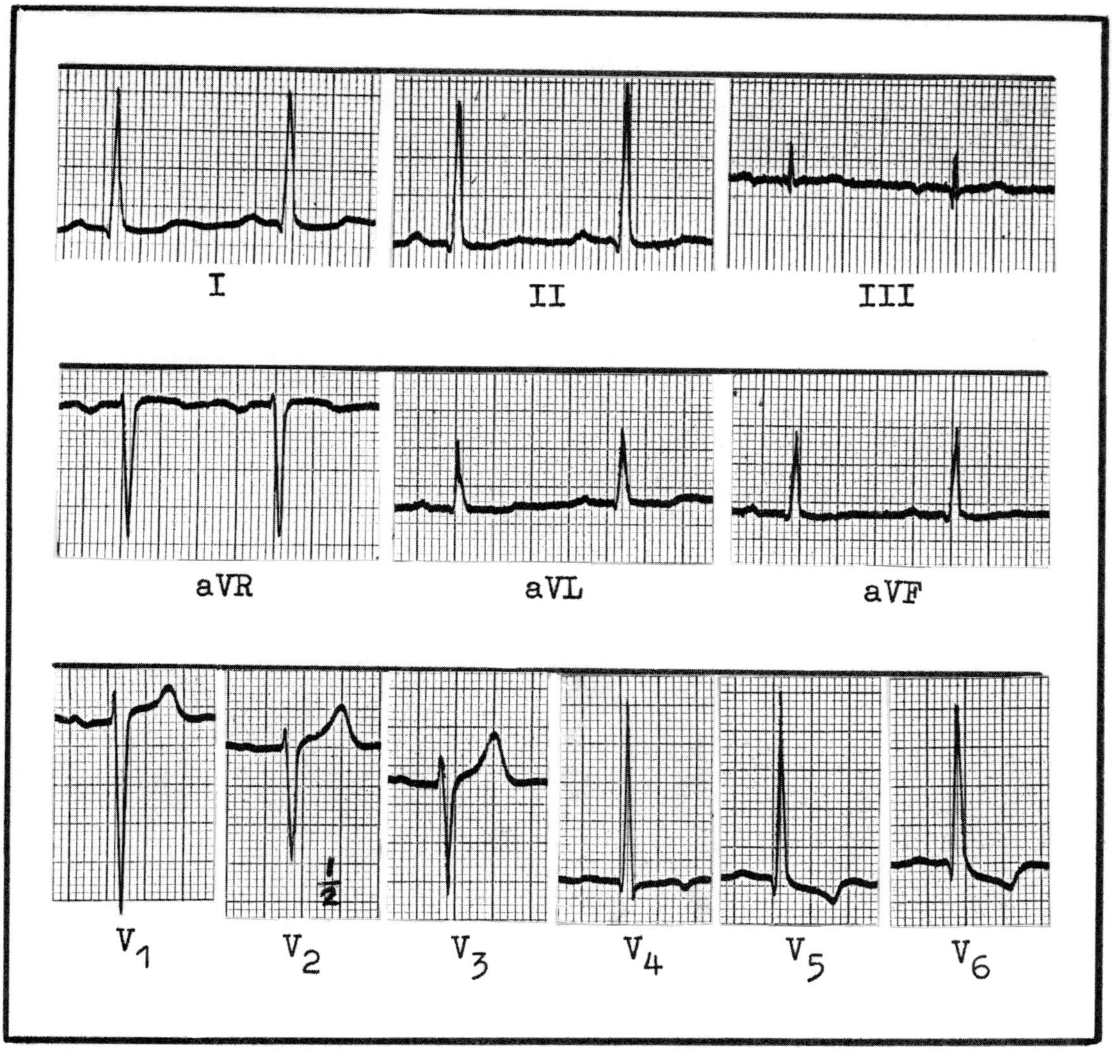

FIGURE 3–18. Left ventricular hypertrophy.

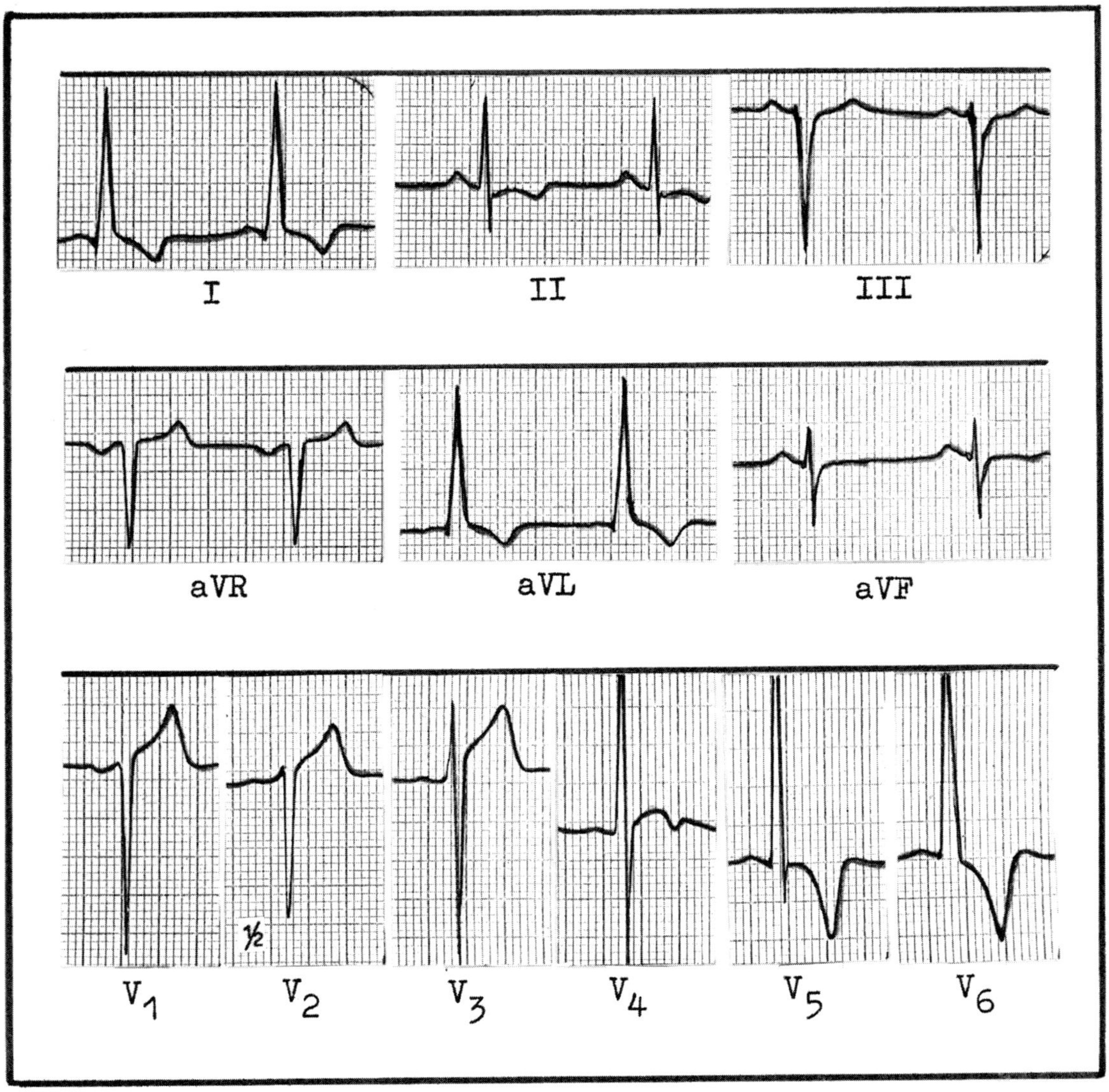

FIGURE 3–19. Left ventricular hypertrophy.

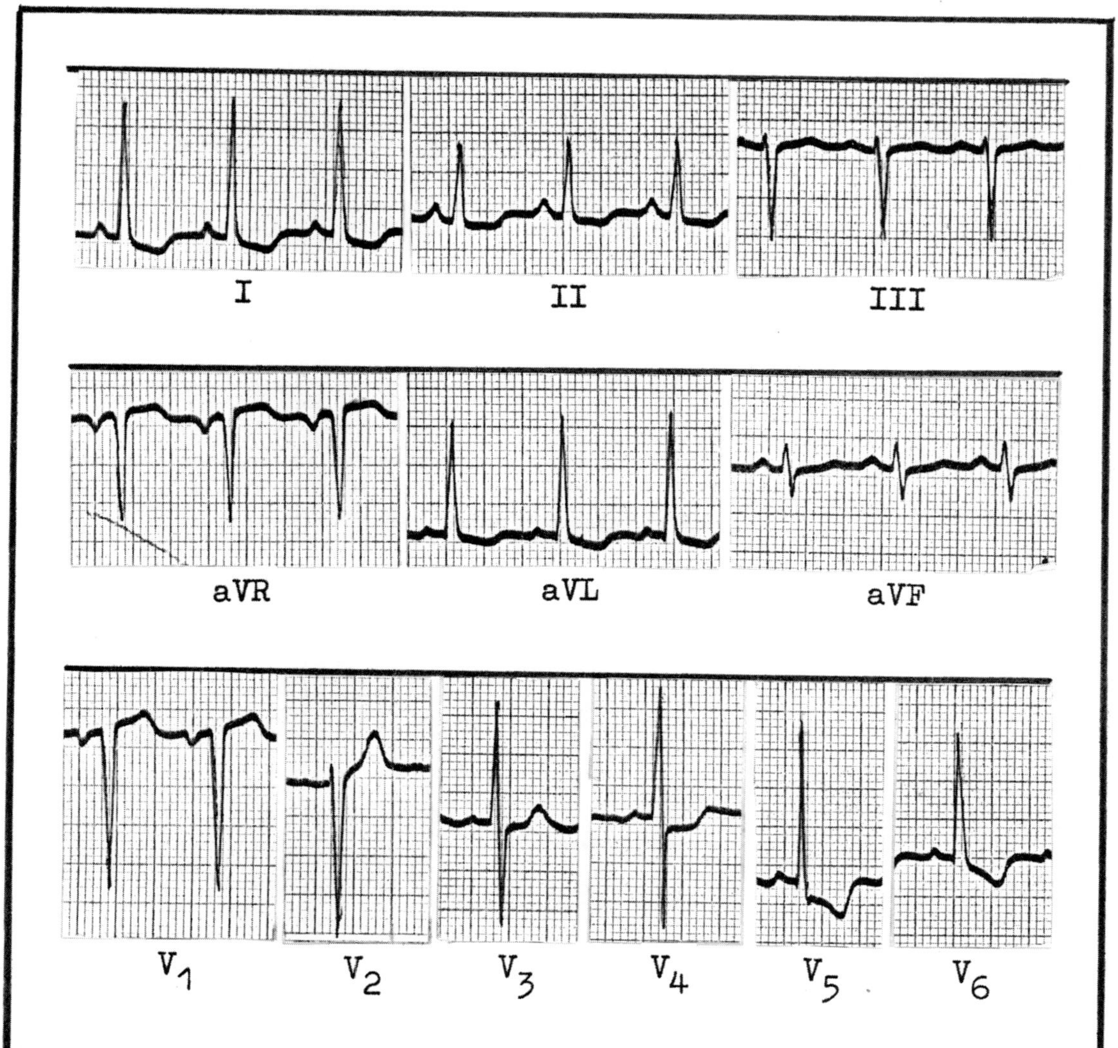

FIGURE 3–20. Left ventricular hypertrophy.

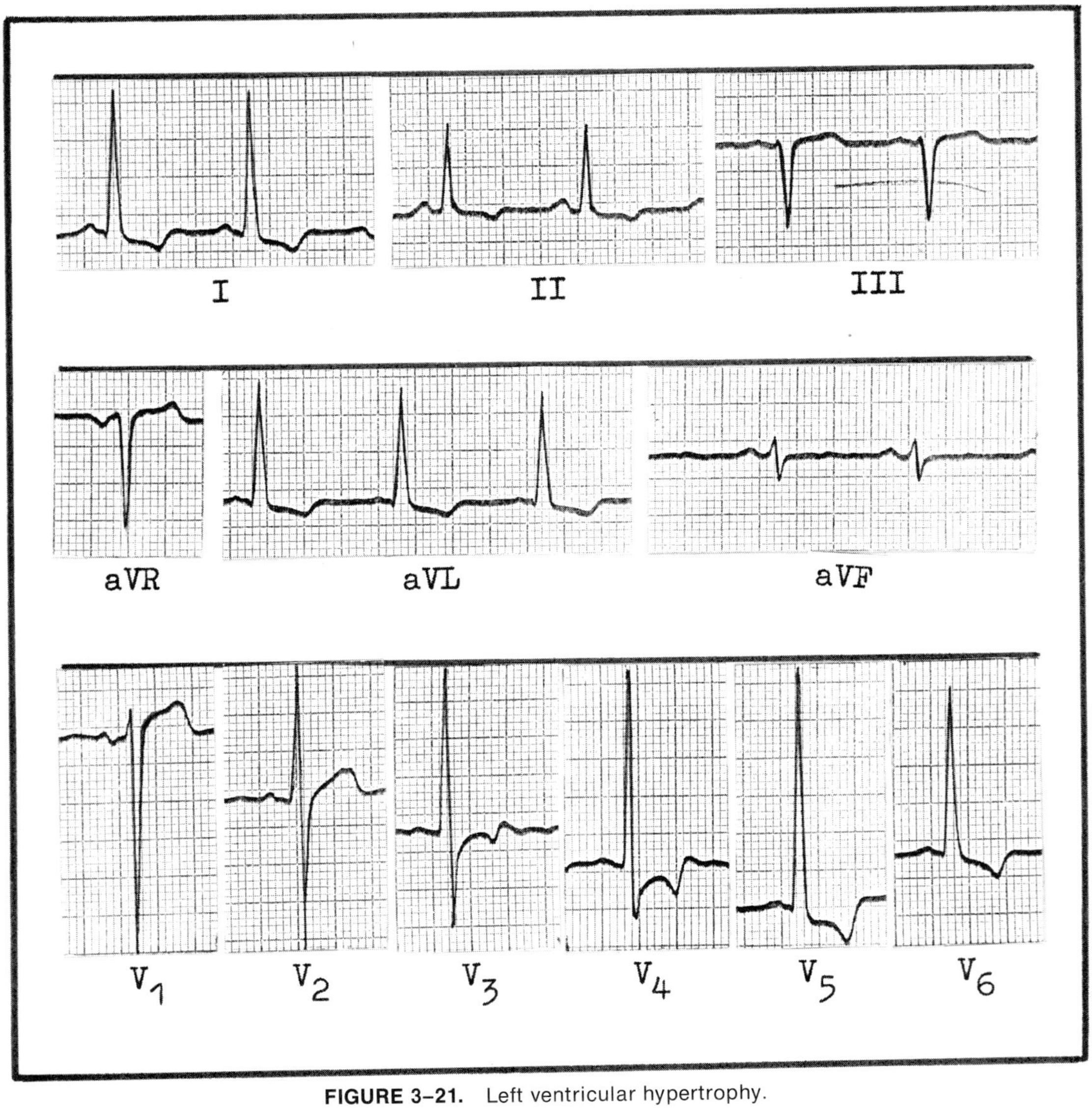

FIGURE 3–21. Left ventricular hypertrophy.

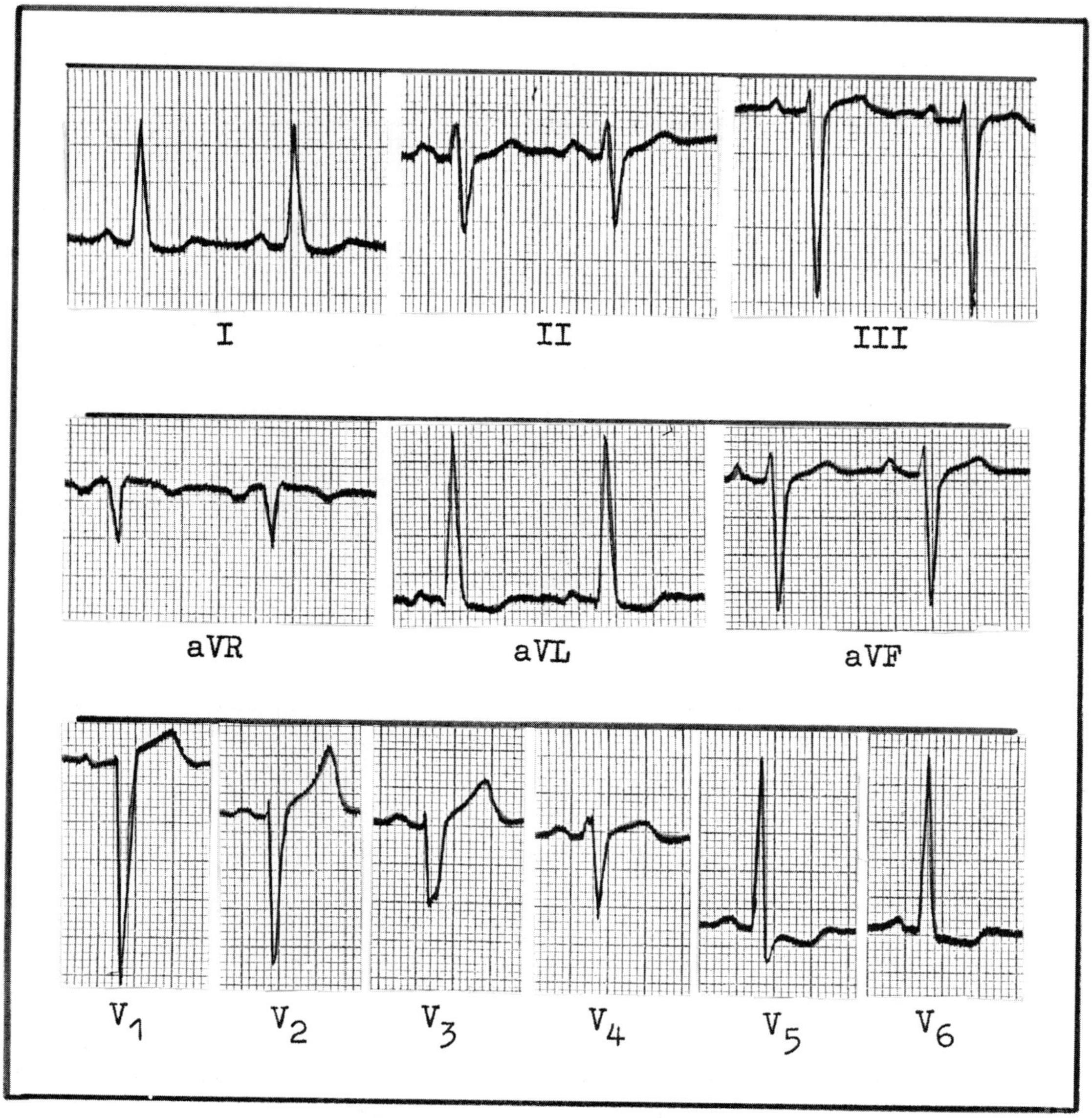

FIGURE 3–22. Left ventricular hypertrophy.

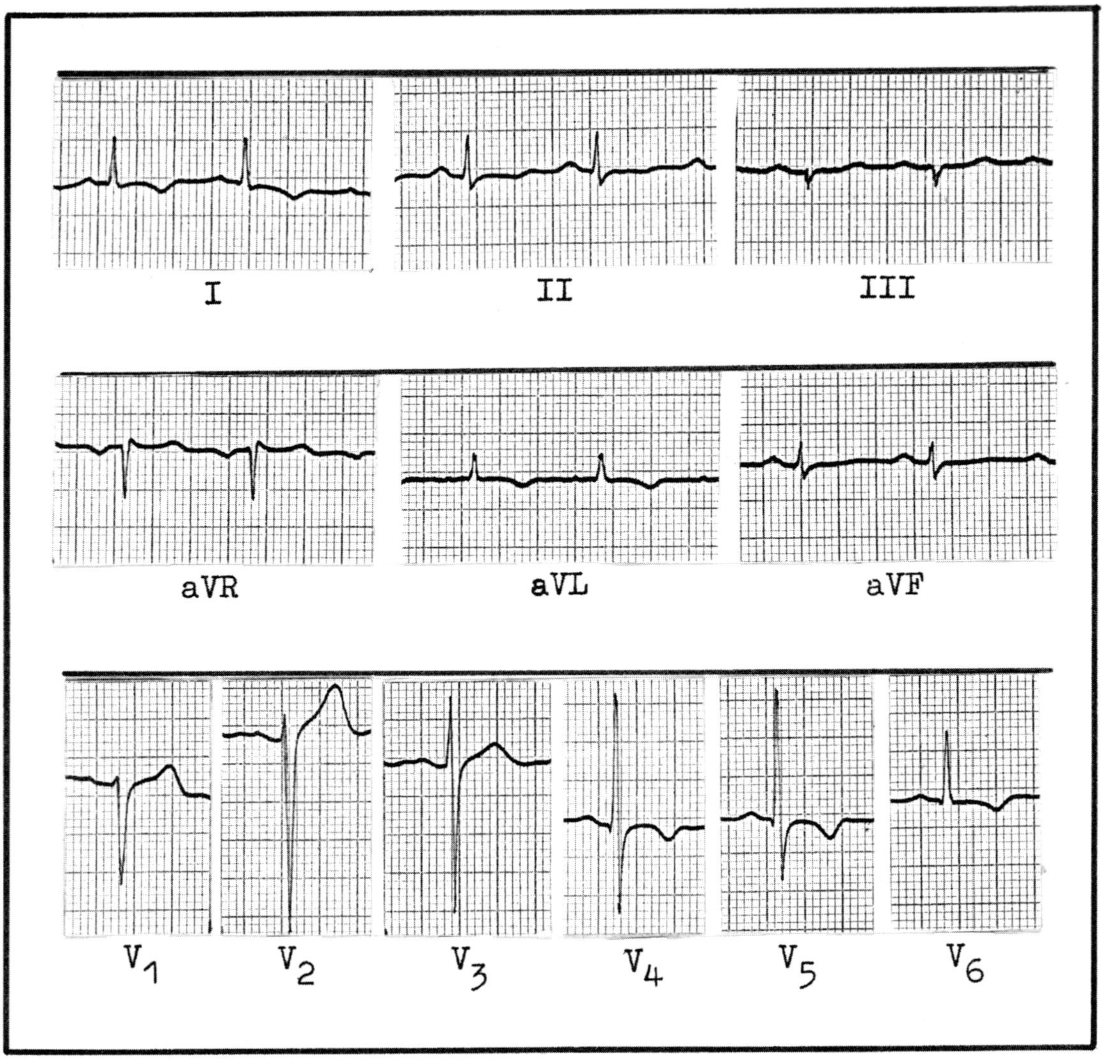

FIGURE 3–23. Left ventricular hypertrophy.

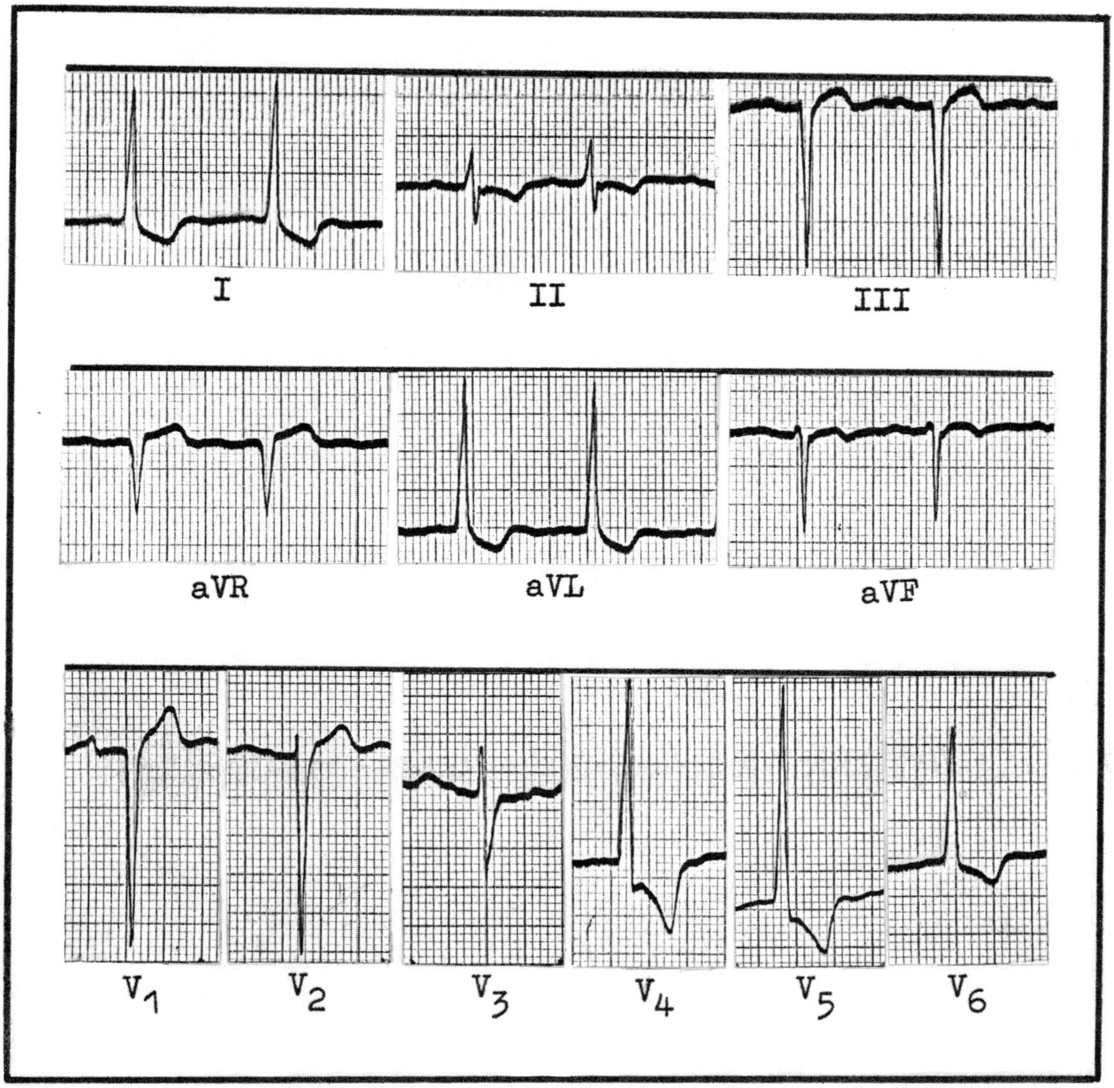

FIGURE 3–24. Left ventricular hypertrophy.

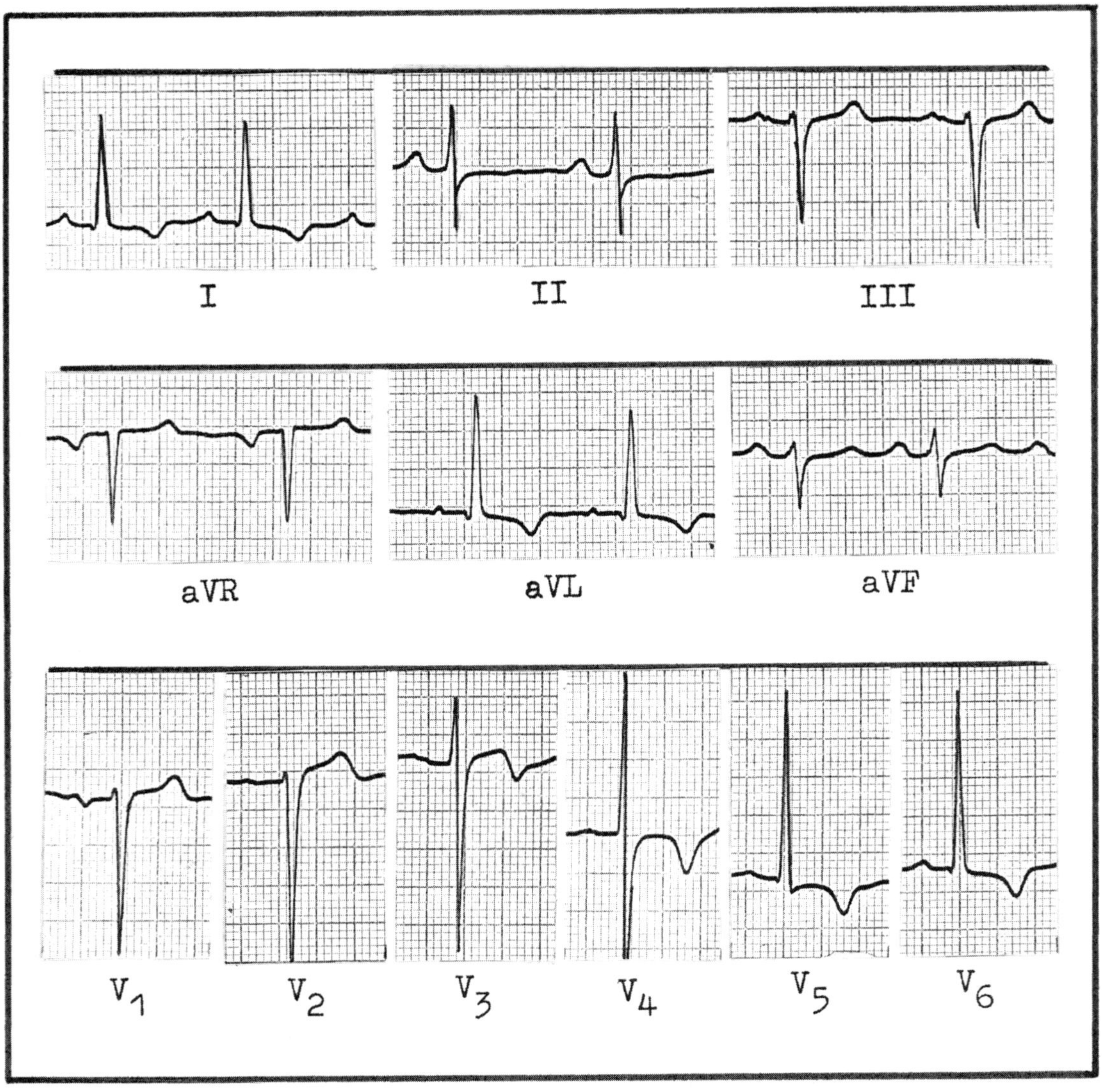

FIGURE 3–25. Left ventricular hypertrophy.

4

REPOLARIZATION (S–T SEGMENT AND T WAVE) ALTERATIONS

Cassette Side 9

NORMAL REPOLARIZATION

This chapter emphasizes the lability of the ventricular repolarization phase (S–T segment and T wave). Reference is also made to atrial repolarization alterations. Repolarization, in contrast to depolarization, is the energy consuming phase, and as such, is much more prone to abnormality under a variety of circumstances. On the other hand, not every S–T segment or T wave which appears abnormal at first is actually abnormal. This will be seen in the "early repolarization" and "juvenile" patterns.

There are many causes of repolarization alterations, some of which are beyond the scope of this course, and more will be described in the future. Prototypes, therefore, are used. For example, digitalis serves as the prototype of drug-induced repolarization changes. The repolarization abnormalities resulting from myocardial infarction have been bypassed, except for an example of ventricular aneurysm, since Chapter 5 is entirely devoted to myocardial infarction. It should be remembered, however, that myocardial infarction is responsible for significant repolarization abnormalities.

The legend to each figure includes textual material to enhance continuity from figure to figure and from subject to subject.

Although this entire chapter is devoted to the repolarization phase of the electrocardiographic cycle, you have actually been studying repolarization in each of the previous three chapters, as noted in Figure 4–1. In the study of the normal electrocardiogram (Chapter 1) you learned that repolarization is studied in its relationship to depolarization (QRS–T angle). In the study of the hypertrophied right

The Normal

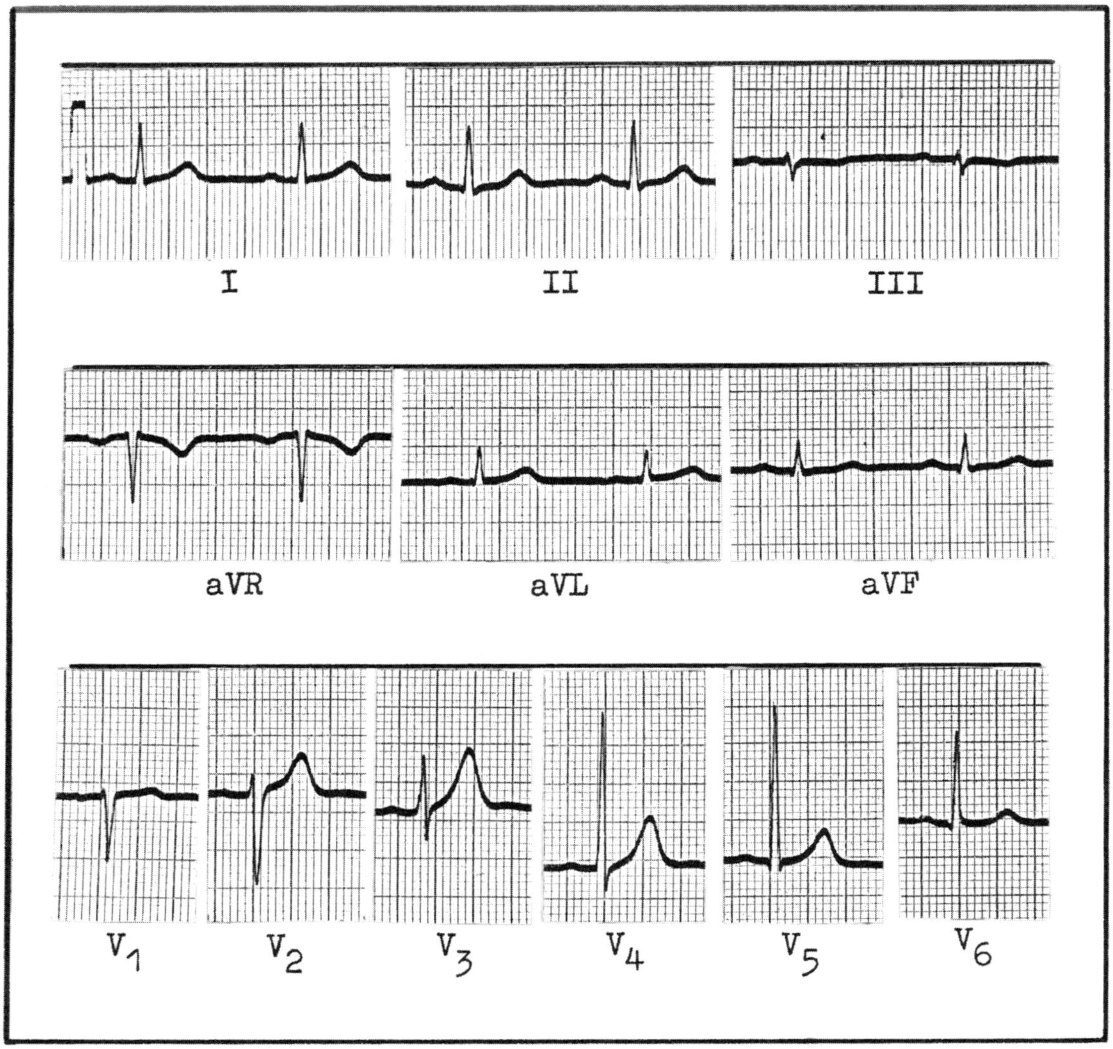

FIGURE 4–1. Normal electrocardiogram. Depolarization of the ventricles is represented by the QRS complexes; repolarization is represented by the S–T segments and T waves. You have actually been studying repolarization throughout the course. In the study of the normal electrocardiogram (Chapter 1) you learned that repolarization is studied in its relationship to depolarization (QRS–T angle). In the study of the hypertrophied right ventricle (Chapter 2) and the hypertrophied left ventricle (Chapter 3) you noted abnormalities in repolarization, abnormal QRS–T angles and abnormal S–T segments.

Review all the features which make this electrocardiogram a normal one. Describe the P waves, P–R intervals, rhythm, QRS complexes, QRS–T angles and S–T segments.

ventricle (Chapter 2) and the hypertrophied left ventricle (Chapter 3) you noted abnormalities in repolarization as criteria for the actual diagnosis (abnormal QRS–T angles and S–T segments). An understanding of Figures 4–1, 4–2 and 4–3 means that Chapters 1, 2 and 3 have been mastered.

Repolarization Abnormalities in Right Ventricular Hypertrophy

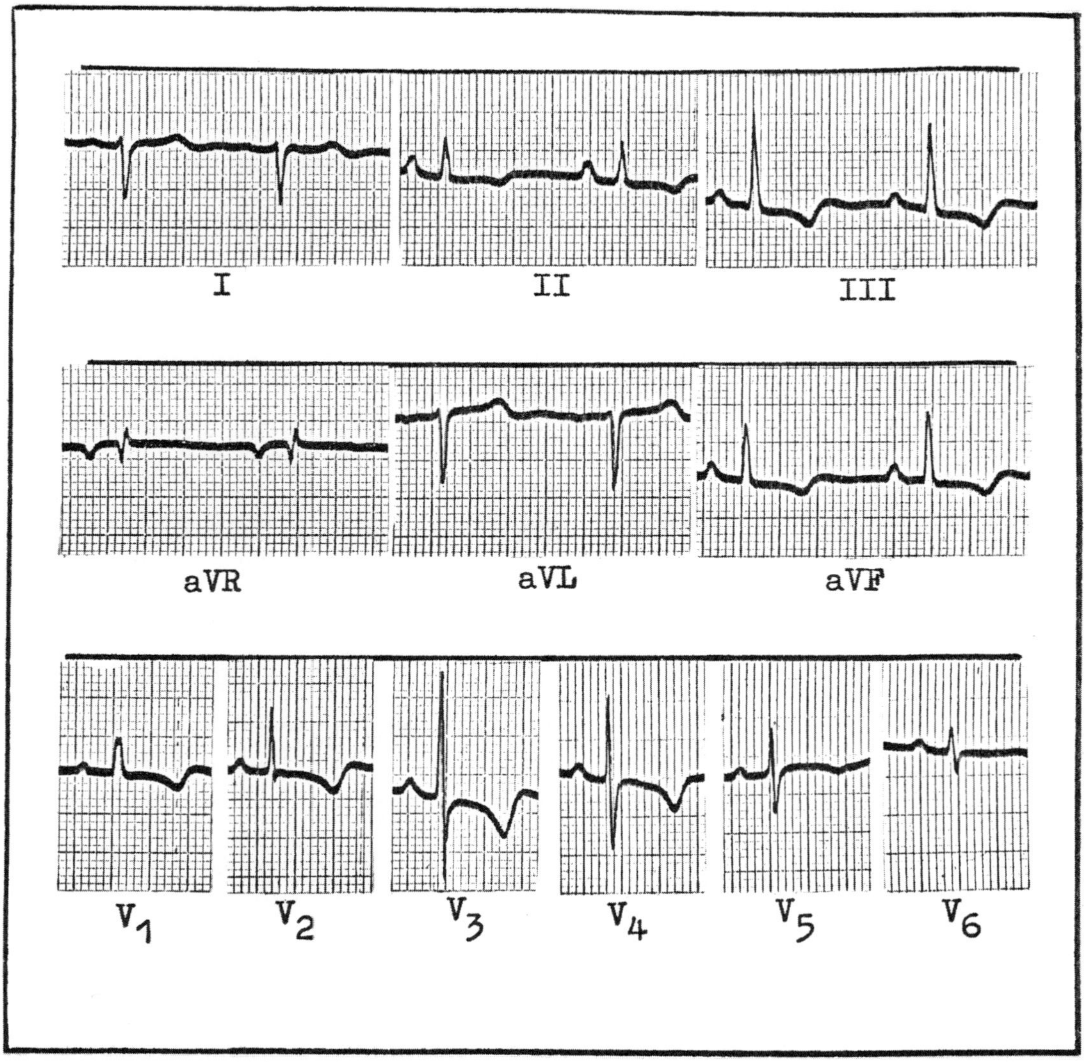

FIGURE 4–2. Right ventricular hypertrophy. Calculate the mean QRS vector and QRS–T angle, and describe the S–T segments. Compare with the normal electrocardiogram in Figure 4–1. If you have any questions as to the characteristics of the hypertrophied right ventricle, especially repolarization abnormalities, take the time to review Chapter 2.

Repolarization Abnormalities in Left Ventricular Hypertrophy

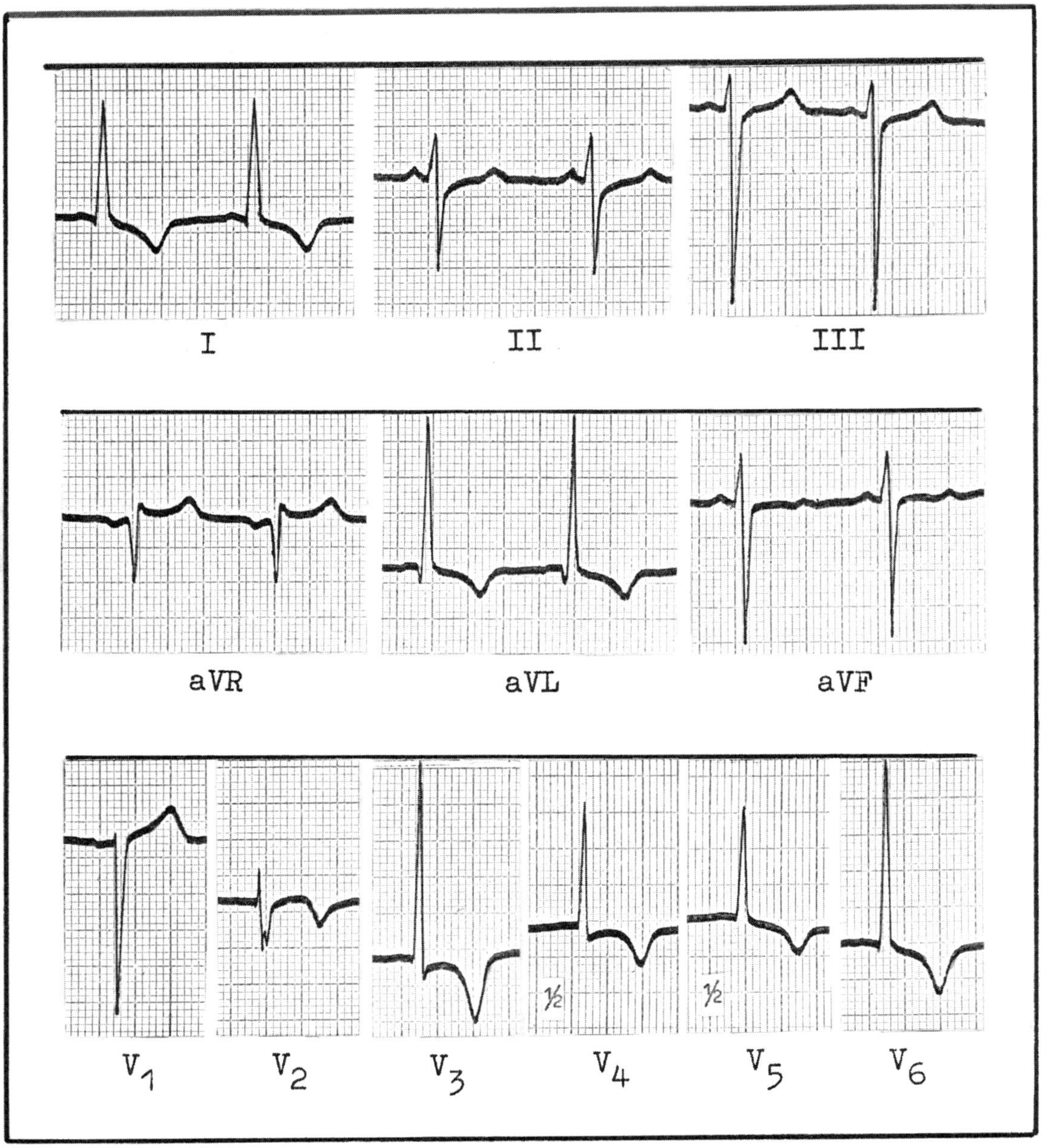

FIGURE 4–3. Left ventricular hypertrophy. Review all the criteria for left ventricular hypertrophy (Chapter 3), especially the repolarization abnormalities.

If you have reviewed and understand the electrocardiograms in Figures 4–1, 4–2 and 4–3, you have actually reviewed all that we have studied hitherto, in Chapters 1, 2 and 3.

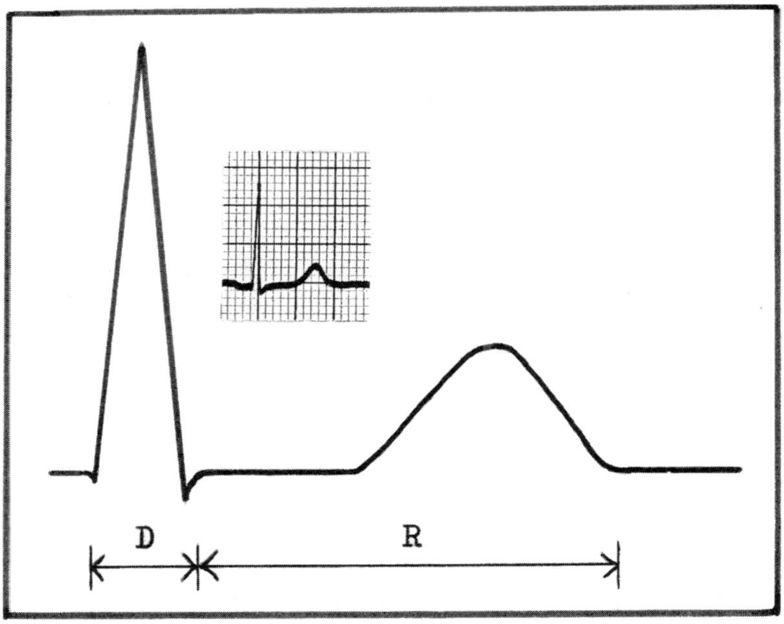

FIGURE 4–4. Electrocardiographic manifestations of ventricular depolarization and repolarization (D and R, respectively).

Depolarization of the ventricles (QRS complex) proceeds from endocardium to epicardium, from the inner areas of the ventricular muscle to the outer areas, and repolarization (S–T segment and T wave), proceeds in the reverse direction, from epicardium to endocardium.

A question should arise: Why is not repolarization, therefore, equal and opposite to depolarization? Why is the T wave *normally* in the same direction as the QRS complex (Fig. 4–4)? In some single muscle strip studies repolarization is indeed opposite to depolarization, the T wave is opposite, in direction, to the QRS complex. In the heart, although many questions have yet to be answered, depolarization and repolarization are not directly opposite processes; they are very different.

1. Depolarization (QRS complex) is a short process.

2. Repolarization (S–T segment and T wave) is a much longer process. There is evidence that repolarization is actually beginning before the end of the QRS complex.

3. Depolarization consumes relatively little energy.

4. Repolarization is the energy consuming phase of the cycle.

Since repolarization is the energy consuming phase it is more prone to abnormality, hence the multiple causes of S–T segment and T wave abnormalities.

Why can repolarization of the ventricles be represented by such different configurations on the electrocardiogram, an S–T segment and a T wave? This again emphasizes how complicated repolarization is and points out a difference between early and late repolarization. There is a known difference in the rate of repolarization from the epicardium to the endocardium.

The S–T segment represents *earlier* repolarization.

The T wave represents *later* repolarization.

Secondary Repolarization Abnormalities

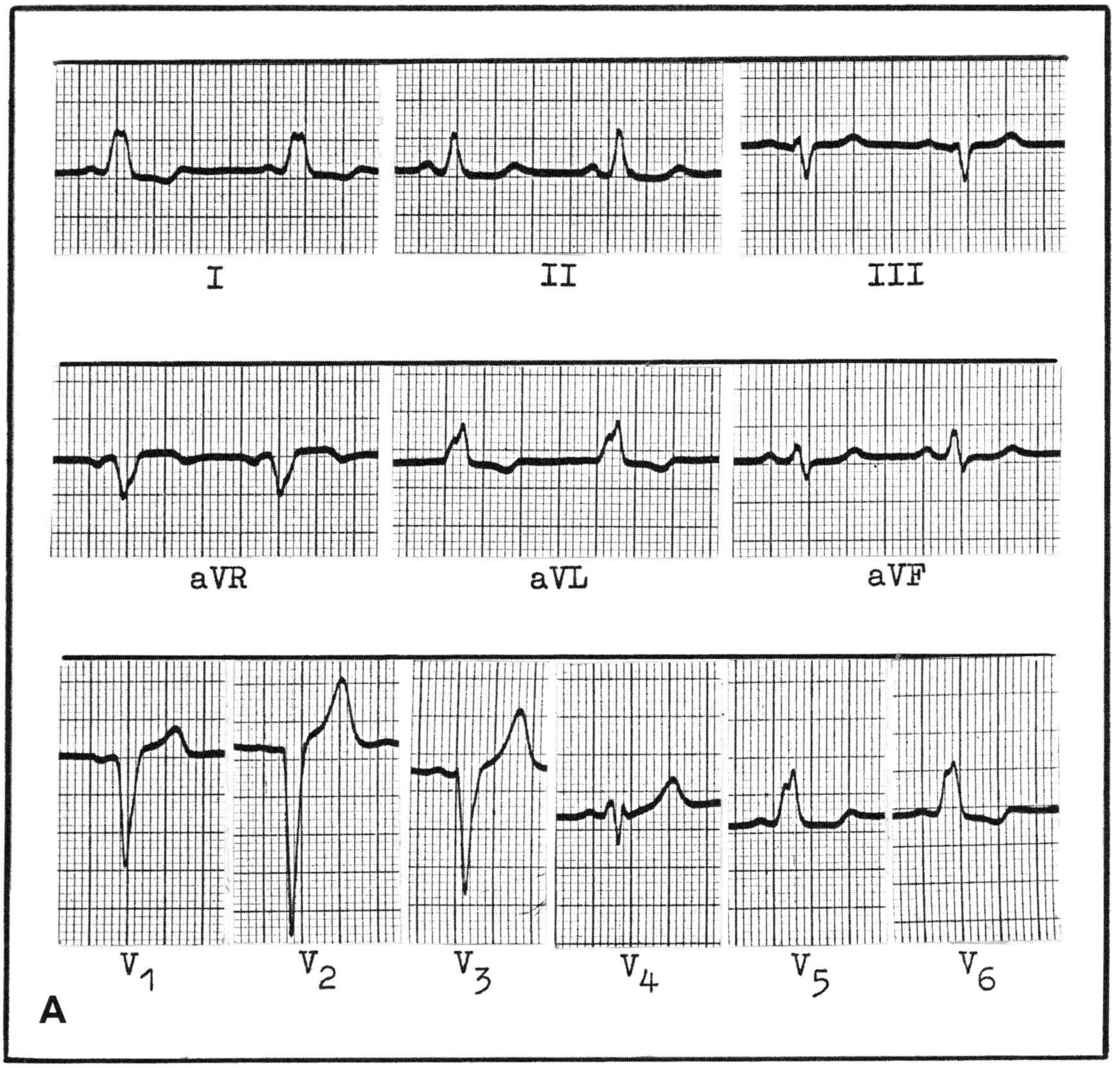

FIGURE 4–5. *A,* This electrocardiogram represents a ventricular conduction disturbance (left bundle branch block), which will be studied later in the course. For the present, note the abnormal width of the QRS complexes and repolarization abnormalities (S–T segment and T wave abnormalities). When repolarization abnormalities are caused by abnormal depolarization, they are known as *secondary* repolarization abnormalities (*secondary* S–T segment and T wave abnormalities). The electrocardiogram in Figure 4–5*B* is from the same patient during normal conduction.

Illustration continued on opposite page.

Repolarization abnormalities may be primary, secondary or both. Figure 4–5*A* illustrates repolarization abnormalities *resulting from abnormal depolarization.* Note the abnormally wide QRS complexes (representing left bundle branch block, to be studied in a later chapter). When repolarization is abnormal because de-

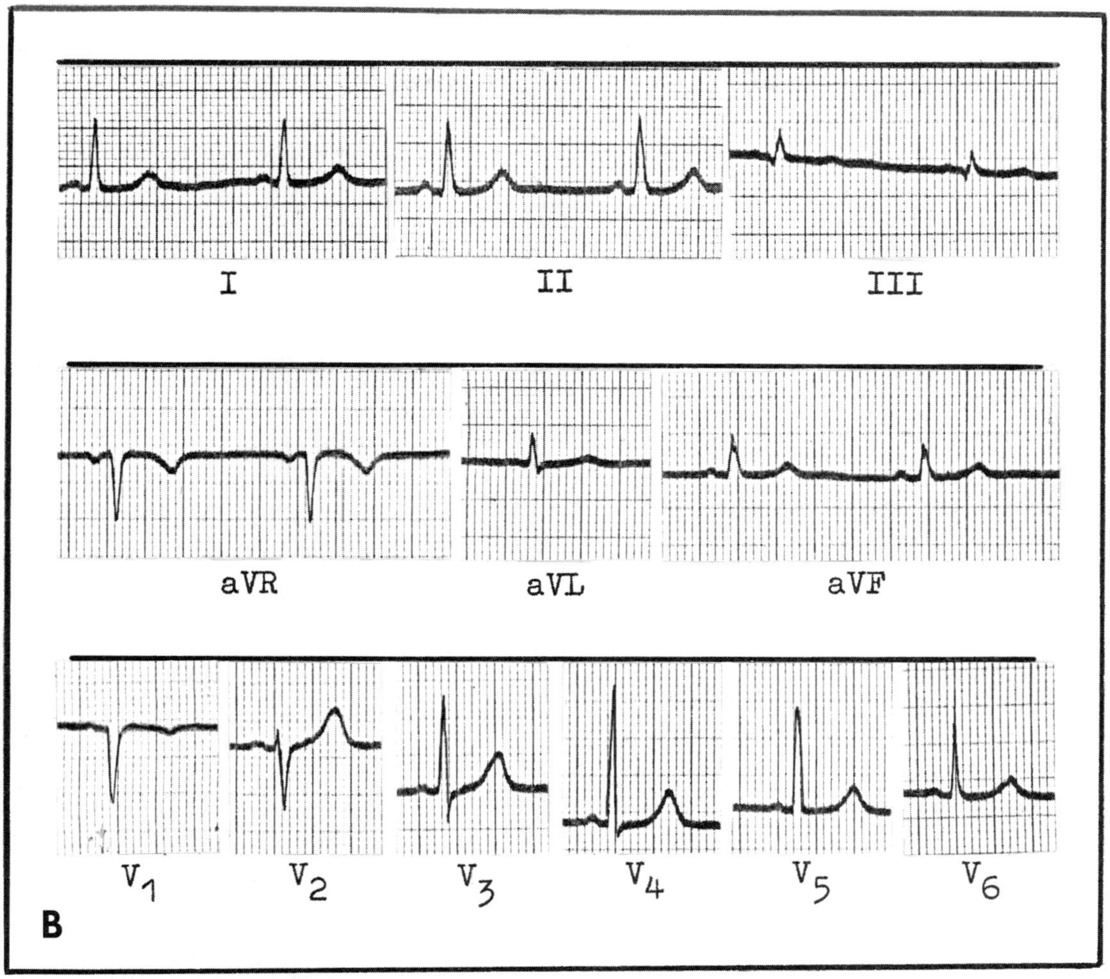

FIGURE 4–5 *Continued. B,* Normal electrocardiogram. Same patient as in Figure 4–5*A.* This electrocardiogram was taken during normal ventricular conduction (normal depolarization with normal QRS complexes) which alternated with abnormal conduction at a critical rate. During this normal depolarization, the repolarization was completely normal. Therefore, the repolarization abnormalities seen in Figure 4–5*A,* following abnormal depolarization, are strictly *secondary* repolarization abnormalities.

polarization is abnormal, the repolarization abnormalities are *secondary*. How do we know that the abnormalities are *secondary* and not *primary* in this patient? Figure 4–5*B* is from the same patient during intermittent *normal* ventricular conduction; the QRS–T angle and S–T segments are entirely normal.

Since patients with *secondary* repolarization abnormalities are not immune to *primary* repolarization abnormalities (abnormalities of repolarization *not due* to abnormalities in depolarization), how do you distinguish between *secondary* and *primary* abnormalities of repolarization in the presence of abnormal depolarization? Several ways have been described, including the calculation of the ventricular gradient, but I have found that serial electrocardiographic tracings yield the best results in the careful follow-up of a patient.

Primary Repolarization Abnormalities

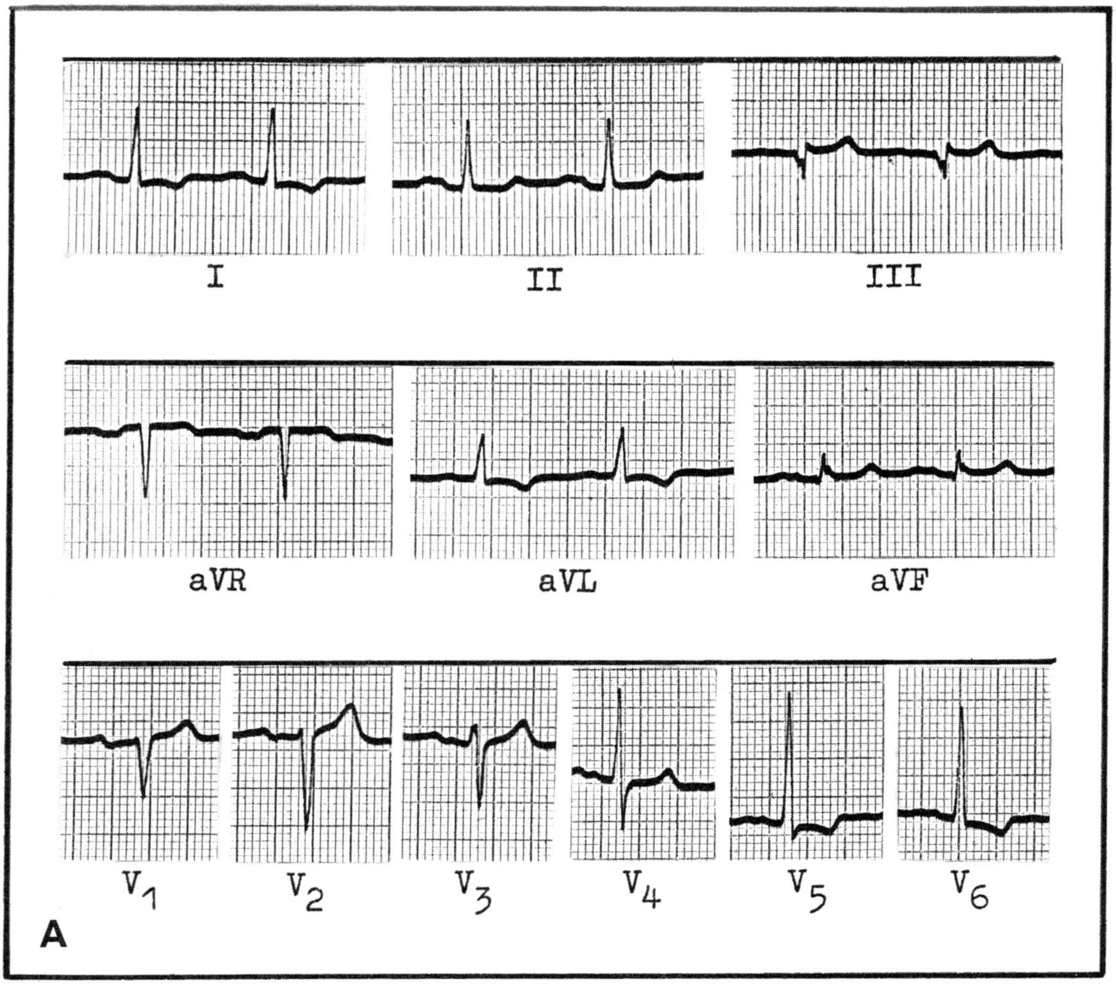

FIGURE 4–6. *A, Primary* repolarization (S–T segment and T wave) abnormalities. When repolarization abnormalities are seen with normal depolarization, they are said to be *primary* (abnormalities due to intrinsic problems in the repolarization phase and not secondary to disordered depolarization). These *primary* abnormalities are often referred to as *non-specific,* unless there is clear evidence as to the specific cause. As previously stated, the phase of repolarization requires increased energy, relative to depolarization, and is more prone to abnormality. There are many causes of *primary* repolarization abnormalities, including a host of metabolic derangements and drug states, in addition to coronary artery disease.

Illustration continued on opposite page.

Figures 4–6A and 4–7 represent *primary* repolarization abnormalities.

The illustrations in Figure 4–6*B* illustrate the rotation of the mean T vector from youth to old age. The "juvenile" pattern is seen in Figure 4–8 with negative T waves in leads V_1 to V_4. This pattern is not infrequently seen in normal healthy young patients well into the third decade

Rotation of Mean T Vector from Youth to Old Age

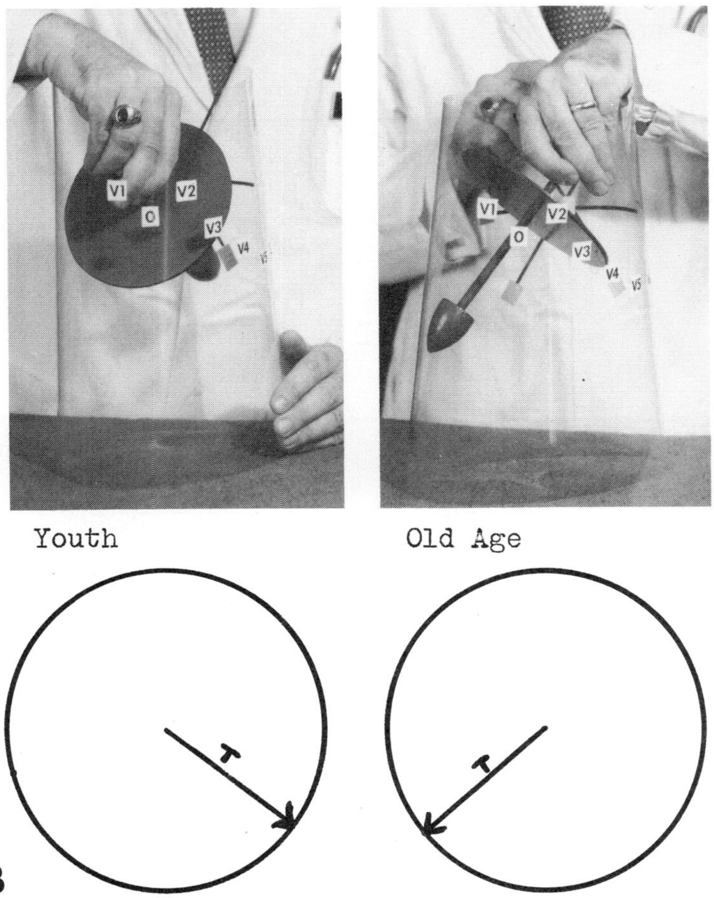

B

FIGURE 4-6 *Continued. B,* Rotation of mean T wave vector from youth to old age. The mean T wave vector in youth is frequently found to be to the *left, inferior* and *posterior,* inscribing a T wave across the chest (see vector model above) as follows: leads V_1, V_2 and V_3 negative, V_4, V_5 and V_6 positive. The T wave may be negative as far as lead V_4. This "juvenile" pattern is illustrated in Figure 4–8.

With increasing age, the mean T vector rotates *rightward* and *anteriorly,* inscribing a T wave across the chest as follows: leads V_1, V_2, V_3 and V_4 positive, V_5 and V_6 negative (see vector model above). This does not always happen; not every elderly patient has negative T waves in V_5 and V_6, nor is it considered normal to have negative T waves in these leads. Many an asymptomatic elderly patient, however, upon being told by an unwary physician that his heart is "ischemic" or "straining" has been prodded into symptoms. You must always treat the patient, not the electrocardiogram detached from the patient.

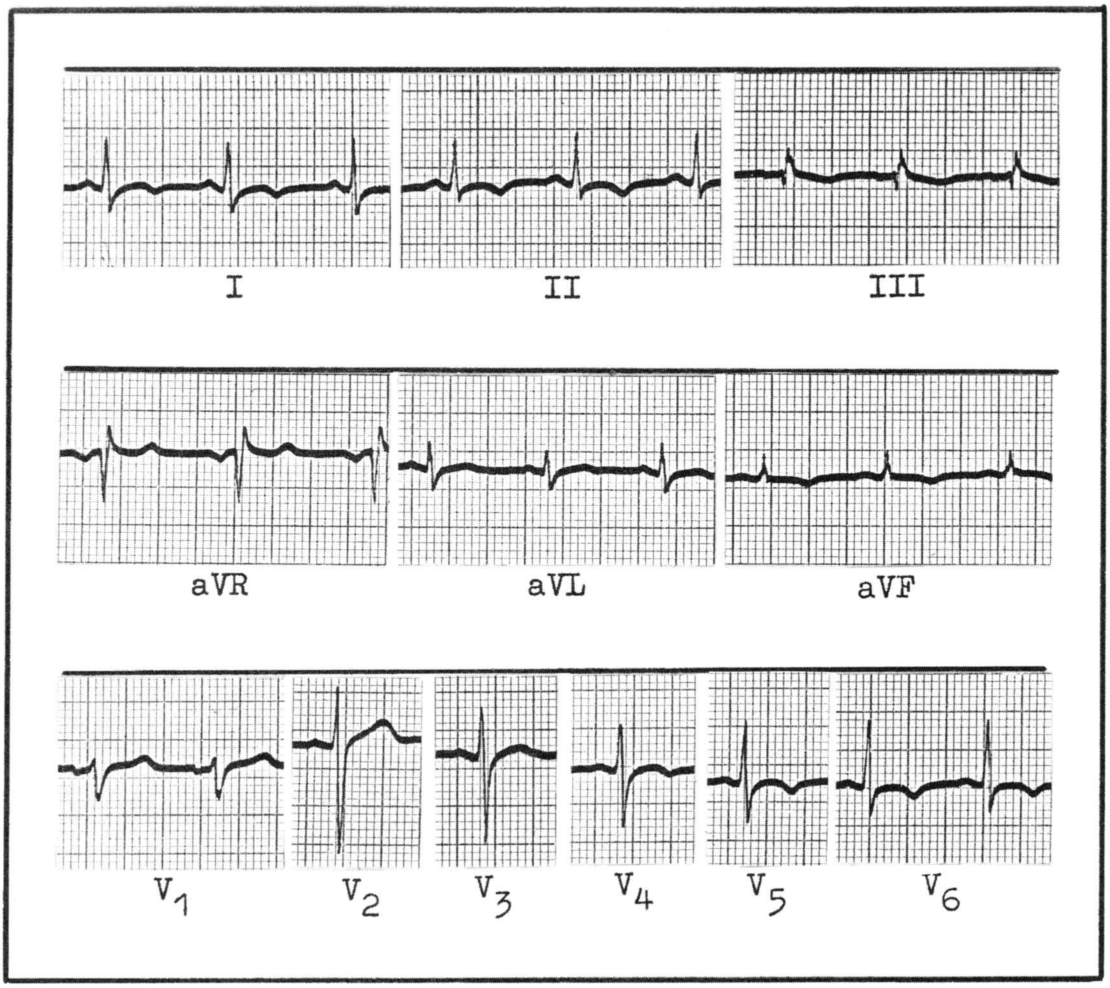

FIGURE 4–7. Wide QRS–T angle. The QRS–T angle is abnormally wide. The term "ischemia" is frequently ascribed to this wide QRS–T angle. The term "strain" is often used for the enlargement of either of the ventricles accompanied by a wide QRS–T angle and S–T segment abnormalities. Some electrocardiographers argue that the word "strain" should not be used without accompanying ventricular enlargement. Both terms, "ischemia" and "strain," as noted earlier, are poor terms in that they give a clinical connotation to a laboratory study.

of life. This emphasizes once again that the electrocardiogram should not be detached from the patient and should not be read without knowing the age of the patient, or without knowledge of pertinent clinical information.

Figure 4–9*B* shows the additive effects of repolarization abnormalities due to a conduction disturbance (left bundle branch block) in addition to previously abnormal repolarization in a patient with a history of myocardial infarction.

"Juvenile" Pattern

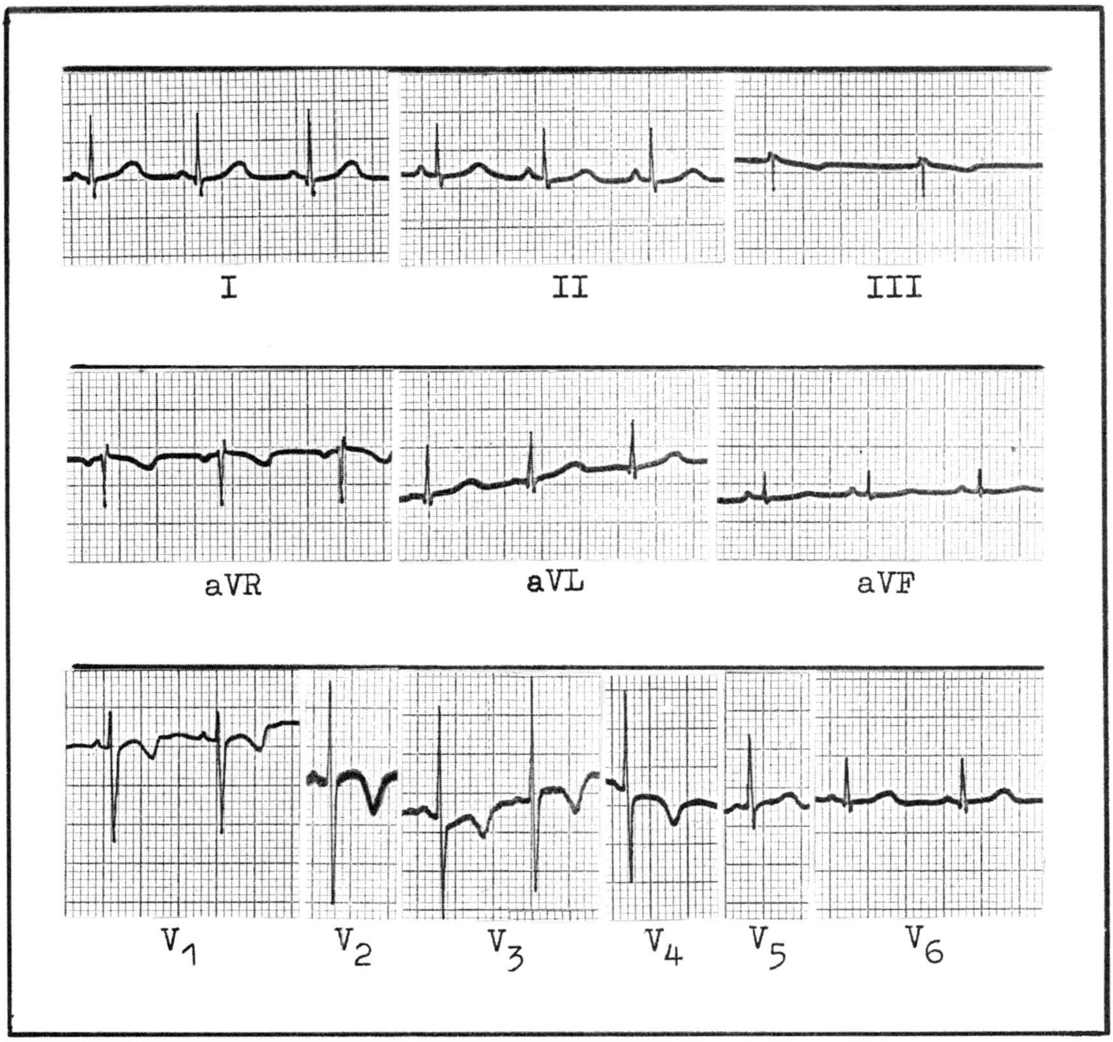

FIGURE 4–8. "Juvenile" pattern in a healthy young patient (refer to the discussion in Figure 4–6*B*). Describe the mean T vector, and contrast with the many normals already seen.

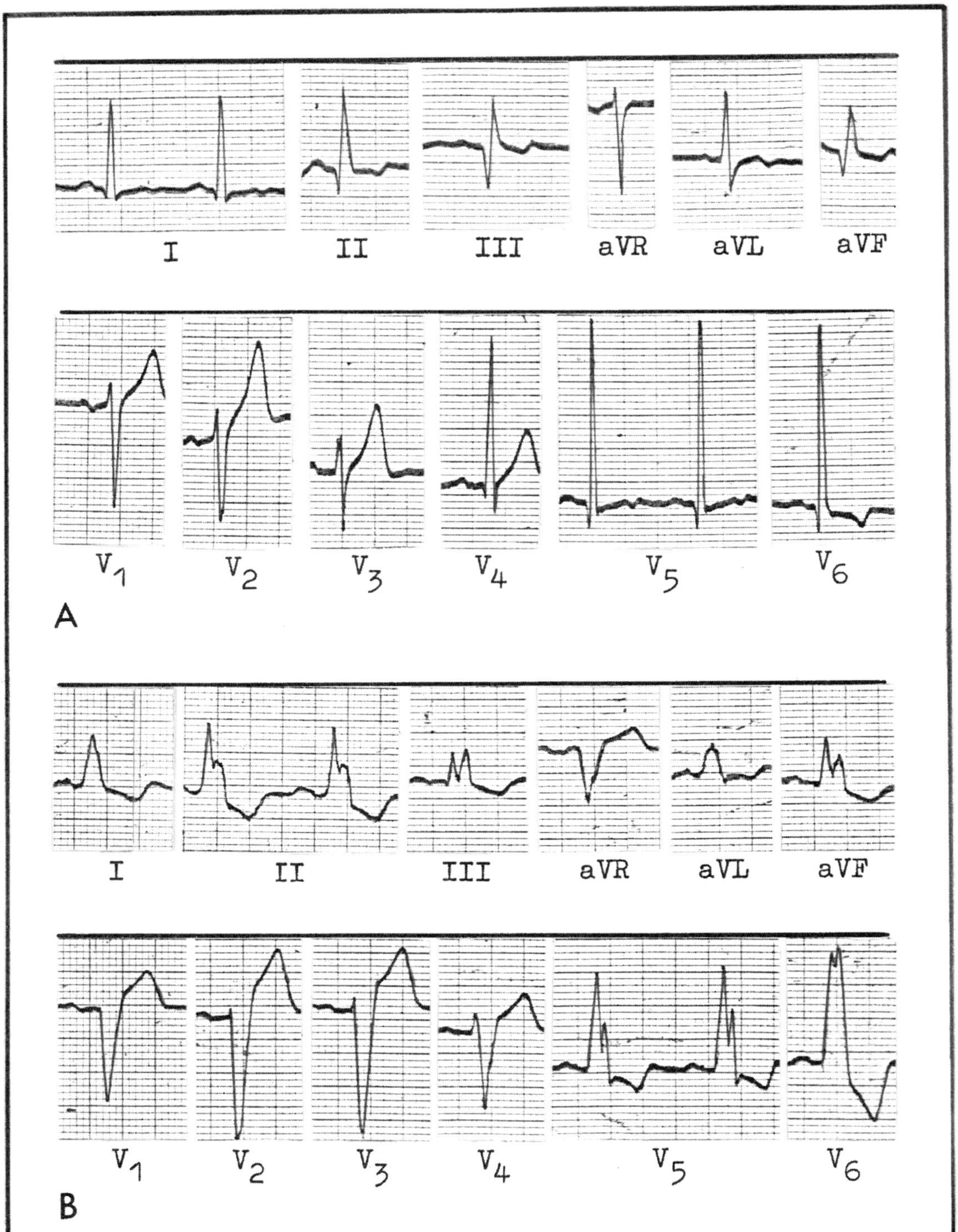

FIGURE 4–9. *A,* Diaphragmatic myocardial infarction (this subject will be studied in the next chapter). For the present, describe the repolarization abnormalities (abnormal S–T segments and T waves). This patient also had left ventricular hypertrophy. *B,* Same patient following the development of a ventricular conduction disturbance (left bundle branch block, to be studied later in this course). Note the markedly widened QRS complexes and the disappearance of the Q waves in leads II, III and aVF. Note also the further changes in repolarization. The repolarization abnormalities due to the left bundle branch block came on top of the previously abnormal repolarization. The best way to appreciate these changes is to know your patients and follow with serial electrocardiograms.

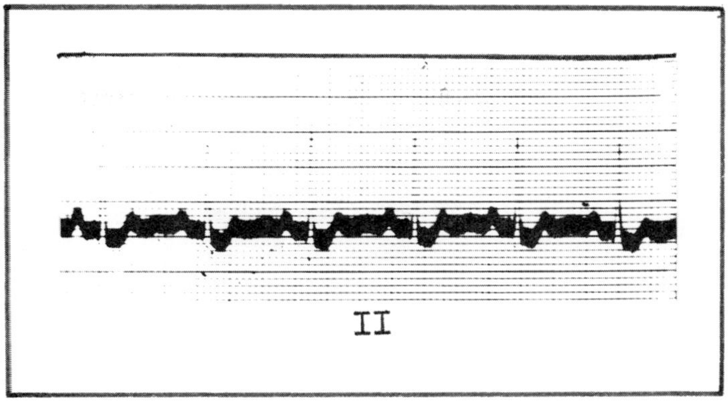

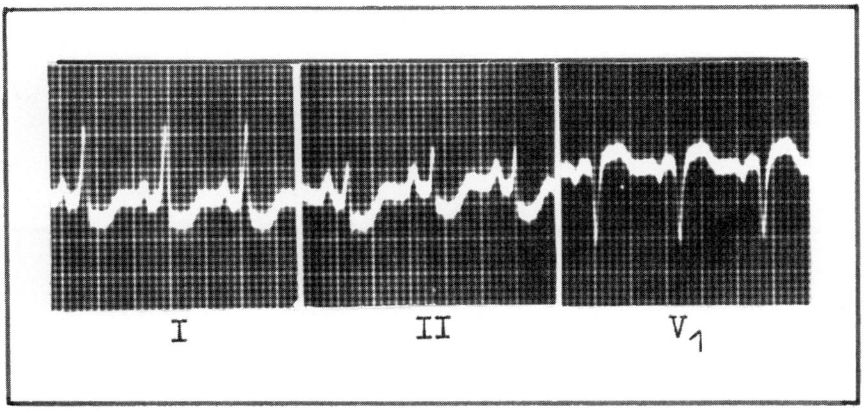

FIGURE 4–10. "Classical" changes on the S–T segments caused by digitalis in two patients. The "classical" changes of digitalis are described as a "fist-like" depression of the S–T segment (as if you were placing your fist in the S–T segment and depressing it), or "paint-brush" inscription (as if you were painting the S–T segment with gradual widening of the paint brush as you approach the S–T segment from the downslope of the R wave), or "scooping" of the S–T segment. The elevation of the S–T segment in lead V_1 represents the same phenomenon as the S–T segment depression in leads I and II.
(Electrocardiograms reduced in size.)

Digitalis Effects on Repolarization

Digitalis has long been known for its effects on ventricular repolarization. The "classical" changes of the S–T segments caused by digitalis are seen in Figures 4–10 to 4–12. These "classical" changes of digitalis are described as a "fist-like" depression of the S–T segment (as if you were placing a fist in the S–T segment and depressing it), or "paint-brush" inscription or "scooping" of the S–T segment. Figures 4–13 to 4–16 are from studies of digitalis effects on repolarization. In spite of the well accepted "classical" changes on early repolarization (S–T segment), the effects on later repolarization (T wave) were just as dramatic. In a substantial number of patients it was not possible to predict which part, or whether the entire phase, of repolarization would be affected (both the S–T segment and the T wave). This again stresses the need to follow each patient very closely without relying on

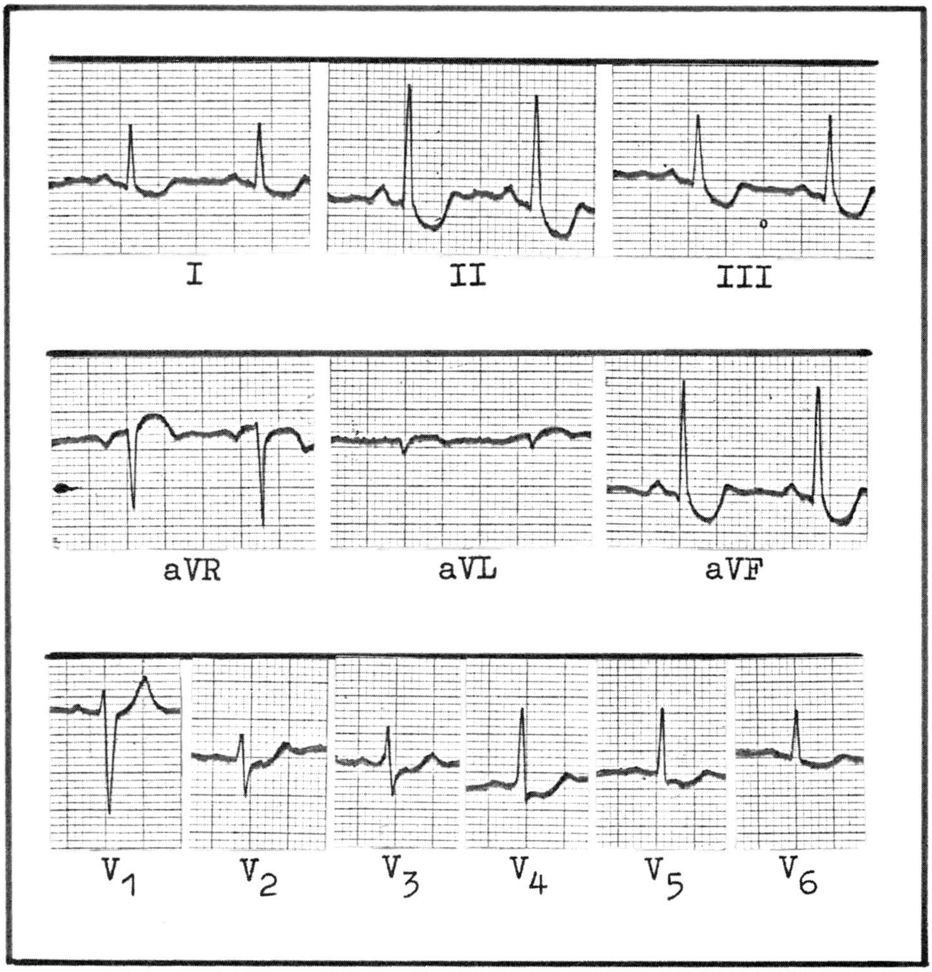

FIGURE 4–11. Review the effects of digitalis on ventricular repolarization.

"predictable" changes. That digitalis could affect the entire phase of repolarization (both the S–T segment and the T wave) was recognized years ago and is seen in Figure 4–17.

Often you will hear that an increase in heart rate will cause a change in repolarization of the ventricles. Figures 4–15 and 4–16 show the effects of digitalis to be more pronounced at the higher rates. Always evaluate critically. Repolarization is not readily predictable. In Figure 4–18 the already abnormal phase of repolarization shows no significant changes despite an increased heart rate.

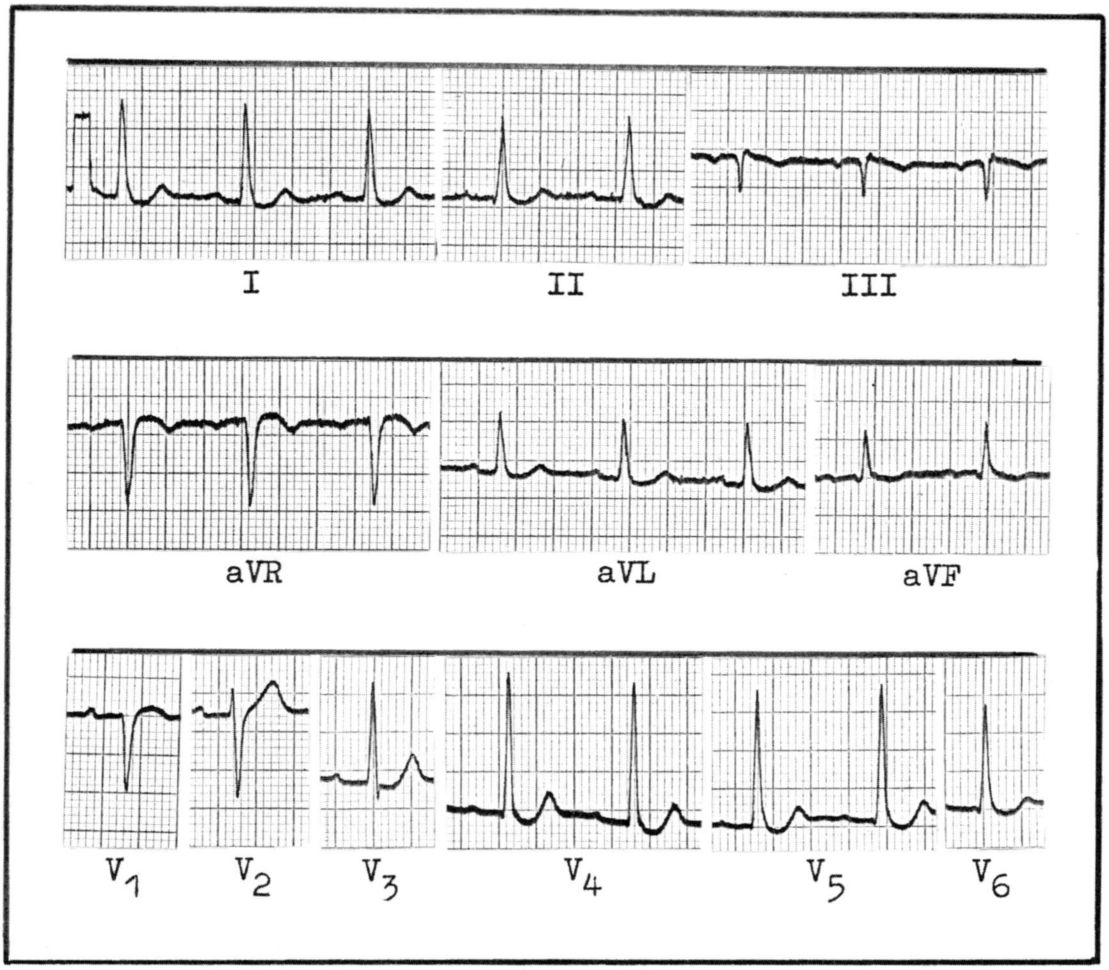

FIGURE 4–12. Patient receiving digitalis. Describe the "classical" changes in the early part of repolarization caused by digitalis and known as "digitalis effects."

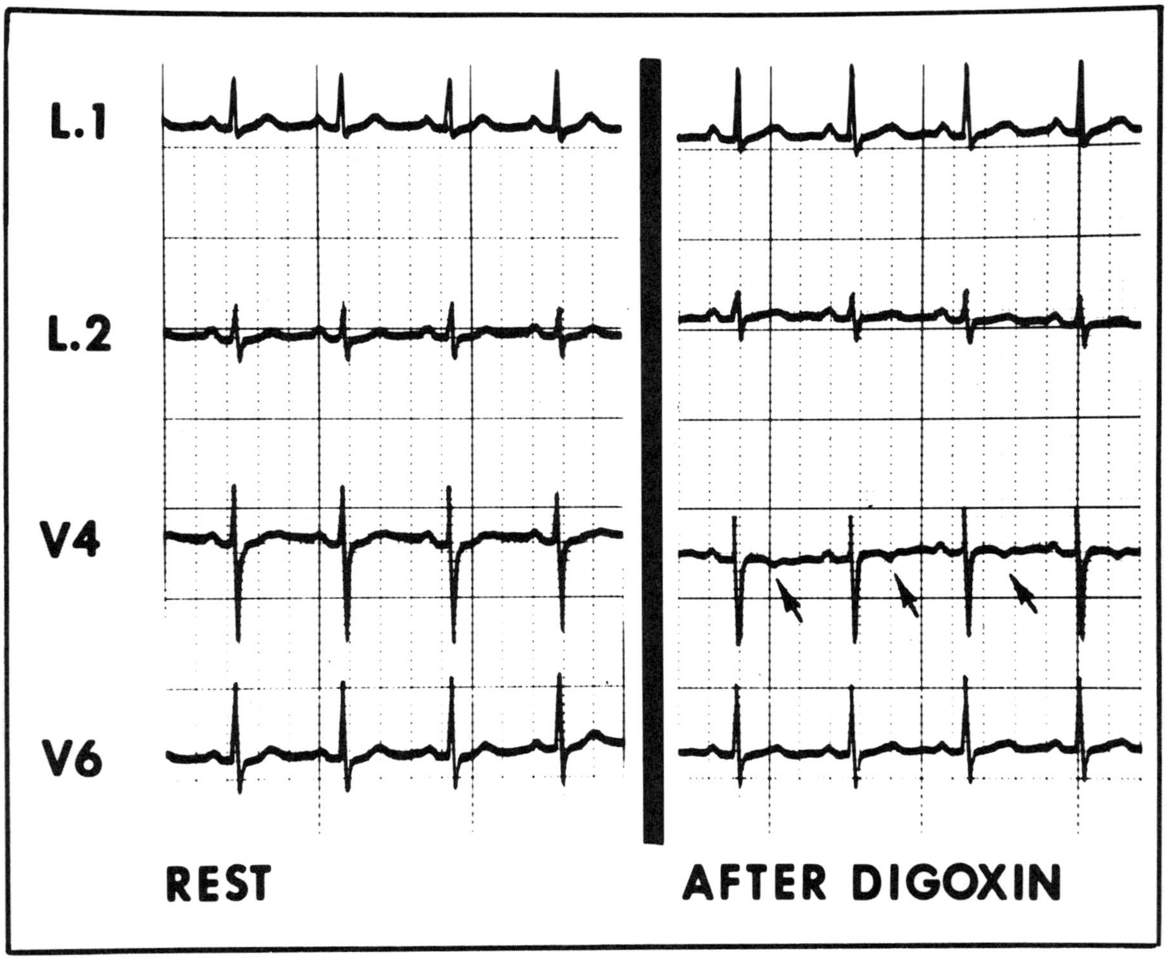

FIGURE 4–13. Repolarization changes due to a digitalis preparation (digoxin). In spite of the "classical" changes ascribed to digitalis on the early part of repolarization (S–T segment), note the effect of a subdigitalizing dose of digoxin on late repolarization (T wave).
(Electrocardiogram reduced in size.)

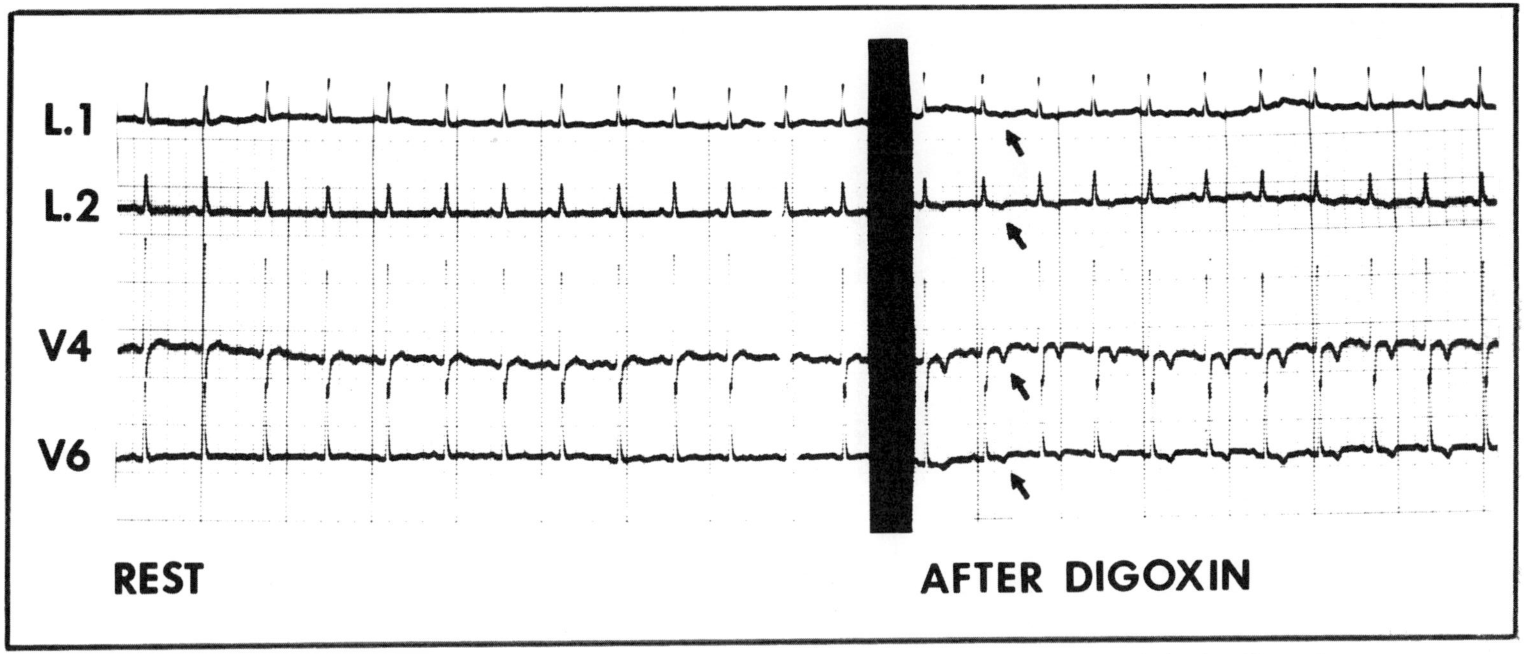

FIGURE 4–14. Repolarization changes due to digitalis. A dramatic effect is seen in late repolarization (T wave) due to a small dose of the digitalis preparation digoxin. There was no other intervention here; the thick black line in the center is where the recording machine was stopped for one hour following the administration of digoxin. It cannot, therefore, be said dogmatically that digitalis affects only the early part of repolarization; the effect on the T waves may be much more marked than the effect on the S–T segments. Repolarization should be dealt with as a unit; the S–T segments and T waves should not be categorically separated. Digitalis may affect one, the other, or both.
(Electrocardiogram reduced in size.)

Cassette Side 10

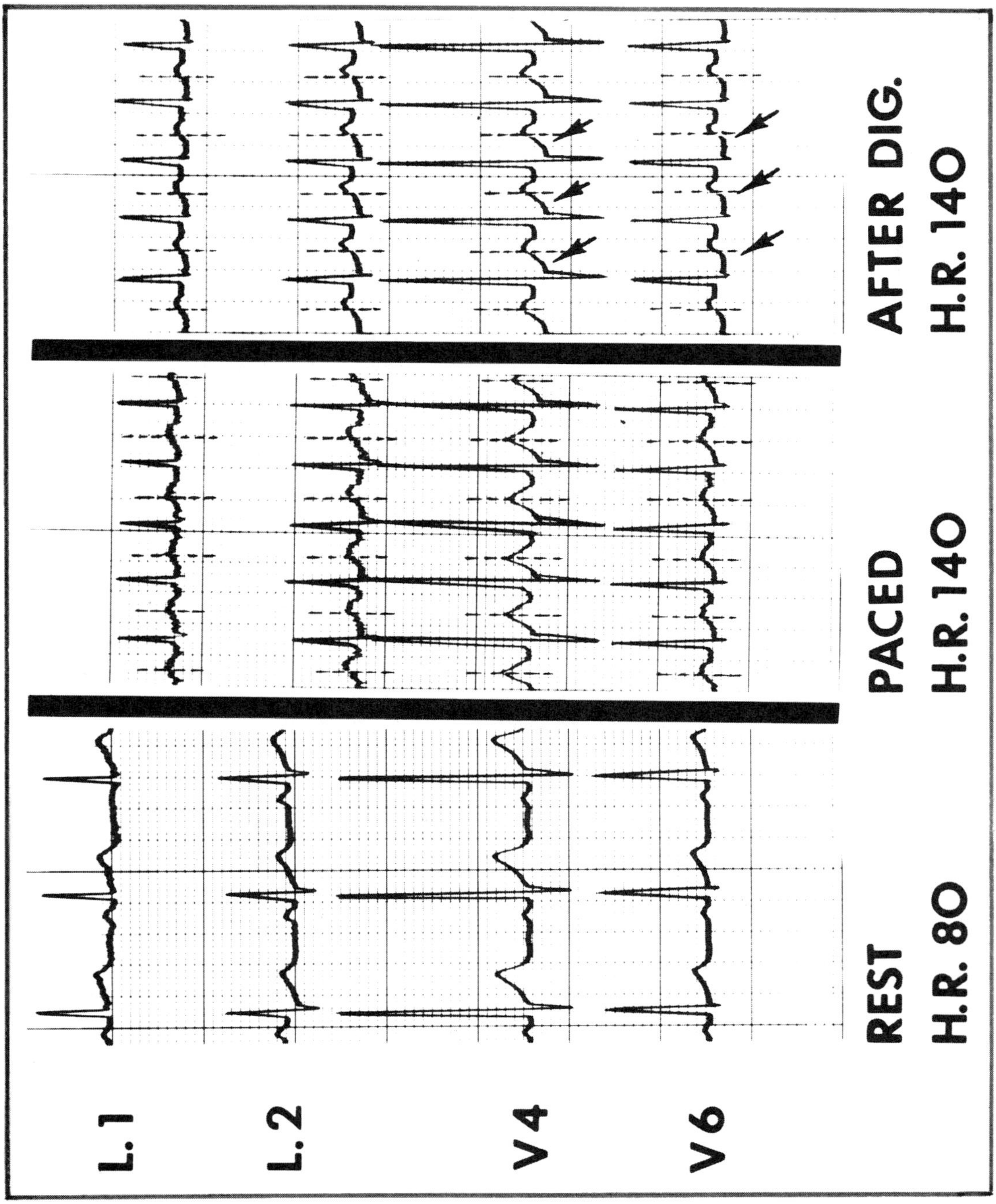

FIGURE 4–15. Repolarization changes due to digitalis. The arrows point to the effects of digitalis on the S–T segments at a given paced heart rate, compared with the same paced heart rate without digitalis. (Electrocardiogram reduced in size.)

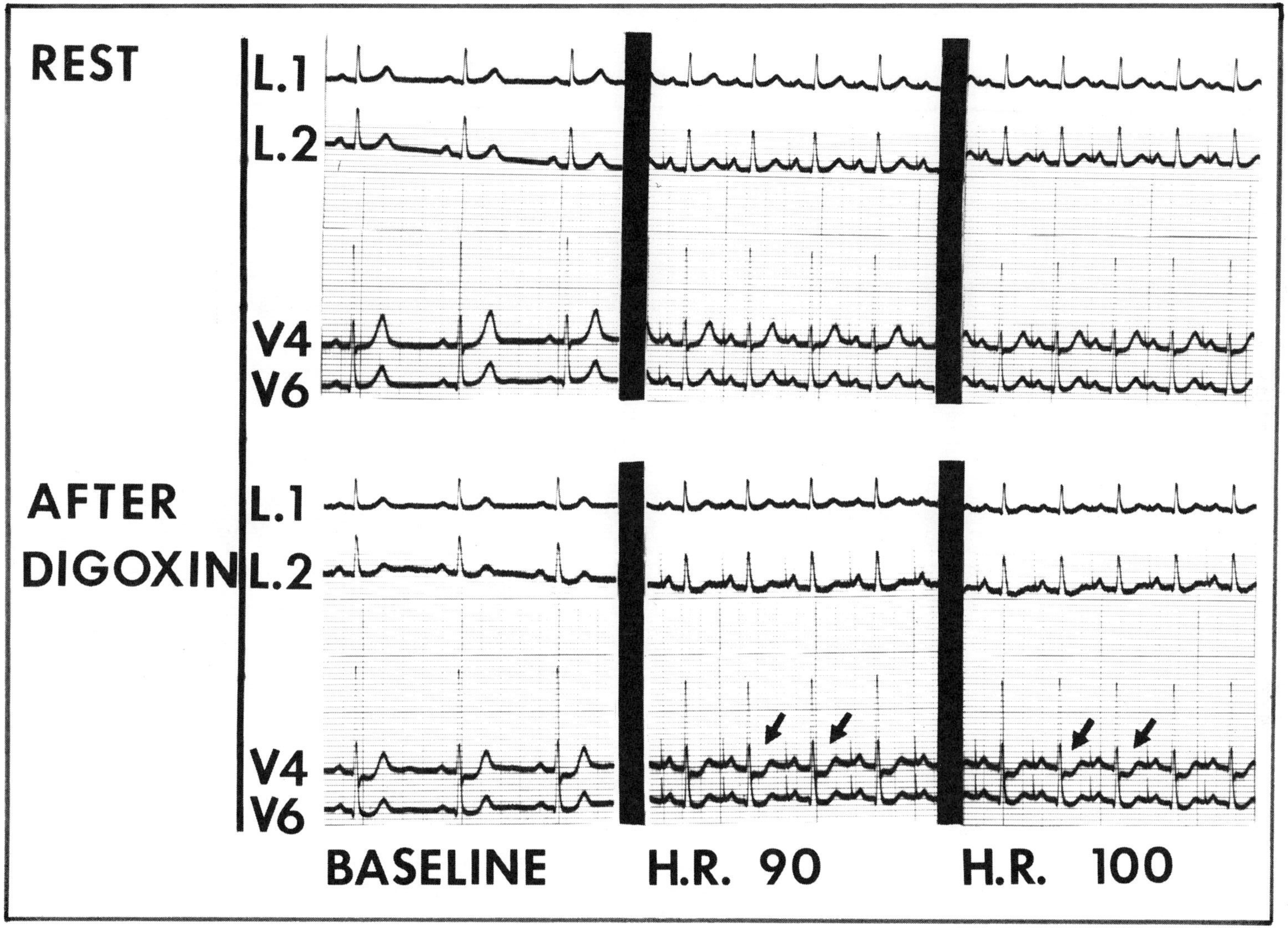

FIGURE 4–16. Digitalis effects on repolarization. Compare the effects of digitalis on each of the paired heart rates, baseline, 90 per minute and 100 per minute.
(Electrocardiogram reduced in size.)

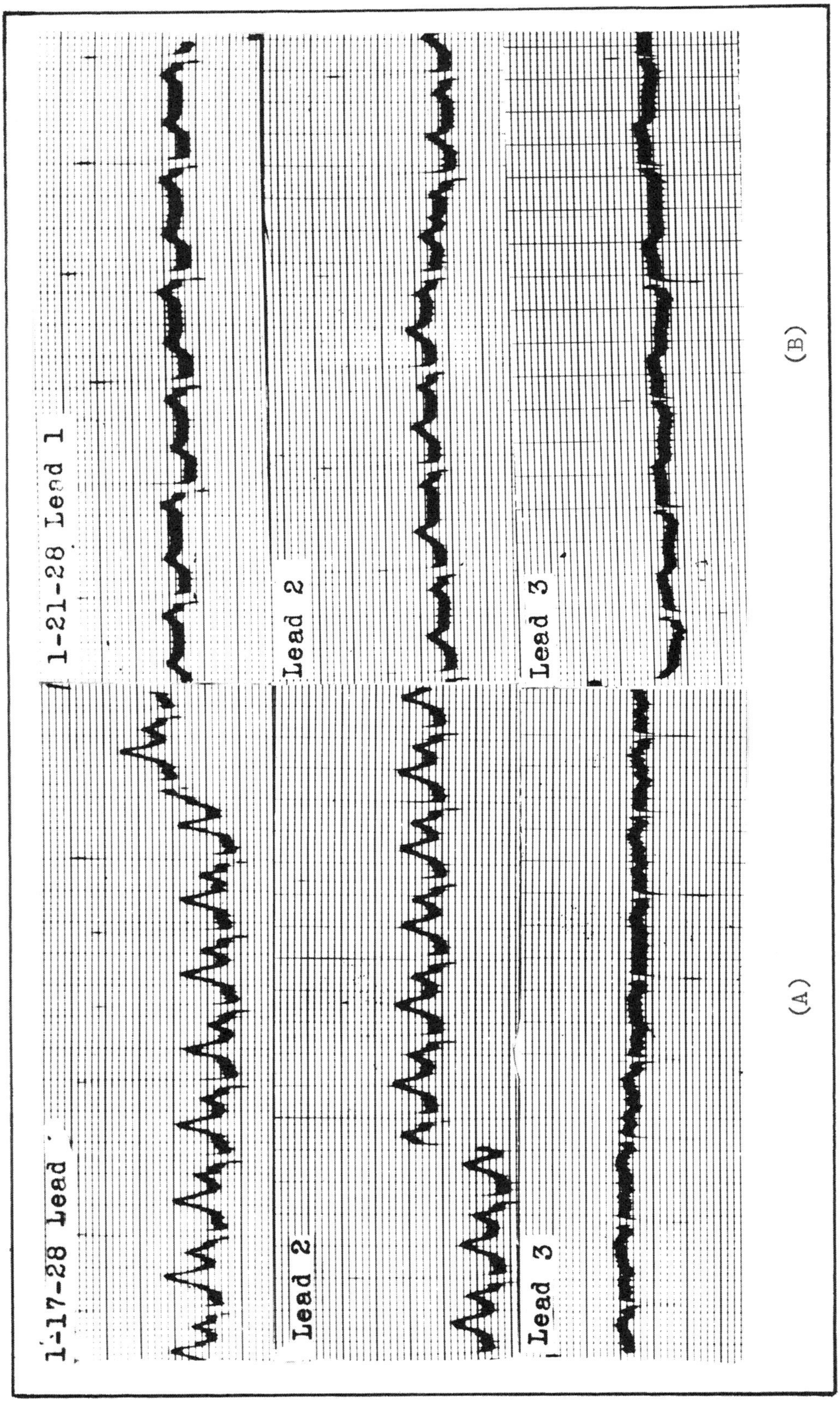

FIGURE 4–17. Before (*A*) and after (*B*) "digitalization." Describe the changes which have occurred during ventricular repolarization (both S–T segment and T wave).

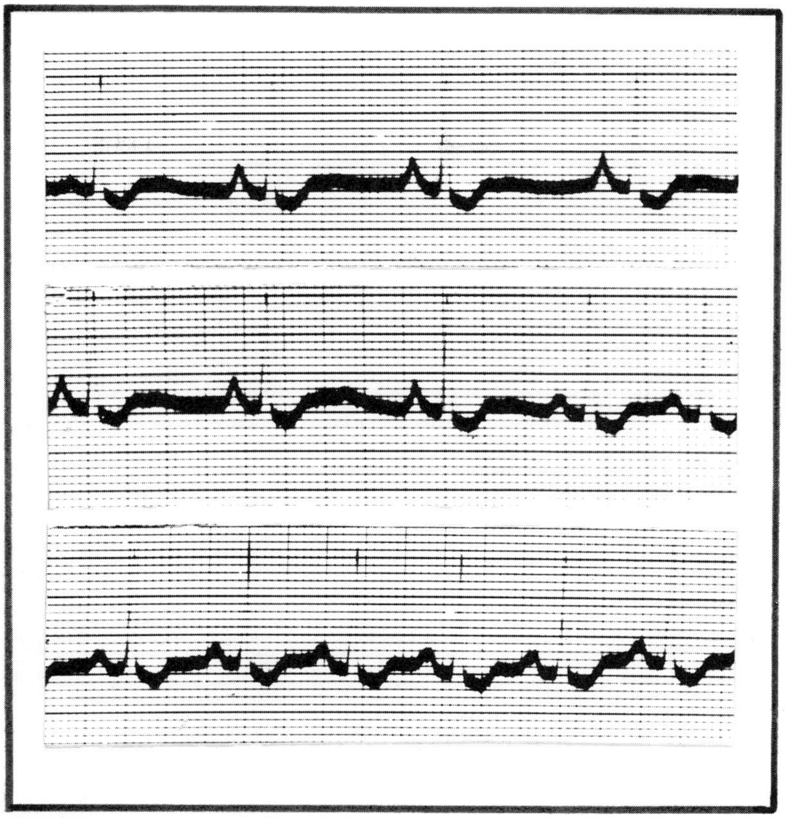

FIGURE 4–18. Repolarization and changes in heart rate. Often you will hear that an increase in heart rate will cause a change in repolarization. You have already seen that the effects of digitalis on repolarization were more pronounced at the higher rates (Figs. 4–15 and 4–16). Always evaluate critically. Repolarization is not readily predictable. In this figure there is no marked change in repolarization in spite of an increased heart rate.

Coronary Heart Disease

Coronary heart disease is a major cause of ventricular repolarization abnormalities. Figure 4–19 shows the effects of activity (Fig. 4–19*B*) on the already abnormal repolarization (Fig. 4–19*A*), in a patient with a history of angina pectoris. Many a patient with a typical history of angina pectoris will have an electrocardiogram with normal ventricular repolarization at rest; this is seen in Figure 4–20*A*, and was seen in multiple resting electrocardiograms. The electrocardiogram of the same patient following a walk from her room to the electrocardiography office is seen in Figure 4–20*B*. Activity (utilizing the patient's normal activity, such as taking a walk), rather than provocative testing, will often yield important information in the *initial* evaluation. This activity did not produce pain, yet the effect on ventricular repolarization is obvious. In Figure 4–21*B* we see the striking S–T segment elevations (lead II), during an episode of chest pain in a patient with a history of angina pectoris principally at rest. You will hear many erudite explanations for it. Remain alert for new information, but remember the old adage that, given the facts, many theories abound. There is nothing categorically explicit about what will be found on the electrocardiogram among a group of patients with the same symptoms. Each patient must be closely followed and any change carefully evaluated. This must be continually emphasized. Some patients with "classical" angina pectoris have been found to have normal appearing coronary arteries (by arteriography). Of even greater interest are the patients with clinical myocardial infarction found to have normal appearing coronary arteries. Much has yet to be learned in this field.

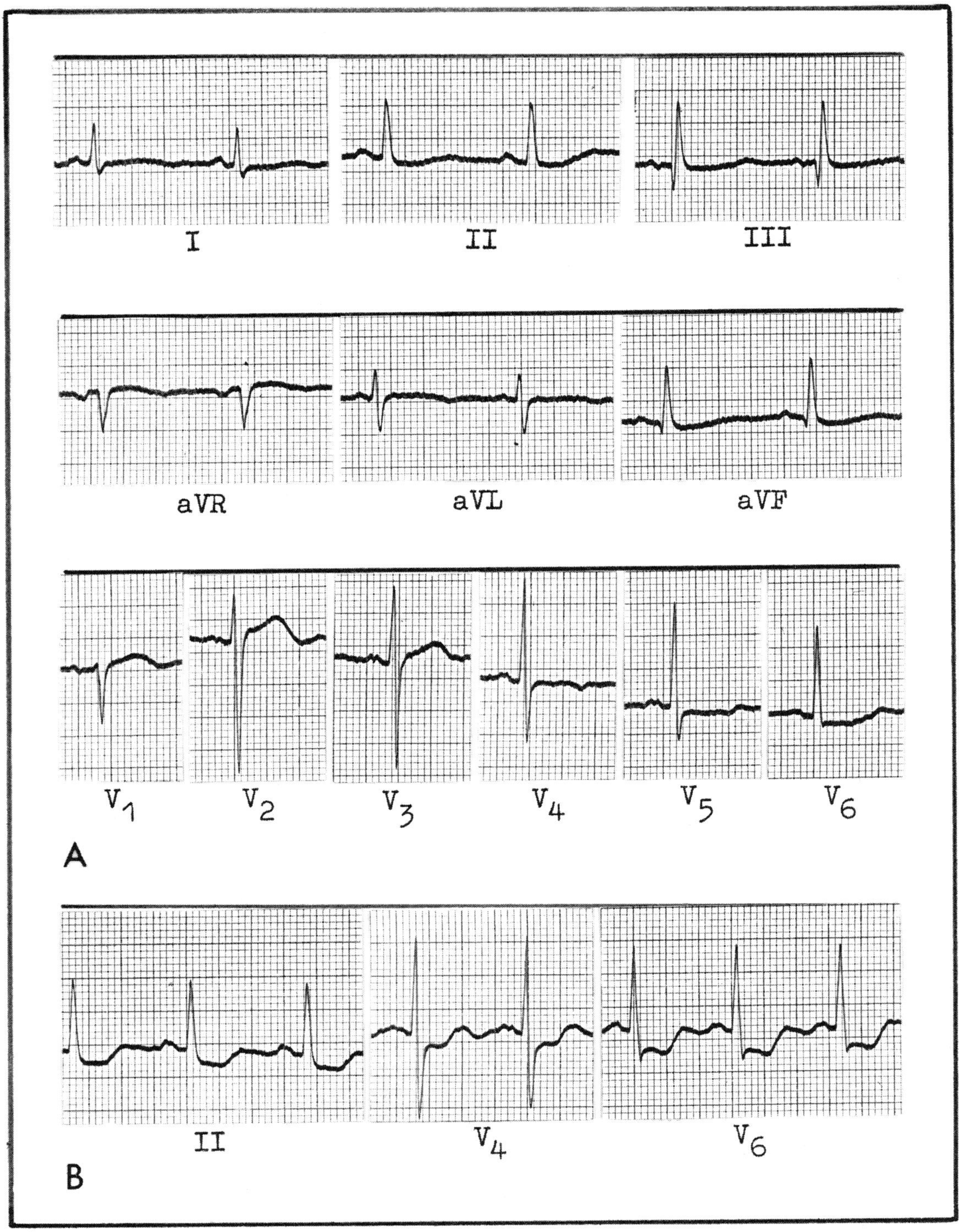

FIGURE 4–19. *A*, Repolarization abnormalities in a patient with a history of angina pectoris. *B*, Following activity, repolarization abnormalities become quite pronounced.

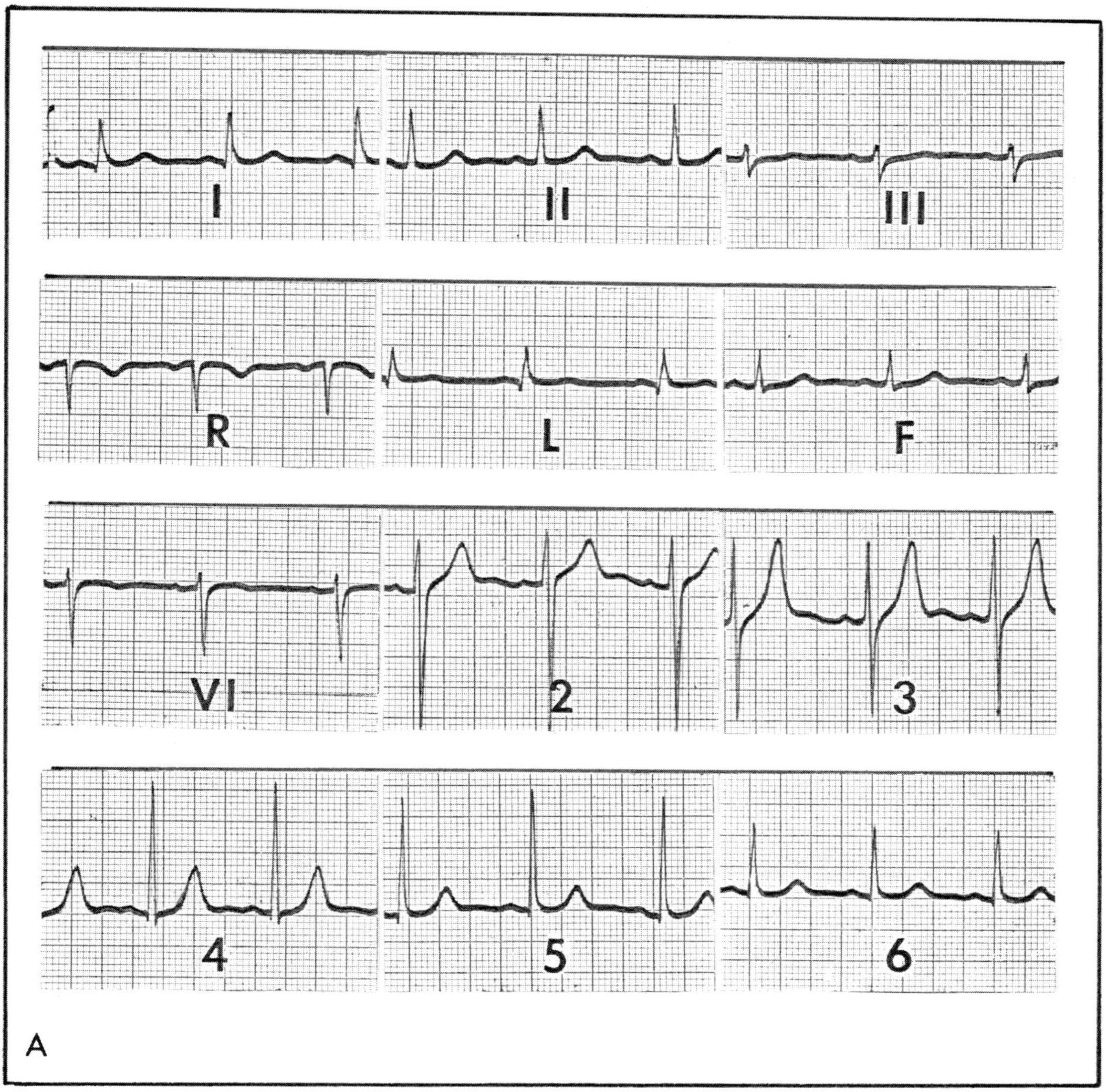

FIGURE 4-20. *A,* Resting electrocardiogram of a patient with a history of angina pectoris. (Electrocardiogram reduced in size.)

Illustration continued on following page.

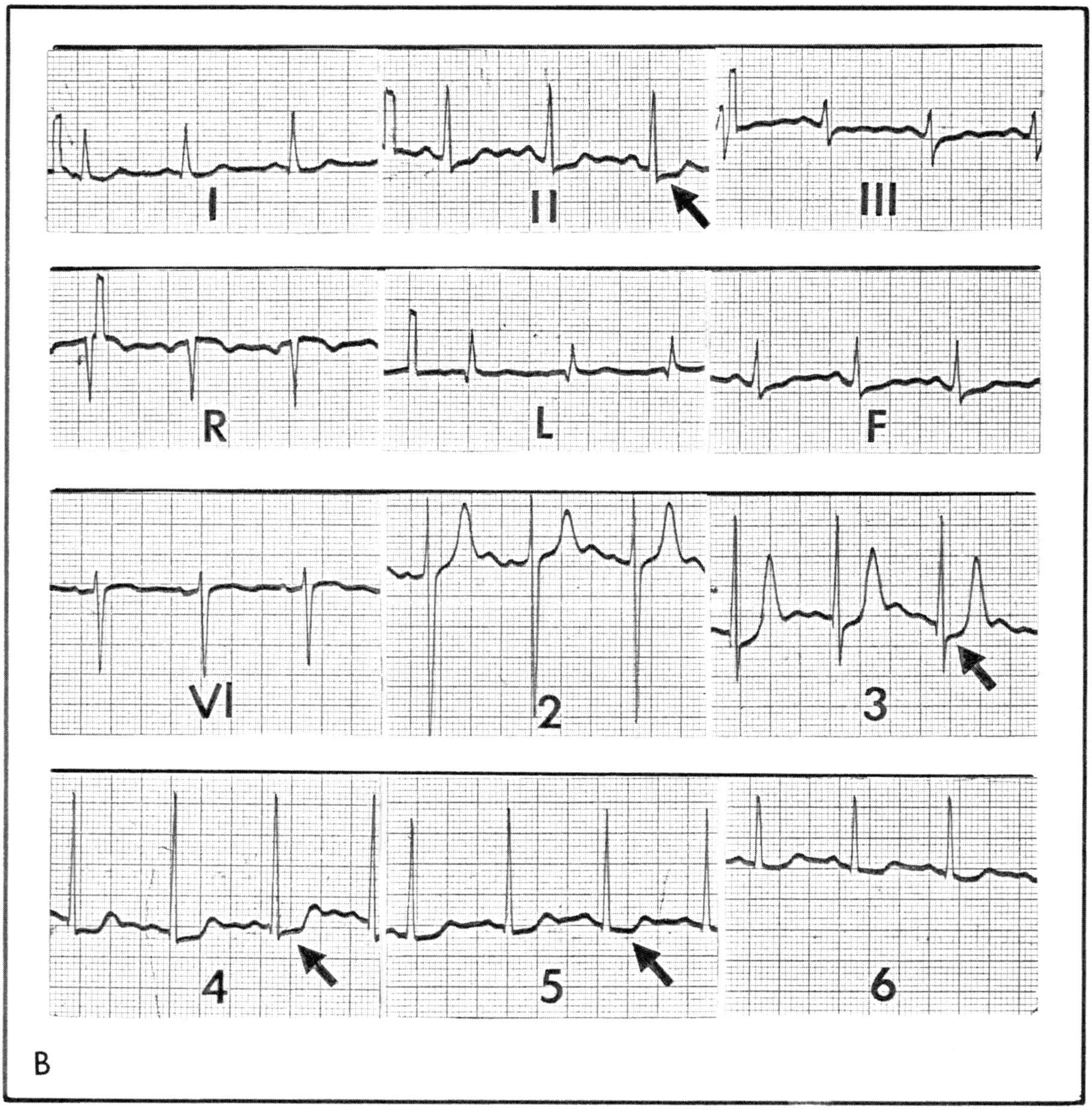

FIGURE 4–20 *Continued.* *B,* Electrocardiogram of same patient as in Figure 4–20*A* following a walk from her room to the electrocardiography office. Activity utilizing the patient's normal activity, such as taking a walk, rather than provocative testing, will often yield important information.
(Electrocardiogram reduced in size.)

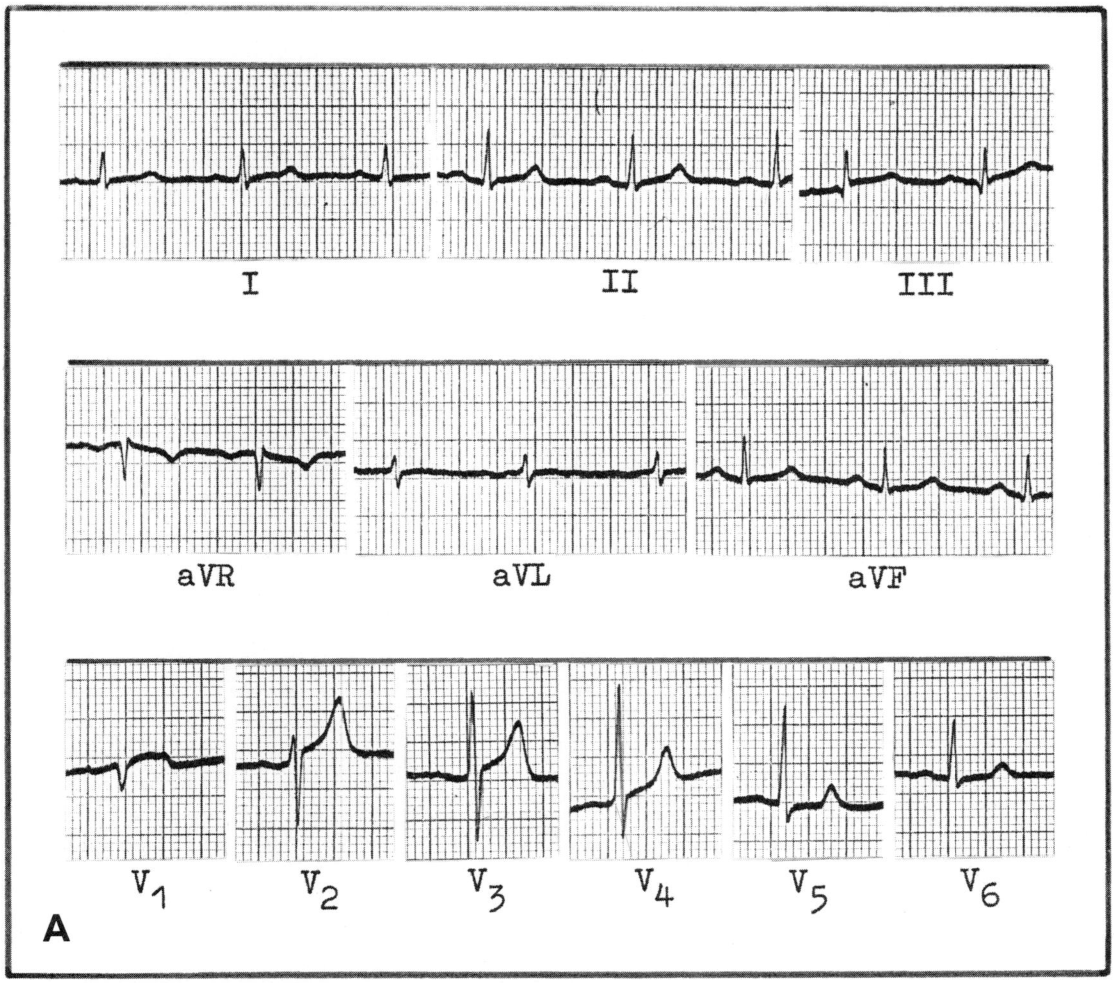

FIGURE 4–21. *A,* Electrocardiogram of a patient with a history of angina pectoris, at rest.

Illustration continued on following page.

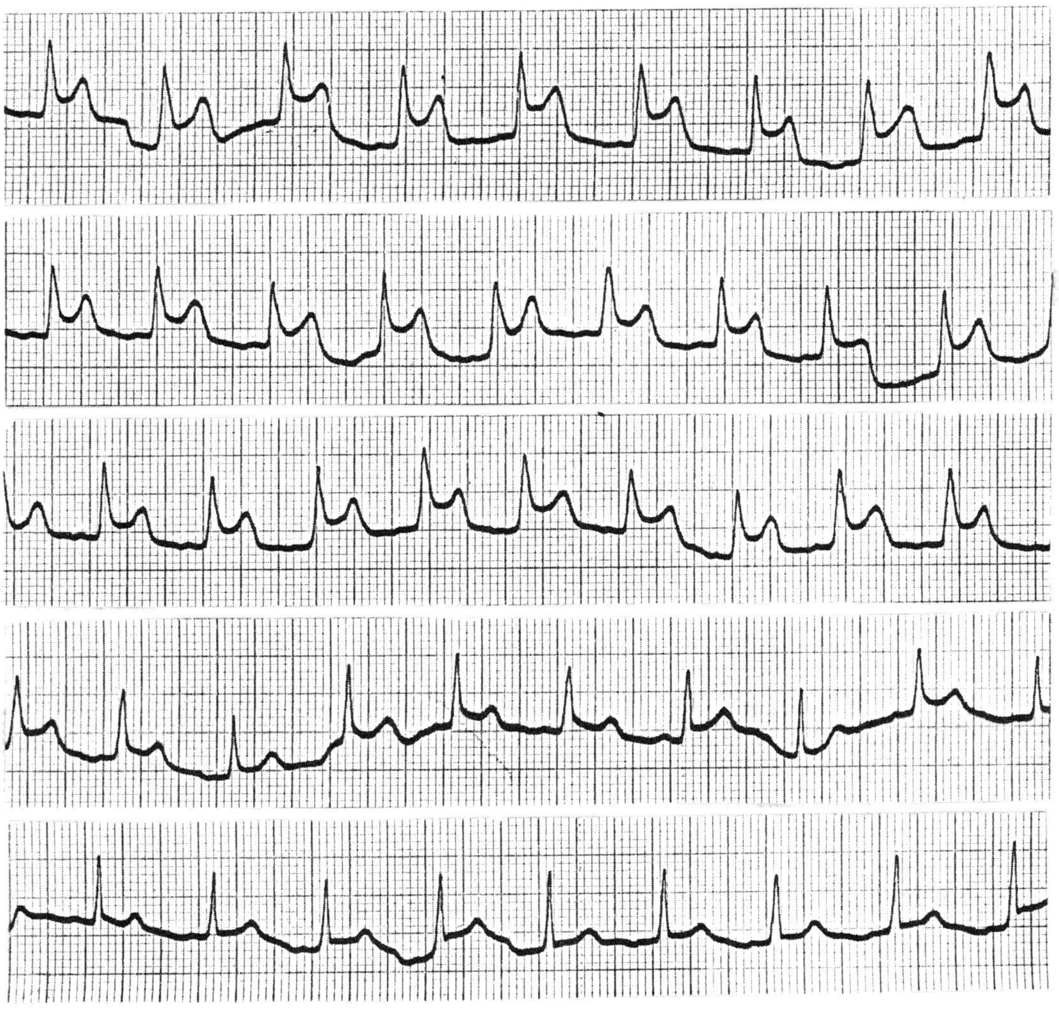

B

FIGURE 4–21 *Continued.* *B,* The electrocardiogram of the same patient as in Figure 4–21*A* during an episode of chest pain at rest, showing a continuous lead II with return of the S–T segments toward normal on subsidence of chest pain. How do these S–T segments differ from the S–T segments in previous electrocardiograms of patients with angina pectoris? You will hear many erudite explanations for it. Remain alert for new information, but remember the old adage that, given the facts, many theories arise. There is nothing categorically explicit about what will be found on the electrocardiogram among a group of patients with the same symptoms. Each patient must be closely followed and any change carefully evaluated.

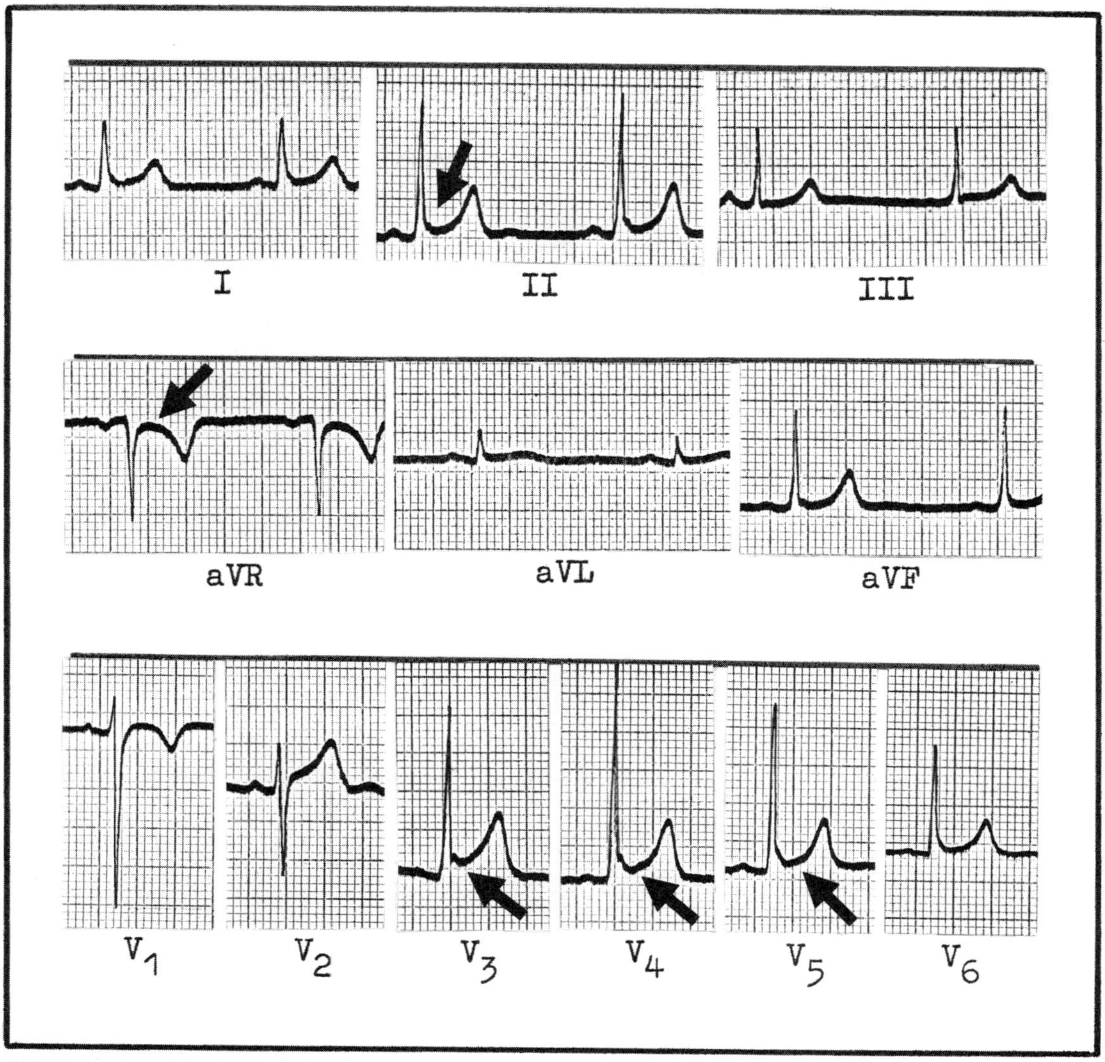

FIGURE 4–22. "Early repolarization" in a normal young patient. This pattern is not infrequently seen in young asymptomatic patients. The S–T segment is elevated (leads II and V_3 to V_5) and depressed (lead aVR) following the orientation of the T wave. The QRS–S-T junction is also displaced. See discussion in text.

Early Repolarization

A common repolarization variant seen in normal young adults is S–T segment displacement usually associated with tall or deep T waves. This pattern (Fig. 4–22) has been known as "early repolarization" and is not considered abnormal. As mentioned earlier, repolarization actually begins before the end of the QRS complex and is reflected in the patients with "early repolarization" by the frequent occurrence of QRS–S-T junction displacement. In these normal patients the mean T and S–T vectors are generally parallel. In Figure 4–22 the S–T segment is elevated (leads II, V_3 to V_5) and depressed (lead aVR) following the orientation of the T wave. Note the displacement of the QRS–S-T junction.

Of importance is the need to distinguish "early repolarization" from the more ominous causes of S–T segment displacement such as pericarditis and myocardial infarction. Distinguishing features of "early repolarization" include:

1. Clinical correlation: the patient is young and well.
2. The S–T segment displacement is associated with increased T wave magnitude.
3. Normal QRS–T angle.
4. The mean T and S–T vectors are generally parallel. The S–T segment is elevated with tall T waves and depressed with deep T waves.

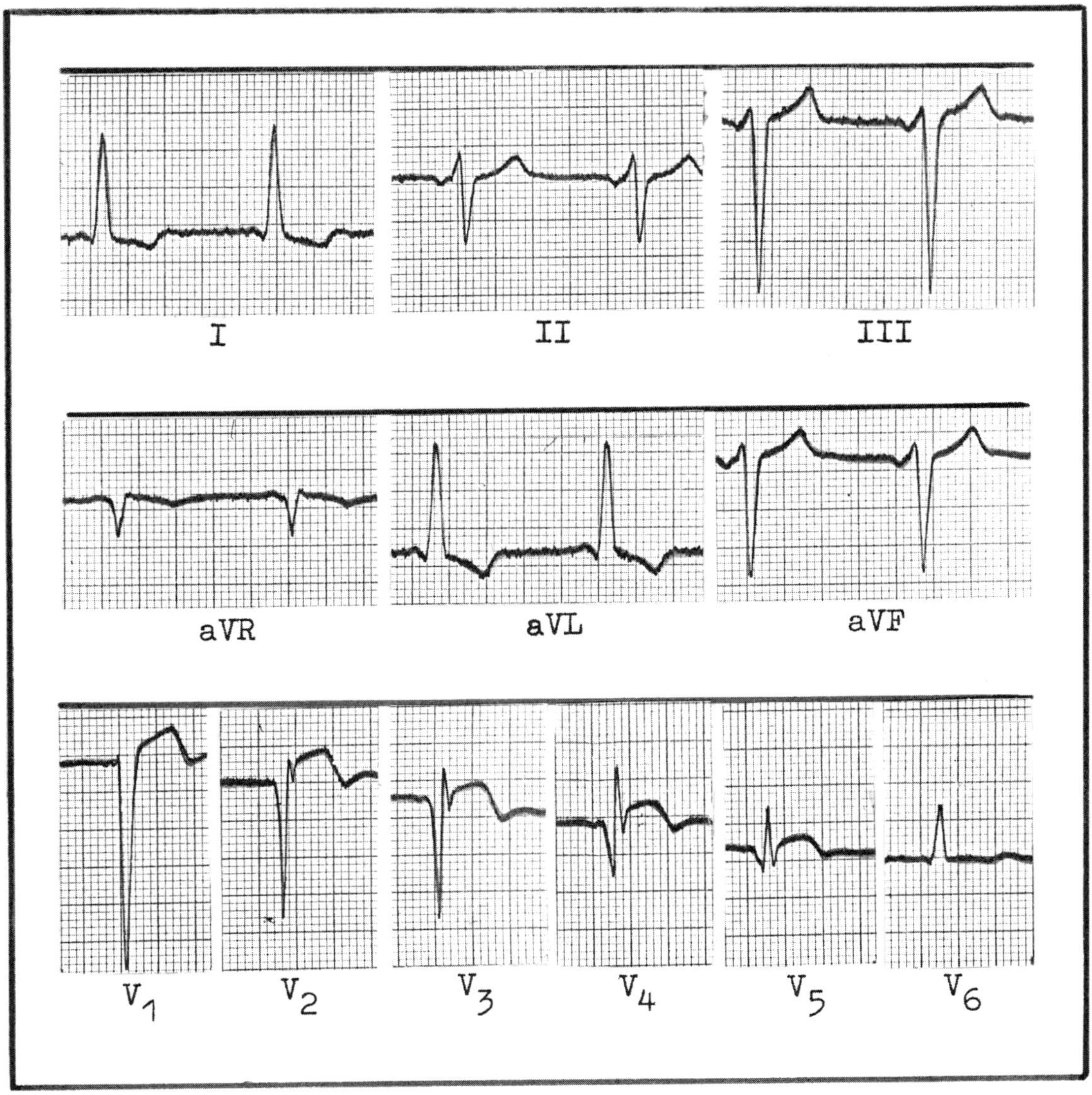

FIGURE 4–23. Repolarization abnormalities due to a ventricular aneurysm in a patient with an old myocardial infarction. See text. This patient also had a very large left ventricle. Note that the rhythm is not sinus.

Ventricular Aneurysm

Figure 4–23, from a patient with a ventricular aneurysm years after a myocardial infarction, illustrates one of the effects of myocardial infarction on ventricular repolarization. The persistent elevation of the S–T segment, described as a persistent "monophasic" curve of injury, represents a ventricular aneurysm, an outpouching of a section of scarred ventricular myocardium. The subject of myocardial infarction will be discussed in Chapter 5.

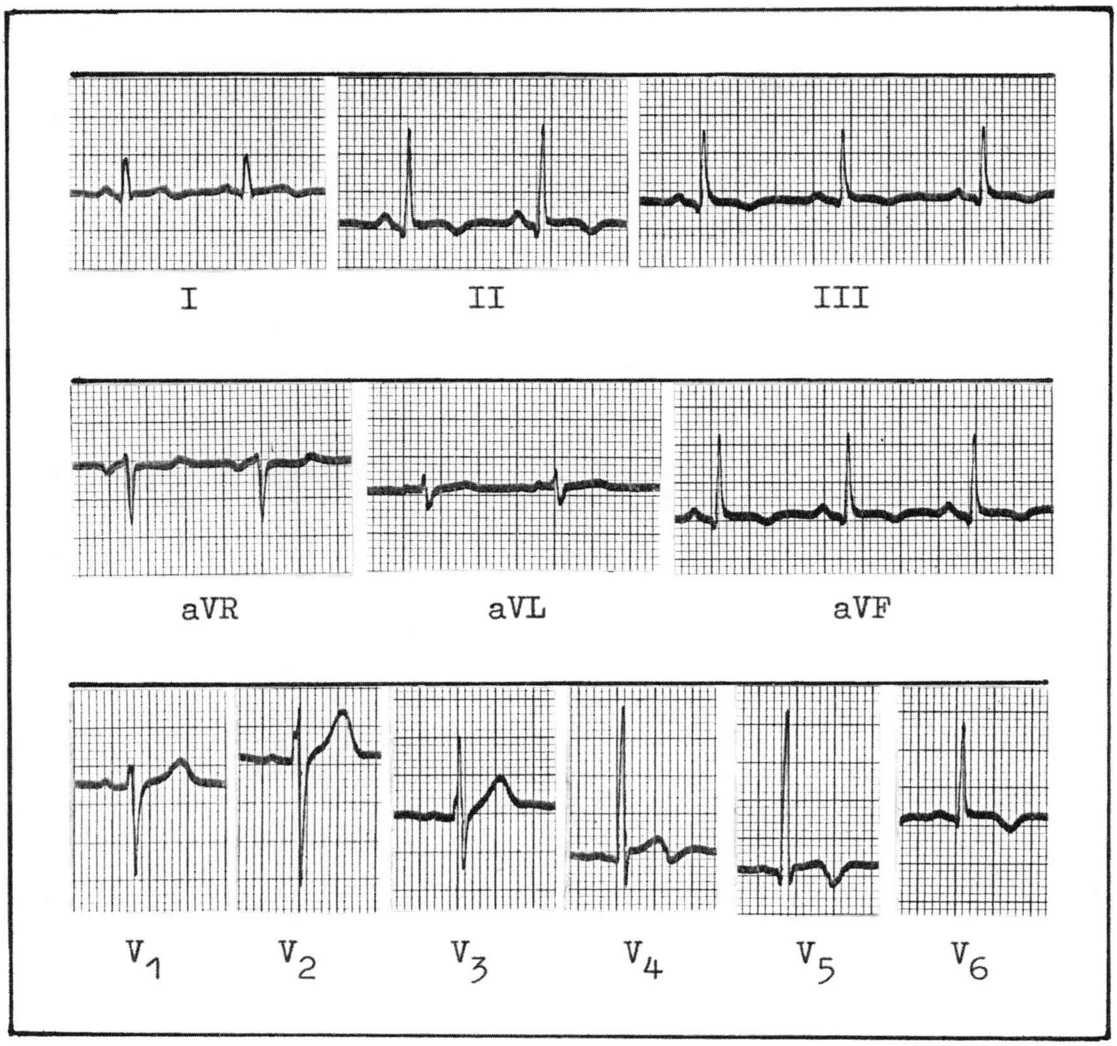

FIGURE 4–24. Repolarization abnormalities in a young patient with pericarditis. See text.

Pericarditis

Repolarization abnormalities in a patient with pericarditis is seen in Figure 4–24. Since the early part (S–T segment) of repolarization is affected, we should expect the abnormality, anatomically, to be in the epicardial area of the heart, nearest the pericardium. Often in the evolutionary serial electrocardiographic tracings the T wave (later repolarization) is also affected. Do not confuse this abnormal, changing, evolving pattern with "early repolarization" (Fig. 4–22) found in many normal, healthy young patients.

Clinical correlation must again be stressed since the pattern seen in Figure 4–24 may not be distinguishable from that of a patient with an acute myocardial infarction.

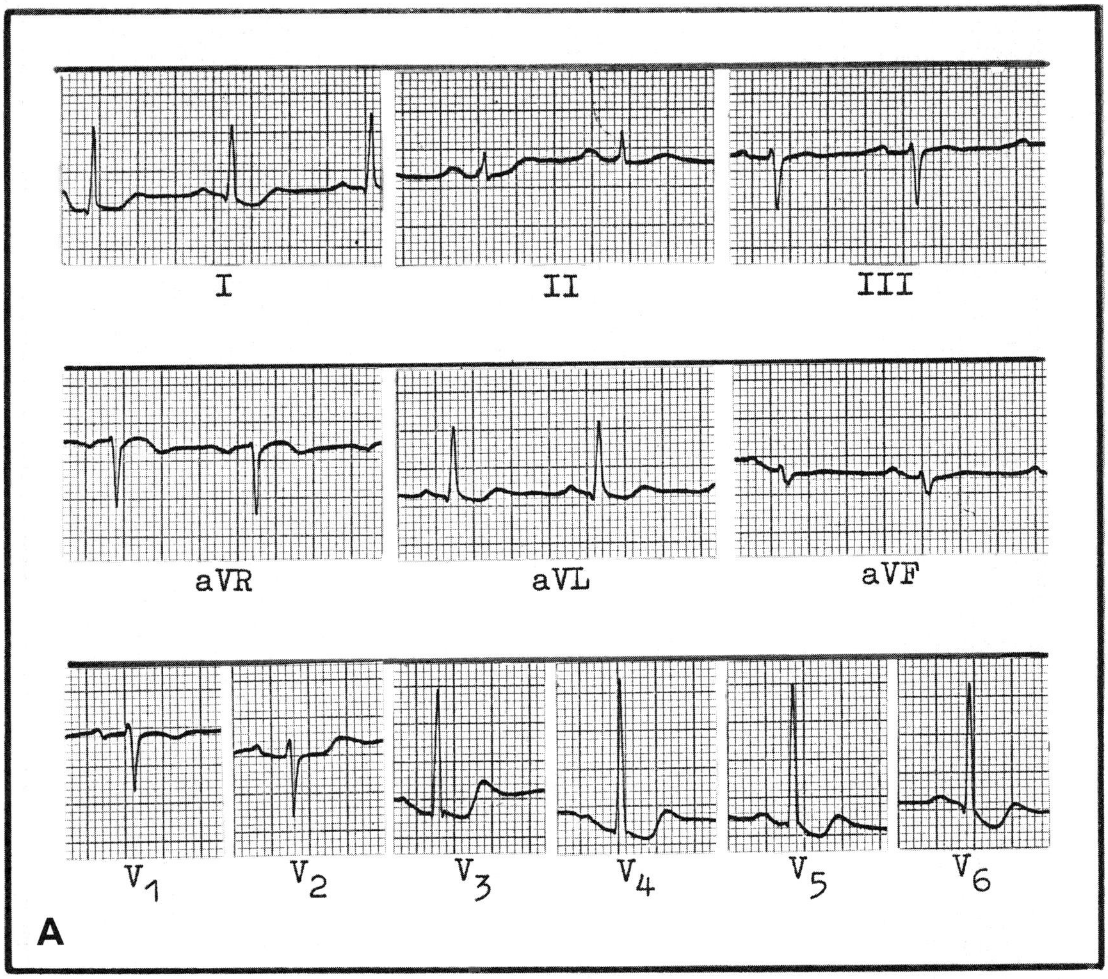

FIGURE 4–25. *A,* Describe the abnormal repolarization.
Illustration continued on opposite page.

Electrolyte Imbalance

Electrolyte imbalance is another common cause of ventricular repolarization abnormalities. If the imbalance is severe, *atrioventricular conduction* as well as *ventricular depolarization* may also be affected, as seen in Figure 4–25*B*. This elderly patient with borderline renal function, whose baseline abnormal electrocardiogram is seen in Figure 4–25*A*, tragically became severely *hyperkalemic*, requiring emergency hospitalization for dialysis.

In comparing Figures 4–25*A* and 4–25*B* note the changes in the:

1. QRS complex (ventricular depolarization).
2. S–T segment and T wave (ventricular repolarization).
3. P–R interval (atrioventricular conduction). The P waves are seen clearly in leads II, III and aVF in Figure 4–25*B*.

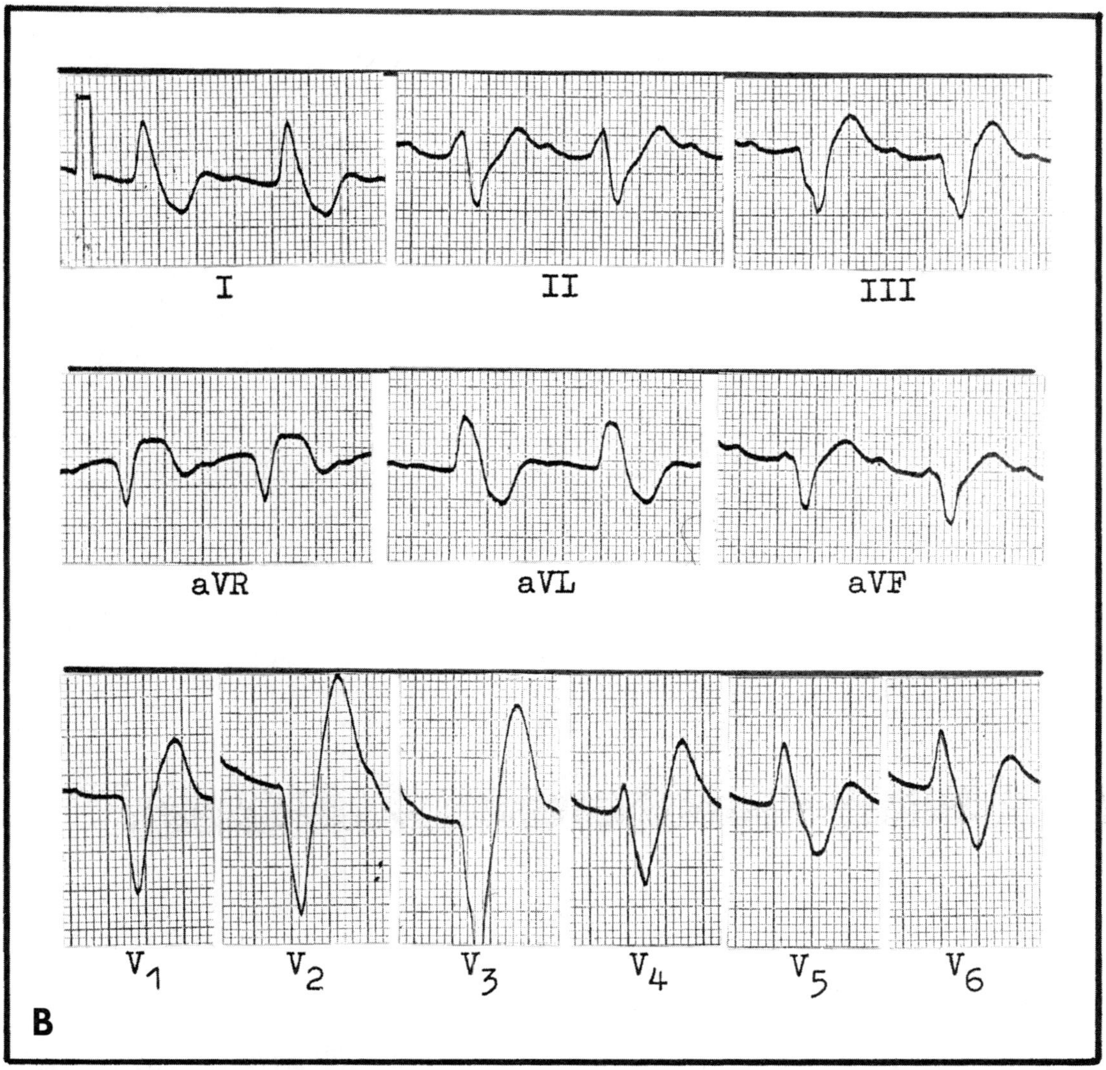

FIGURE 4–25 *Continued.* *B,* Hyperkalemic state in patient whose prior electrocardiogram was seen in Figure 4–25*A*. Describe the additional abnormalities seen here during repolarization, as well as during depolarization and atrioventricular conduction.

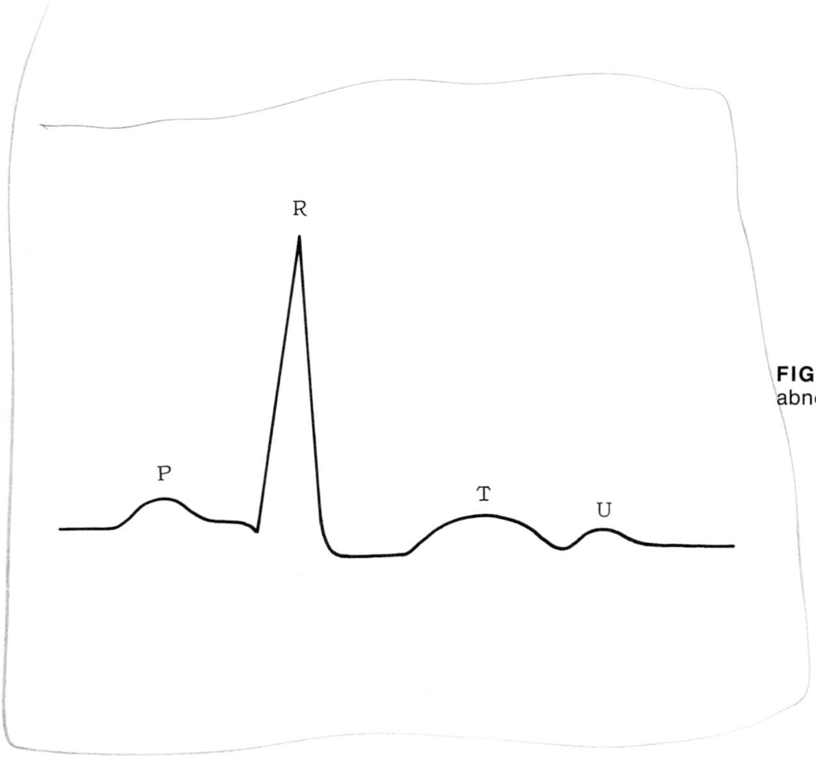

FIGURE 4–26. Electrocardiographic abnormalities with hypokalemia.

Hypokalemia may produce striking electrocardiographic abnormalities, such as depression of the S–T segment, lowering and flattening of the T wave and appearance of a U wave (Fig. 4–26). In Figure 4–27 there appears to be a prolonged Q–T interval in leads II, III, aVR and aVF. Leads V_2 and V_3, however, reveal the hypokalemic U wave on the descending limb of a flattened T wave.

It might be argued that the T wave is notched and that the Q–T interval is really prolonged, both of which may be seen in hypokalemia. Close electrocardiographic follow-up of the patient, while correcting the deficiency, would reveal that both the T and the U waves are present here. With improvement, the T wave gradually becomes taller and the U wave gradually disappears.

Figure 4–28 reveals the striking *prolongation of the Q–T interval* in a patient with long-standing *hypocalcemia*. The heart rate of the patient is 84 per minute. At this rate the Q–T interval should be 0.34 sec., rather than 0.48 sec., as seen here. Refer back to Chapter 1 for the relationship between the Q–T interval and the heart rate. *Hypercalcemia* is often represented electrocardiographically by a short Q–T interval. There is an inverse relationship between the Q–T interval and the level of serum calcium.

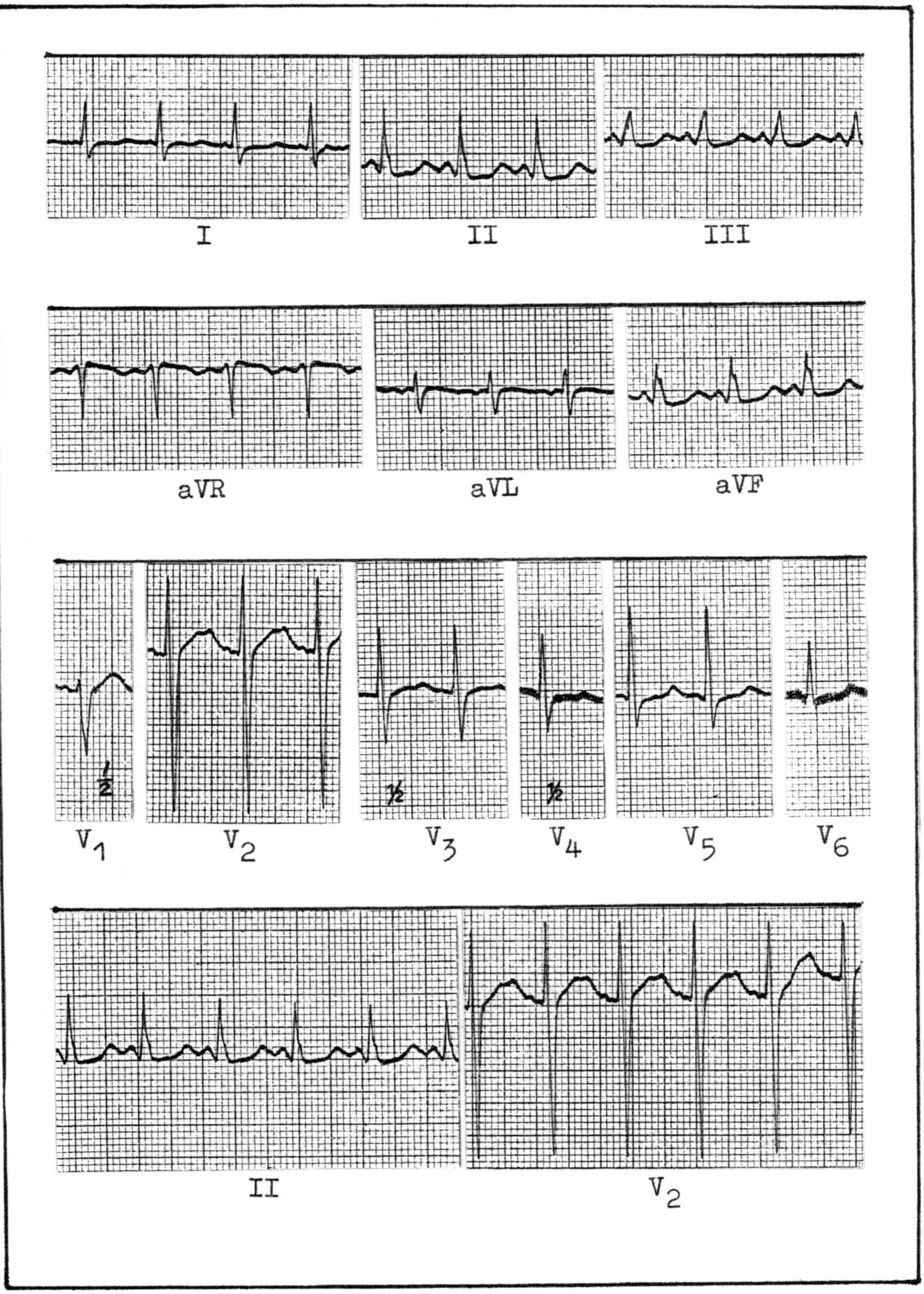

FIGURE 4–27. Hypokalemia in a patient with sinus tachycardia. See text. Leads V_1, V_3 and V_4 are one half standard.

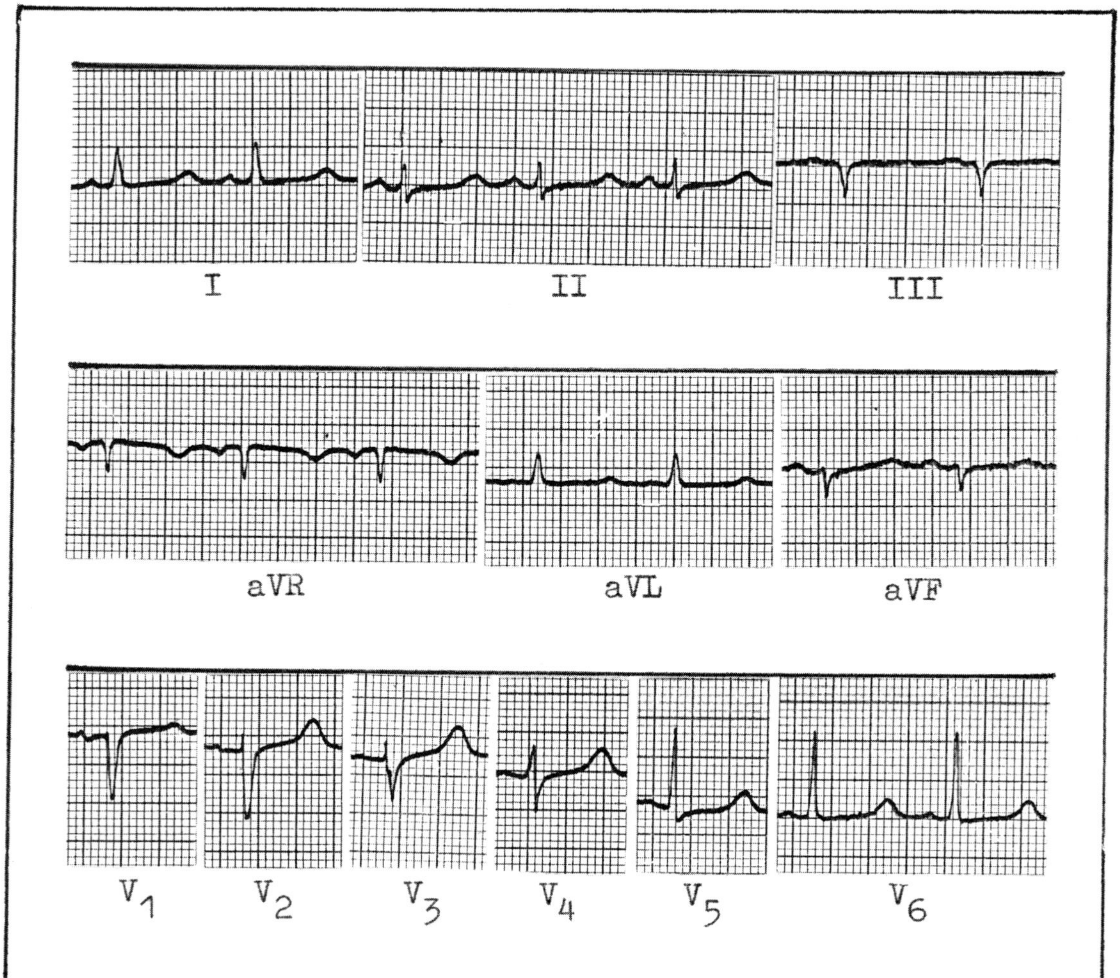

FIGURE 4–28. Hypocalcemia of long standing in an elderly patient. See text.

Atrial Enlargement

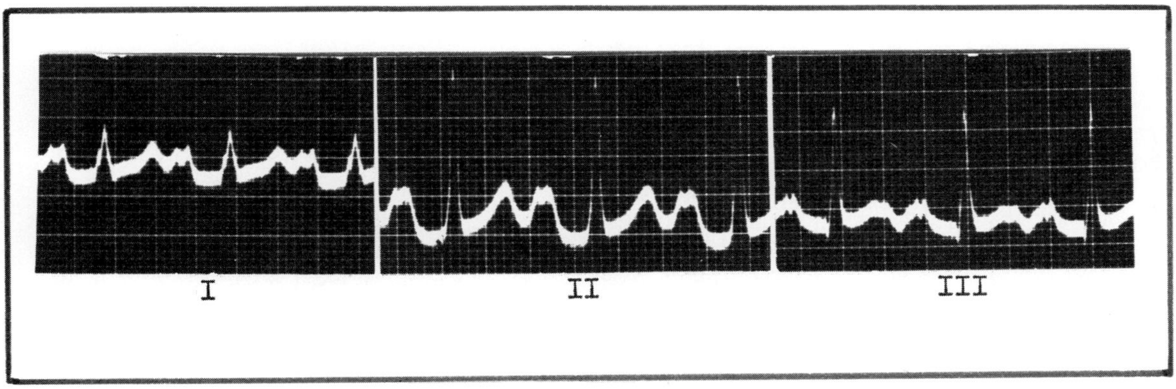

FIGURE 4–29. Left atrial enlargement and first degree atrioventricular block in a patient with mitral stenosis. See text.
(Electrocardiogram slightly enlarged.)

ATRIAL REPOLARIZATION

Although the subject of this chapter is repolarization of the ventricles, atrial repolarization must not be neglected. This is usually not evident on the clinical electrocardiogram because the P wave itself is relatively small and is quickly followed by the prominent QRS complex. Under special circumstances parts of the atrial repolarization phase may be seen as in Figure 4–29. There is:

1. Atrial enlargement. Note the size of the P wave in lead II.

2. A wide P–R interval, first degree atrioventricular block, which gives us the opportunity to see an abnormally depressed "S–T segment" of the P wave. Normal atrial repolarization does not produce an S–T segment depression of this magnitude (lead II).

Always look for abnormalities in atrial repolarization; you may find clues not seen anywhere else in the electrocardiogram. An example of this is seen in Figure 4–30, which is a precordial lead in a patient with myocardial infarction involving the atria. The patient had evidence of myocardial infarction, including elevated blood enzyme levels. No Q waves nor ventricular repolarization abnormalities developed. The only striking change was the depressed "S–T segment" of the P wave. Among the causes of abnormal atrial repolarization are: atrial enlargement, pericarditis involving the atria, myocardial infarction involving the atria, manipulation and injury to the atria during open heart surgery.

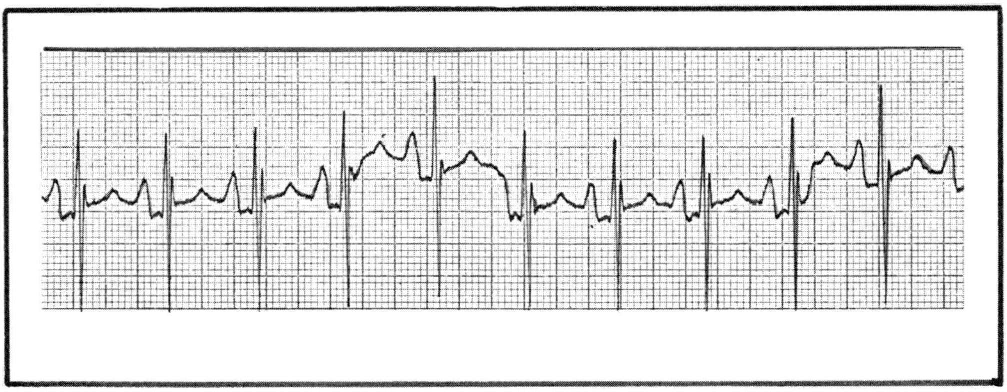

FIGURE 4–30. Abnormal atrial repolarization in a patient with myocardial infarction involving the atria. See text.

"MARCH OF THE ARROWS" CONCEPT

The emphasis in this course has always been on the concept rather than on memorized patterns and normal values. Since the study of ventricular repolarization is so closely related to coronary heart disease, the "march of the arrows" concept (Fig. 4–31) will be introduced at this point, prior to the actual study of myocardial infarction. The natural history of coronary heart disease may be considered according to this concept. The assumption is made that at least 40 per cent of functioning myocardium is needed for asymptomatic, full activity (this is only an assumption; it may or may not be accurate). The 100-per cent starting point represents birth. As a person matures and ages, the arrows continue to march inexorably toward the 0 point.

Panel A (Fig. 4–31A). A man had reached the age of 95 years with 50 per cent of his myocardium fibrosed. He had been asymptomatic, that is, with no chest pain nor shortness of breath. He did not run around a football field but did whatever a 95 year old man wished to do. At postmortem examination his heart was small and the coronary arteries were markedly narrowed, but not occluded. Many were amazed that he had been able to function so well with so much myocardial destruction.

Panel B (Fig. 4–31B). A 50 year old man was asymptomatic until he suffered a myocardial infarction a year ago. He never recovered fully and has continued to have both angina pectoris and shortness of breath on effort. There was enough myocardial destruction resulting from the infarct to cross the bar at 40 per cent. The arrows have continued to march with time and symptoms have been progressive.

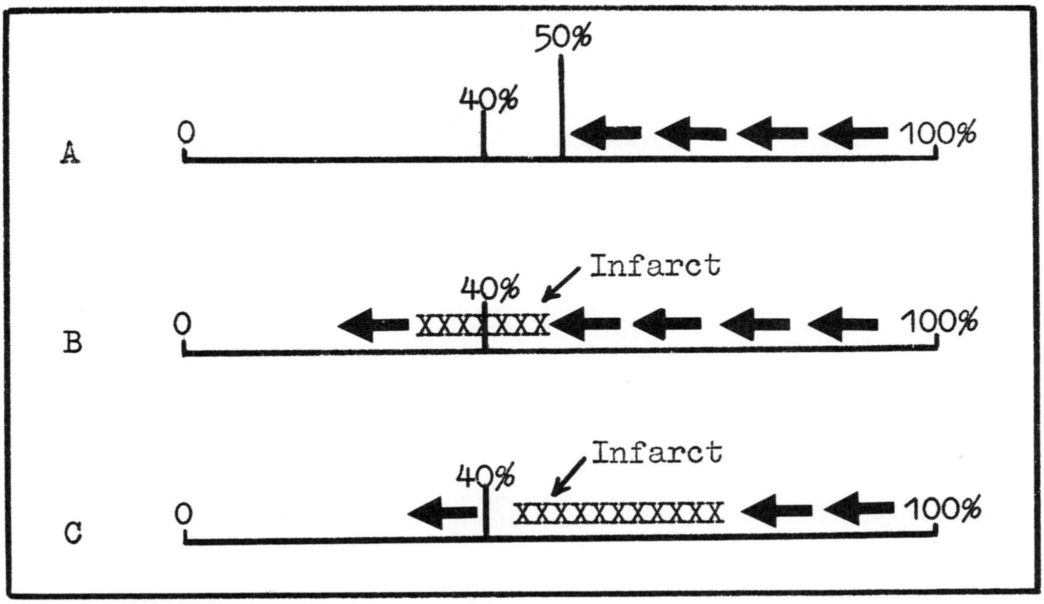

FIGURE 4–31. The "march of the arrows" concept in coronary heart disease. See text.

Panel C (Fig. 4–31C). A 60 year old man had had a massive myocardial infarction at age 58. He recovered fully and was asymptomatic for about one year. During the following year he began to experience both chest pain and shortness of breath. This panel shows that the infarction caused substantial myocardial destruction, but the bar at 40 per cent had still not been crossed. The crossing took place at a later date coinciding with the onset of symptoms. The infarction hastened the process.

This concept, which may be applied to other organ systems, and which permits you to see change in an orderly fashion, may appear oversimplified; it is. The process is far more complex, and hidden within it are the secrets of aging. There are those who stand at a podium and give you all the answers; I am merely raising some of the questions. Why does one individual proceed so rapidly along the path to disaster while another has relatively little difficulty? Where are you along this road?

We have discussed a number of entities affecting repolarization; you will learn many more as you continue with electrocardiography. Based on the material learned to date you will now analyze Figures 4–32 to 4–40.

REVIEW ELECTROCARDIOGRAMS (FIGURES 4–32 TO 4–40)

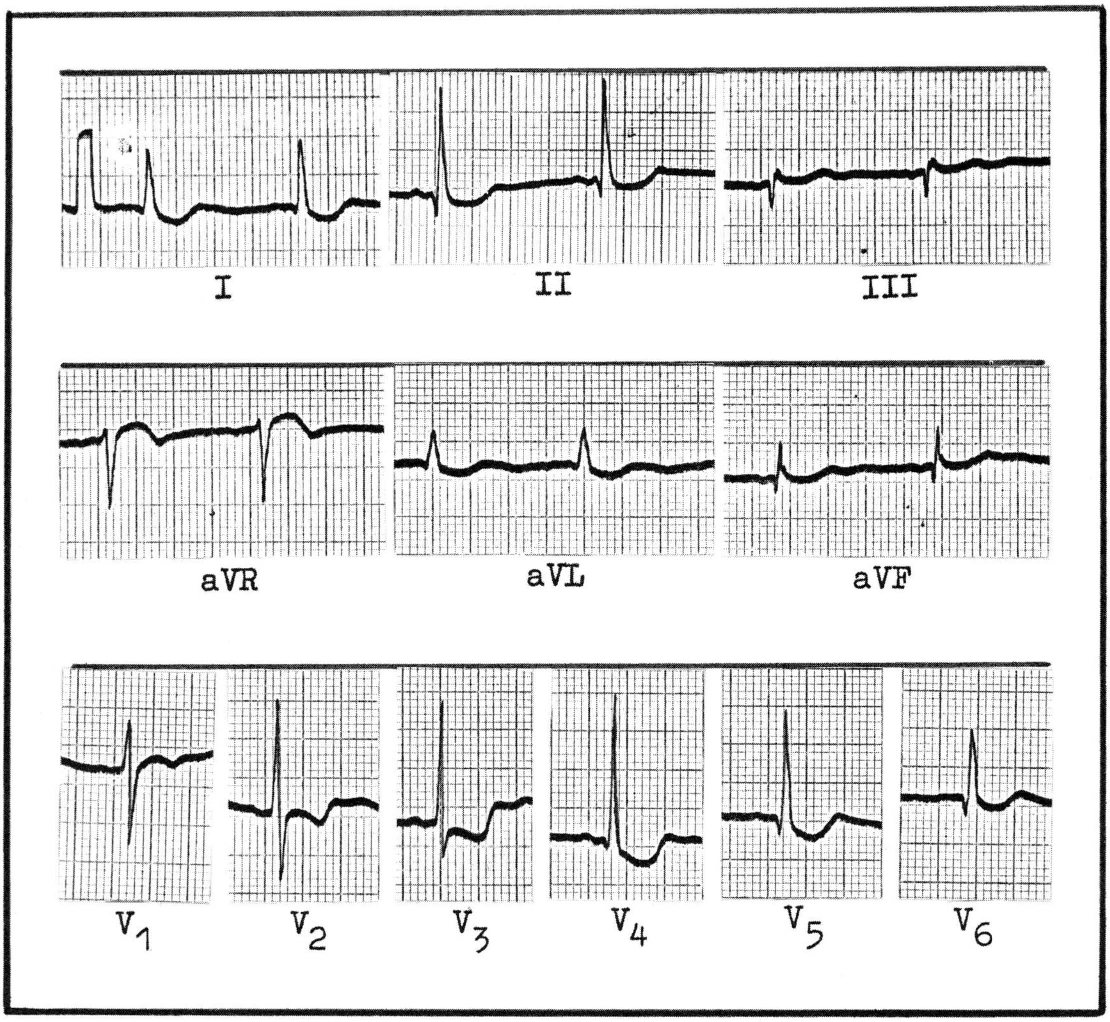

FIGURE 4–32. Describe the repolarization abnormalities. Can you state with absolute certainty, from this one electrocardiogram, that all the repolarization abnormalities are due to digitalis?

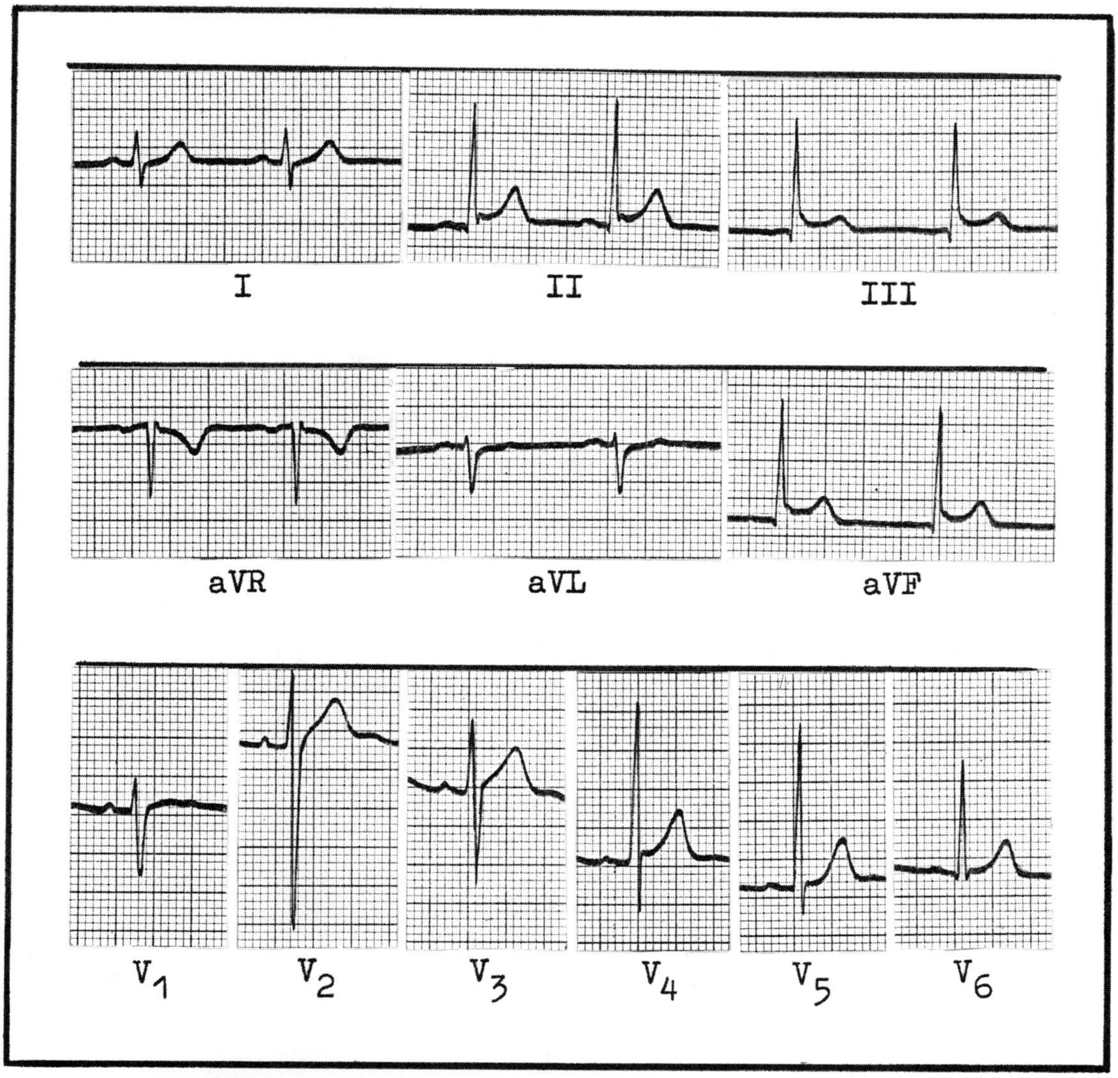

FIGURE 4–33. Analyze this electrocardiogram from a healthy 18 year old student.

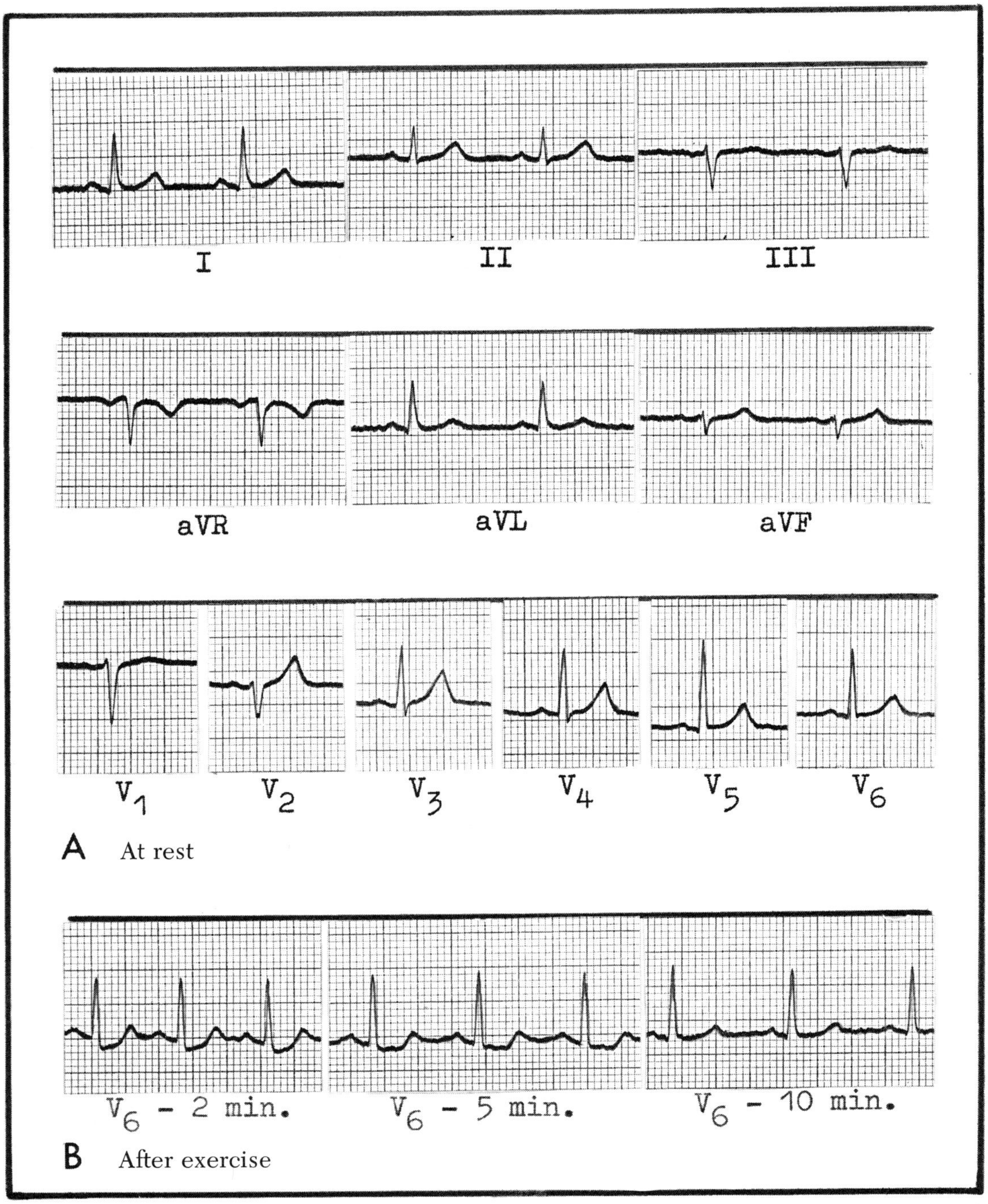

FIGURE 4–34. *A,* At rest; *B,* after exercise. What changes have occurred in repolarization after exercise in this patient with a history of angina pectoris?

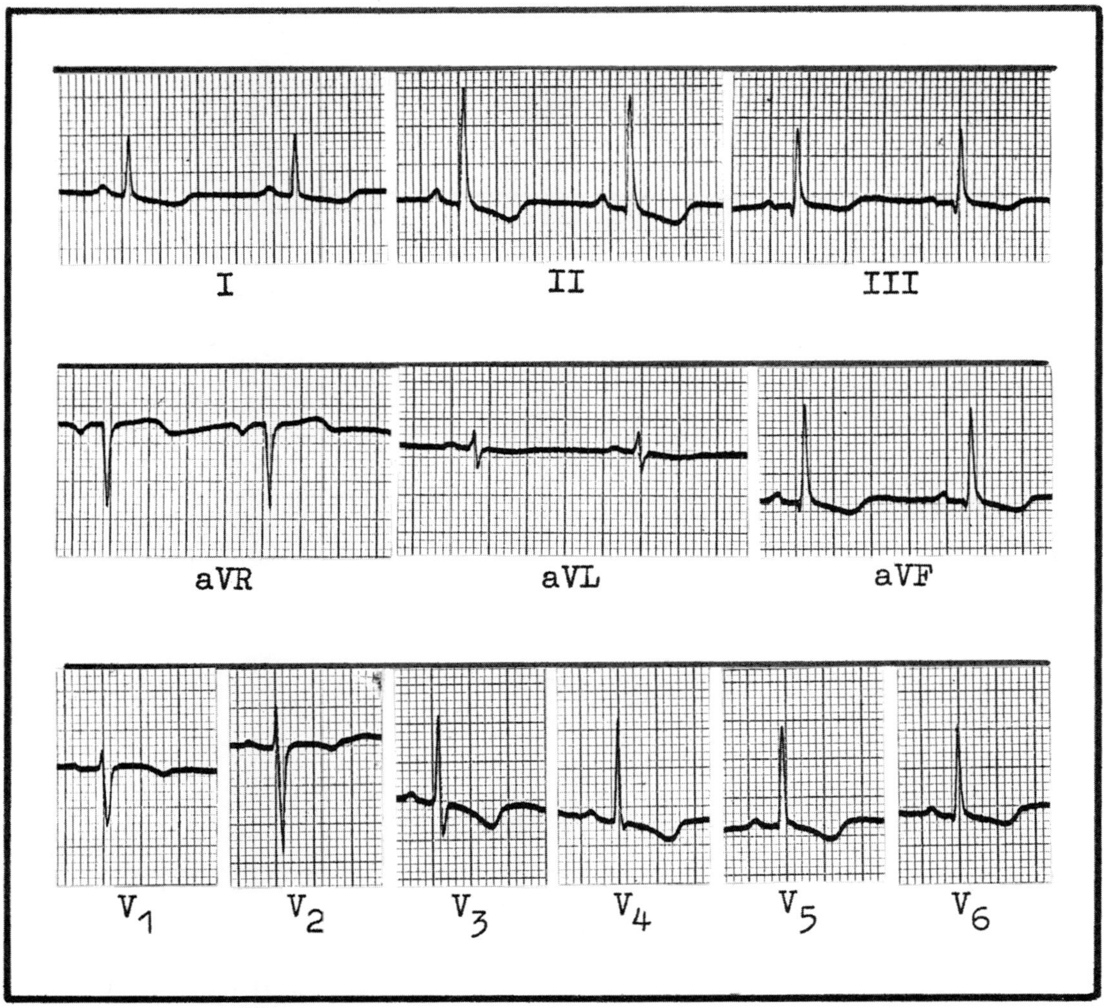

FIGURE 4-35. Abnormal repolarization (nonspecific) in a middle-aged, asymptomatic patient with a normal sized heart. This patient may have coronary heart disease; the diagnosis, however, should not be made from the electrocardiogram alone.

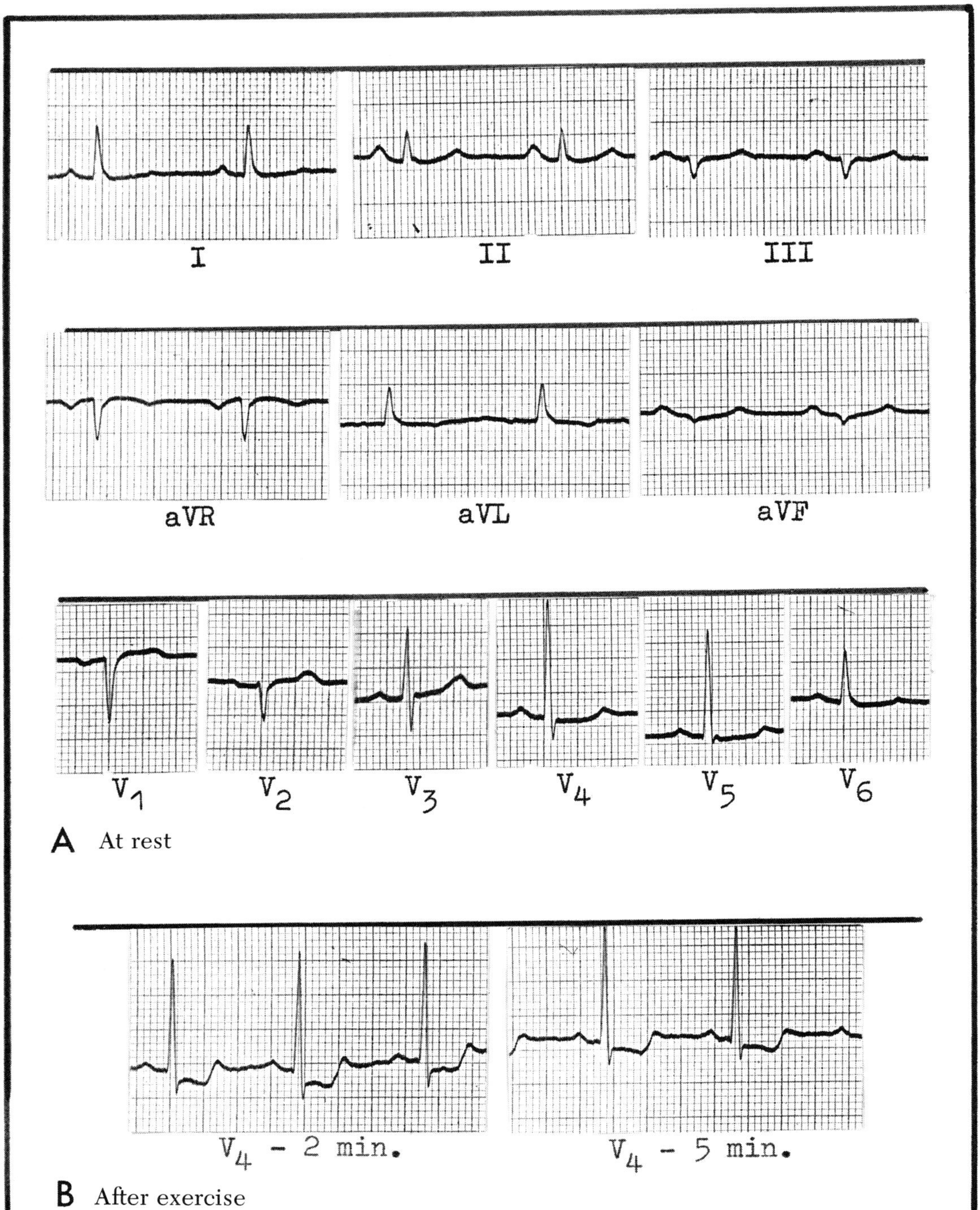

FIGURE 4–36. *A,* At rest; *B,* after exercise. What changes have occurred following activity in this patient with a history of coronary heart disease?

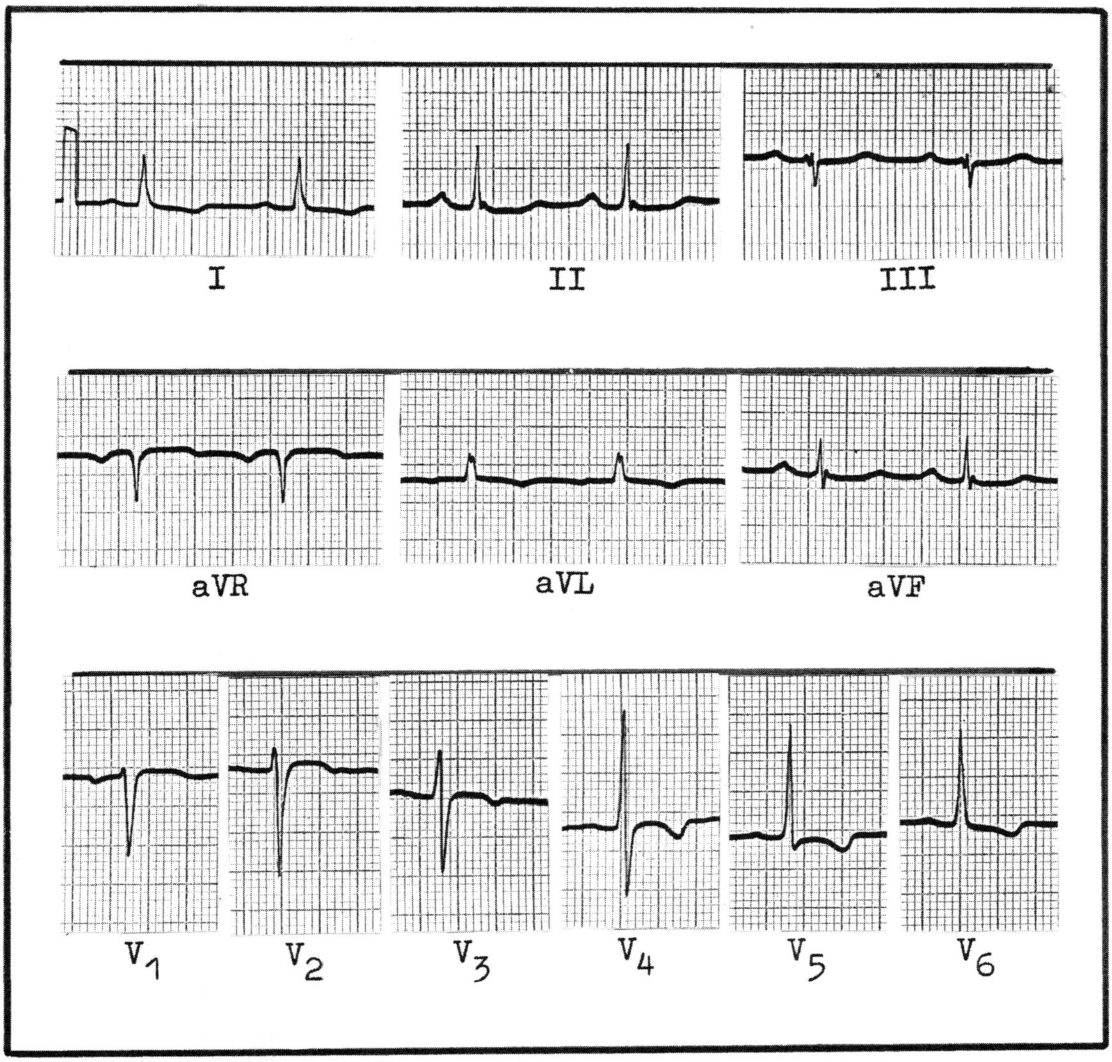

FIGURE 4–37. Abnormal repolarization (nonspecific) in a middle-aged, asymptomatic patient with a normal sized heart.

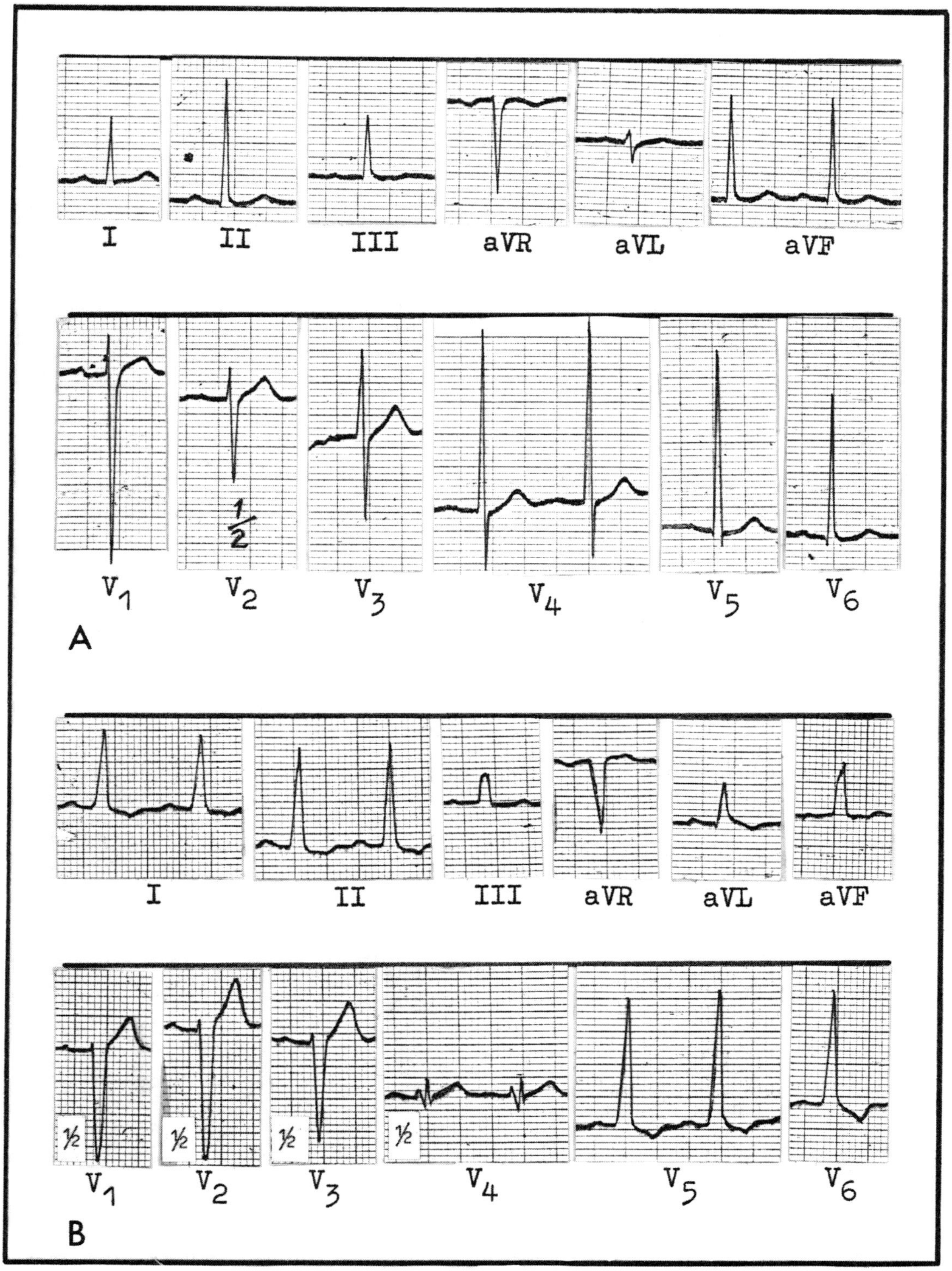

FIGURE 4–38. What changes are seen as this patient alternates between "normal" conduction and left bundle branch block (a ventricular conduction disturbance)? Are the S–T segment and T wave abnormalities in *B primary* or *secondary*?

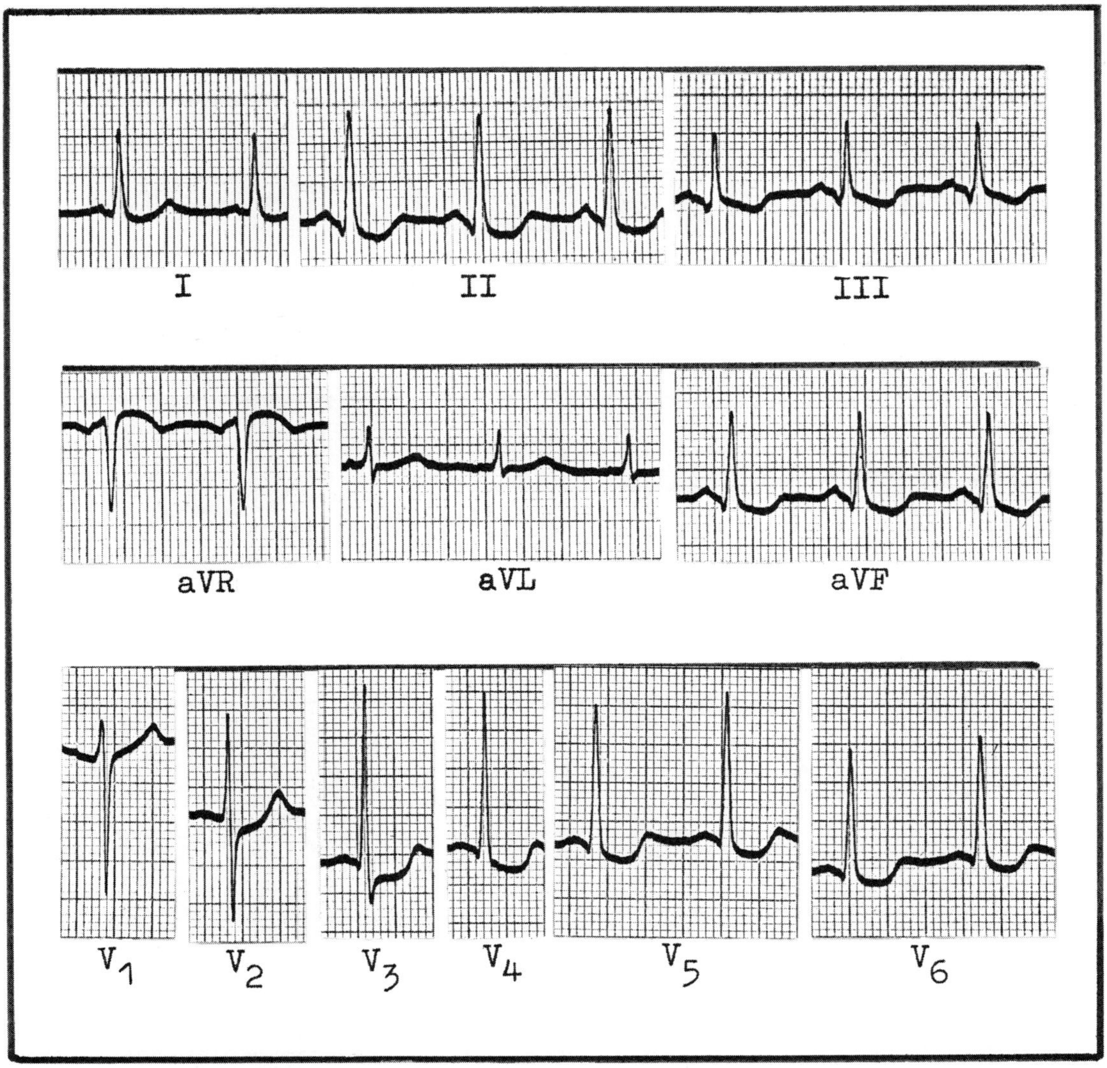

FIGURE 4–39. Repolarization abnormalities in a patient on digitalis. Judging from this one electrocardiogram, was the electrocardiogram prior to digitalization normal?

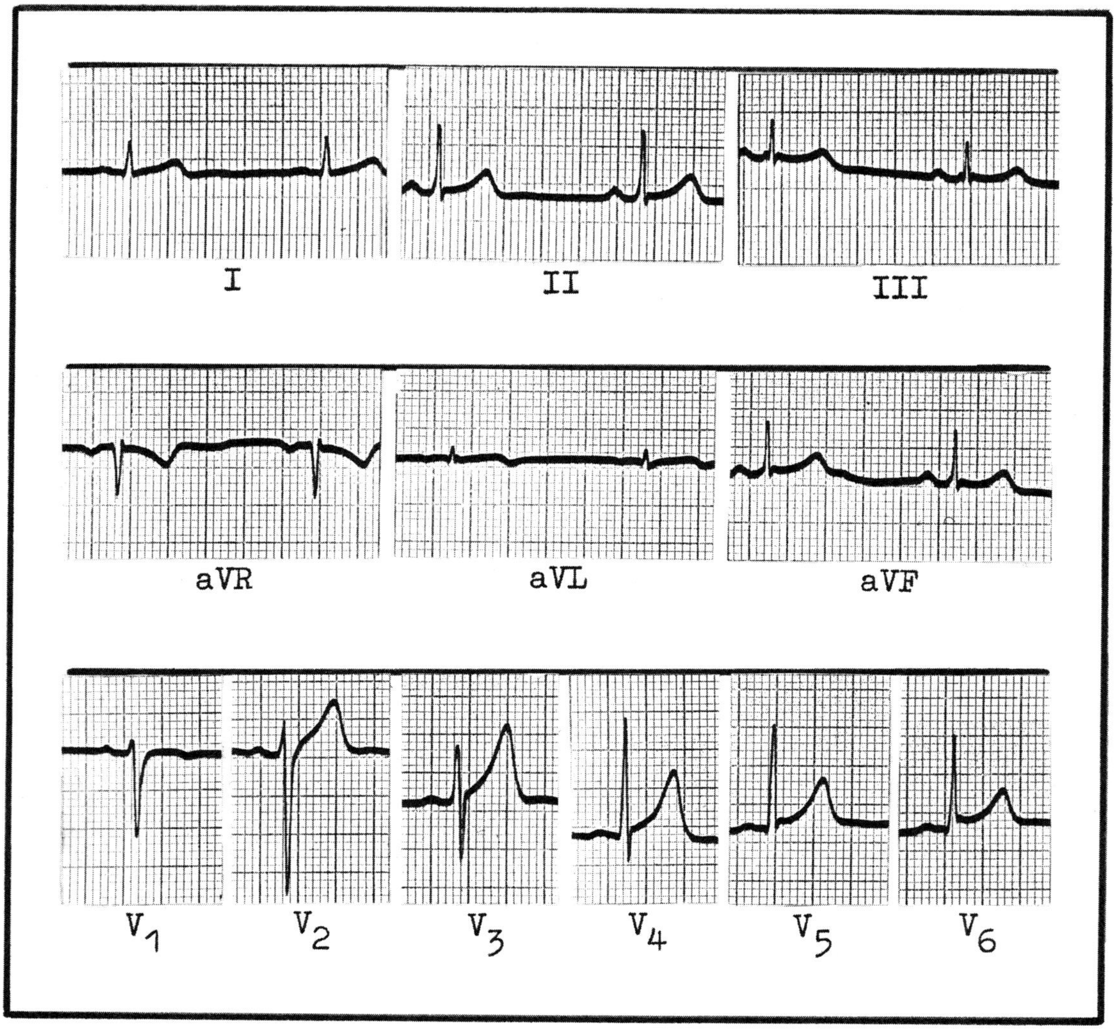

FIGURE 4–40. "Early repolarization" in a normal young man.

5

MYOCARDIAL INFARCTION

Cassette Side 11

MYOCARDIAL INFARCTION—INTRODUCTION AND A FEW WORDS OF CAUTION

Nowhere in the entire study of electrocardiography should the failings of the clinical electrocardiogram be emphasized more than in the study of myocardial infarction. Nowhere have diagnoses been made with such erudition and such explicitness, only to be shown to be completely wrong on examination of the heart. Myocardial infarction, from the smallest infarct to the most extensively scarred heart, may be manifest on the clinical electrocardiogram by:

1. No abnormalities.
2. "Nonspecific" abnormalities.
3. "Classical" abnormalities.

Especially does this problem arise in the case of multiple infarctions. Which came before which and where are they located? Conceivably, the balance of vectorial forces resulting from multiple infarctions may deceptively "normalize" the electrocardiogram.

There are three "nevers" which must always be kept in mind.

1. Never finalize the age of an infarct from a single electrocardiogram.

2. Never prognosticate as to the outcome of the myocardial infarction from a single electrocardiogram. So many patients with normal electrocardiograms are ill, while others with the most striking electrocardiographic abnormalities are well clinically. The electrocardiogram in a state of flux, such as occurs with infarction of the heart, should be studied sequentially. Always ask for serial electrocardiograms.

3. Never allow the electrocardiogram to be anything more than an adjunct to the practice of medicine, as has already been stressed. It can never replace clinical acumen.

With these limitations in mind, the "classical" findings associated with myocardial infarction will now be studied. These "classical" electrocardiographic patterns are shown in Figure 5–1. The early electrocardiographers were wont to illustrate these electrocardiographic patterns associated with infarction of the heart as follows: the *Q wave, elevated S–T segment* and *inverted T wave*. The Q wave

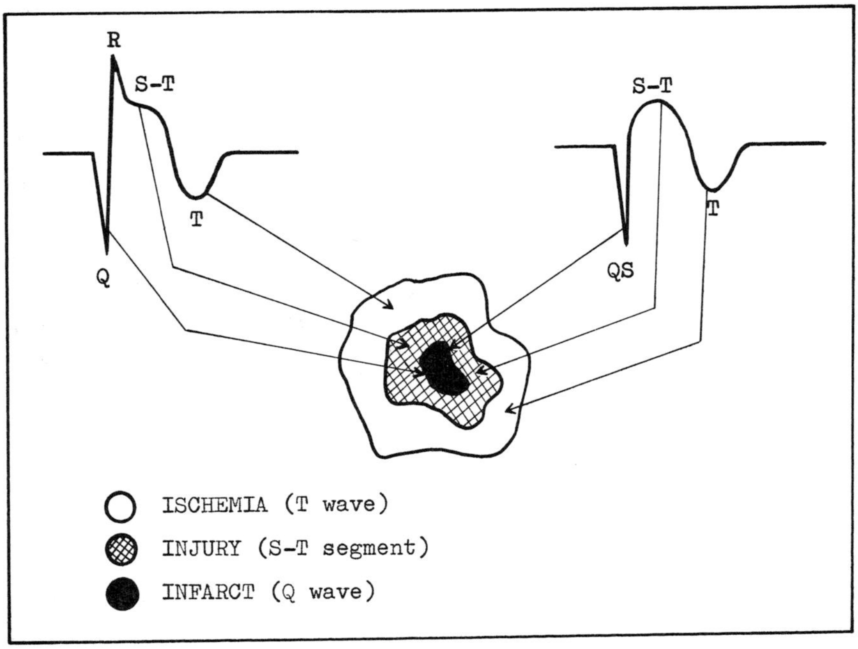

FIGURE 5–1. "Classical" electrocardiographic patterns of myocardial infarction.

(or QS complex, if there was no R wave) represented infarction, the elevated S–T segment signified injury, and the inverted T wave, ischemia. The accompanying diagram would show a dead zone surrounded by zones of injury and ischemia.

A myocardial infarction is not, however, needed to show all the "classical" findings of infarction. The electrocardiographic tracing in Figure 5–2 was recorded during an electrocardiographically monitored therapeutic pericardiocentesis. The arrows point to the two complexes recorded when the tip of the needle "touched" the epicardium. Obviously, this did not represent myocardial infarction, although all the features described were present. As soon as the needle was withdrawn a minute distance, the normal processes ensued. We are using this example in spite of the fact that it could be argued that we are dealing with a different process. Depolarization and repolarization were altered because of epicardial "touching" of the heart. This example is offered merely to show that a myocardial infarc-

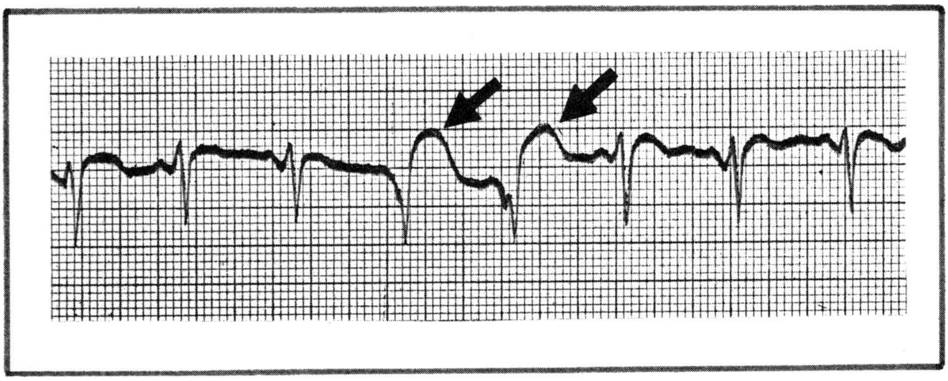

FIGURE 5–2. Electrocardiogram during pericardiocentesis.

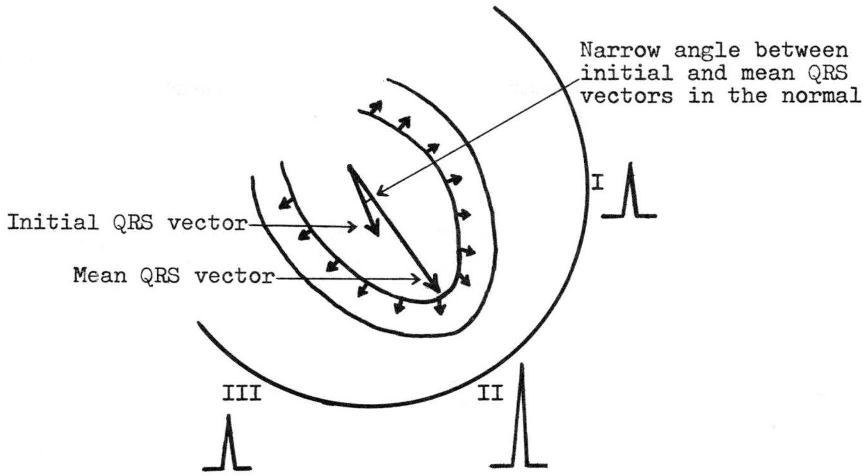

FIGURE 5–3. Narrow angle between the initial QRS vector (initial 0.04 sec. vector) and mean QRS vector (the entire 0.08 sec. vector) in the normal.

tion is not needed to produce all the "classical" electrocardiographic manifestations.

On a vectorial basis, infarction of the heart may be studied as follows:

A. Initial QRS vector abnormalities—the formation of the Q wave.

B. Repolarization abnormalities (abnormalities of the S–T segment and T wave).

C. Terminal QRS vector abnormalities.

Before beginning the study of initial QRS vector abnormalities, and the formation of the Q wave, turn to Figure 5–3. This illustration, of the left ventricle, shows the relationship between the initial QRS vector (the first 0.04 sec. vector) and the mean QRS vector (the mean vector of the entire QRS complex, the 0.08 sec. vector) in the *normal*. The mean QRS vector in the normal is to the left and inferior (Chapter 1) and depolarization of the ventricles, as already seen, proceeds from endocardium to epicardium. If we study the initial QRS vector, the first 0.04 sec. vector of the QRS (the first part of the QRS, written within one small box on the

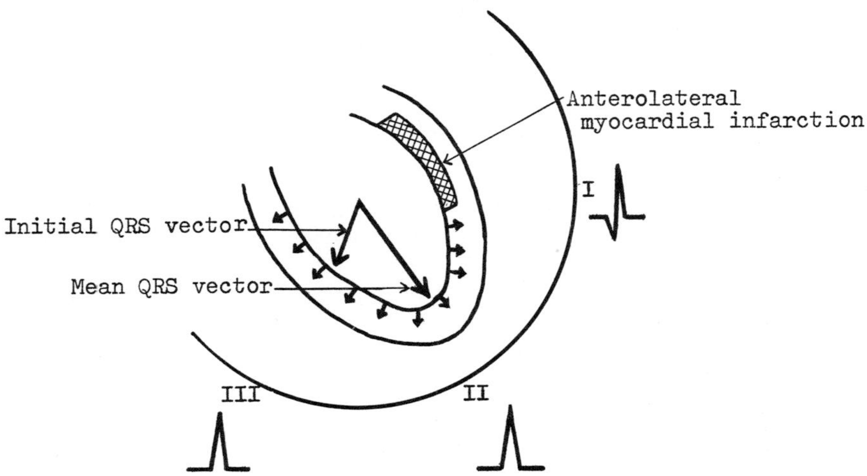

FIGURE 5–4. Disturbance of the initial QRS vector as a result of myocardial infarction.

electrocardiogram), we find that the angle between it and the mean QRS vector is *narrow*.

EFFECTS OF MYOCARDIAL INFARCTION

A. Initial QRS Vector Abnormalities —The Formation of the Q Wave in Myocardial Infarction

Although an area of left ventricular myocardium is infarcted (Fig. 5–4, shaded area), the *mean QRS vector* may not be changed. Compare Figures 5–3 and 5–4. Due to the interference with early depolarization caused by the infarct, there is a shift of the *initial* vector. The small arrows in Figure 5–4, representing the initial vector, tend to summate *away* from the area of infarction. This example shows an infarct which is on the anterolateral surface of the heart; the initial vector faces *away* from lead I, hence the Q wave.

The Q wave *does not* represent a "hole" in the heart; it represents initial vectorial forces going away from the electrode at the point of recording. The Q wave of significance is frequently at least 0.04 sec. in duration (one small box) and from one fourth to one third the size of the QRS complex.

Note: The diagram in Figure 5–4 (as well as the diagrams in other chapters) is presented to explain a concept and may not represent strict anatomic accuracy. For example, the infarction in this diagram is shown to be on the endocardial surface of the heart. Some good experimental evidence shows that there must be some epicardial involvement with the infarction in order to have Q waves. Of importance is the concept; once you learn the concept you can incorporate new information with greater ease.

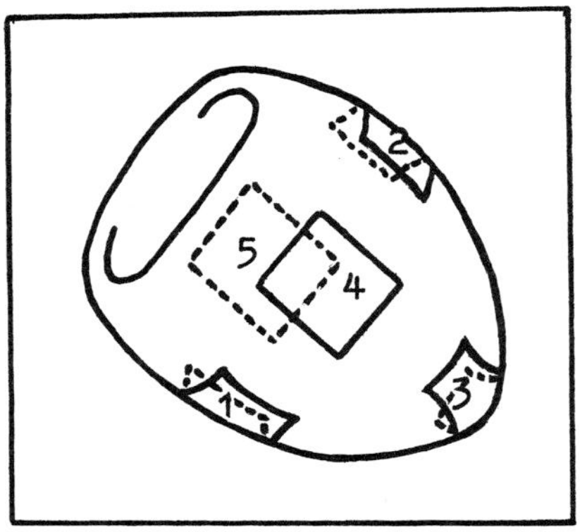

FIGURE 5–5. Division of the left ventricle into five regions, as shown by Grant, where infarction may occur. These regions are as follows:
1. Diaphragmatic or inferior.
2. Anterolateral.
3. Apical.
4. Strictly anterior or anteroseptal.
5. Strictly (true) posterior.

(Redrawn from J. R. Beckwith, *Grant's Clinical Electrocardiography*. New York, Blakiston Division, McGraw-Hill Book Company, 1970. Used by permission.)

The left ventricle is divided into five regions, as illustrated in Figure 5–5, where infarction may occur.

Overlapping is, however, more the rule than the exception. For ease of understanding the concept we will study infarction of the left ventricle since this site is most prone to infarction. That is not to say that infarcts do not occur in the right ventricle or in the atria. In Chapter 4 you studied an electrocardiogram in which the only electrocardiographic sign of myocardial infarction was abnormal atrial repolarization.

An initial QRS vector pointing away from some area of the left ventricle reveals an infarct in that area.

1. Diaphragmatic or inferior myocardial infarction is seen in Figure 5–6*B* and diagrammed in Figure 5–6*A*. The initial QRS vector faces away from the diaphragmatic area of the heart, hence there are Q waves in leads II and III.

2. Anterolateral myocardial infarction is illustrated in Figure 5–7. The initial QRS vector, pointing away from the anterolateral myocardial infarction, produces Q waves in leads I and aVL.

3. In Figure 5–8*B*, Q waves are present in leads I, II, III and aVF. A question should arise. Did one myocardial infarction produce these abnormalities (such as an apical infarct, diagrammed in Fig. 5–8*A*), or are they the result of *more than one infarction at different times*? Figure 5–8*C* was taken just prior to the infarction which brought about the changes seen in Figure 5–8*B*. Close patient follow-up and serial electrocardiograms are of great help.

Text continued on page 204.

1. Diagraphmatic or Inferior Myocardial Infarction

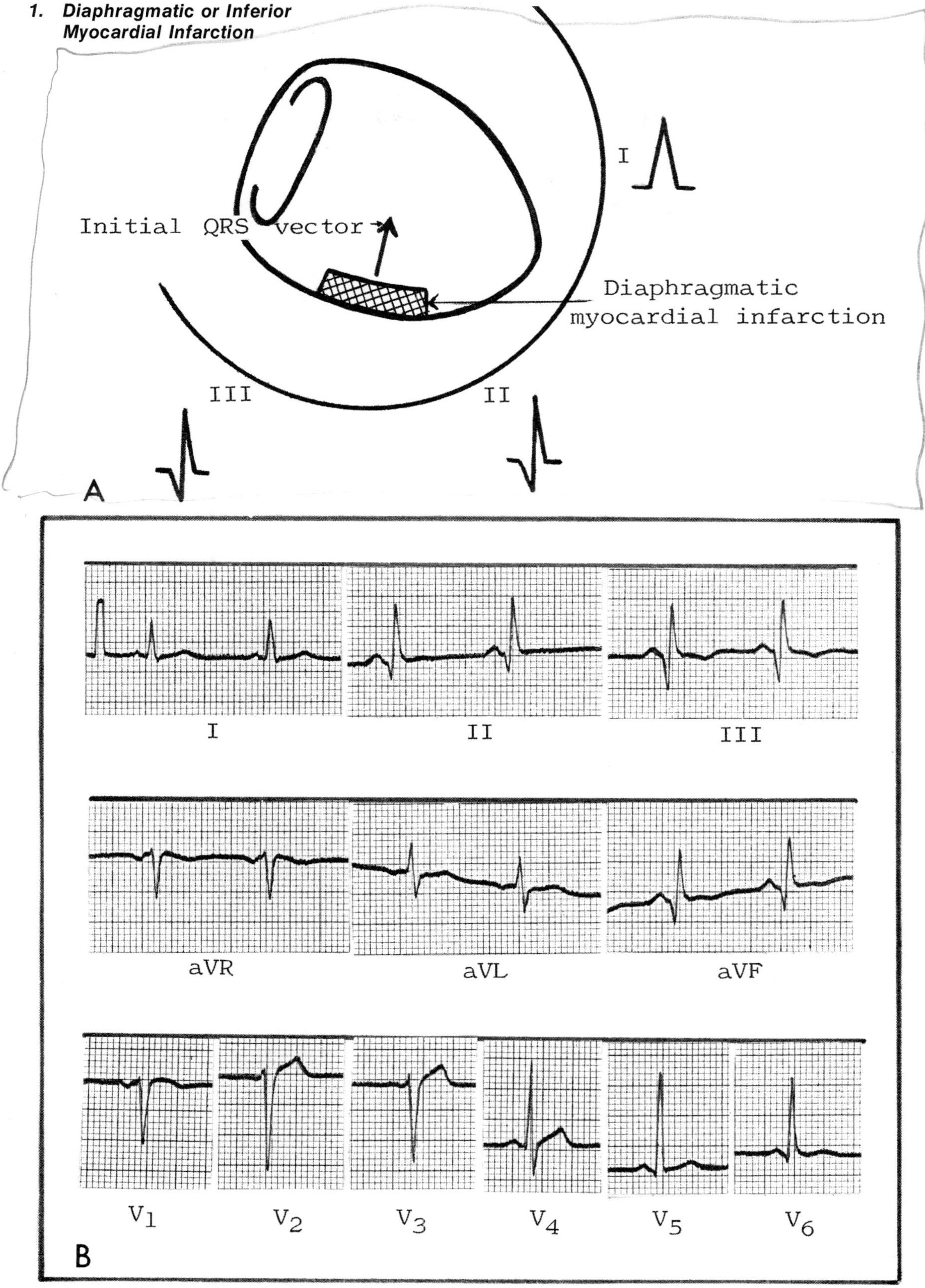

FIGURE 5–6. Diaphragmatic myocardial infarction. Q waves are seen in leads II and III since the initial vector of depolarization faces away from these leads.

2. *Anterolateral Myocardial Infarction*

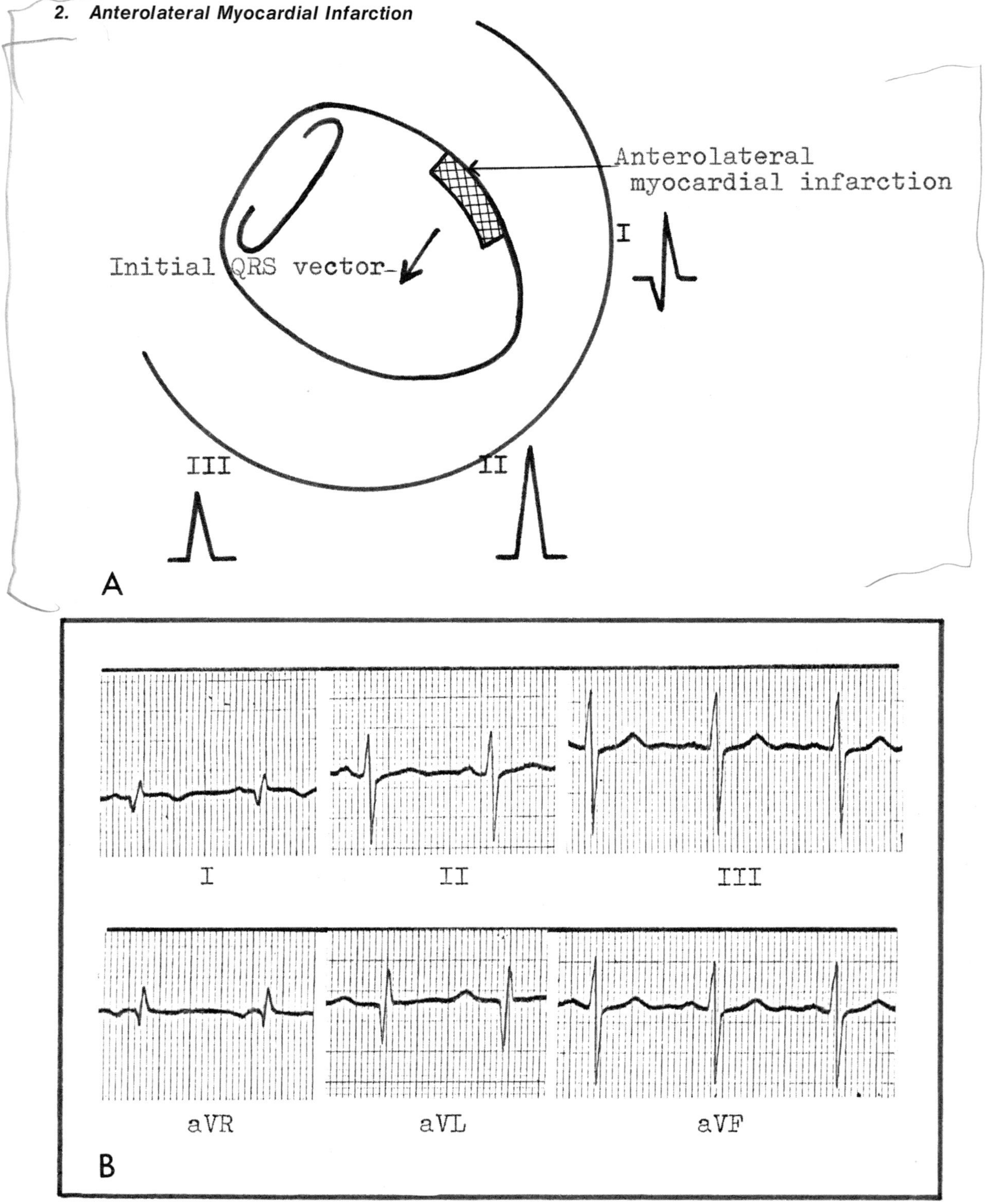

FIGURE 5–7. Anterolateral myocardial infarction. The initial QRS vector, pointing away from the anterolateral myocardial infarction, produces Q waves in leads I and aVL and sometimes, depending on the vectorial direction, in leads V_5 and V_6.

3. Apical Myocardial Infarction

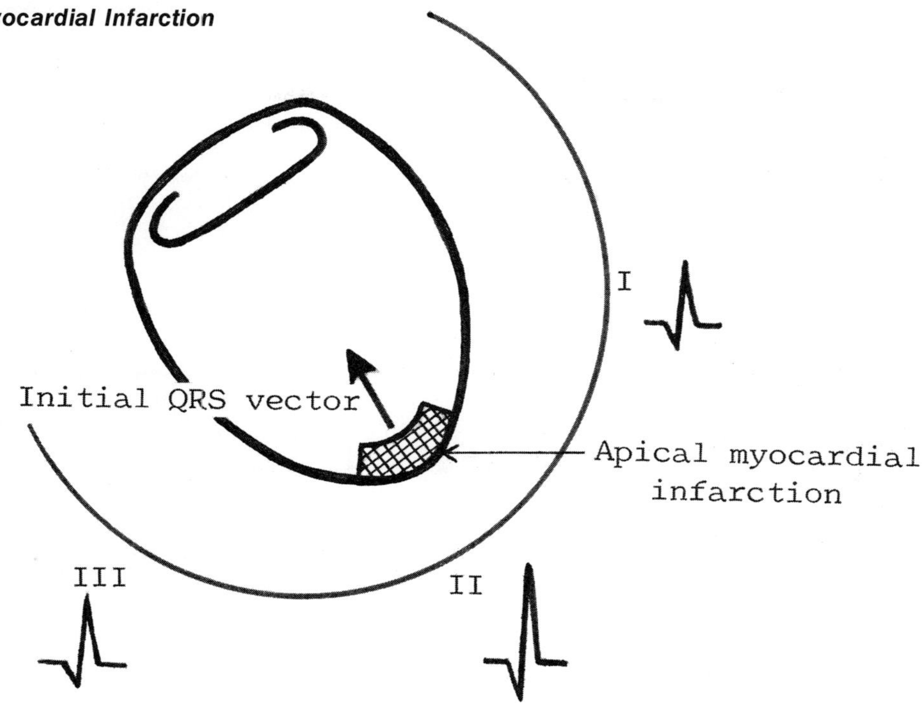

A

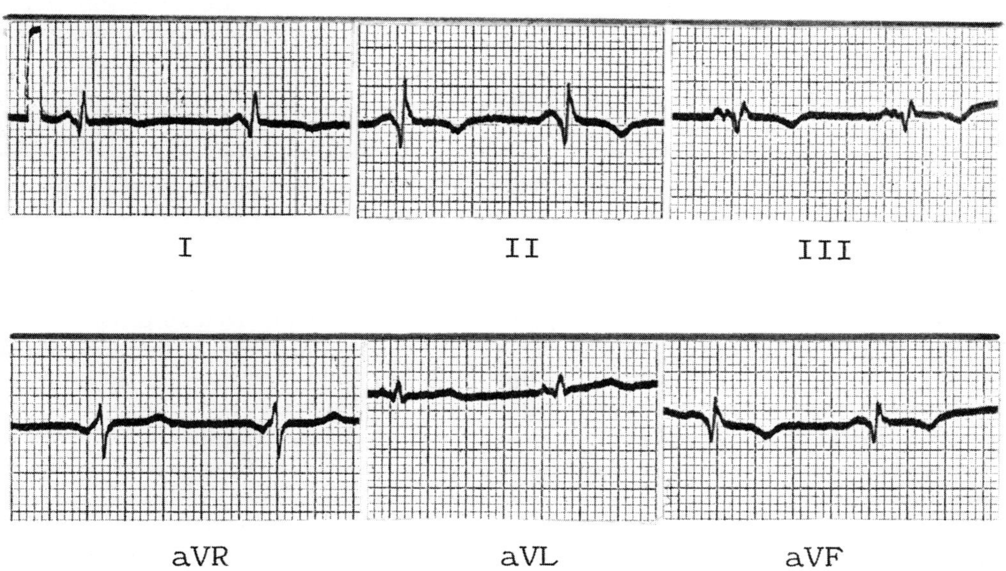

B

FIGURE 5–8. *A* and *B,* Apical myocardial infarction. The initial QRS vector, pointing away from the apical myocardial infarction and from leads I, II and III, produces Q waves in all three leads. The question arises: did one myocardial infarction produce these abnormalities, or are they the result of more than one infarction at different times? See Figure 5–8*C*.

Illustration continued on following page.

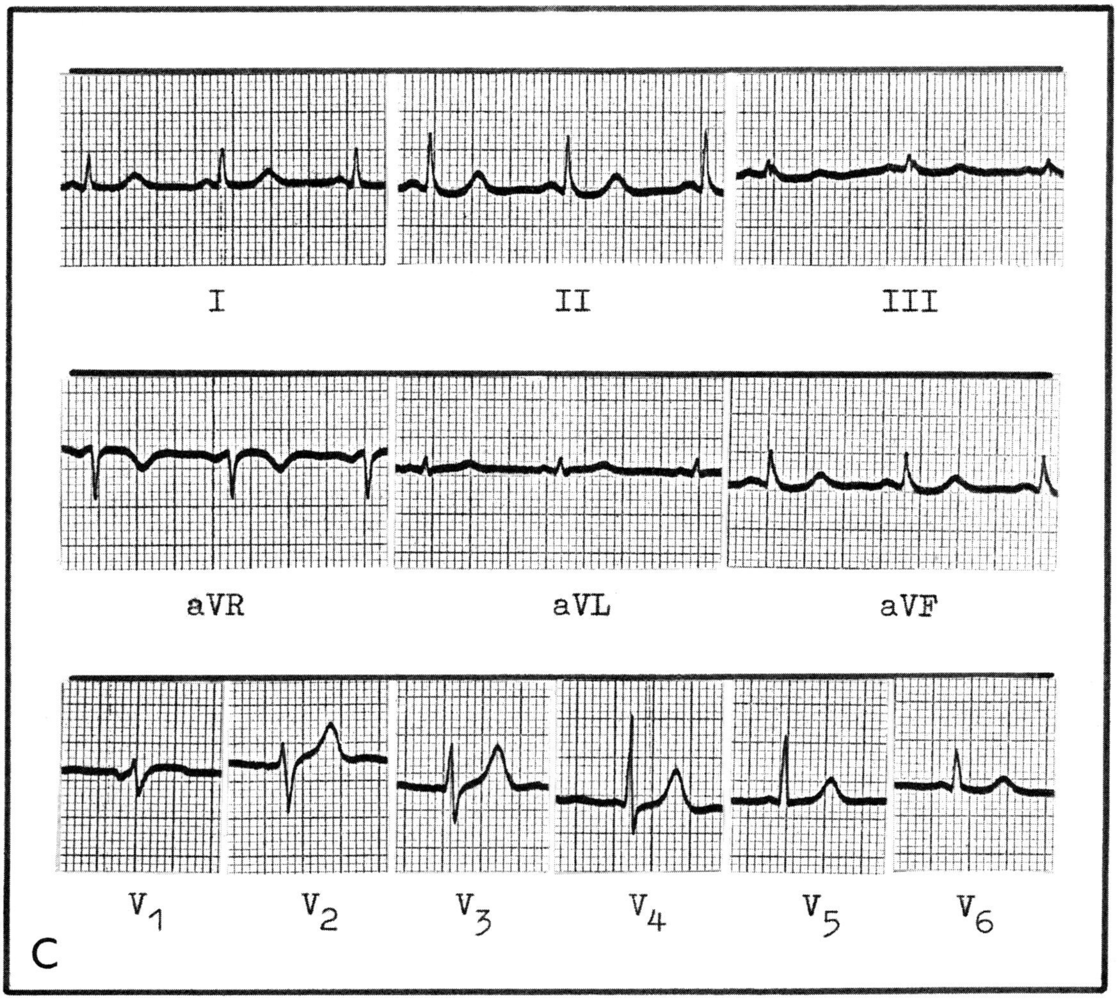

FIGURE 5–8 *Continued.* *C,* Electrocardiogram just prior to the infarction which brought about the changes seen in Figure 5–8*B*. The only way to answer the question posed in Figure 5–8*B* is to follow the patient clinically and have serial electrocardiograms.

4. The strictly anterior or anteroseptal myocardial infarction is seen in Figure 5–9*B* and diagrammed in Figure 5–9*A*. The initial vector of depolarization, the initial QRS vector, faces posteriorly, inscribing Q waves in leads V_1 to V_3, without producing significant Q waves in the frontal plane leads.

Cassette Side 12

5. Figure 5–10*B* is from a patient with an old strictly posterior and a new diaphragmatic-lateral myocardial infarction. The initial QRS vector is anteriorly oriented, away from the posterior area of the heart. Note that the R wave in lead V_1 is the main ventricular deflection. In Chapter 2 you learned that an R wave, which is the main ventricular deflection in lead V_1, should make you include in the differential diagnosis:

a. Right ventricular hypertrophy.

b. Strictly, or true, posterior wall myocardial infarction.

c. Right bundle branch block (RSR′).

d. Preexcitation (Wolff-Parkinson-White) syndrome.

There may or may not be Q waves in the other leads, depending on the vectorial orientation of the initial QRS vector, associated with the strictly (true) posterior myocardial infarction. Q waves in the other leads, in addition to repolarization abnormalities, may represent damage in

4. *Strictly Anterior or Anteroseptal Myocardial Infarction*

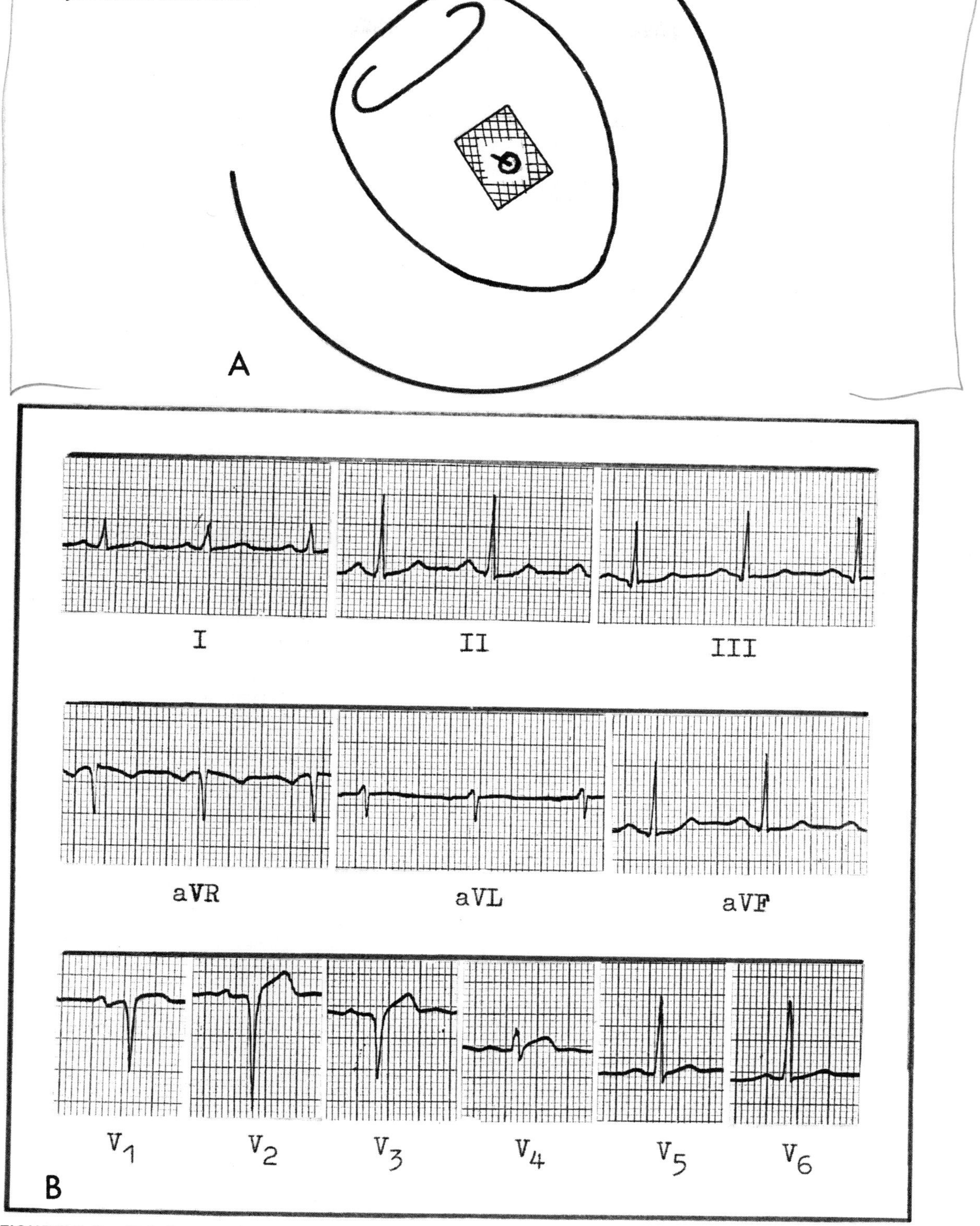

FIGURE 5–9. Strictly anterior or anteroseptal myocardial infarction. The initial vector of depolarization, the initial QRS vector, faces posteriorly, inscribing Q waves in leads V_1 to V_3, without significant Q waves in the frontal plane leads.

5. Strictly (True) Posterior Myocardial Infarction

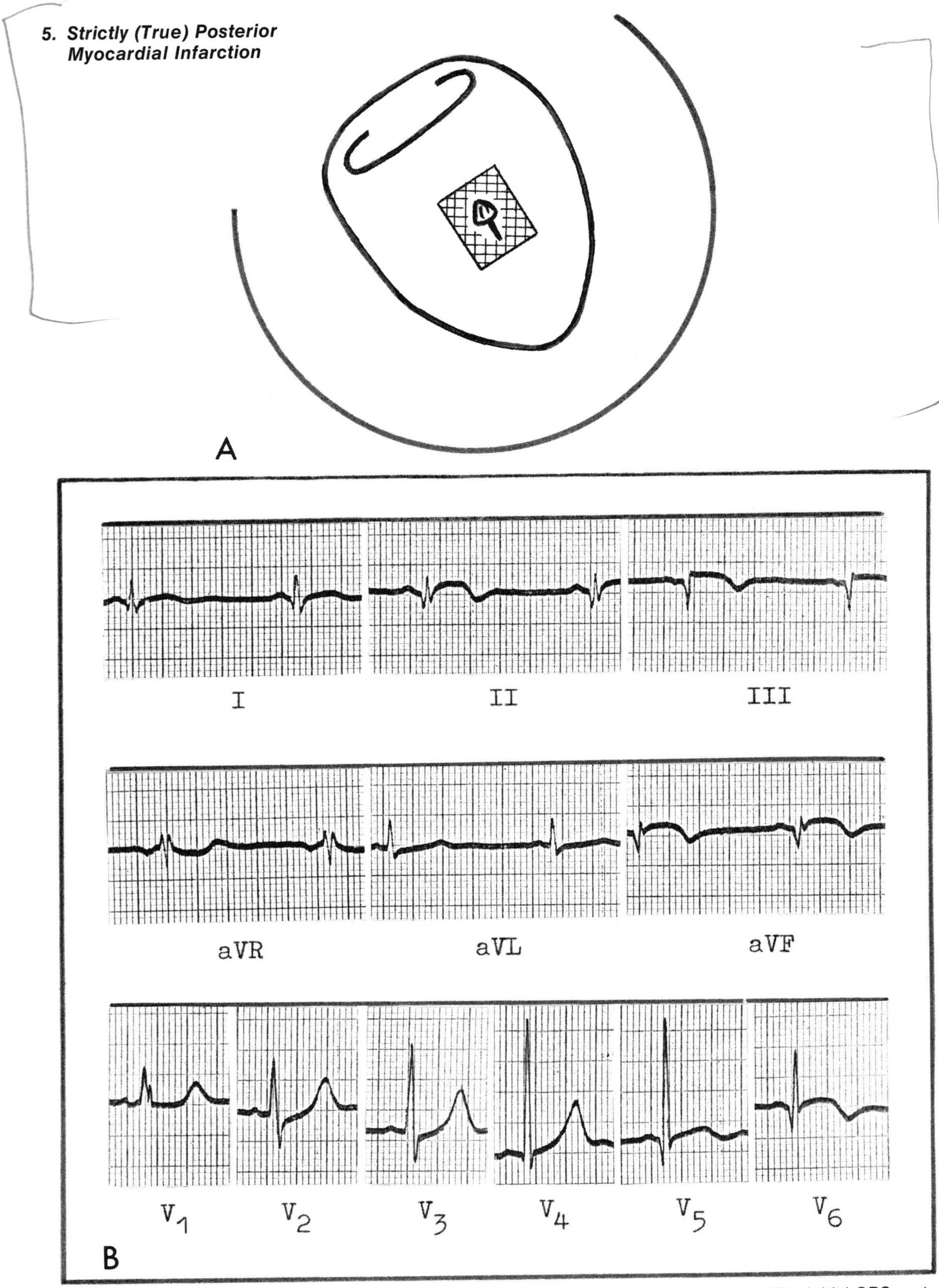

FIGURE 5–10. Old strictly posterior and new diaphragmatic-lateral myocardial infarction. The initial QRS vector is anteriorly oriented, away from the posterior area of the heart. Note that the R wave in lead V_1 is the main ventricular deflection.

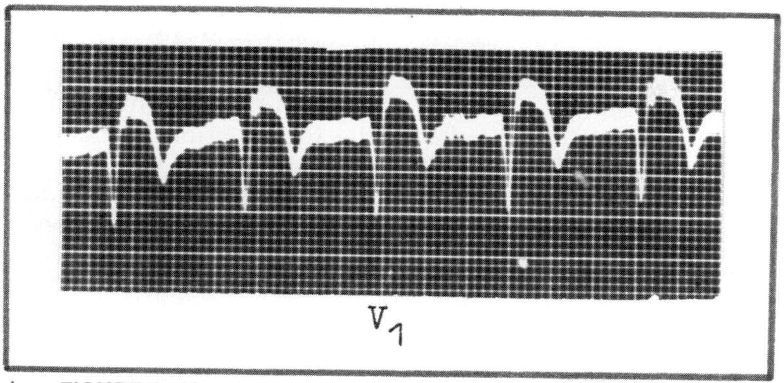

FIGURE 5–11. Anterior or anteroseptal myocardial infarction. (Electrocardiogram enlarged for clarity.)

other parts of the heart having occurred at other times, as in Figure 5–10*B*.

Figure 5–11 is from a patient with strictly anterior or anteroseptal myocardial infarction, a diagnosis made decades ago. Much credit is due the early electrocardiographers who recognized the Q wave and repolarization abnormalities as signs of myocardial infarction. They carefully correlated clinical-pathological findings and made the most of what they had to work with.

Do not wager your inheritance on an *exact* correlation between the electrical and anatomic location of the infarct. Keep in mind that the findings on the clinical electrocardiogram are the result of the balancing of vectorial forces. Much depends on the forces prior to infarction, often unknown in a given patient. It also becomes more and more difficult to localize the site with each ensuing infarct. It is so vital to study each problem carefully with serial electrocardiograms, observing changes as they occur. You must know your patients and their clinical histories since Q waves may be found in conditions other than myocardial infarction, as in cardiomyopathy, ventricular hypertrophy, left bundle branch block, the Wolff-Parkinson-White syndrome and the hemiblocks. In addition, Figure 5–16 illustrates Q waves in a normal patient.

B. Ventricular Repolarization Abnormalities (Abnormalities of the S–T Segment and T Wave)

The S–T segment and T wave represent the early to late repolarization phase of the ventricles (epicardium to endocardium) and are sensitive indicators of the state of the myocardium.

The altered state of early (S–T segment) repolarization in acute myocardial infarction, the current of injury, is reflected in a mean S–T vector oriented *toward* the site of infarction, opposite to the initial QRS vector (Q wave). Late repolarization results in a mean T vector of the same orientation as the initial QRS vector. In summary, in acute myocardial infarction, the Q wave and T wave are of the same orientation and opposite to the S–T segment. This is seen in Figure 5–12.

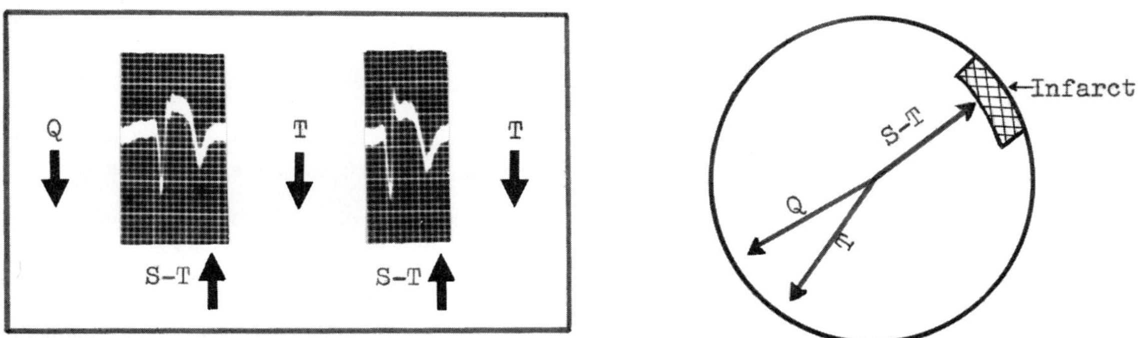

FIGURE 5–12. Acute anterior myocardial infarction (lead V_1) showing the abnormal depolarization and repolarization.
(Electrocardiogram reduced in size.)

Three sets of serial electrocardiograms will be presented—Figures 5–13 (*A* to *E*), 5–14 (*A* to *D*) and 5–15 (*A* to *C*). Descriptive text material has been added to the legend of each electrocardiogram for continuity.

1. All three patients are alive and *well*, two of the three more than five years after the myocardial infarction.
2. The electrocardiographic "extent" of the infarct varies. The patient whose electrocardiograms appear the most foreboding (Fig. 5–13) is the most active of the three.
3. The three "nevers" mentioned in the introduction to this chapter must be kept in mind.
4. The evolutionary changes in depolarization (Q wave) and repolarization (S–T and T) are illustrated.
5. The importance of serial electrocardiograms is obvious from these sets.

Text continued on page 220.

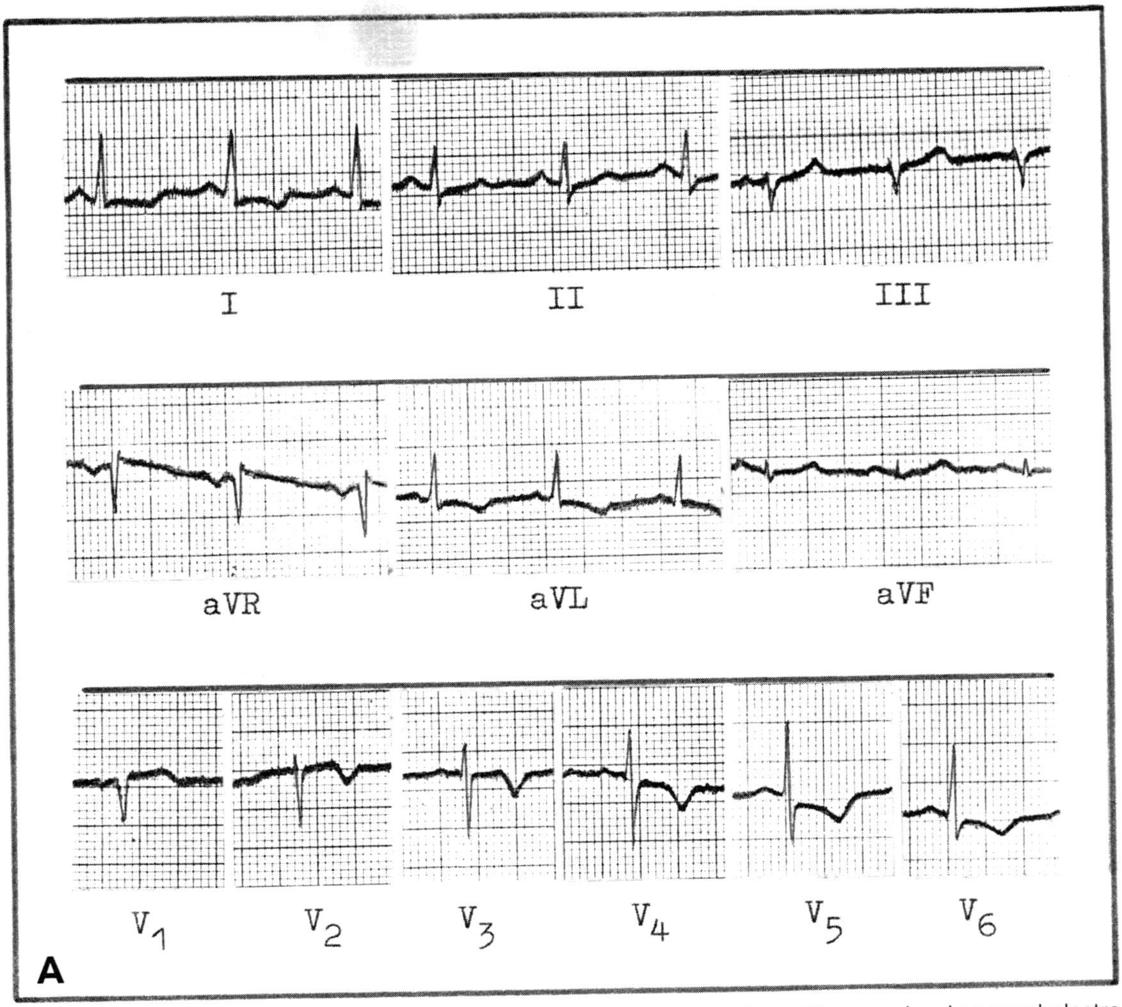

FIGURE 5–13. *A,* Onset of chest pain in a previously asymptomatic patient with a previously normal electrocardiogram. Describe the abnormalities noted here.

A number of terms have been used to describe the evolutionary electrocardiographic changes associated with myocardial infarction—hyperacute (minutes to hours to days), acute (hours to days to weeks), subacute or recent (weeks to months) and old (stabilized, months to years after infarction). As you can readily see, there is much overlap and these terms can be misleading. A good way to time an infarct is to carefully follow your patients clinically and with serial electrocardiograms. To reemphasize the importance of serial tracings several sets are presented.

The above electrocardiogram was taken one week before clear and unequivocal evidence of myocardial infarction was evident. What could this mean?

Illustration continued on opposite page.

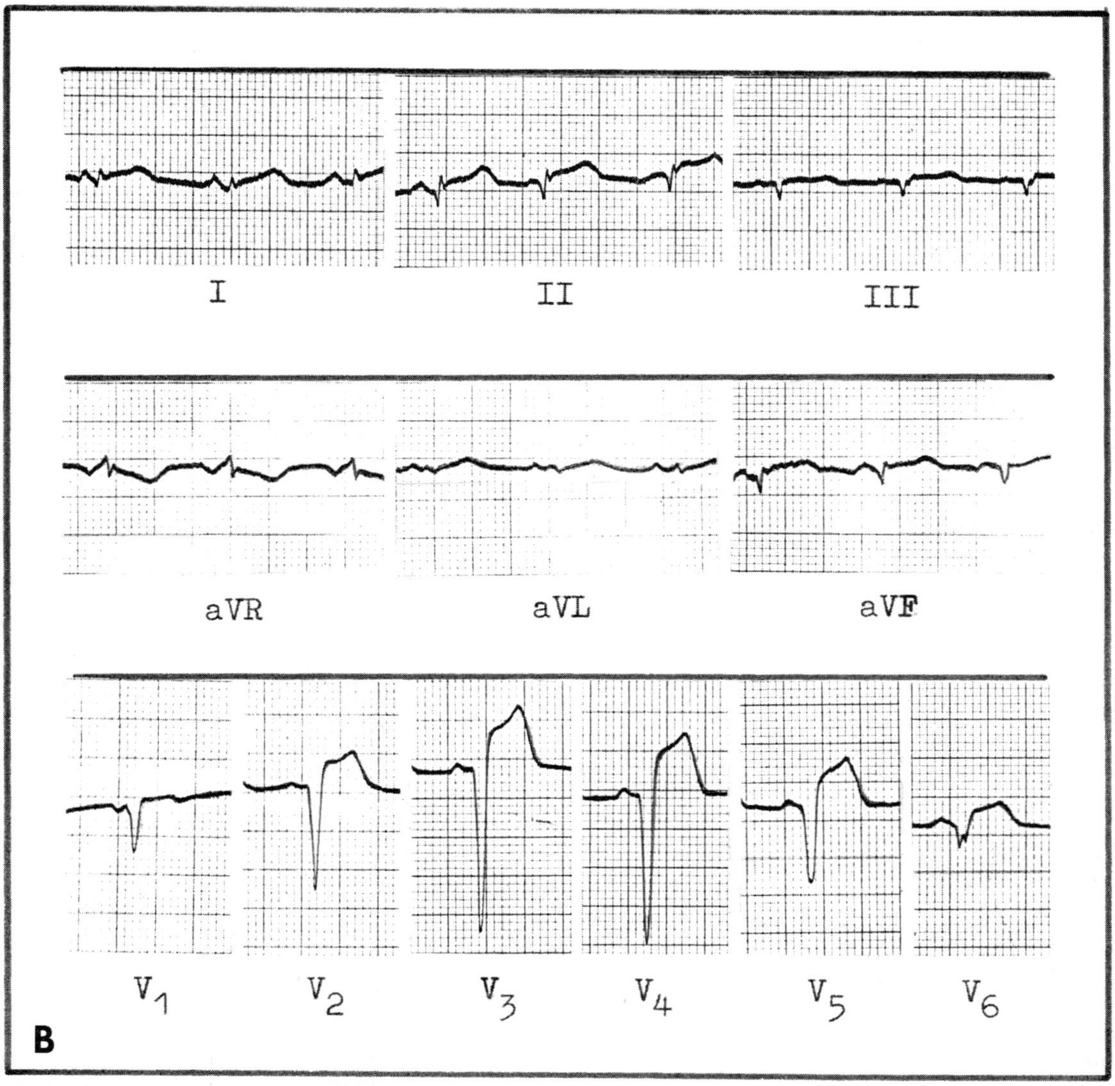

FIGURE 5–13 *Continued. B,* Following onset of "crushing" chest pain in the same patient. Blood enzymes became abnormal at this time. Although the patient was treated as if he had a myocardial infarction following the previous tracing (taken one week earlier with the blood enzymes remaining normal for the entire week), this stage was not prevented. Describe the depolarization (Q wave) and repolarization (S–T segment and T wave) abnormalities.

Illustration continued on following page.

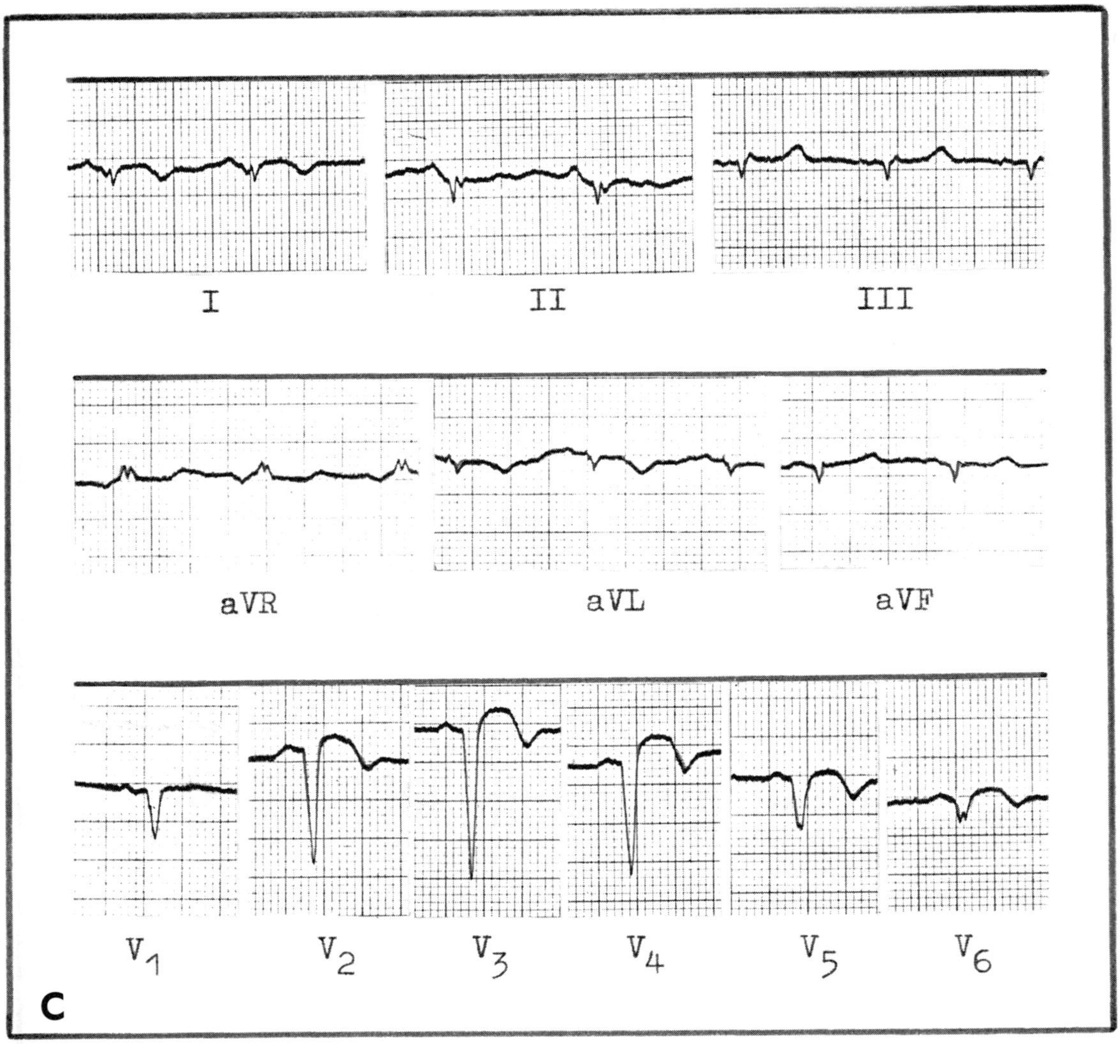

FIGURE 5–13 *Continued.* *C,* Evolutionary changes in acute myocardial infarction (one week after the electrocardiogram in Figure 5–13*B*). The chest pain had subsided. Compare each lead with those in the previous electrocardiograms and describe the serial changes.

Illustration continued on opposite page.

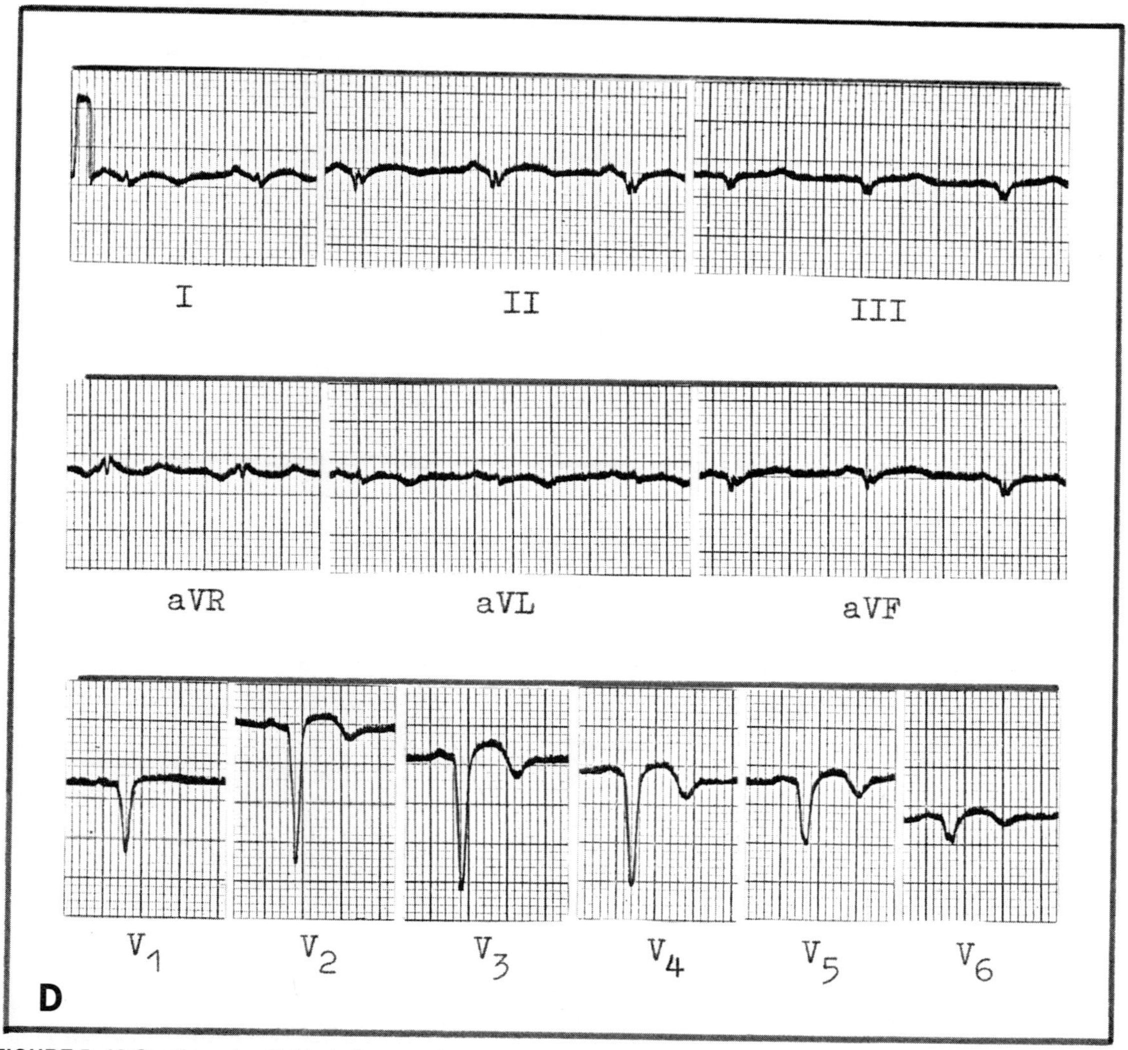

FIGURE 5–13 *Continued.* *D,* Evolutionary changes in acute myocardial infarction (three days after electrocardiogram in Figure 5–13*C*).

Illustration continued on following page.

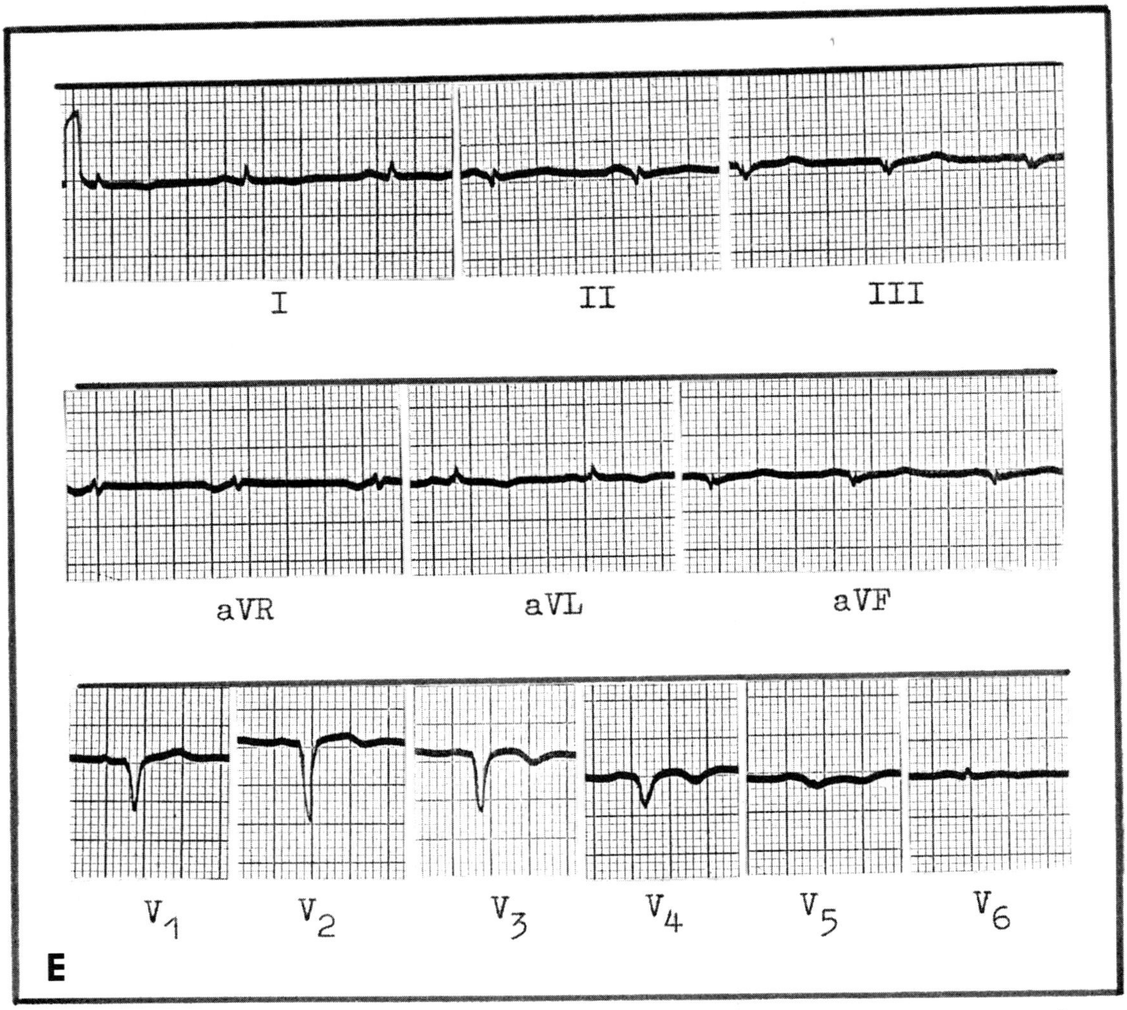

FIGURE 5–13 *Continued.* *E,* Stabilized electrocardiogram obtained a year and a half after the electrocardiogram in Figure 5–13*D*. The patient is presently asymptomatic and active in business. Review and carefully analyze this entire series. Could you predict an asymptomatic, active patient from these "terrible-looking" electrocardiograms, indicating an "extensive infarction, covering a large area of myocardium?" Remember the dictum that the patient is to be treated, not the electrocardiogram.

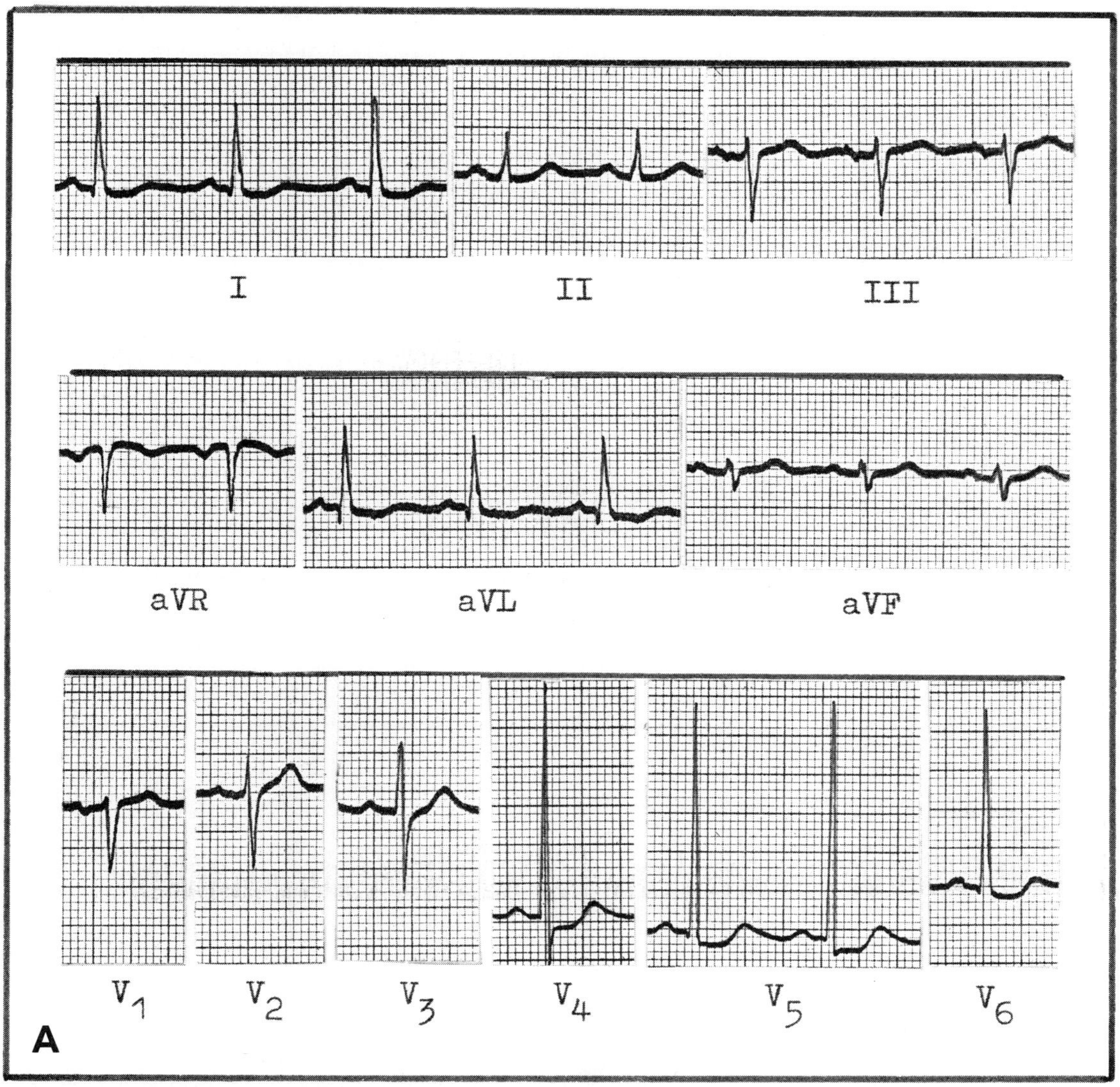

FIGURE 5–14 *A.* Onset of intermittent chest pain in a previously asymptomatic patient. Describe the repolarization abnormalities. Are there any significant Q waves? Criteria for left ventricular hypertrophy?

Just as with the previous patient (Figures 5–13*A, B, C, D* and *E*), this patient was treated as if he had a myocardial infarction, in spite of the normal blood enzymes and abatement of chest pain, for an entire week.

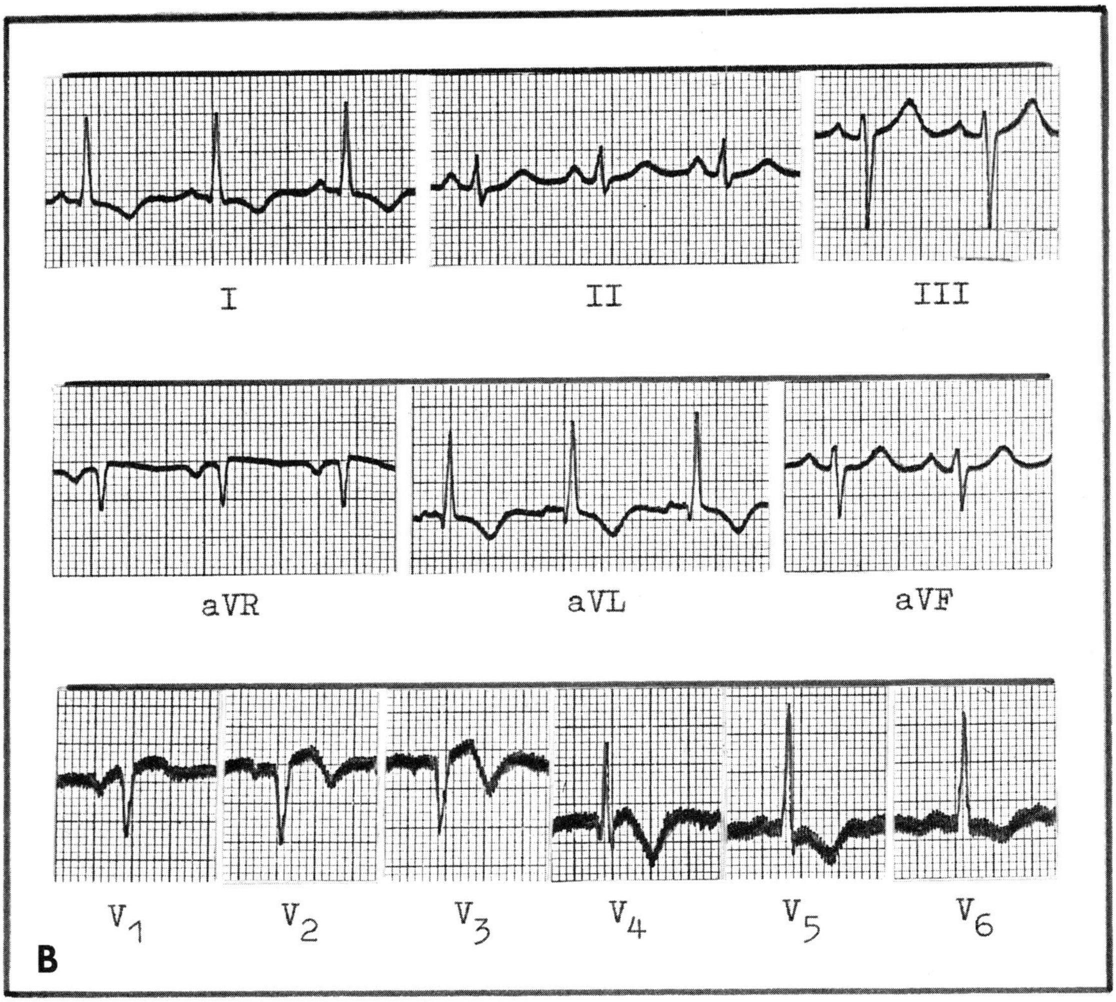

FIGURE 5–14 *Continued.* *B,* Electrocardiogram one week after the electrocardiogram in Figure 5–14*A.* Although under treatment, the patient experienced "crushing" chest pain and blood enzymes became abnormal. Describe the abnormalities in depolarization (Q waves) and repolarization (S–T segments and T waves).

Illustration continued on opposite page.

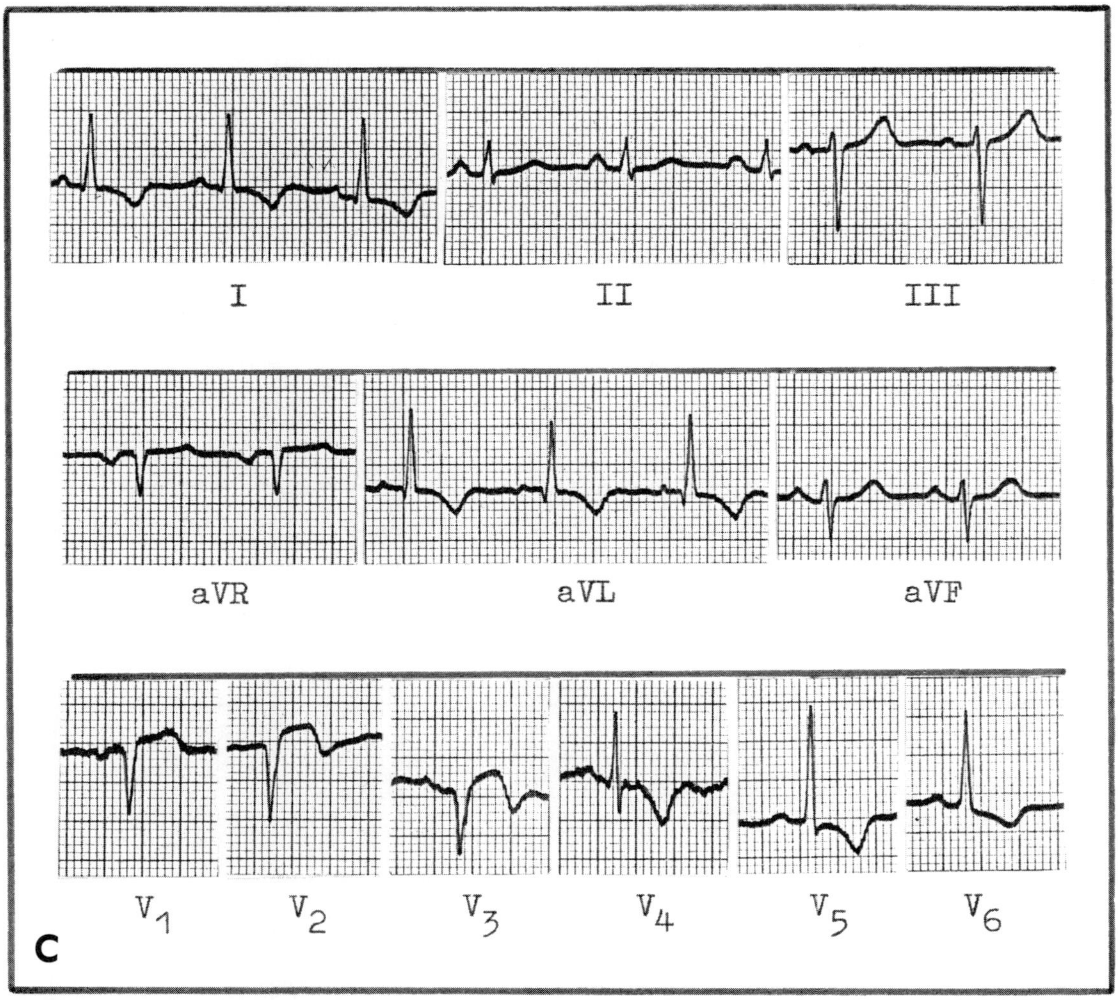

FIGURE 5–14 *Continued.* *C,* Evolutionary changes in strictly anterior or anteroseptal infarction one week after the electrocardiogram in Figure 5–14*B*. Describe.

Illustration continued on following page.

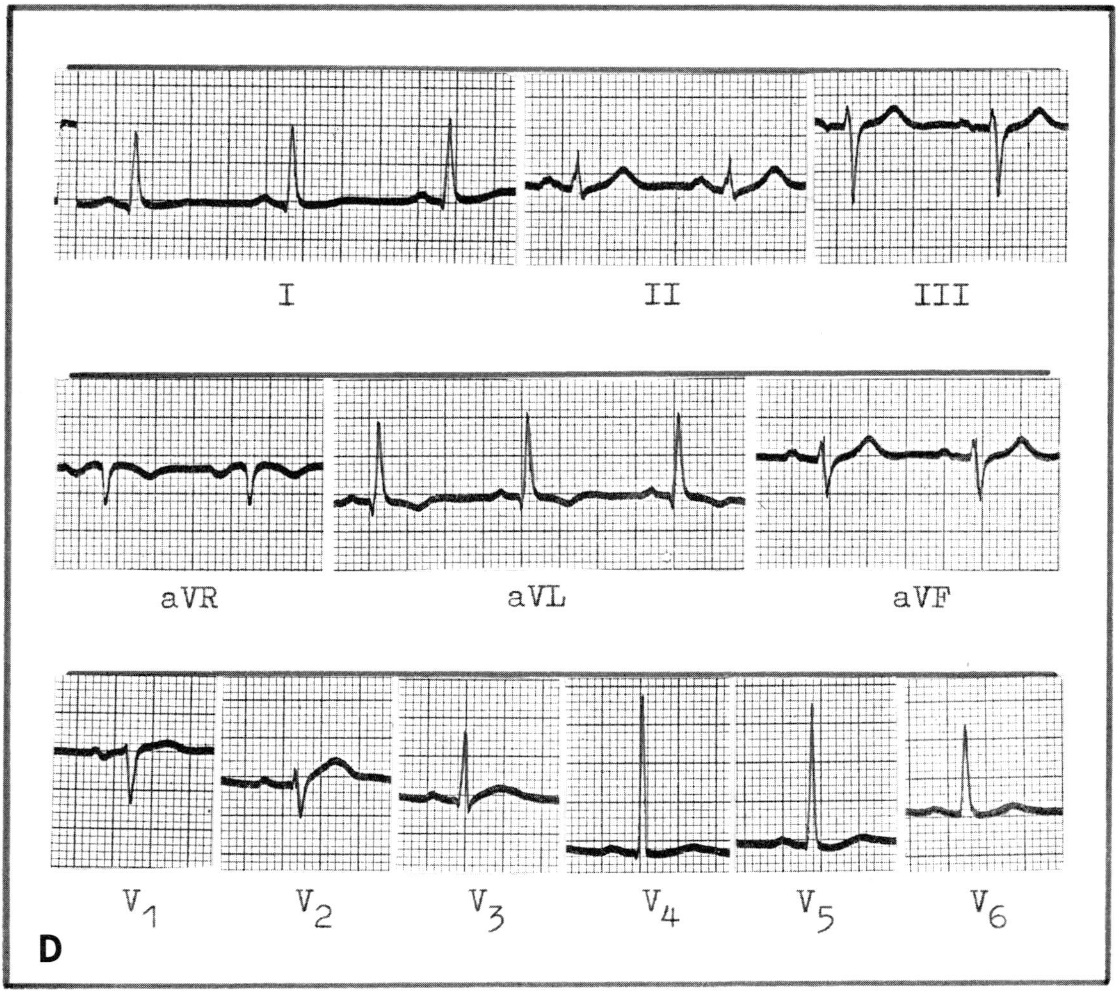

FIGURE 5–14 *Continued.* *D,* Electrocardiogram *three years* after the electrocardiogram in Figure 5–14*C.* Any sign of the infarct? Are you surprised? Could you make the diagnosis of anteroseptal myocardial infarction if you did not have the serial electrocardiograms?

Cassette Side 13

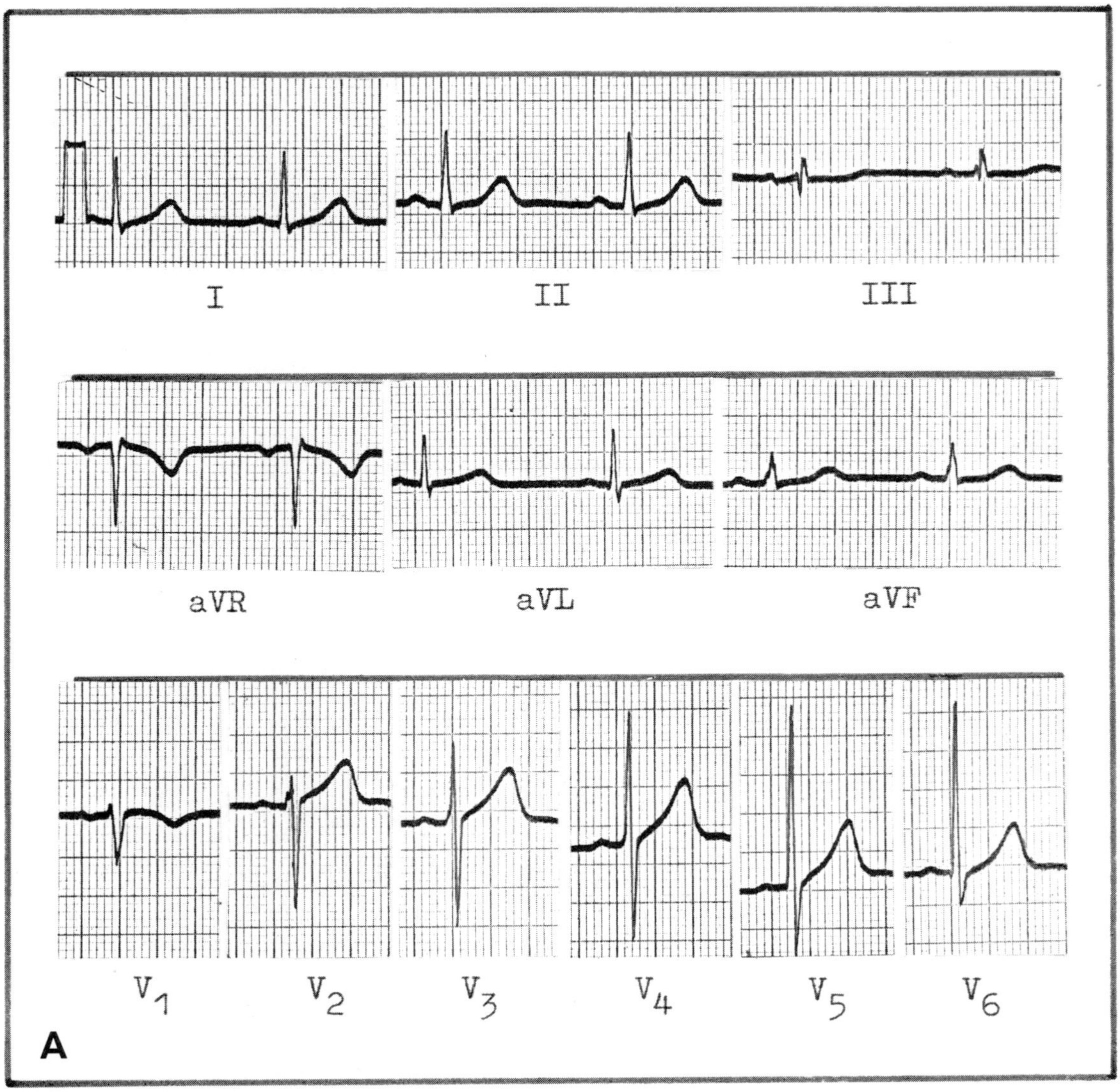

FIGURE 5–15. *A*, Baseline electrocardiogram in a patient who subsequently developed a myocardial infarction (Figures 5–15*B* and *C*).

Illustration continued on following page.

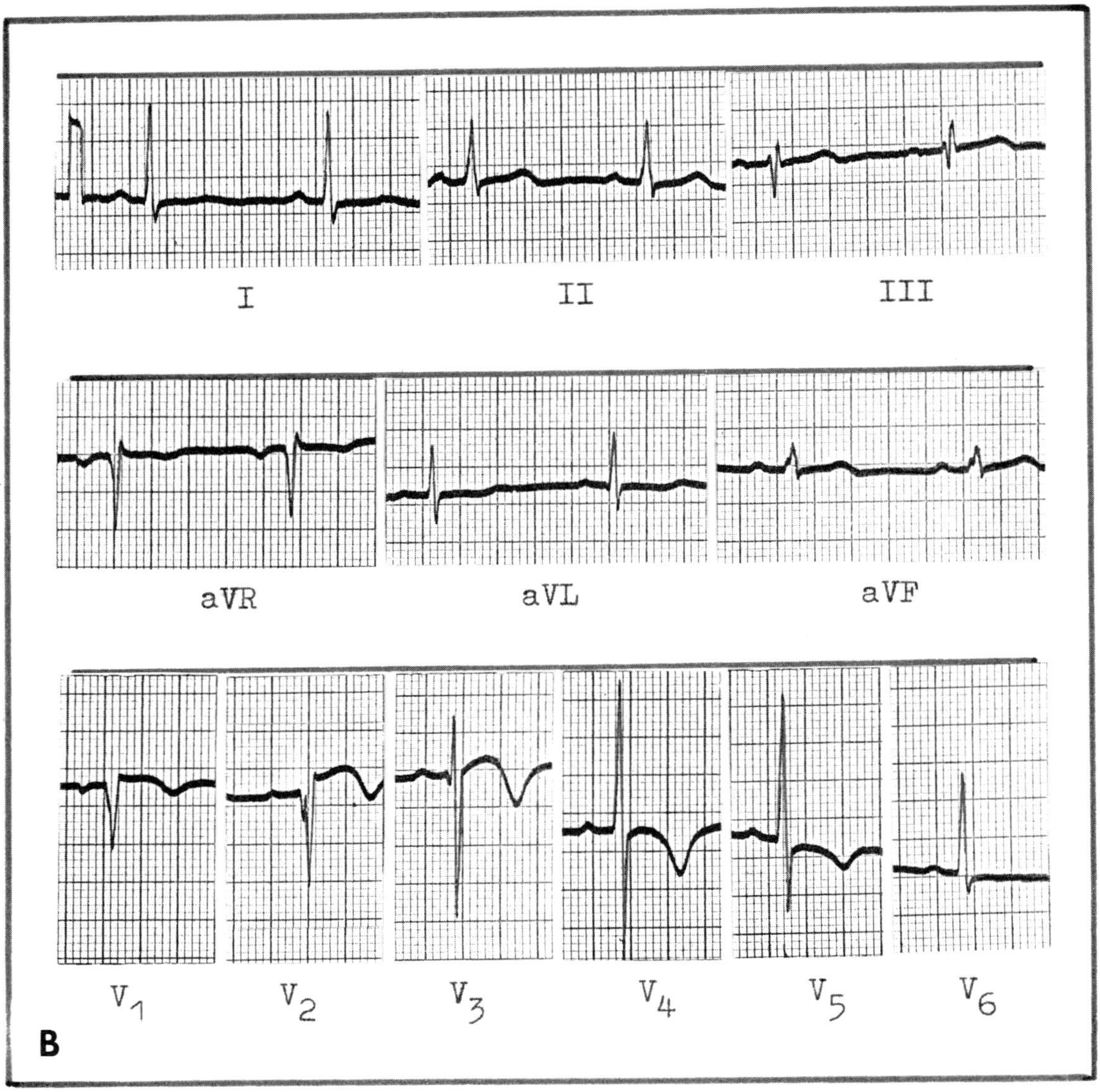

FIGURE 5–15 *Continued.* *B,* Strictly anterior or anteroseptal myocardial infarction in same patient as in Figure 5–15*A*. Describe abnormalities.

Illustration continued on opposite page.

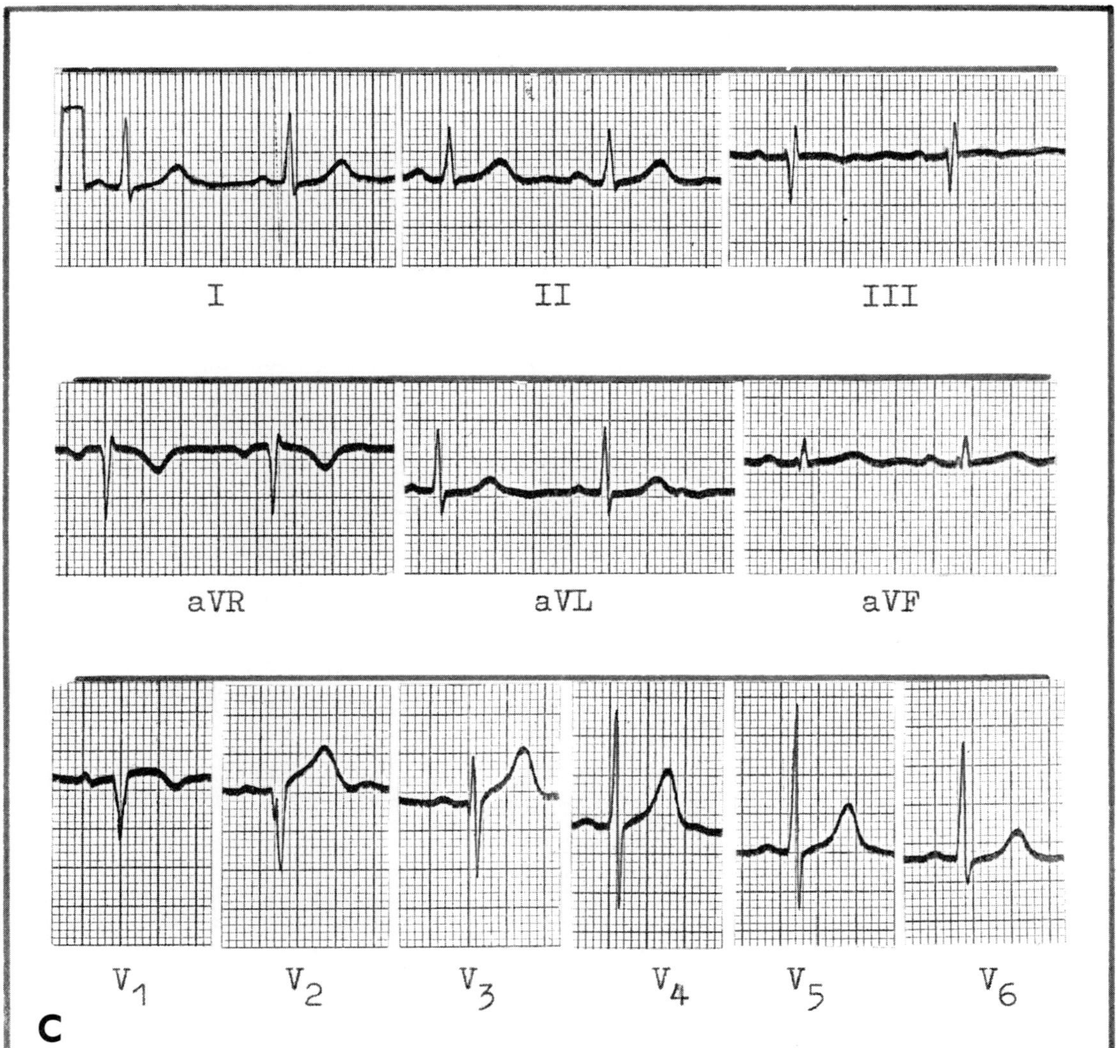

FIGURE 5–15 *Continued.* *C,* Stable electrocardiogram one year after the electrocardiogram in Figure 5–15*B*. Review this series and describe the changes.

These cases (Figures 5–13, 5–14 and 5–15) emphasize the need for serial tracings. Very few things of value will come to you accidentally. You must know what to look for; you must search to find.

Note that in lead V_3 there is an initial Q wave in the presence of a predominantly *negative* QRS complex. This is known as a pre-transitional Q wave and is never normal. In this electrocardiogram it represents the anteroseptal infarction. It may also be found in cardiomyopathy and in the hemiblocks.

Not all Q waves signify infarction of the heart, even though the Q wave is "significant." Figure 5–16 shows lead III in a normal patient. The Q wave in lead III may vary in size with respiration in a normal person due to slight vectorial shifts during respiration. This figure illustrates why it is not advisable to make the

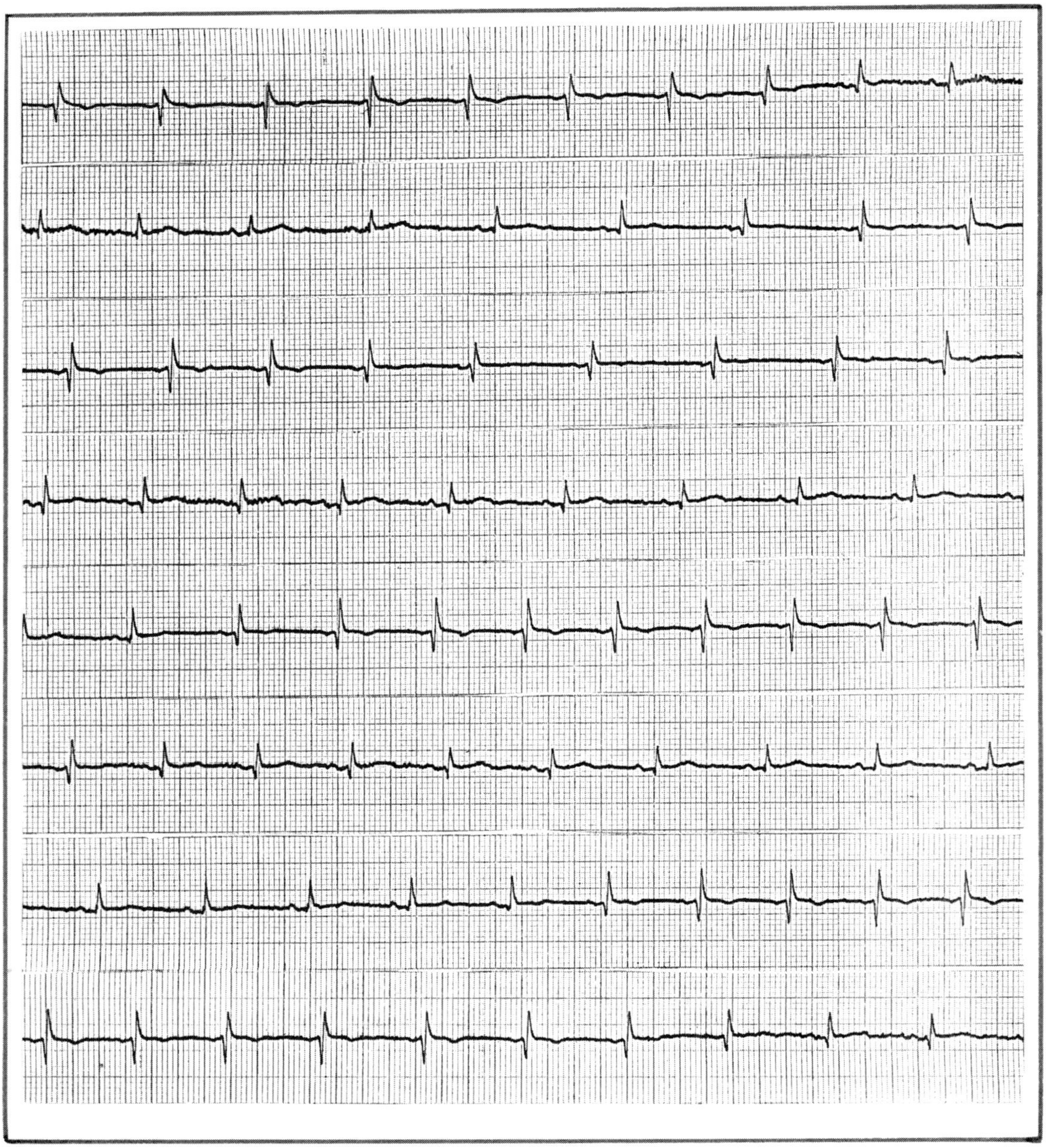

FIGURE 5–16. Q waves in lead III in a normal patient. The Q wave in lead III may vary in size with respiration in a normal person, due to slight shifts in the vectorial forces during respiration. (Electrocardiogram reduced in size.)

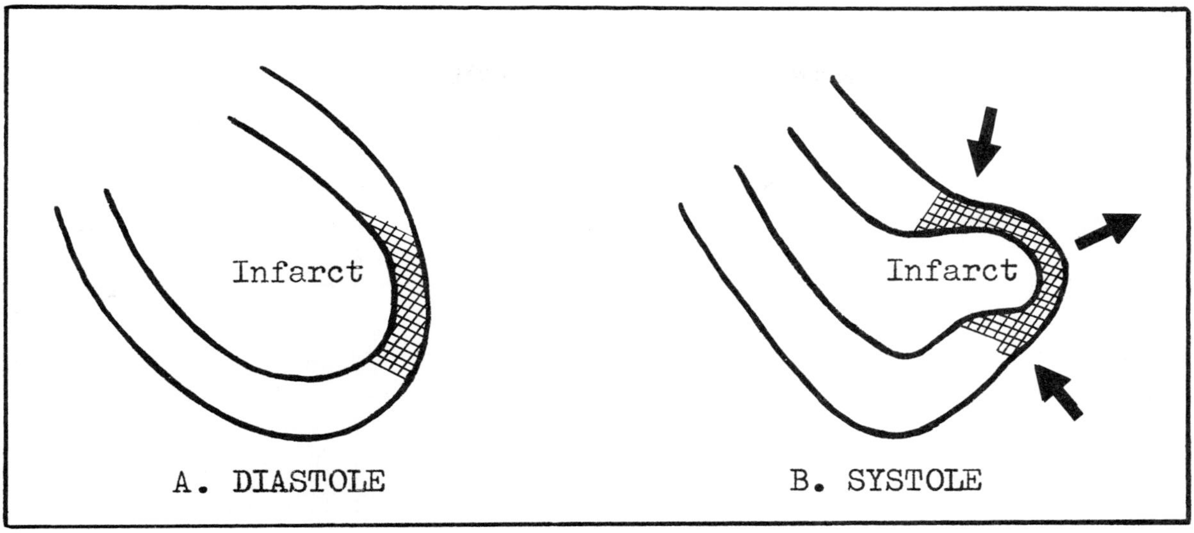

FIGURE 5–17. Ventricular aneurysm. The scarred area of myocardium, following infarction, is not able to beat synchronously with the remainder of the ventricle. During systole, with ventricular contraction, this area bulges outward with "paradoxical" motion.

diagnosis of myocardial infarction from a single electrocardiogram with a "significant" Q wave in lead III. Conversely, this *does not* mean that a Q wave in lead III may not be the result of a myocardial infarction. How may serial electrocardiograms be of help?

Figure 5–18 is from a patient with a ventricular aneurysm years after a myocardial infarction. The *persistent* elevation of the S–T segment, described as a persistent "monophasic" curve of injury, represents a ventricular aneurysm, an outpouching of a section of scarred ventricular myocardium, illustrated in Figure 5–17. During systole, with ventricular contraction, this area bulges outward with "paradoxical" motion. Paradoxical motion is also frequently seen during acute infarction. Paradoxical motion of the normal myocardium at the rim of the aneurysm may explain the elevated S–T segment in both acute myocardial infarction and ventricular aneurysm. A completely satisfactory explanation, however, has not been given. Only serial electrocardiograms will tell you the age of an elevated S–T segment. A favorite examination question is to show an electrocardiogram which appears to indicate an acute myocardial infarction. Once you diagnose this "acute" infarction with certainty, the examiner will show you an identical electrocardiogram taken years before. Always ask for comparison electrocardiograms.

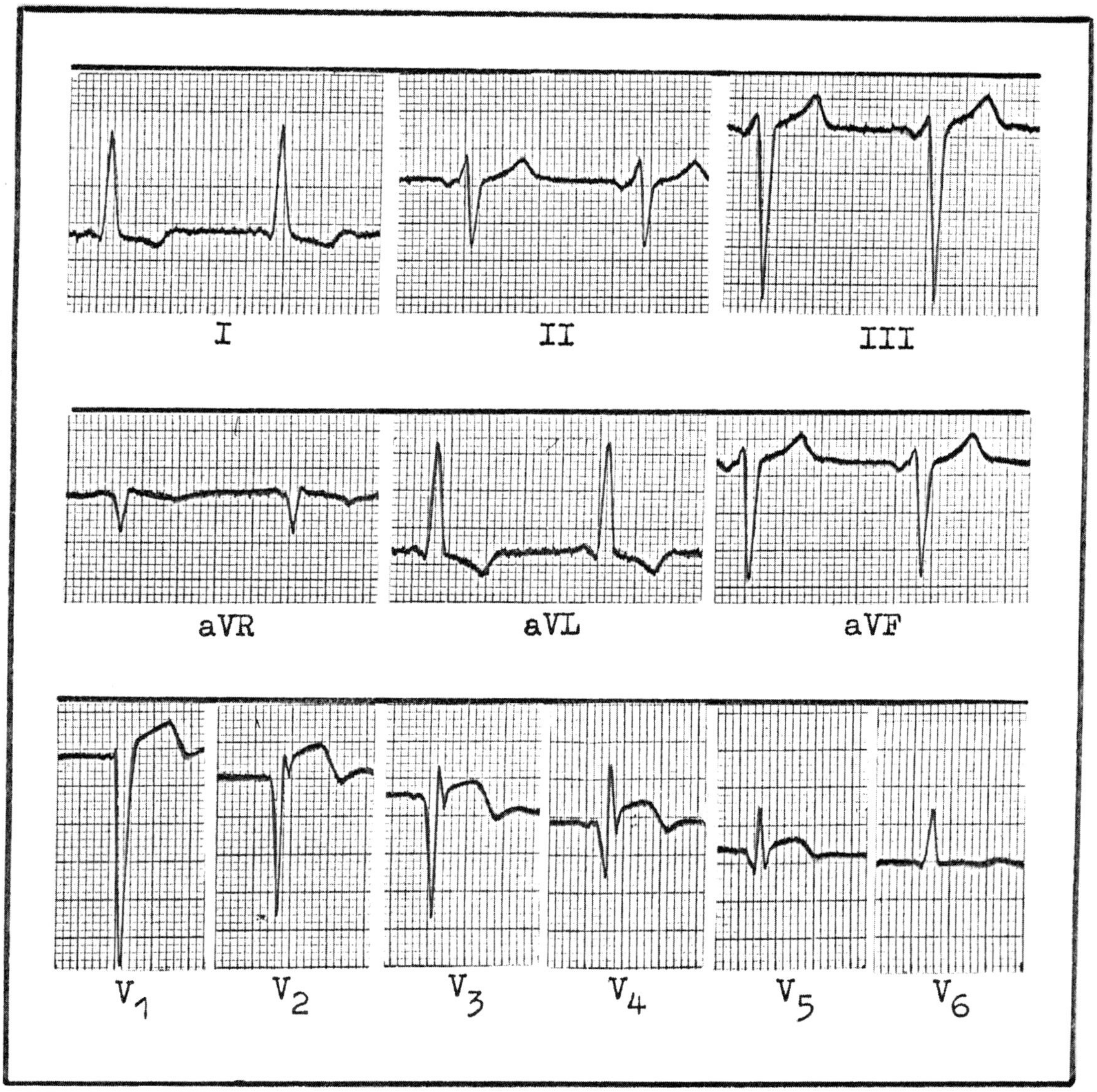

FIGURE 5–18. Ventricular aneurysm in a patient with an old myocardial infarction. This patient also had a very large left ventricle. Note that the rhythm is not sinus.

"Subendocardial" Infarction

Clinical evidence of infarction of the heart (by history, physical examination and enzyme abnormalities) is frequently encountered without Q waves on the electrocardiogram. It had been thought that when the subendocardium of the heart was infarcted the only electrocardiographic manifestations might be repolarization (S–T and T) abnormalities.

Significant experimental evidence has shown that if the parts of the heart responsible for the *second half* of the QRS complex are infarcted there is no formation of Q waves, although the area of infarction may be extensive. The only electrocardiographic manifestations seen are often only terminal QRS changes and repolarization abnormalities.

Although it may be misleading, the term "subendocardial" infarction will be used in this course because of common usage. Anterior subendocardial infarction is illustrated in Figures 5–19 (*B, C, D*) and 5–20; posterior subendocardial infarction is illustrated in Figure 5–21.

As noted earlier, there may not be exact electrical and anatomic correlation. Multiple combinations may be seen in spite of logical localizations and interpretations. The clinical picture of infarction should be quite clear before an electrocardiogram is labeled "subendocardial" infarction, since these repolarization abnormalities, although striking, may be nonspecific.

Text continued on page 229.

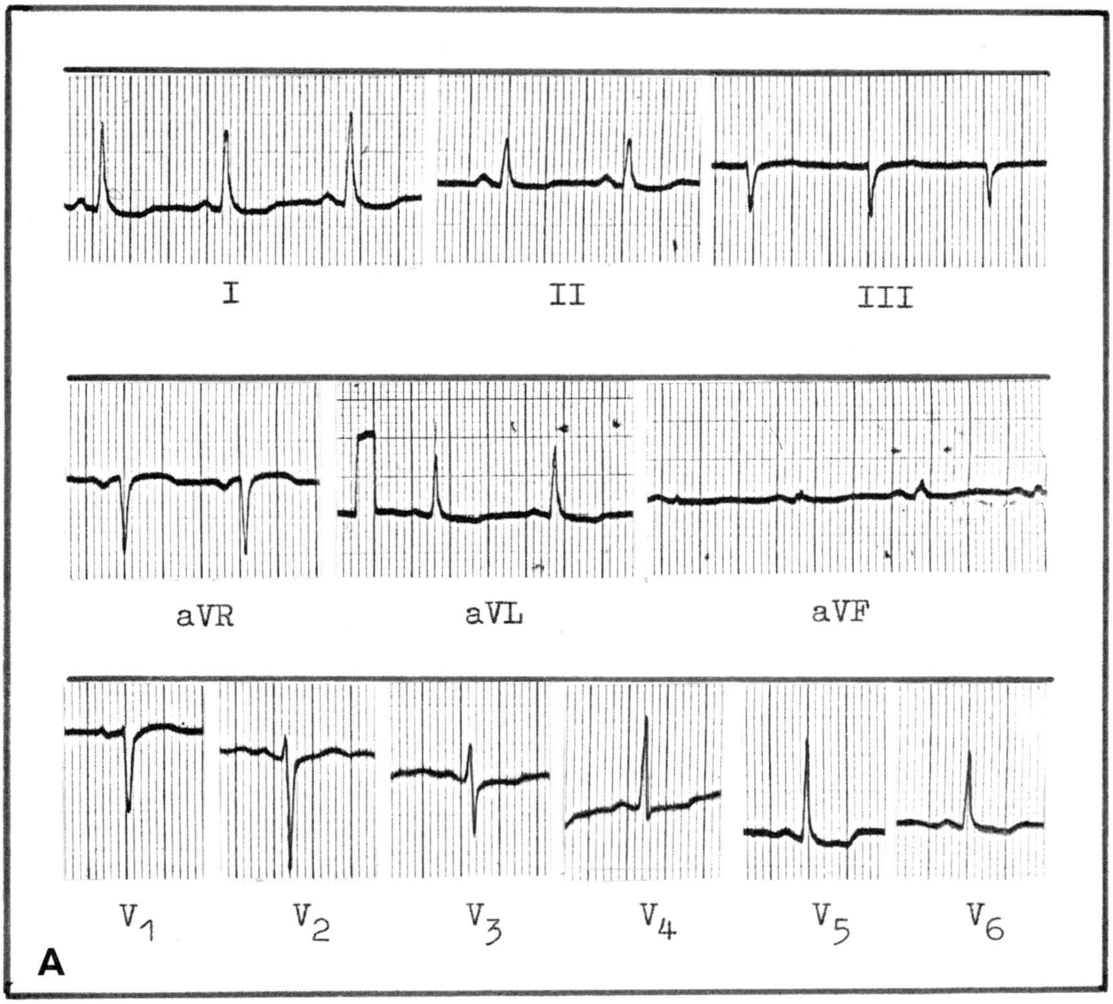

FIGURE 5–19. *A,* Baseline electrocardiogram prior to onset of subendocardial infarction. Is it normal?

Illustration continued on following page.

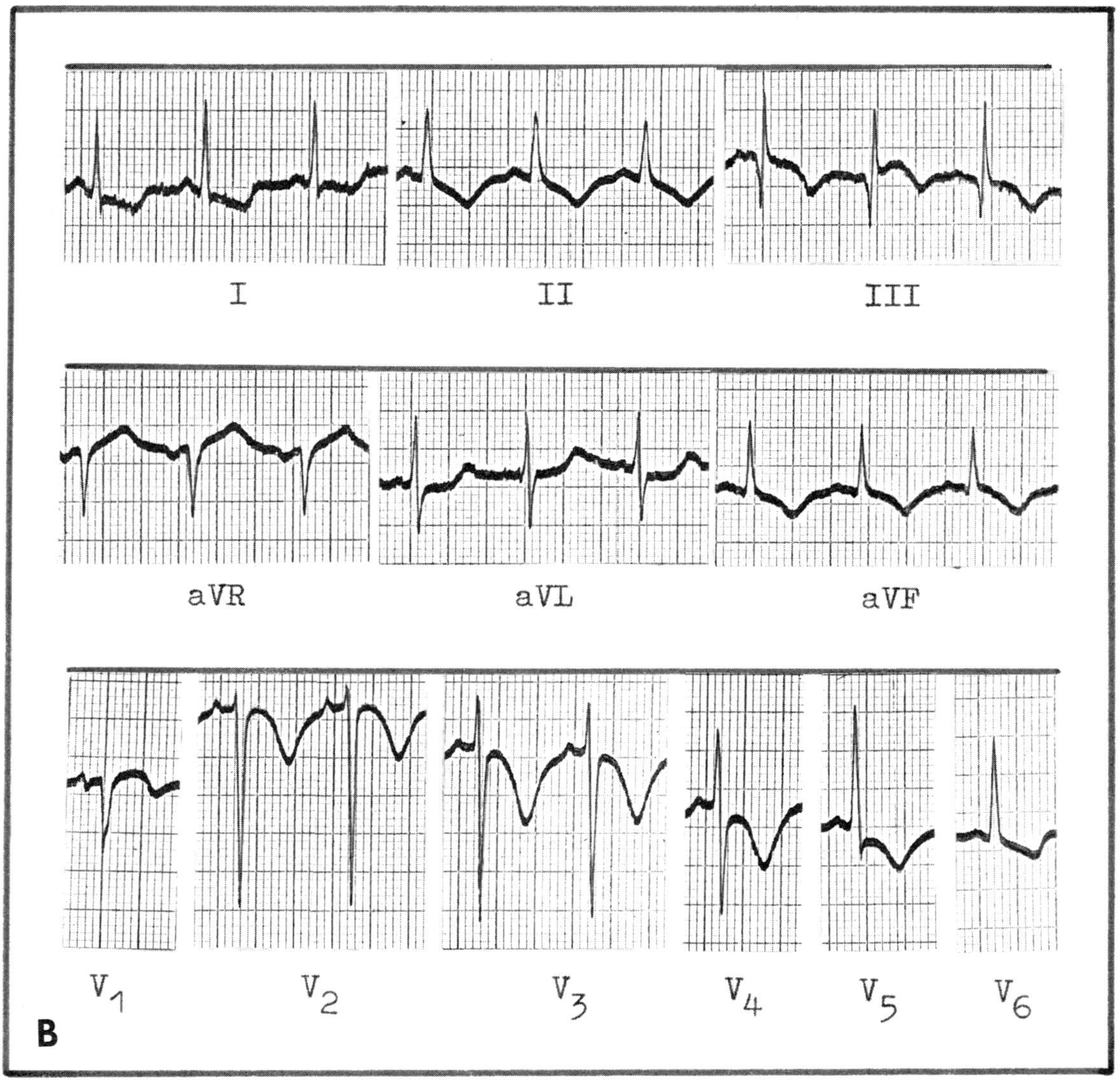

FIGURE 5–19 *Continued.* *B,* Electrocardiogram following onset of clinical evidence of myocardial infarction. As noted in the text, the clinical picture of infarction should be quite clear before an electrocardiogram is labelled "subendocardial" infarction, since these repolarization abnormalities, although striking, may be nonspecific. Note that in the precordial leads the mean T vector faces *away* from the anterior wall of the heart, *away* from the anterior subendocardial infarction.

Illustration continued on opposite page.

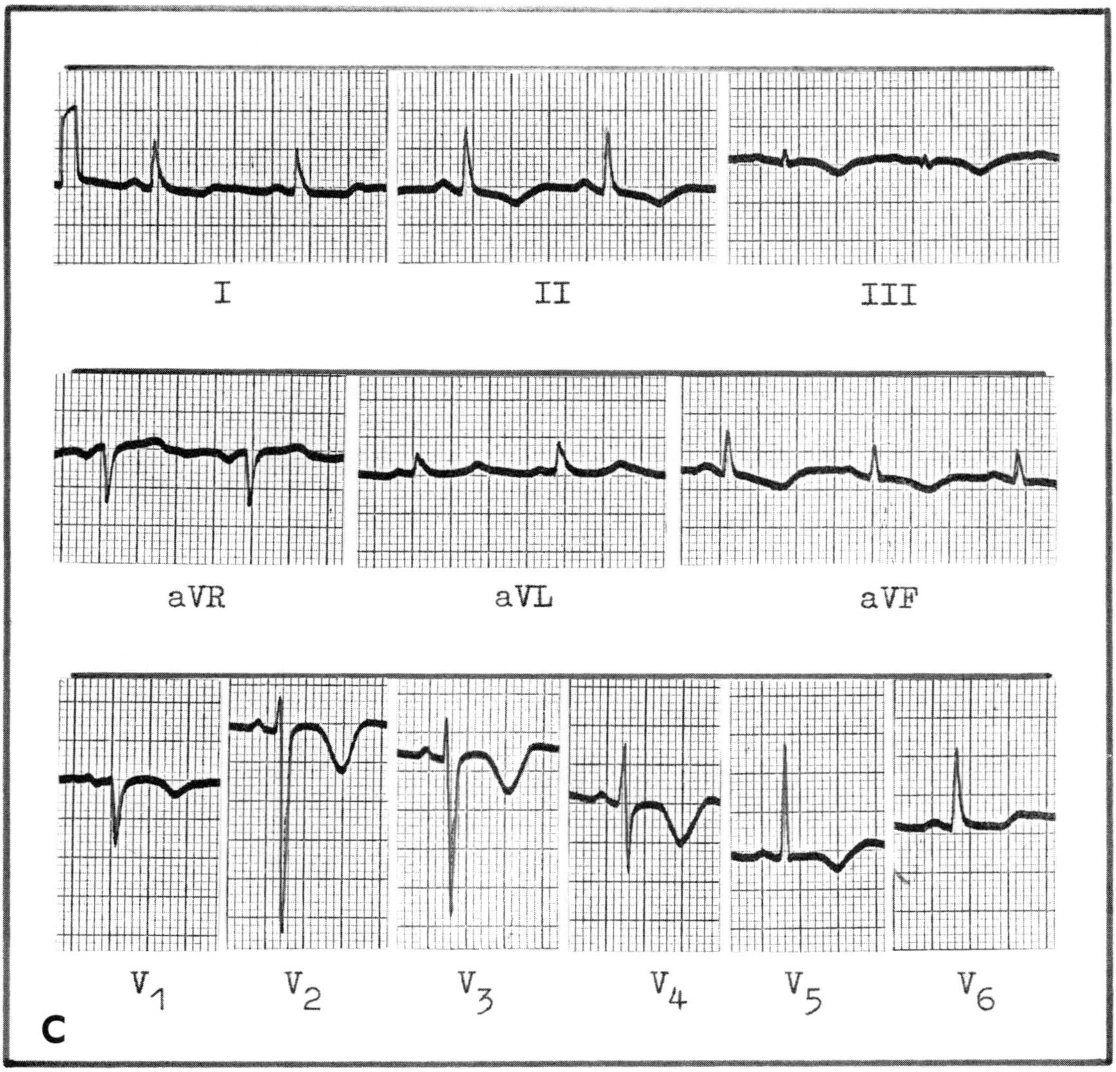

FIGURE 5–19 *Continued.* *C,* Serial changes in subendocardial infarction. Are there any significant Q waves?

Illustration continued on following page.

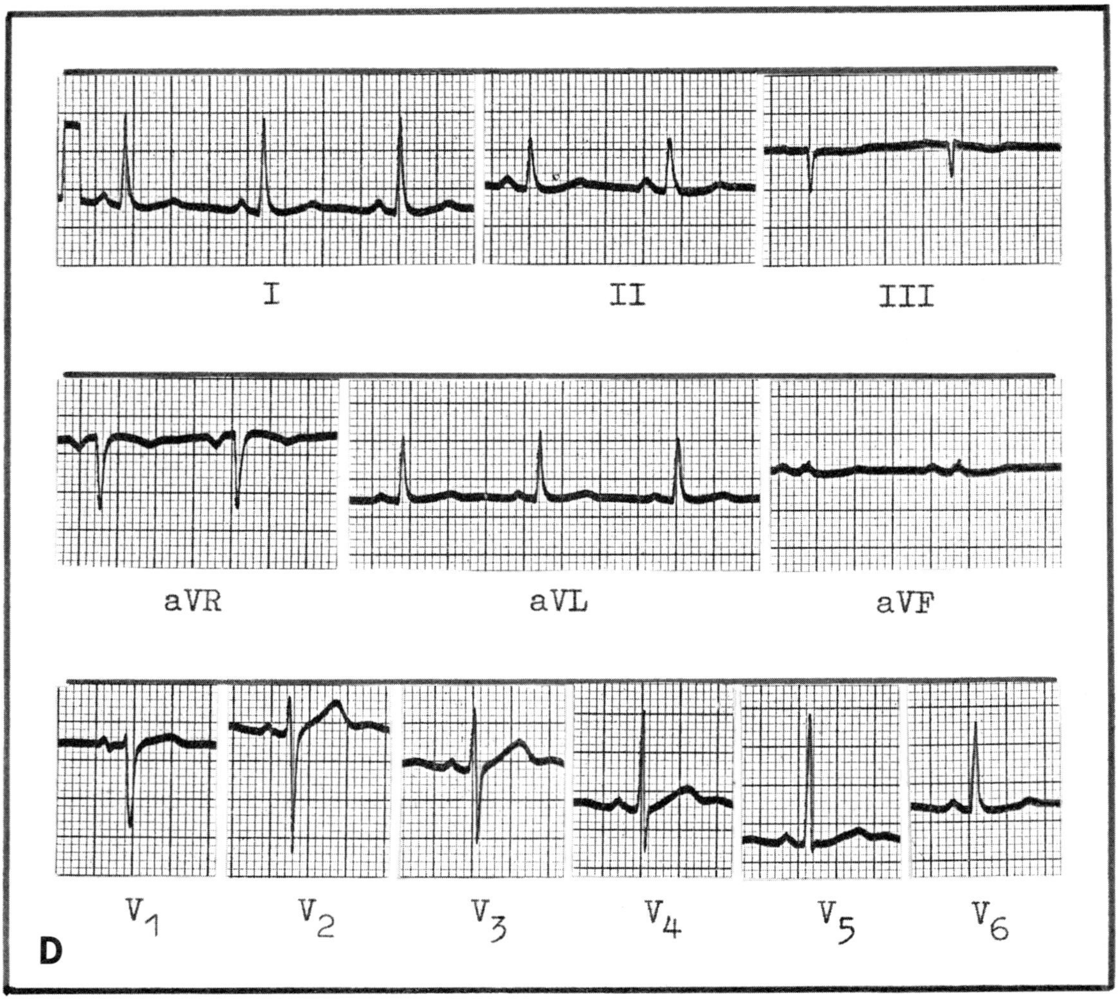

FIGURE 5–19 *Continued.* *D,* Stable electrocardiogram 2½ years after the electrocardiogram in Figure 5–19*C*. Describe the striking changes in the precordial leads.

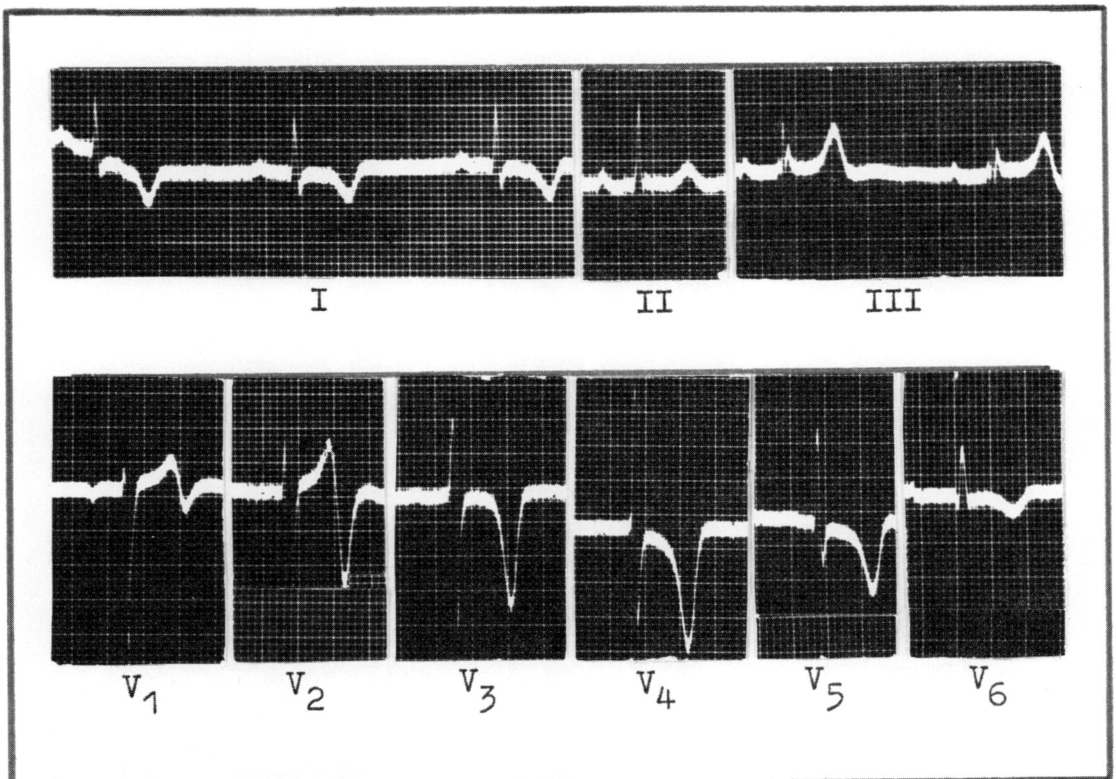

FIGURE 5–20. Subendocardial (anterior) infarction. Myocardial infarction, without Q waves, was recognized many years ago. The biphasic T waves in leads V_1 and V_2, as well as the depth of T wave inversion, are highly suggestive of myocardial infarction.
(Electrocardiogram reduced in size.)

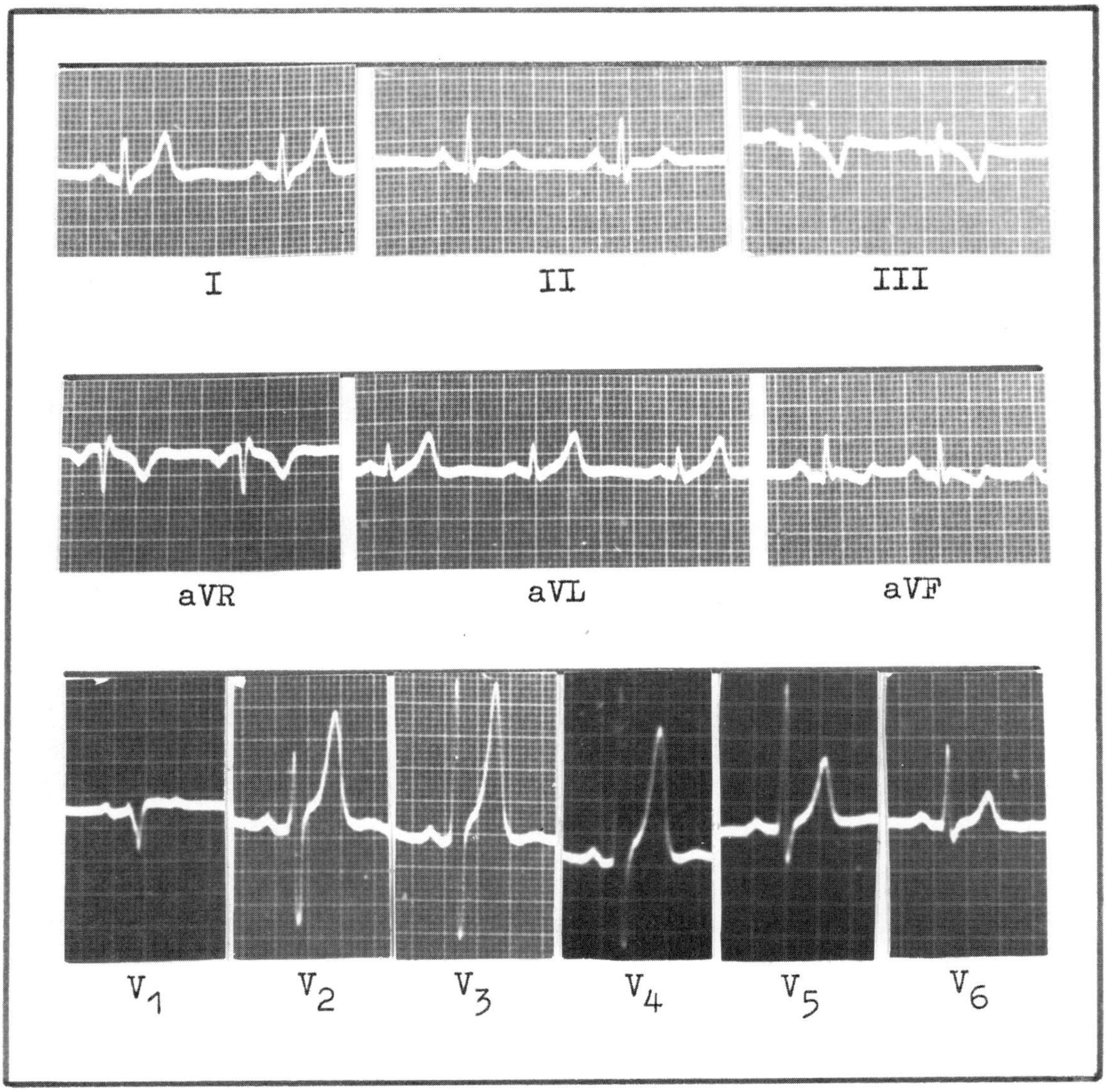

FIGURE 5–21. Subendocardial (posterior) infarction. The mean T vector faces *away* from the infarction in the posterior wall. Again, you must be certain that infarction is present clinically, since similar changes may be caused by electrolyte imbalance.
(Electrocardiogram reduced in size.)

C. Terminal QRS Vector Abnormalities

In examining for electrocardiographic alterations associated with myocardial infarction it has been customary to look for an abnormal initial QRS vector (Q wave) and abnormal repolarization (S–T and T abnormalities). Multiple examples have been seen in the preceding electrocardiograms. Terminal QRS vector abnormalities associated with myocar-

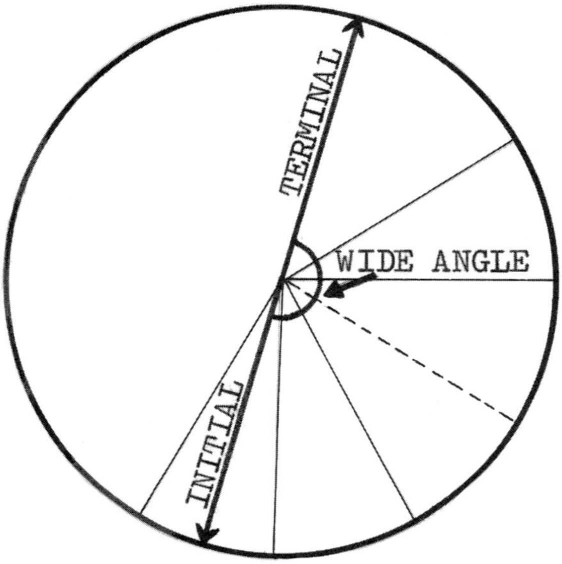

A

Wide angle between initial and terminal QRS vector.

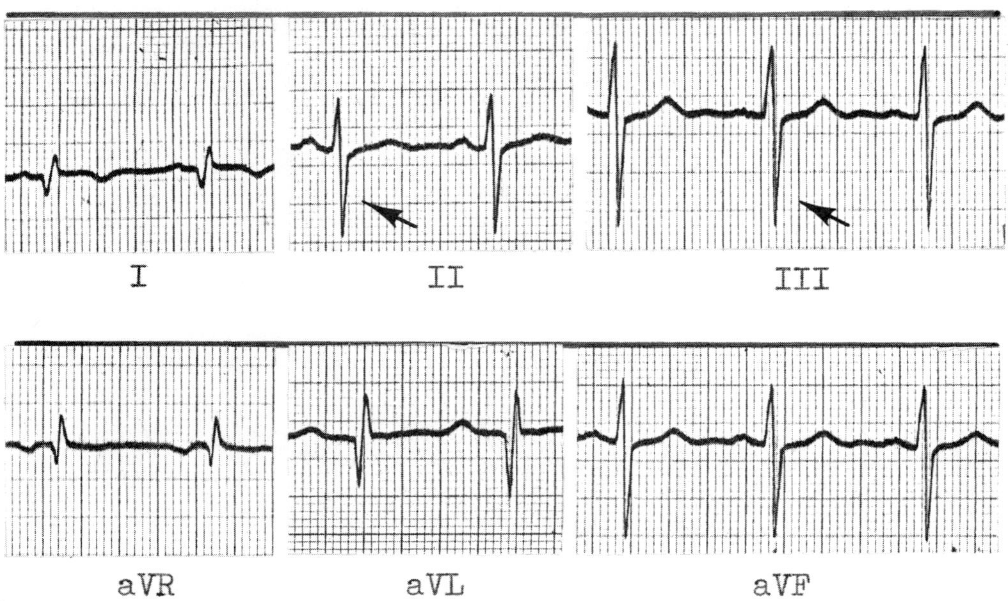

B

FIGURE 5–22. Anterolateral myocardial infarction with leftward shift of the terminal QRS vector. The left axis deviation of the QRS vector will be discussed in the section on hemiblocks in Chapter 6. The arrows in leads II and III point to the deep S waves in leads II and III signifying a terminal QRS vectorial shift to the left.

dial infarction have received less attention, unfortunately; every electrocardiogram should be inspected for these changes. Figure 5–22 reveals the Q waves in leads I and aVL of an anterolateral infarction. Of great importance is also the fact that the terminal QRS vector shifted leftward as a result of the infarct, creating a wide angle between the initial and terminal QRS vectors. This had "classically" been called peri-infarction block due to anterolateral myocardial infarction. Carefully inspect the electrocardiograms prior to infarction to be certain that the terminal vectorial abnormalities were not present *before* the infarct. This is especially true in anterolateral myocardial infarction because left axis deviation is often found to antecede the infarction. If left axis deviation existed prior to the infarction, obviously the infarction cannot be implicated in its cause.* Again serial electrocardiographic tracings are of great help.

Figure 5–23 illustrates the terminal QRS vectorial changes following diaphragmatic myocardial infarction. This QRS alteration is under investigation.

*This left axis deviation will be discussed in the section on hemiblocks in Chapter 6.

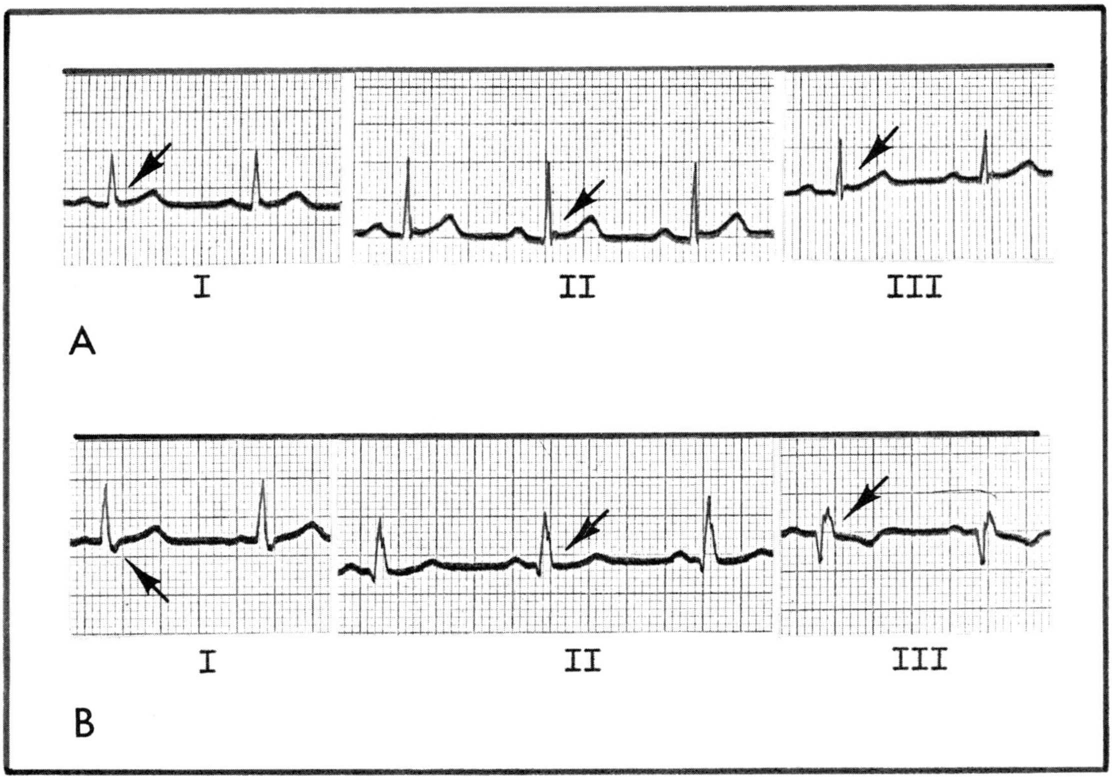

FIGURE 5–23. *A*, Baseline electrocardiogram. *B*, Diaphragmatic myocardial infarction. In addition to the Q waves in leads II and III note the terminal QRS vectorial change in all three leads (arrows).

REVIEW ELECTROCARDIOGRAMS

Before beginning the analysis of Figures 5–24 to 5–48, the rest of the electrocardiograms in this chapter, review the basic concepts of myocardial infarction. Included are several sets of serial electrocardiograms not too frequently seen.

Figures 5–25*A* and 5–25*B* are from a patient with dextrocardia before and after an anterior wall myocardial infarction. Review the mean P vector of dextrocardia in Chapter 1. Note—in the third panel of Figure 5–25*A*, marked V_1 to V_6—the R waves across the precordium are decreasing in magnitude.* When the leads are placed on the right side, rather than on the left side, of the chest the leads appear properly placed (fourth panel). Study this set; all the features of dextrocardia are included.

*This may be confused with the "poor R wave progression" associated with myocardial damage, ventricular hypertrophy and some conduction disturbances.

Figures 5–28 and 5–30 are from patients with diaphragmatic myocardial infarction and disturbances of the atrioventricular conduction system. This is not uncommon in myocardial infarction. Aspects of the atrioventricular conduction system will be discussed in Chapter 6.

Figures 5–43*A* and *B* are from a patient with a history of an old diaphragmatic myocardial infarction who developed right bundle branch block with right axis deviation and a new massive myocardial infarction. This entity, known as bifascicular block (left posterior hemiblock plus right bundle branch block), will be discussed in Chapter 6.

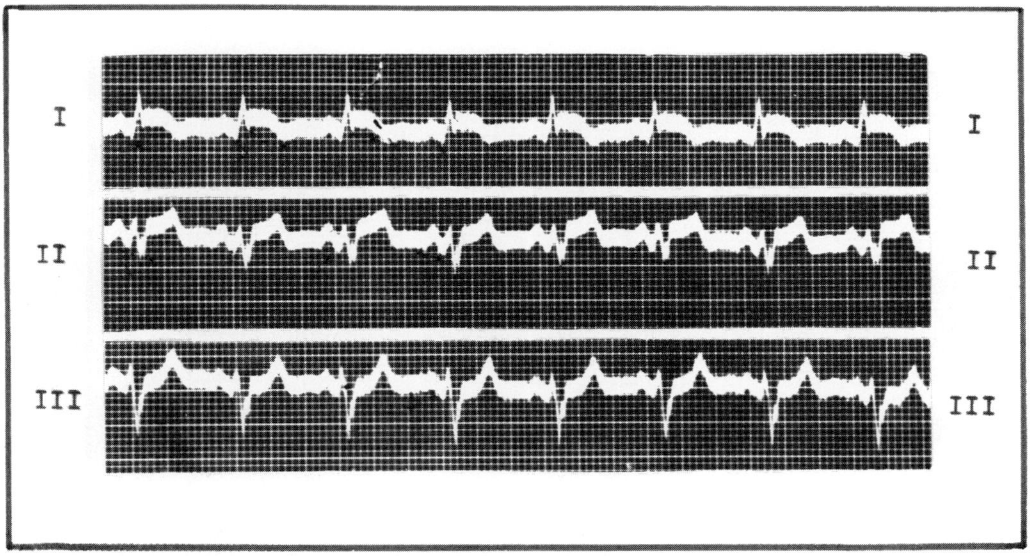

FIGURE 5–24. Anterior myocardial infarction. This electrocardiogram was taken when the patient was experiencing chest pain, with clinical evidence of myocardial infarction. Describe. (Electrocardiogram reduced in size.)

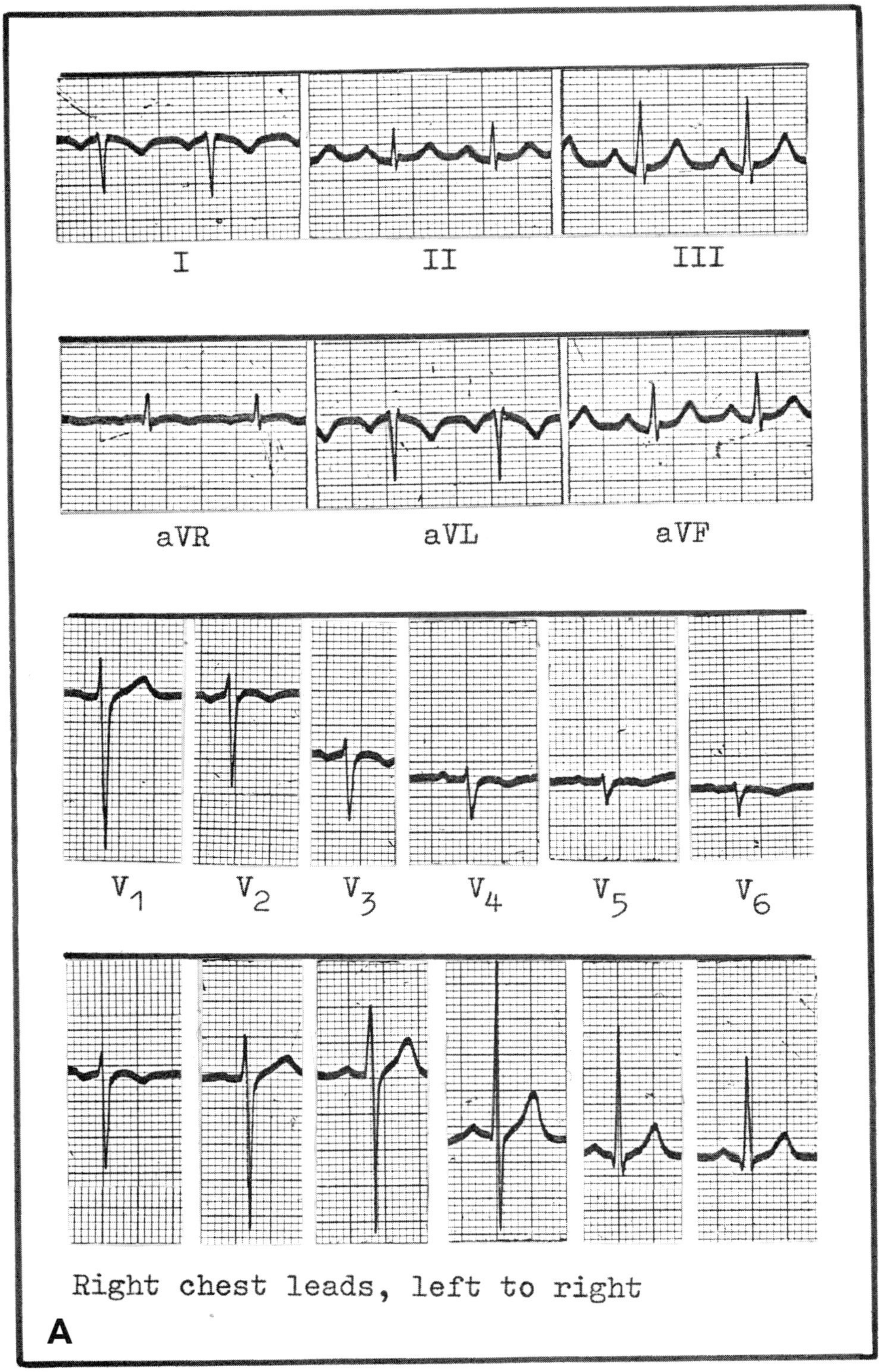

FIGURE 5–25. *A,* Dextrocardia. This is the baseline electrocardiogram. Before proceeding to Figure 5–25*B*, review the mean P vector of dextrocardia in Chapter 1.

Illustration continued on opposite page.

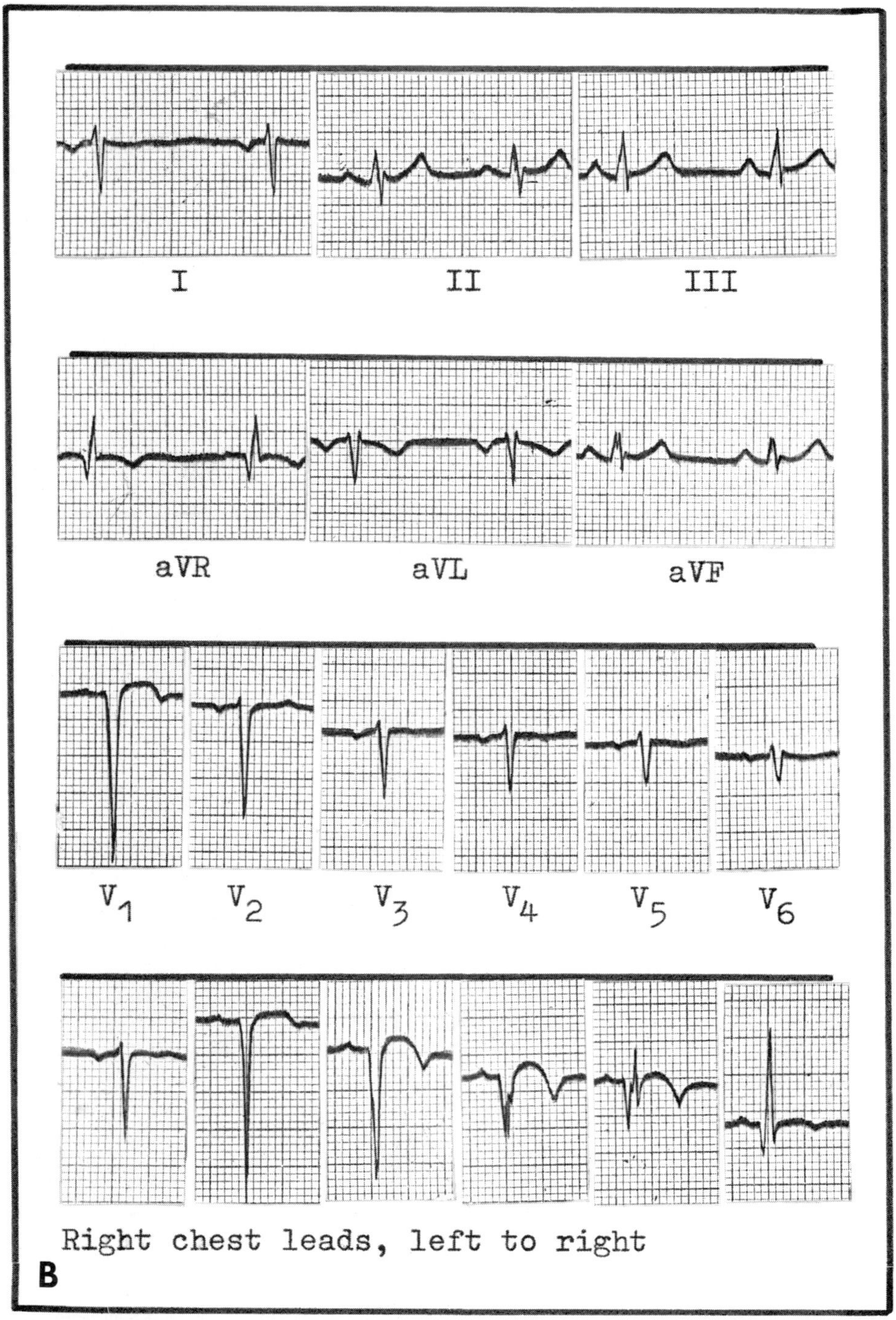

FIGURE 5–25 *Continued.* *B,* Dextrocardia. This is the same patient as in Figure 5–25*A* following an anterior wall myocardial infarction. Explain the findings.

Cassette Side 14

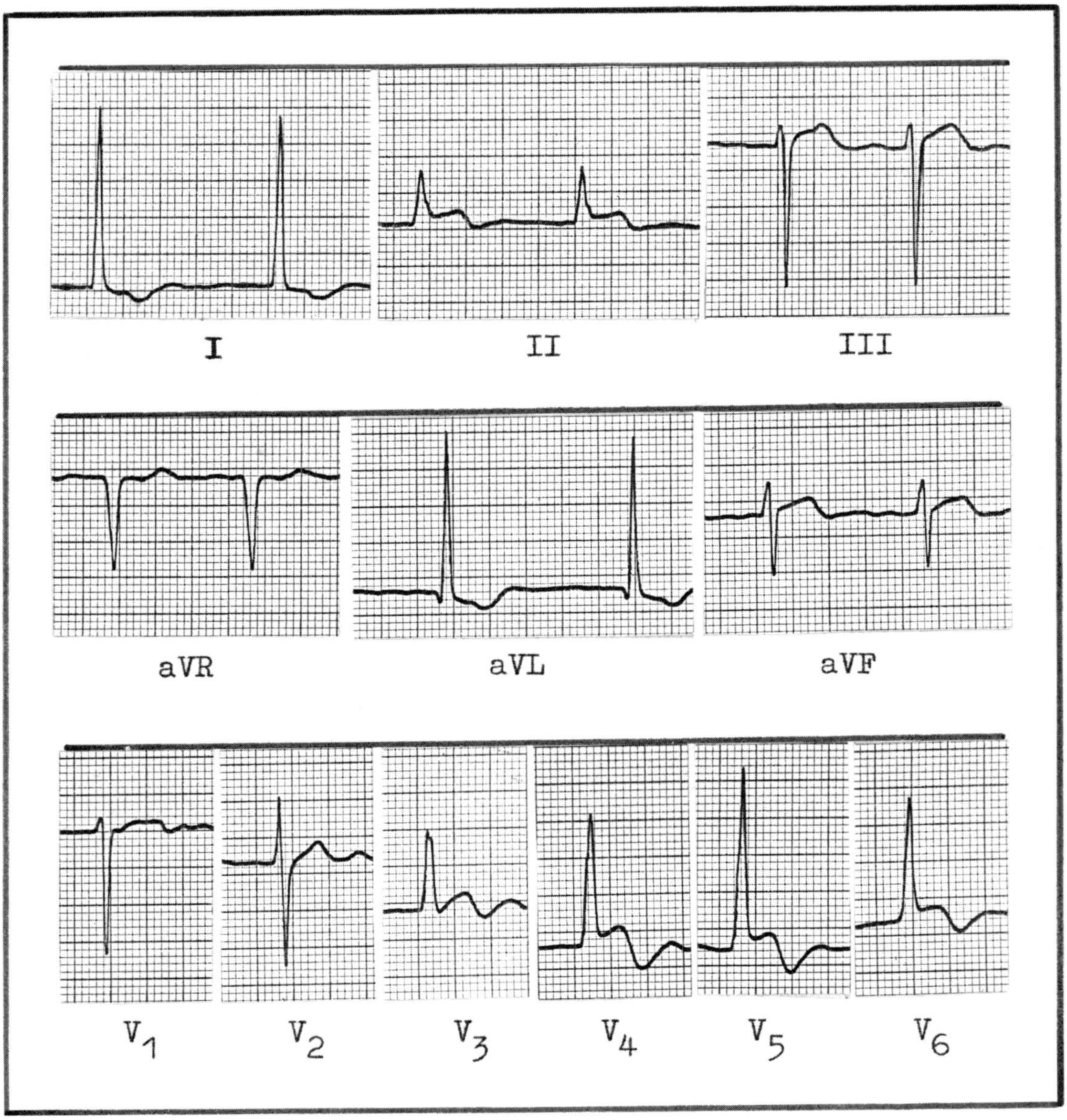

FIGURE 5–26. Ventricular aneurysm in an elderly patient with an enlarged left ventricle and atrial fibrillation. Could you make a diagnosis of myocardial infarction on the basis of Q waves? This pattern has been stable in this patient for about five years following acute myocardial infarction. How would you treat this patient if you did not know him and he walked into your office complaining of chest pain and exhibited this electrocardiogram?

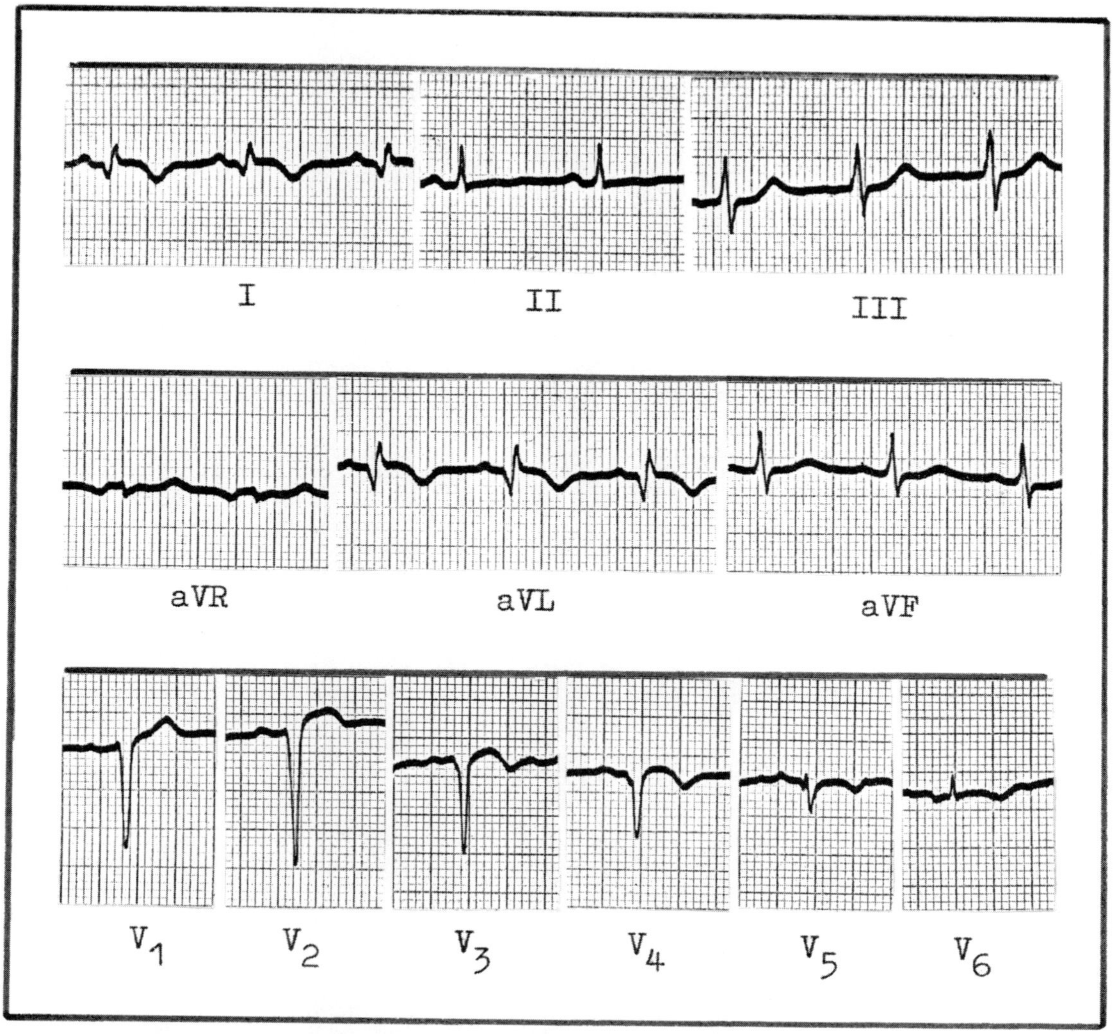

FIGURE 5–27. Ventricular aneurysm following myocardial infarction. This is a stable pattern many months after the acute infarction.

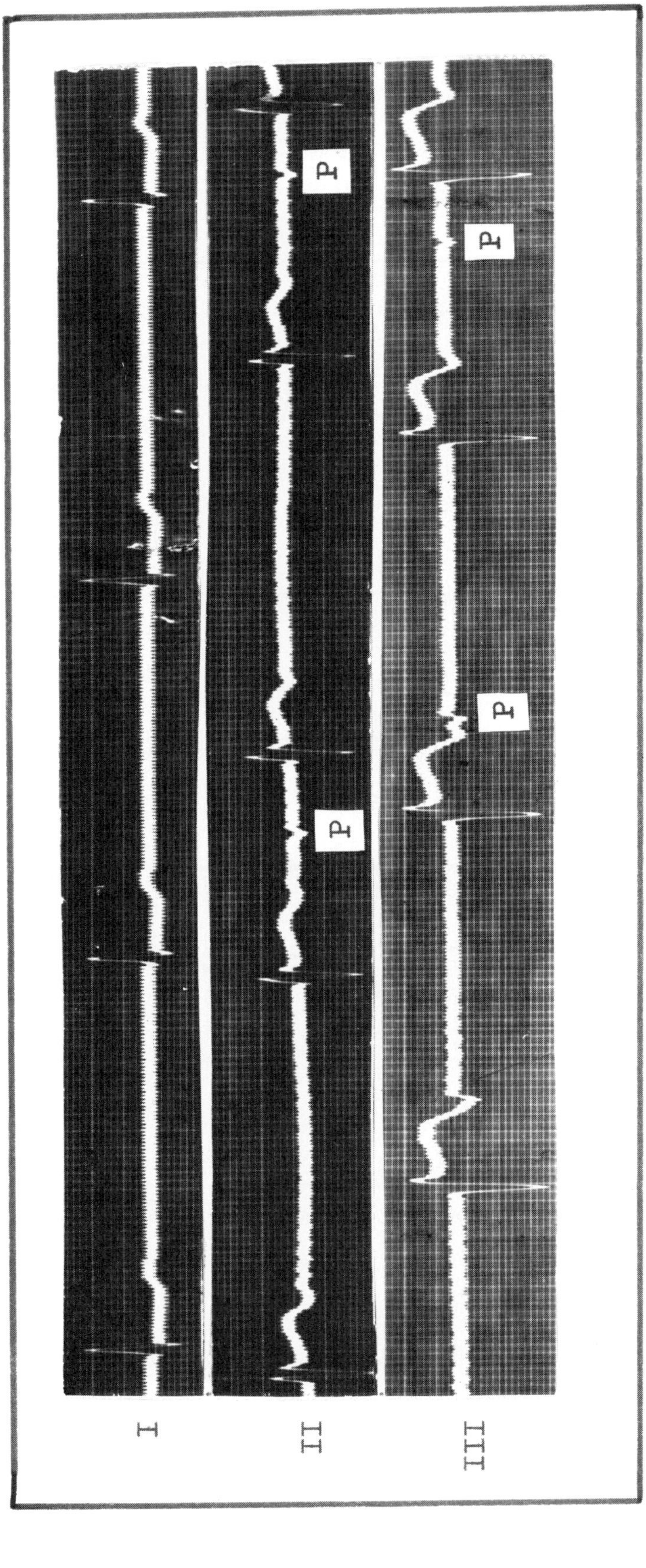

FIGURE 5–28. Diaphragmatic myocardial infarction. Why is the rhythm irregular? The P waves, where seen, are indicated in leads II and III. This is not uncommon in myocardial infarction.

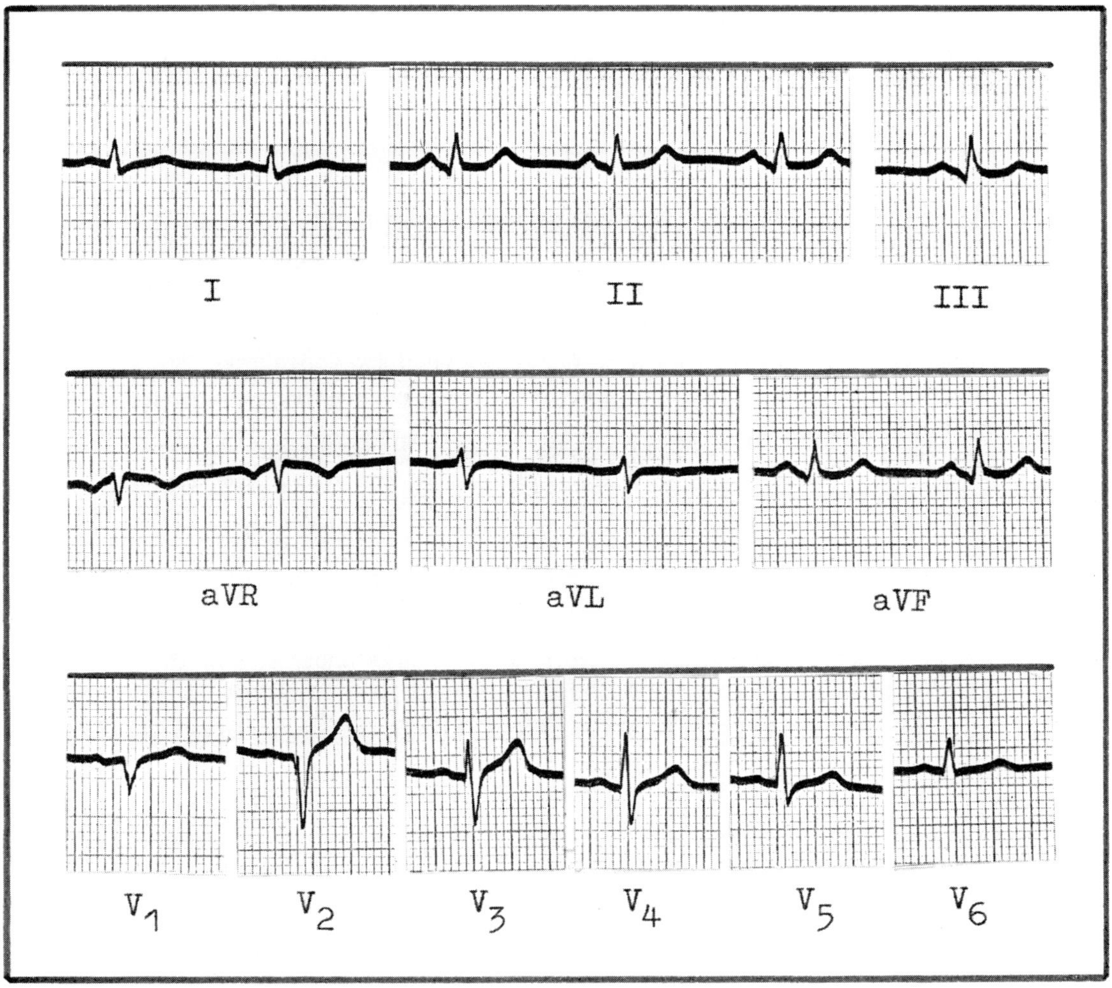

FIGURE 5–29. Anteroseptal or strictly anterior myocardial infarction in a patient with a history of old diaphragmatic myocardial infarction.

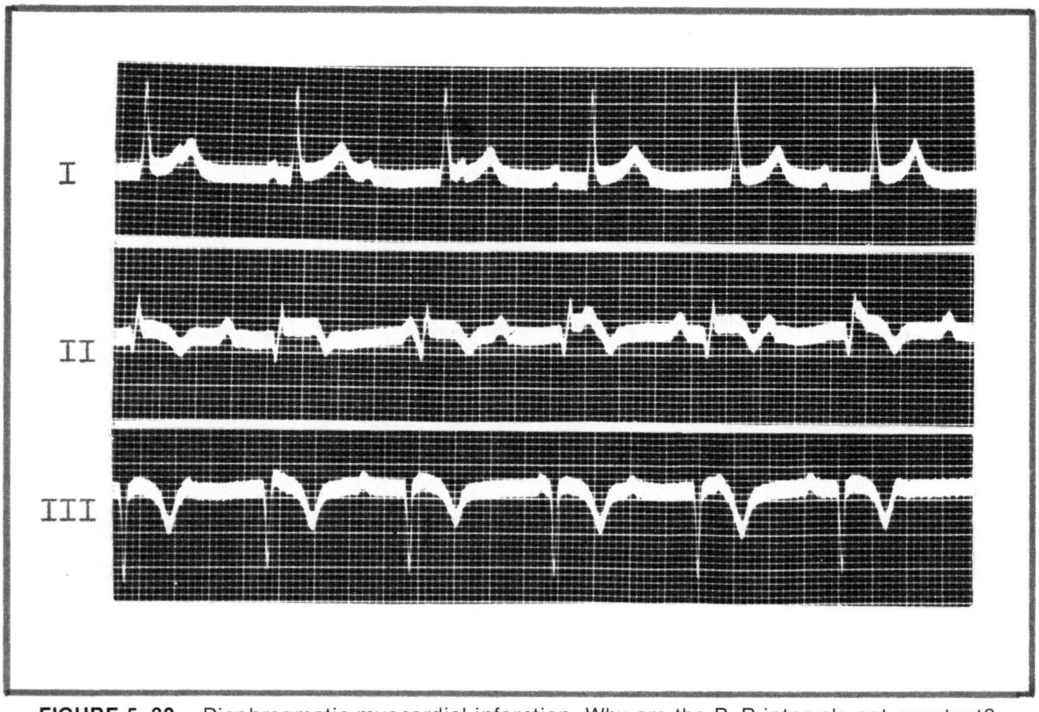

FIGURE 5–30. Diaphragmatic myocardial infarction. Why are the P–R intervals not constant? (Electrocardiogram reduced in size.)

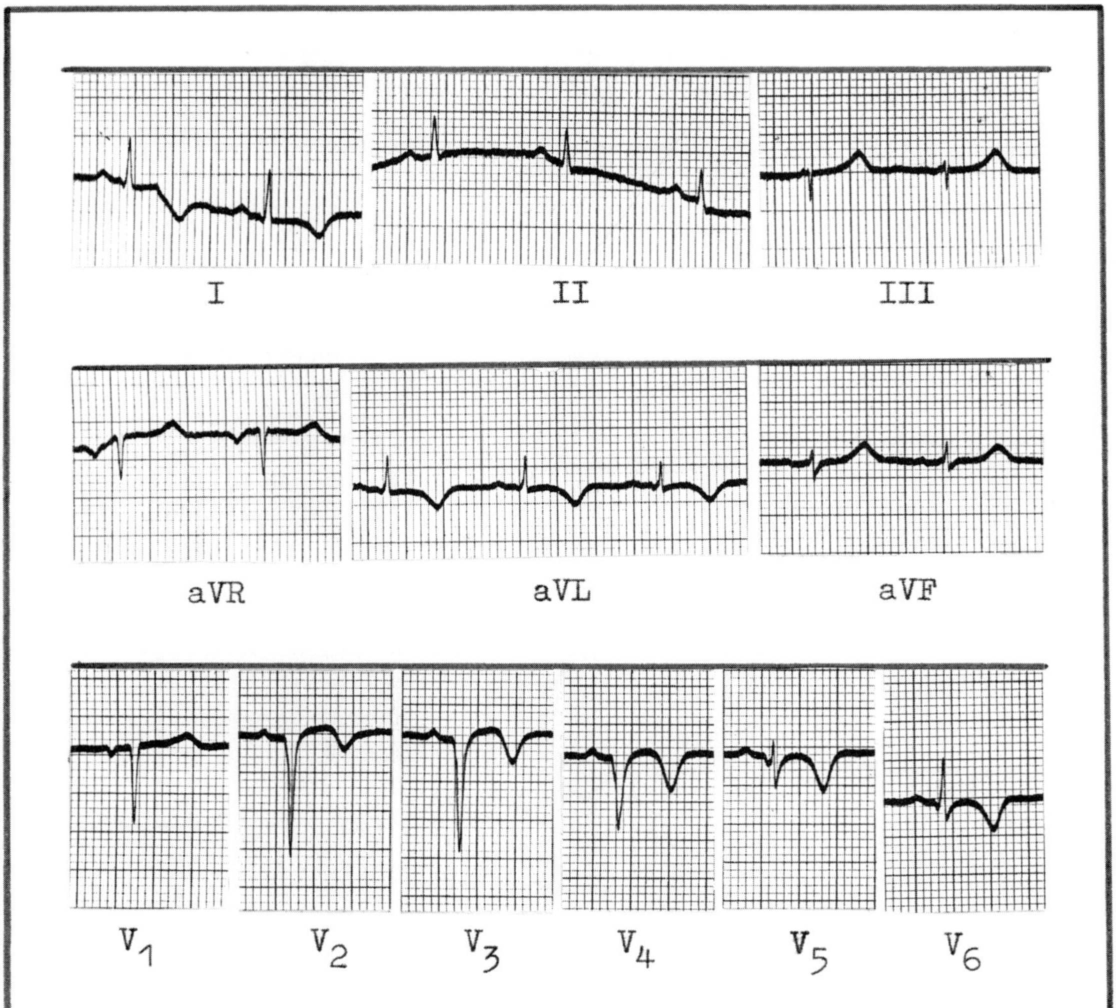

FIGURE 5–31. Anterior myocardial infarction. Could you make this diagnosis without the chest leads?

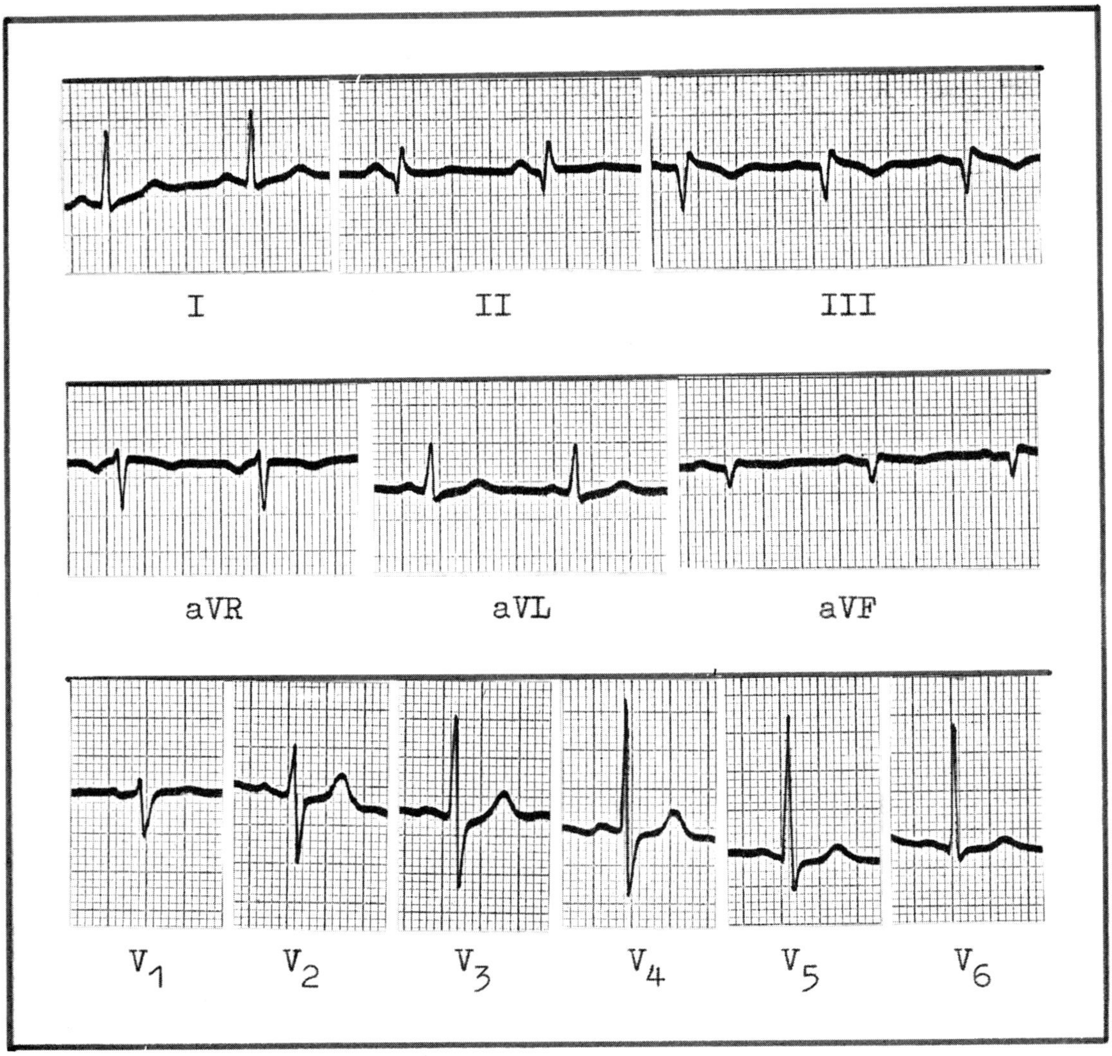

FIGURE 5–32. Diaphragmatic myocardial infarction.

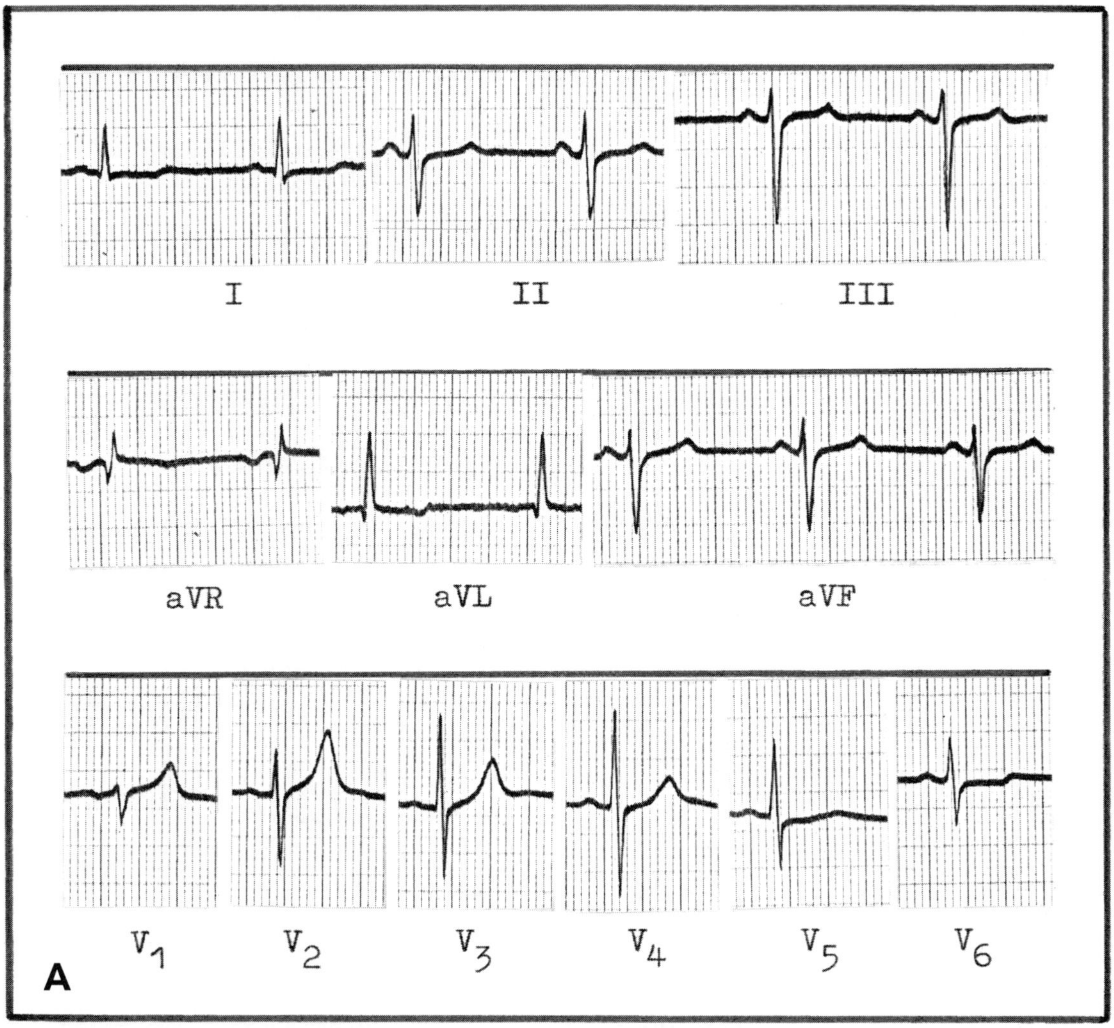

FIGURE 5–33. *A,* Baseline electrocardiogram prior to myocardial infarction. Describe the abnormalities.
Illustration continued on following page.

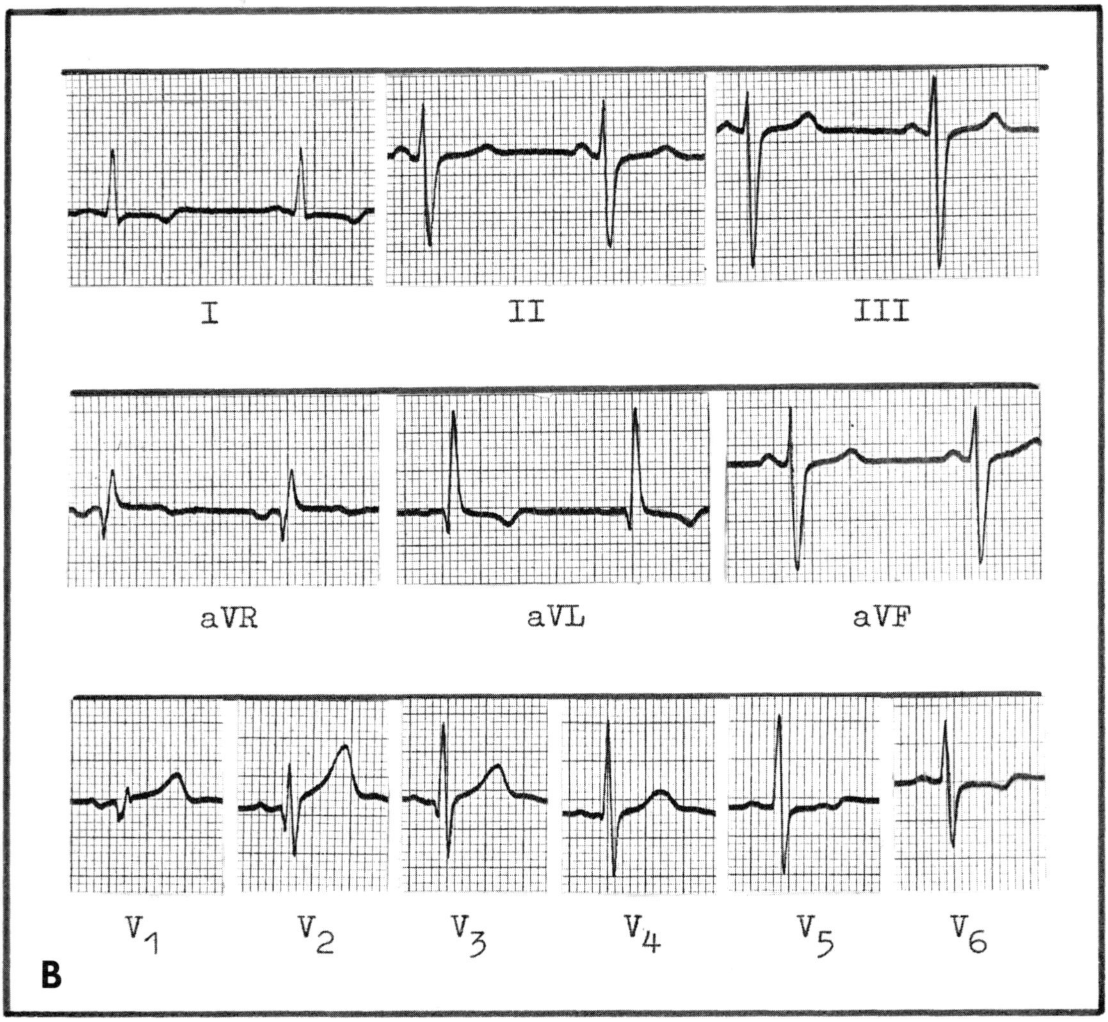

FIGURE 5–33 *Continued.* *B,* Same patient as in Figure 5–33*A* following anteroseptal myocardial infarction.

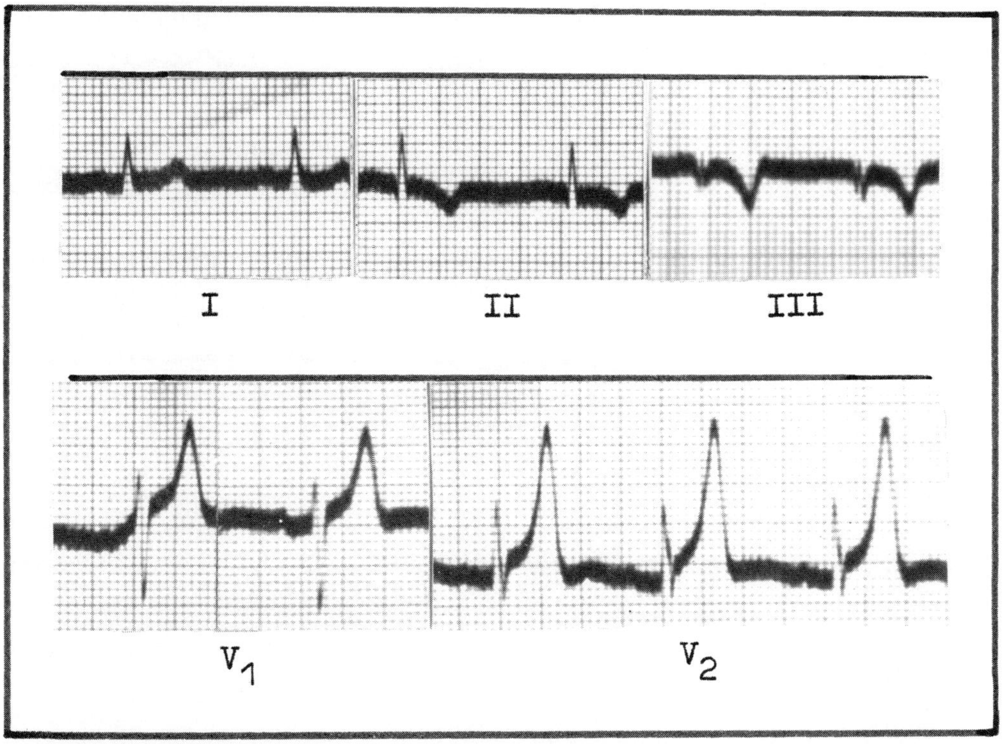

FIGURE 5–34. Patient with clinical evidence of myocardial infarction. In addition to deep Q waves in lead III and smaller Q waves in lead II, there is marked peaking of the T waves in leads V_1 and V_2. Where was the infarct?
(Electrocardiogram enlarged for clarity.)

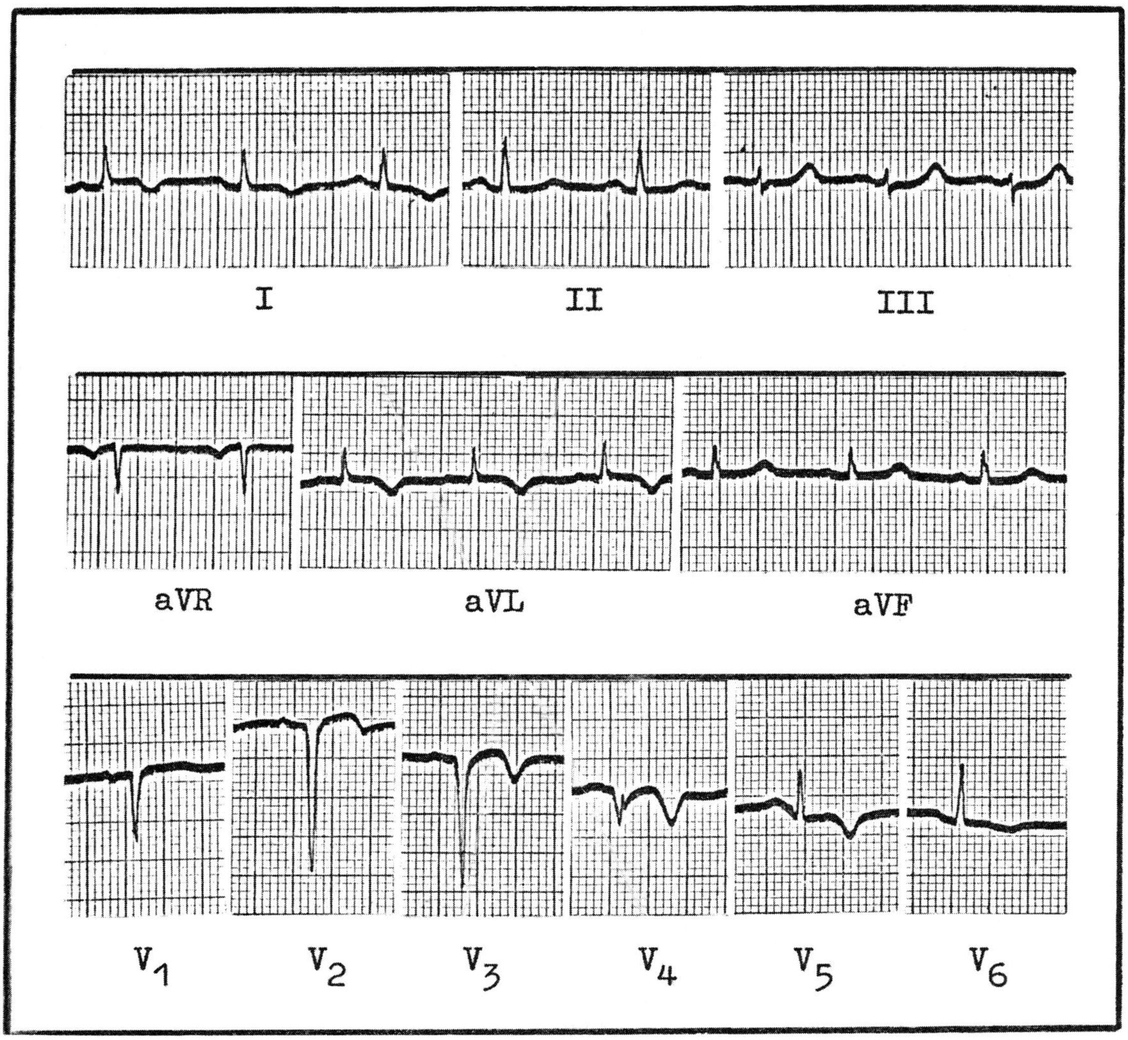

FIGURE 5–35. Anterior myocardial infarction. Explain the absence of Q waves in the frontal plane leads.

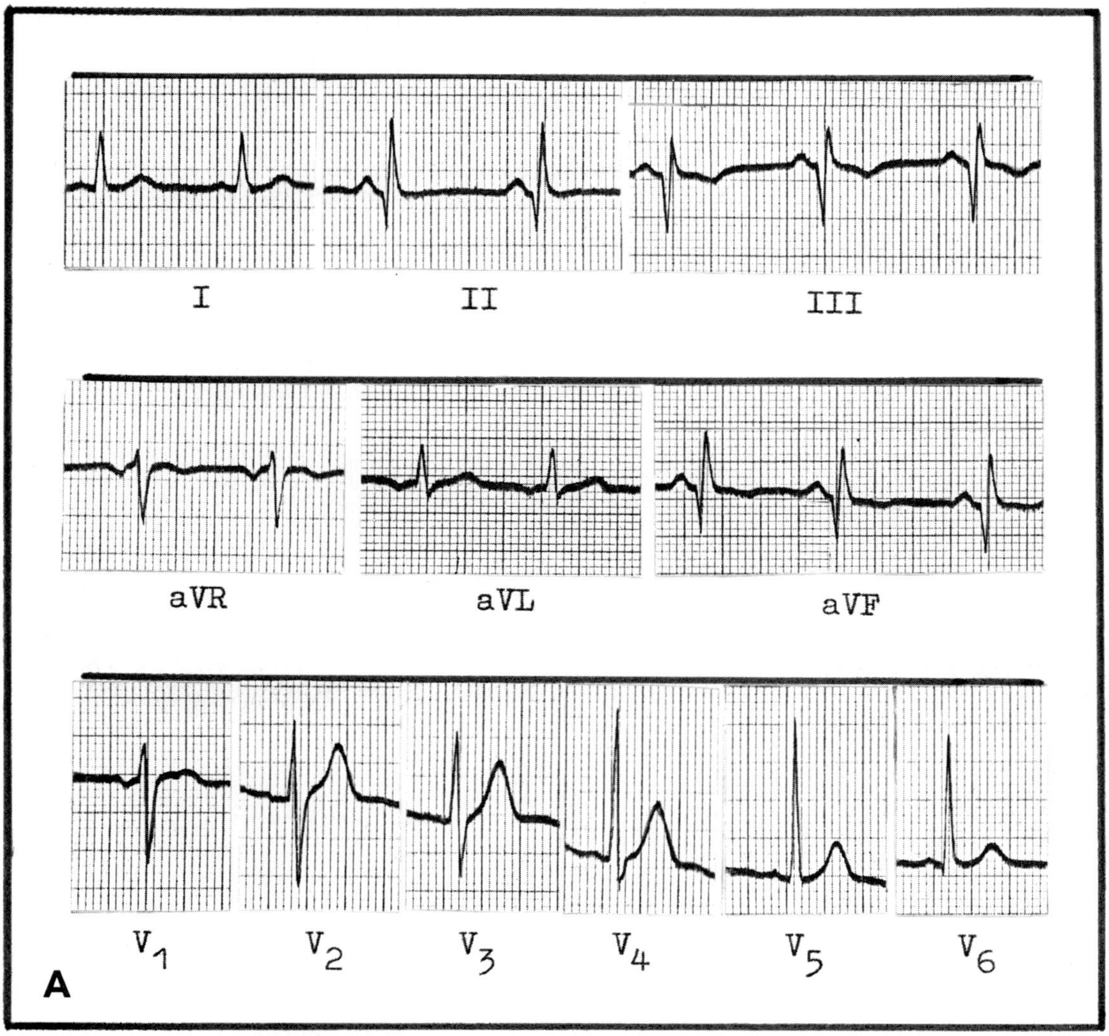

FIGURE 5–36. *A,* Diaphragmatic myocardial infarction.

Illustration continued on following page.

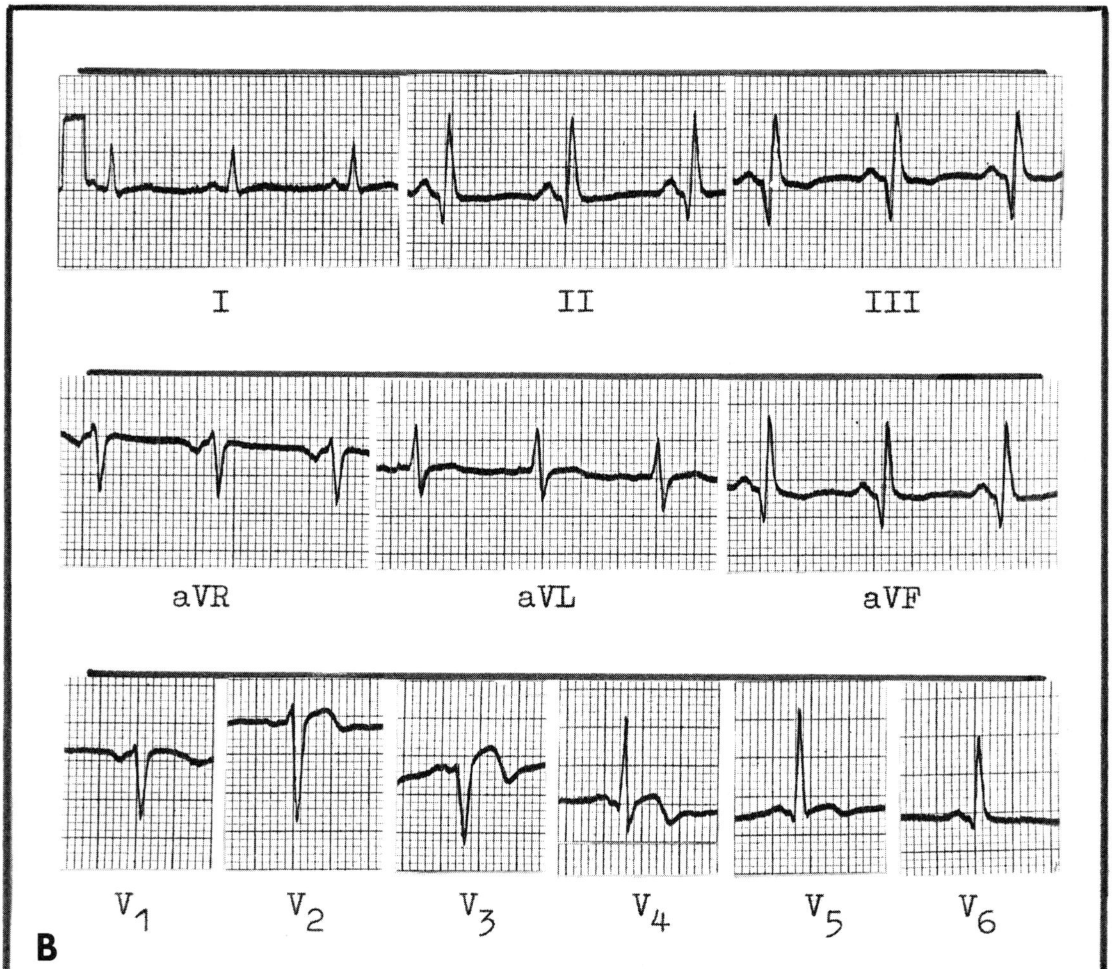

FIGURE 5–36 *Continued.* *B,* Same patient as in Figure 5–36*A* following development of an anteroseptal myocardial infarction. Without the comparison tracings, how would you determine which infarct came before which?

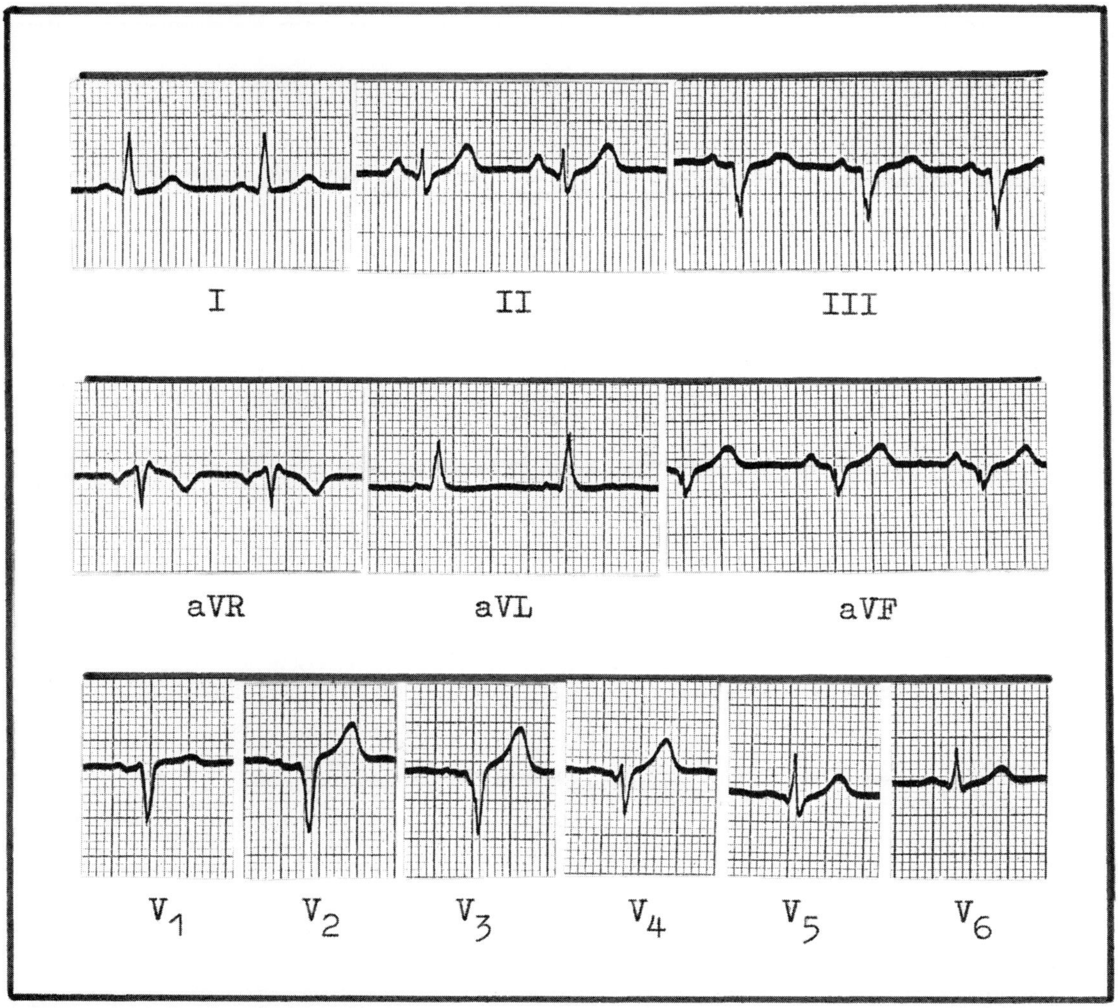

FIGURE 5–37. Infarction of the heart involving the anterior and diaphragmatic areas. Were these changes the result of one or more than one myocardial infarction?

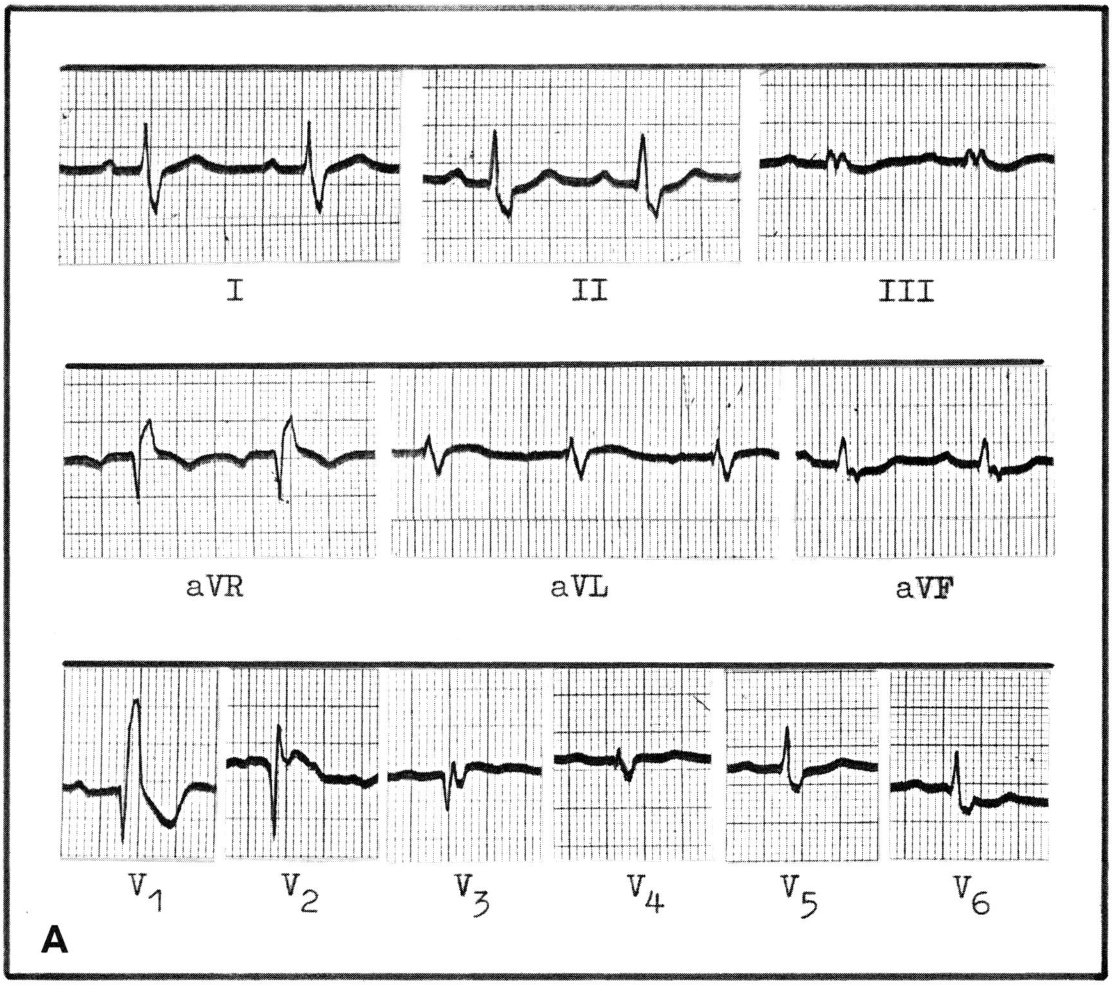

FIGURE 5–38. *A,* Anteroseptal myocardial infarction in a patient with right bundle branch block.
Illustration continued on opposite page.

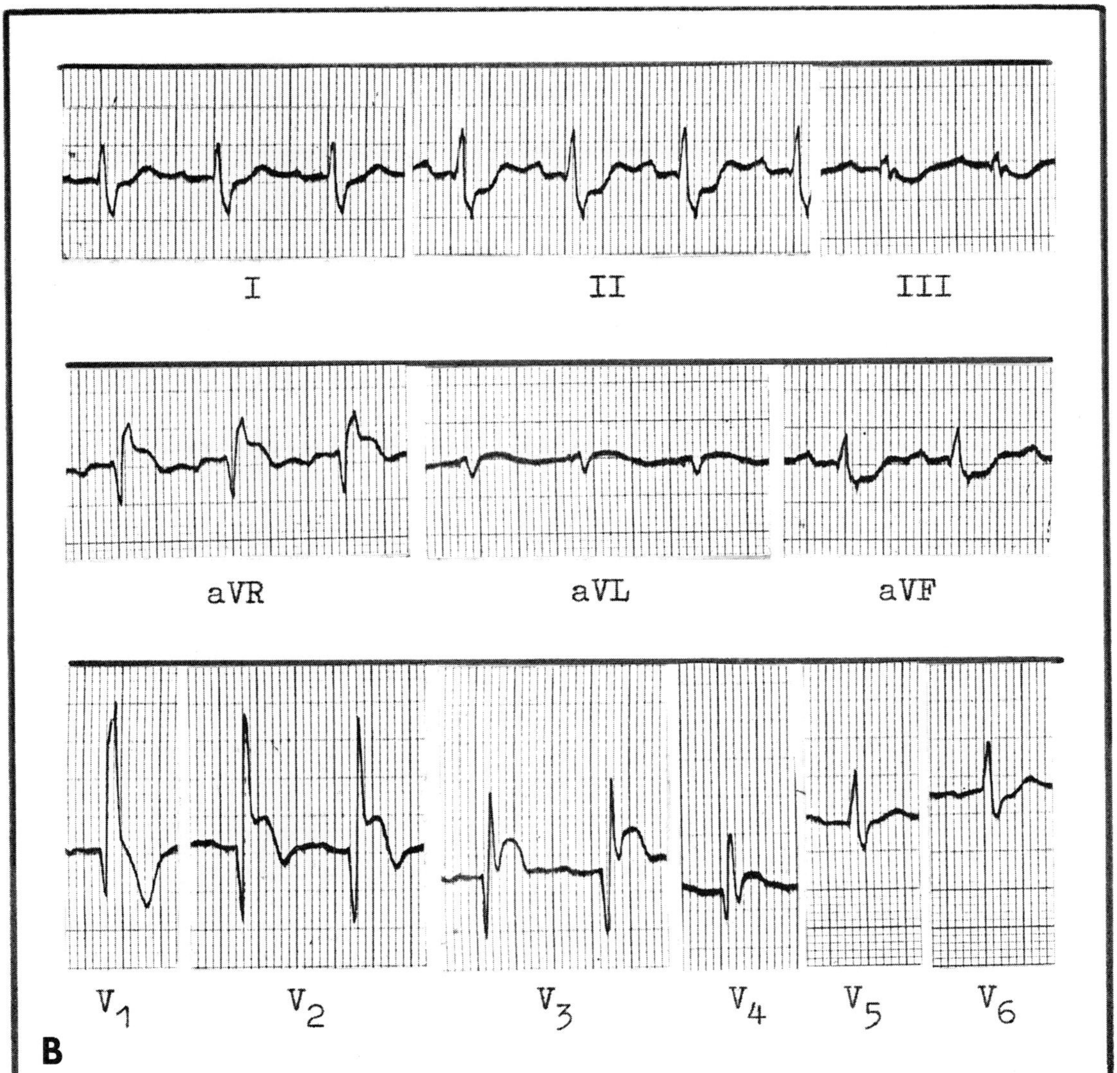

FIGURE 5–38 *Continued.* *B,* Acute myocardial infarction in same patient as in Figure 5–38*A.* Is it possible to have a new myocardial infarction in the area of the old infarction?

Illustration continued on following page.

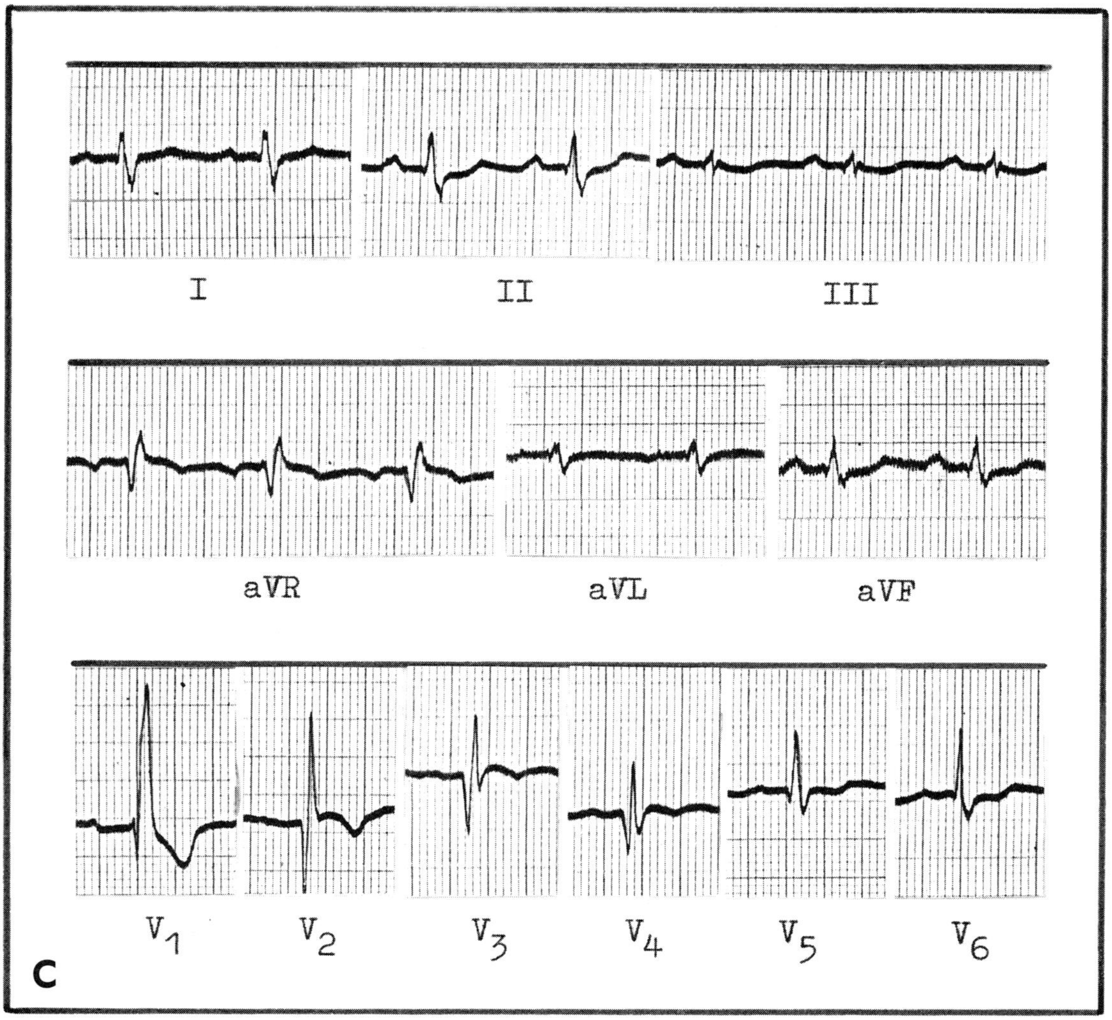

FIGURE 5–38 *Continued.* *C,* Evolutionary changes during recovery from the infarct seen in Figure 5–38 *B.*

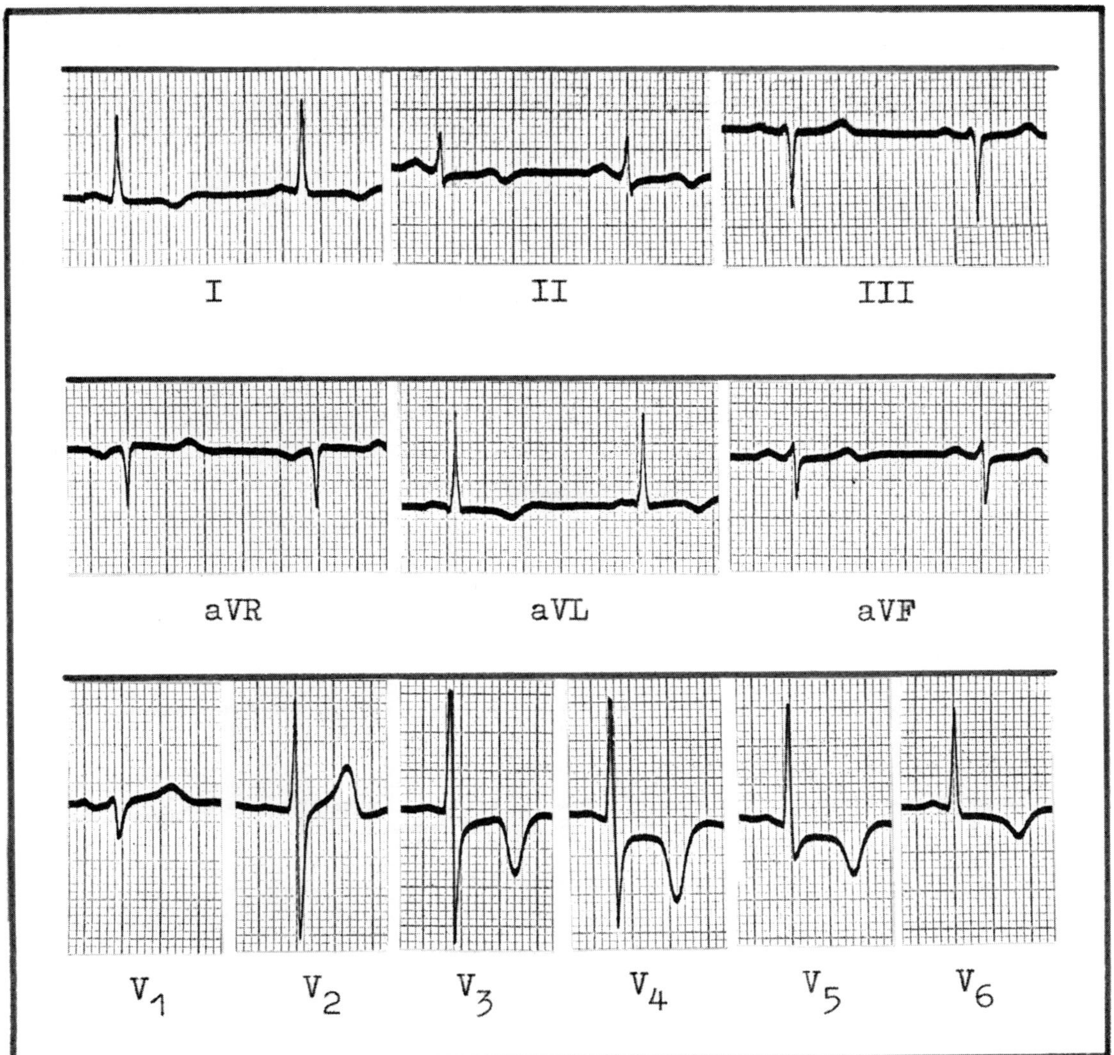

FIGURE 5–39. Anterior or anterolateral subendocardial infarction. If there were no clinical evidence of myocardial infarction, could you make the diagnosis on the basis of the repolarization abnormalities?

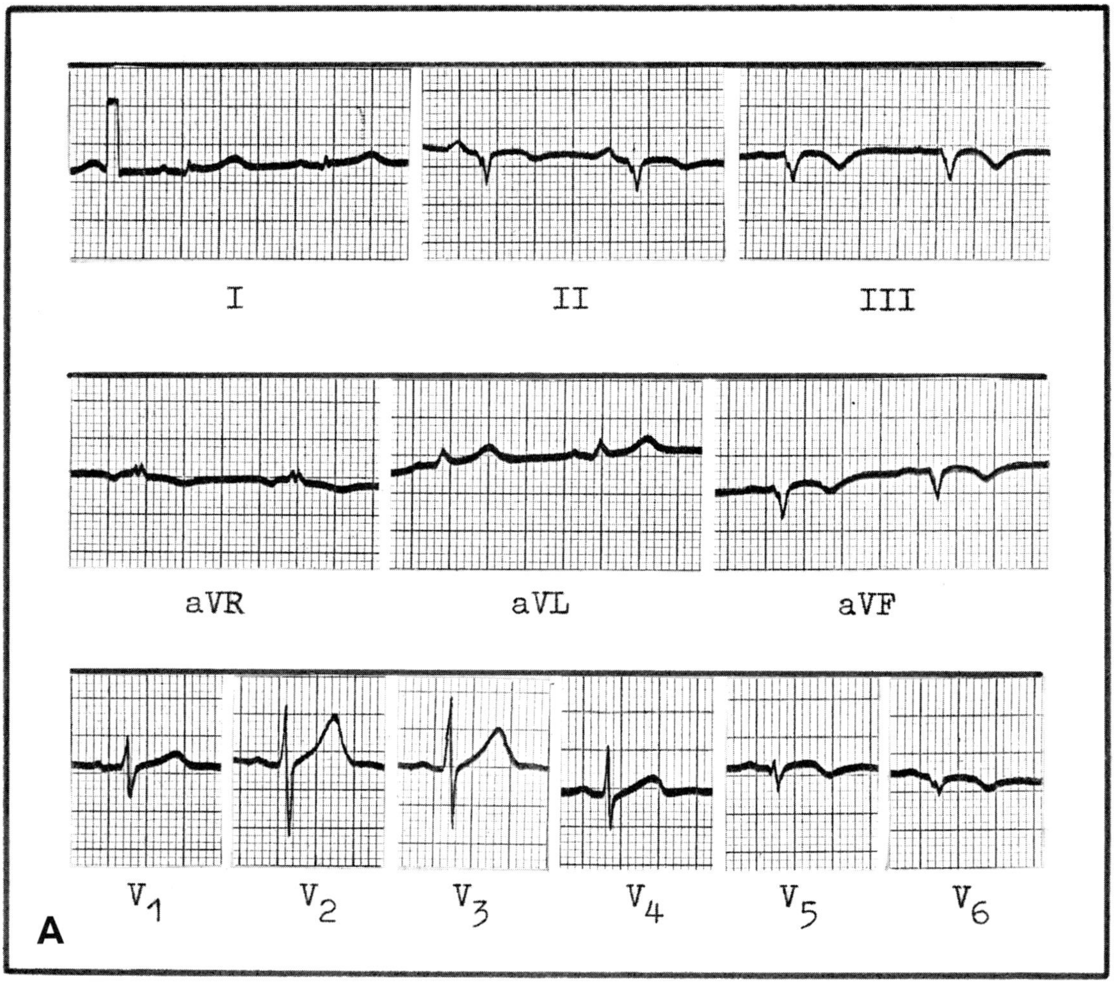

FIGURE 5–40. *A,* Evolving changes during recovery from myocardial infarction. Note Q waves in leads II, III, aVF, V_5 and V_6.

Illustration continued on opposite page.

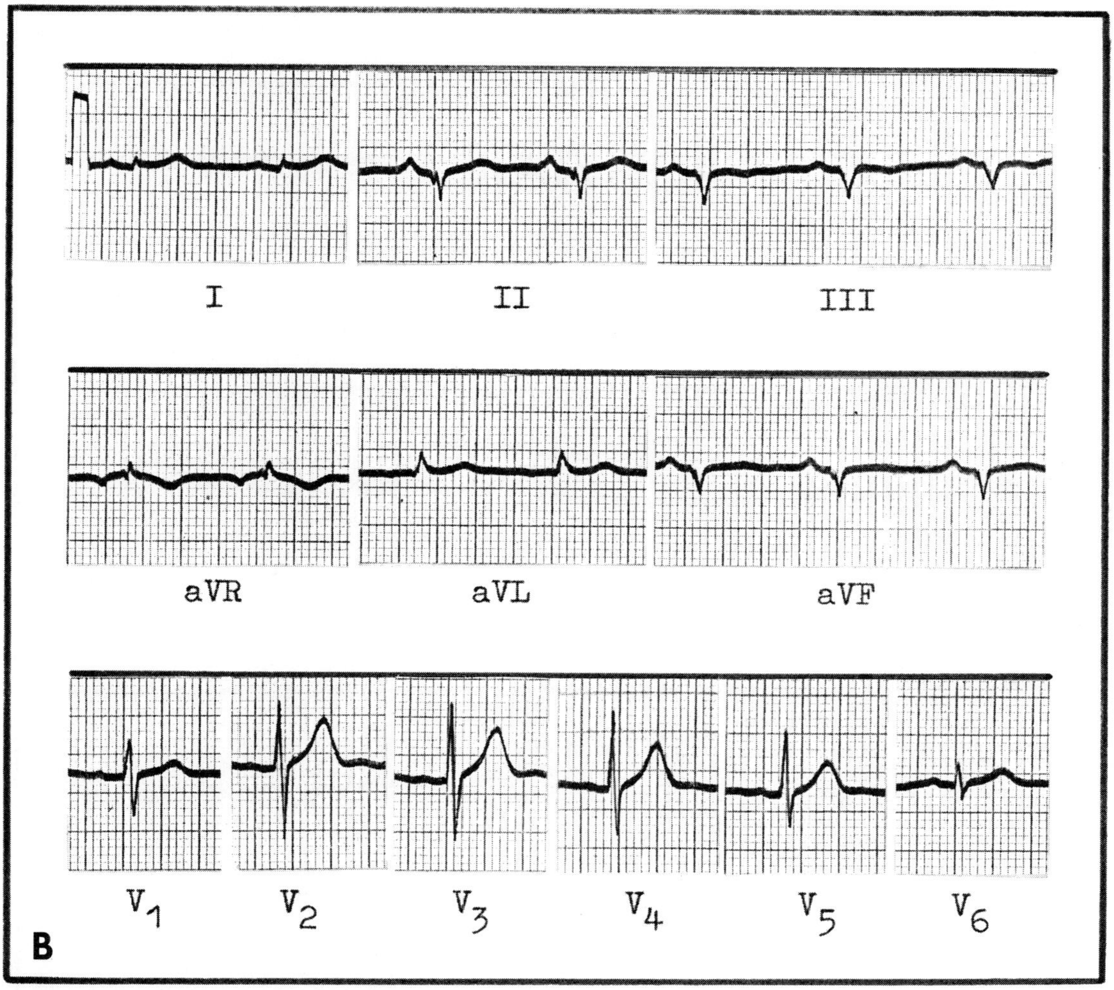

FIGURE 5–40 *Continued.* *B,* Two months following the electrocardiogram in Figure 5–40*A.* What happened to the Q waves in leads V_5 and V_6? Do Q waves have to be permanent? Did the infarct change location?

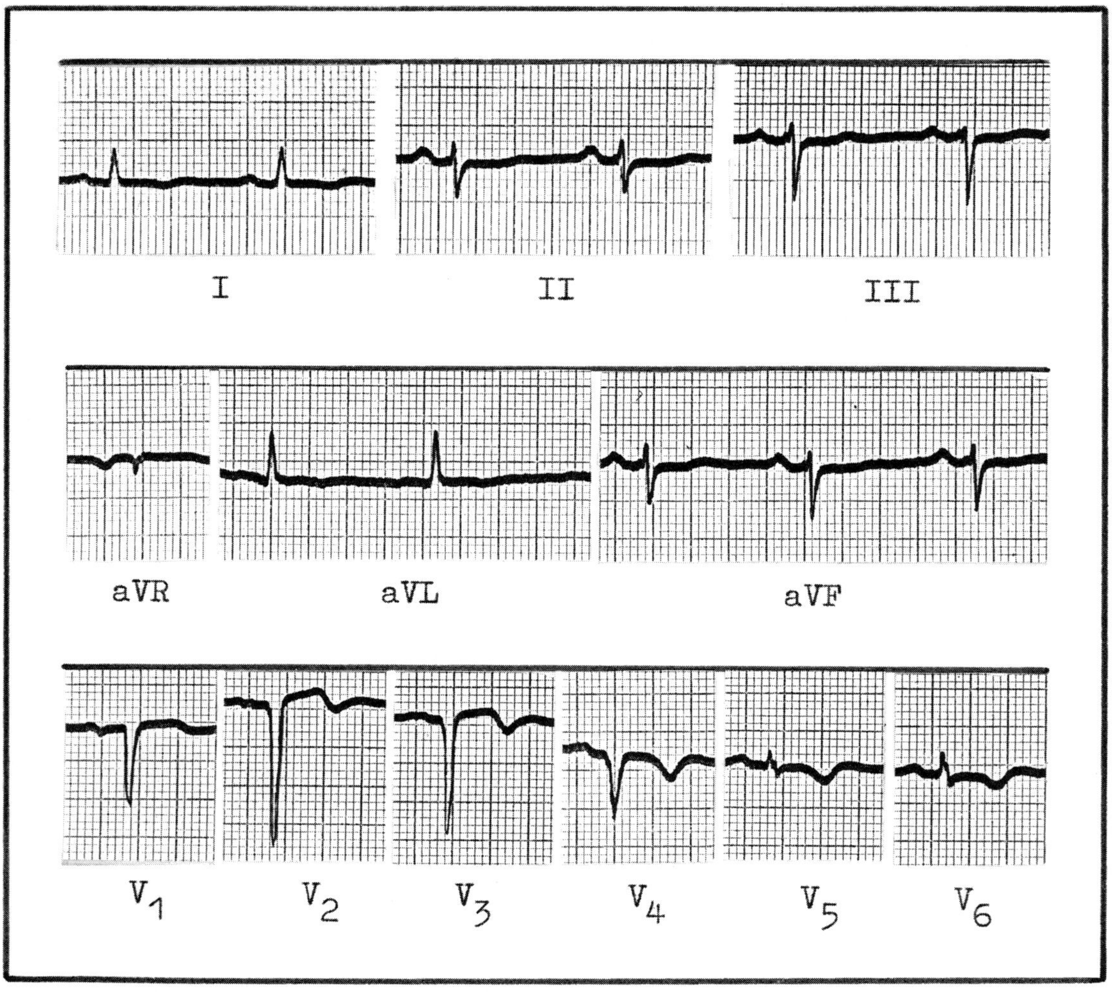

FIGURE 5–41. Anterior or anteroseptal myocardial infarction. Any other abnormalities?

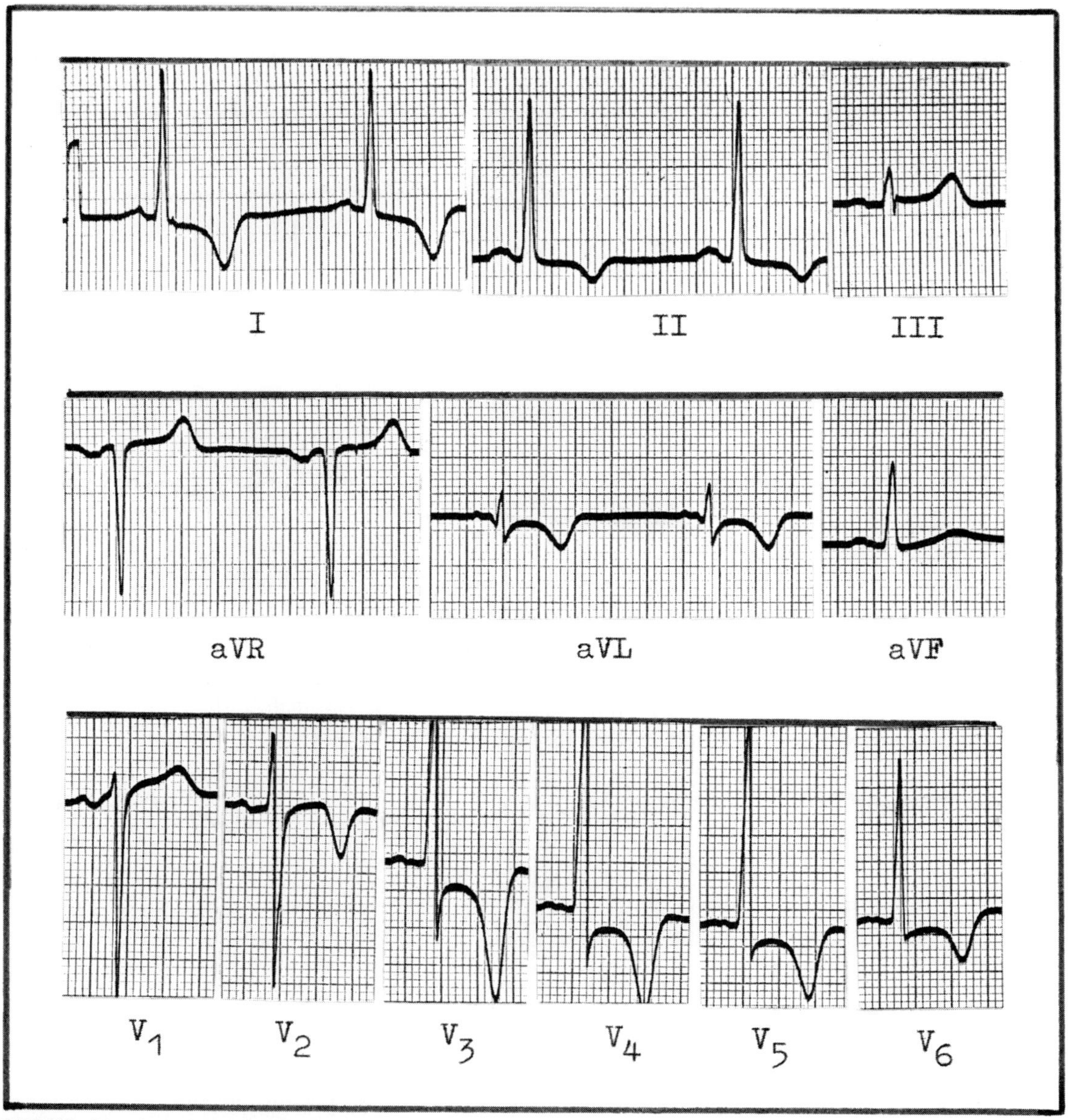

FIGURE 5–42. Anterior subendocardial infarction. If you did not have clinical evidence of infarction, what would be your differential diagnosis?

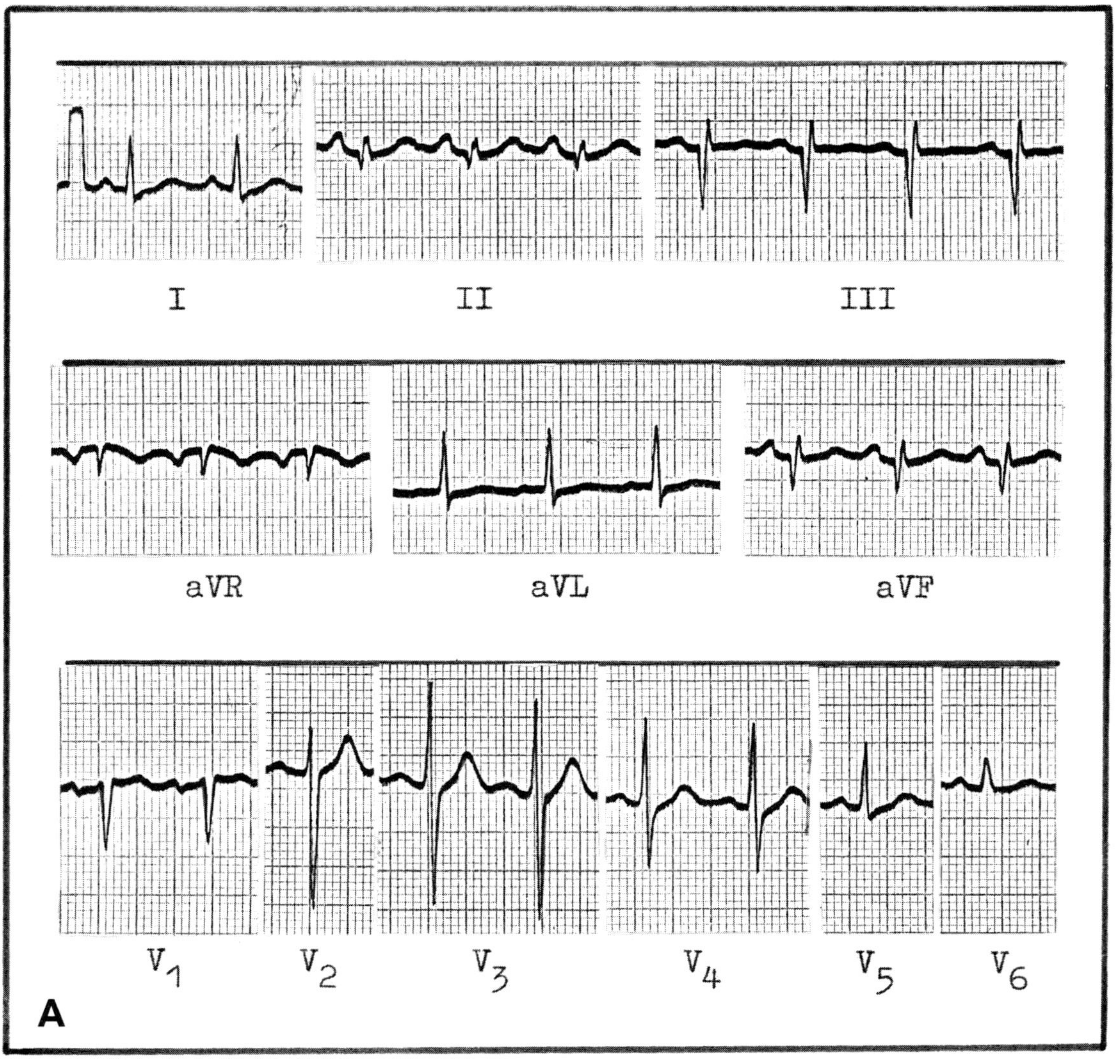

FIGURE 5–43. *A,* Diaphragmatic or inferior myocardial infarction.

Illustration continued on opposite page.

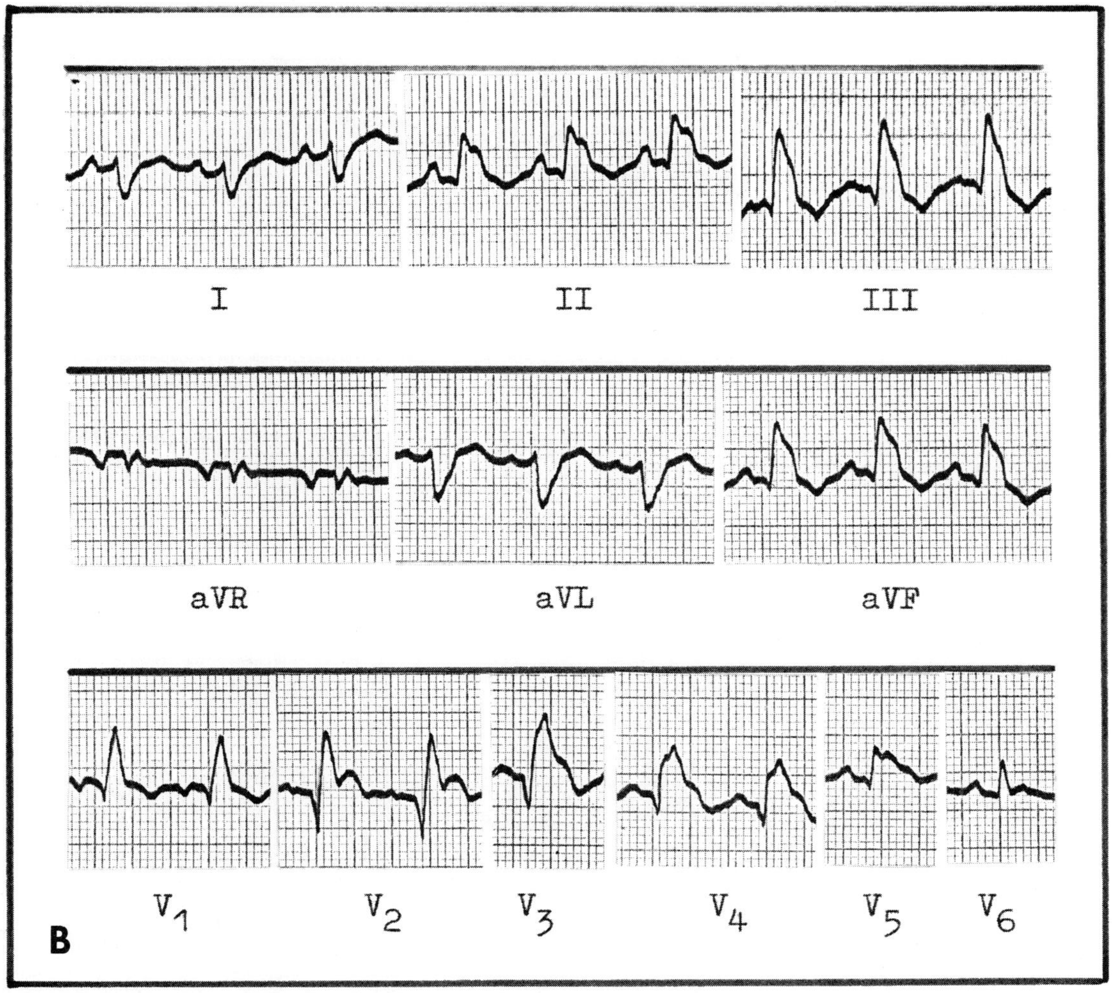

FIGURE 5–43 *Continued.* *B,* Same patient as in Figure 5–43*A,* who presented with crushing chest pain with evidence of myocardial infarction. Note the changes which have occurred in both depolarization and repolarization of the ventricles, especially the onset of right bundle branch block and Q waves in leads V_1 to V_5. The right bundle branch block plus the right axis deviation (left posterior hemiblock) is known as bifascicular block and will be studied in the next chapter.

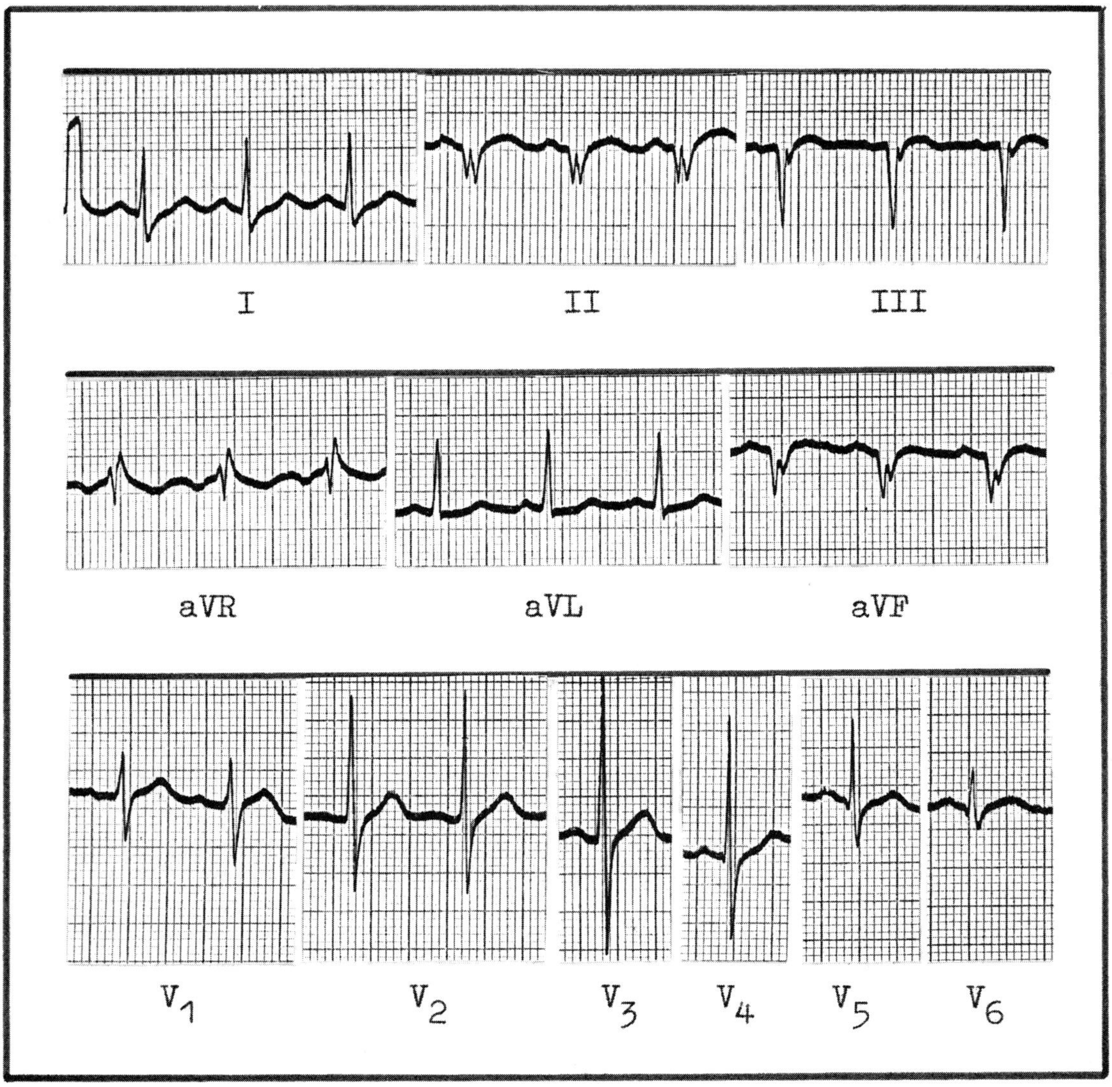

FIGURE 5–44. Inferior–posterior myocardial infarction.

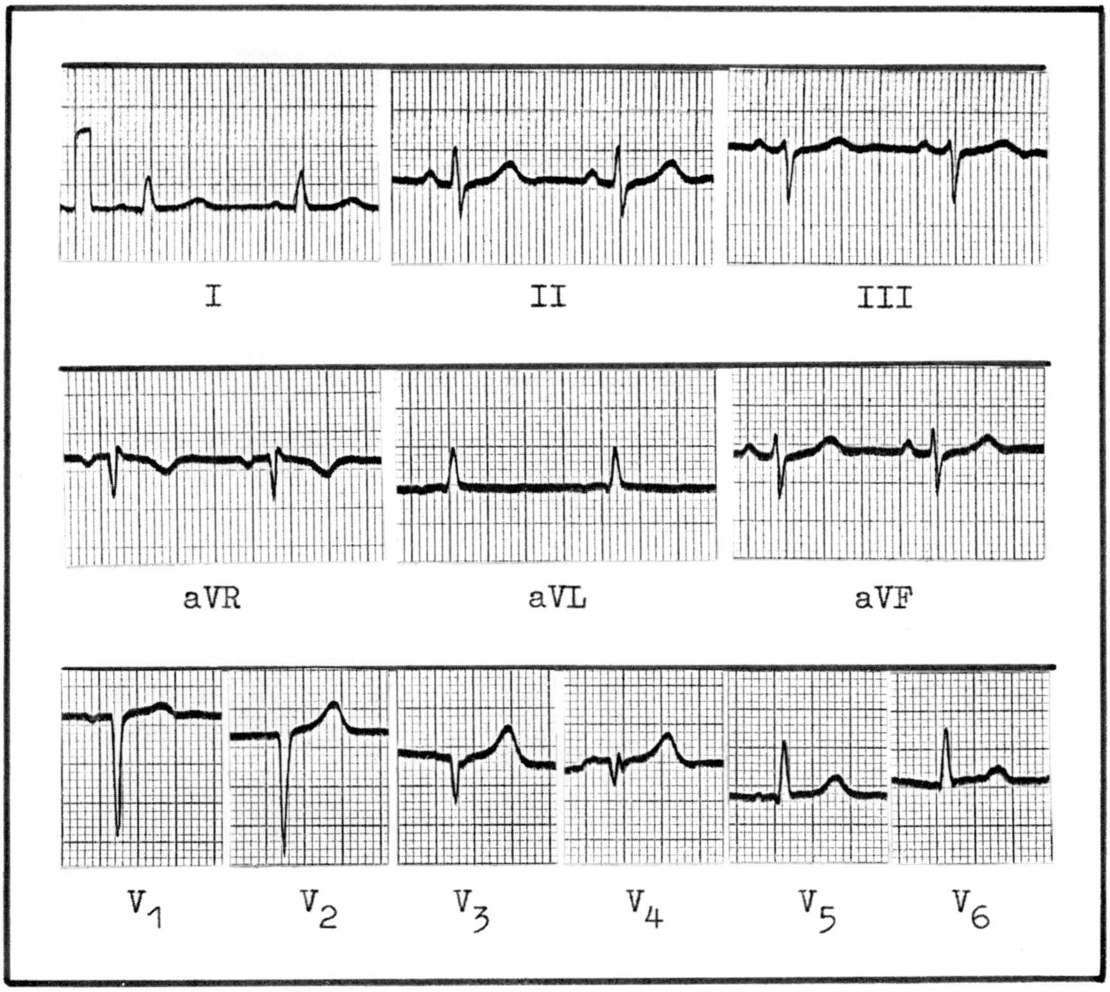

FIGURE 5–45. Anterior or anteroseptal myocardial infarction.

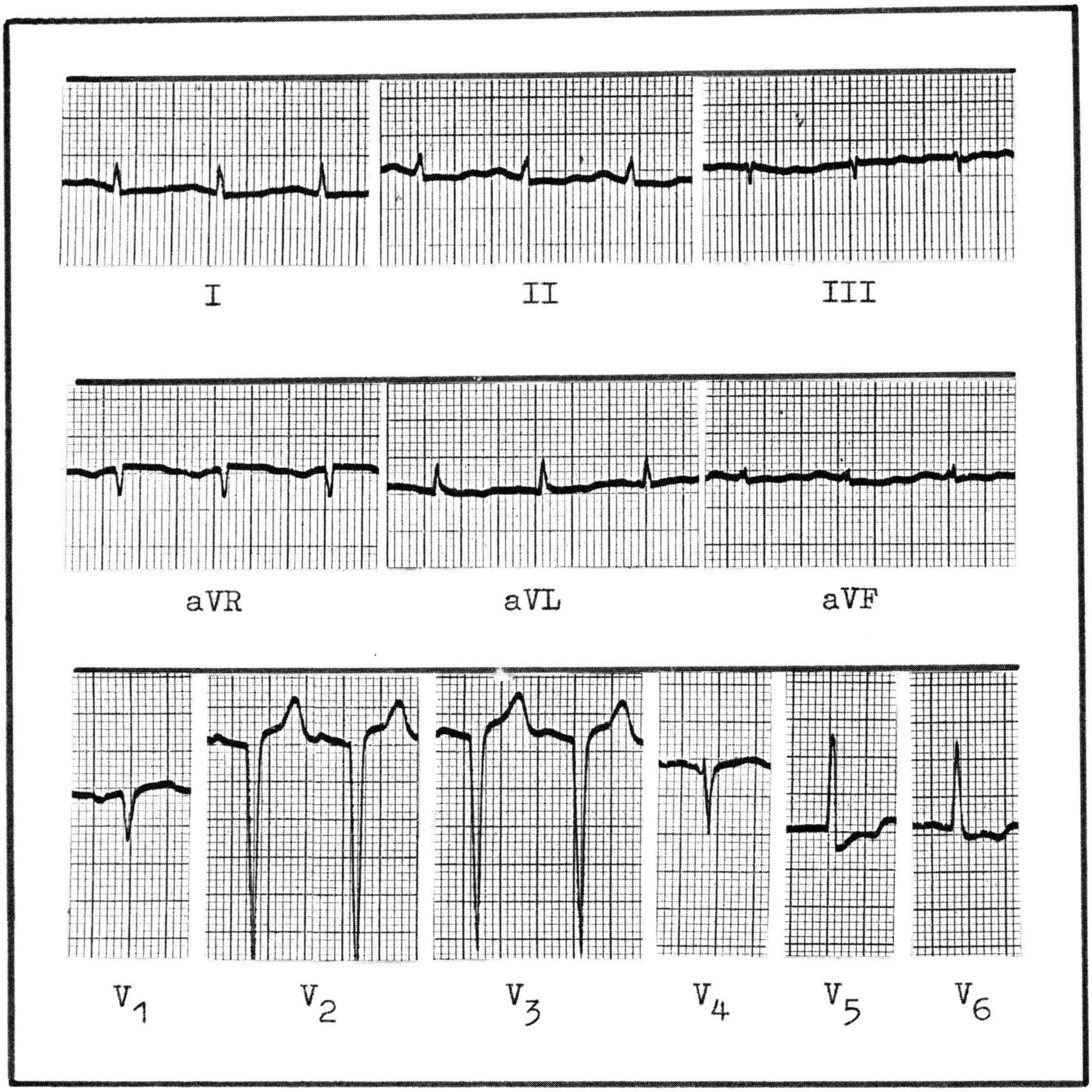

FIGURE 5–46. Anterior myocardial infarction. Why are the deflections (QRS) in leads I, II, III, aVR, aVL and aVF so small in a patient with a known large left ventricle? Review Chapter 3.

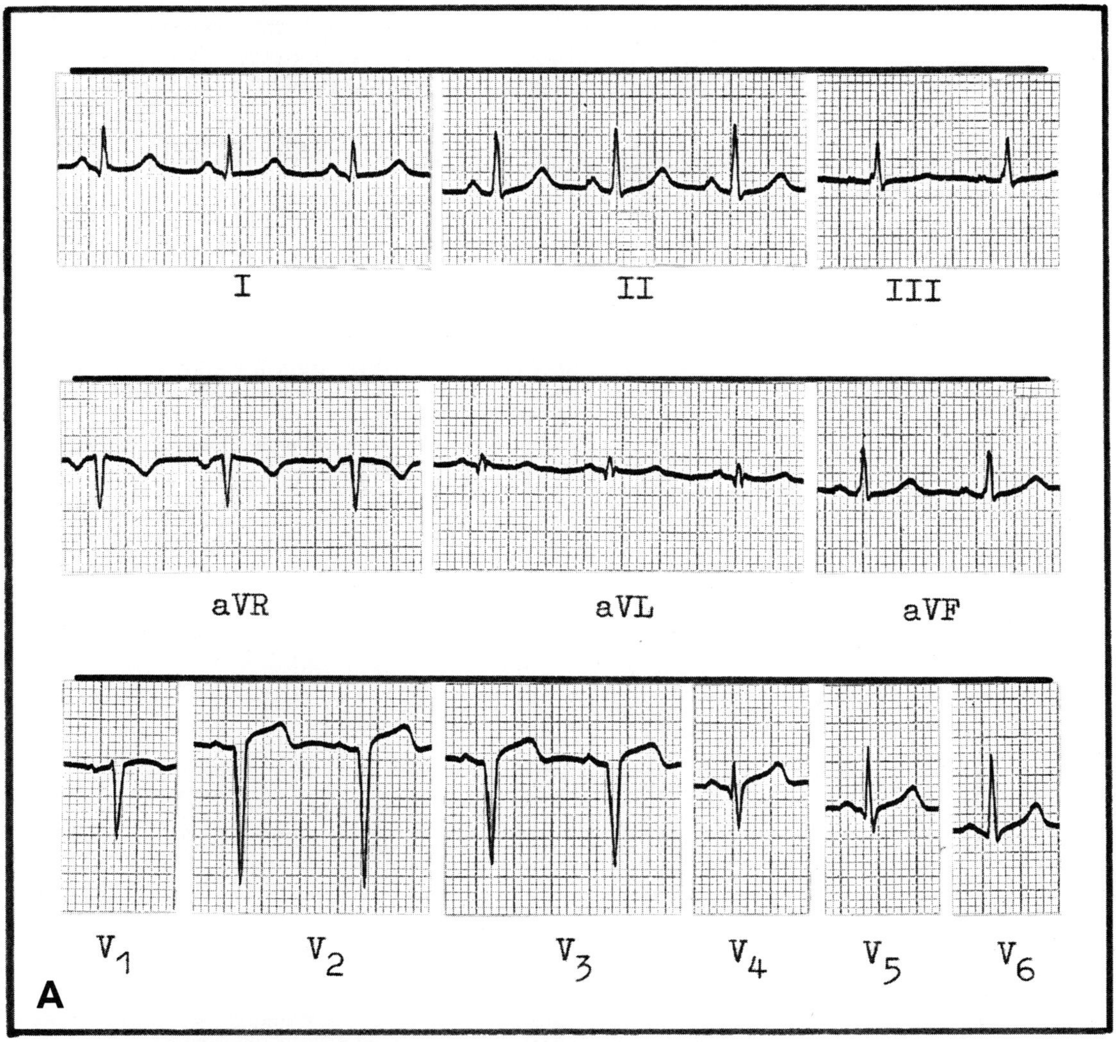

FIGURE 5–47. *A,* Anterior myocardial infarction. What is the age of the infarct?
Illustration continued on following page.

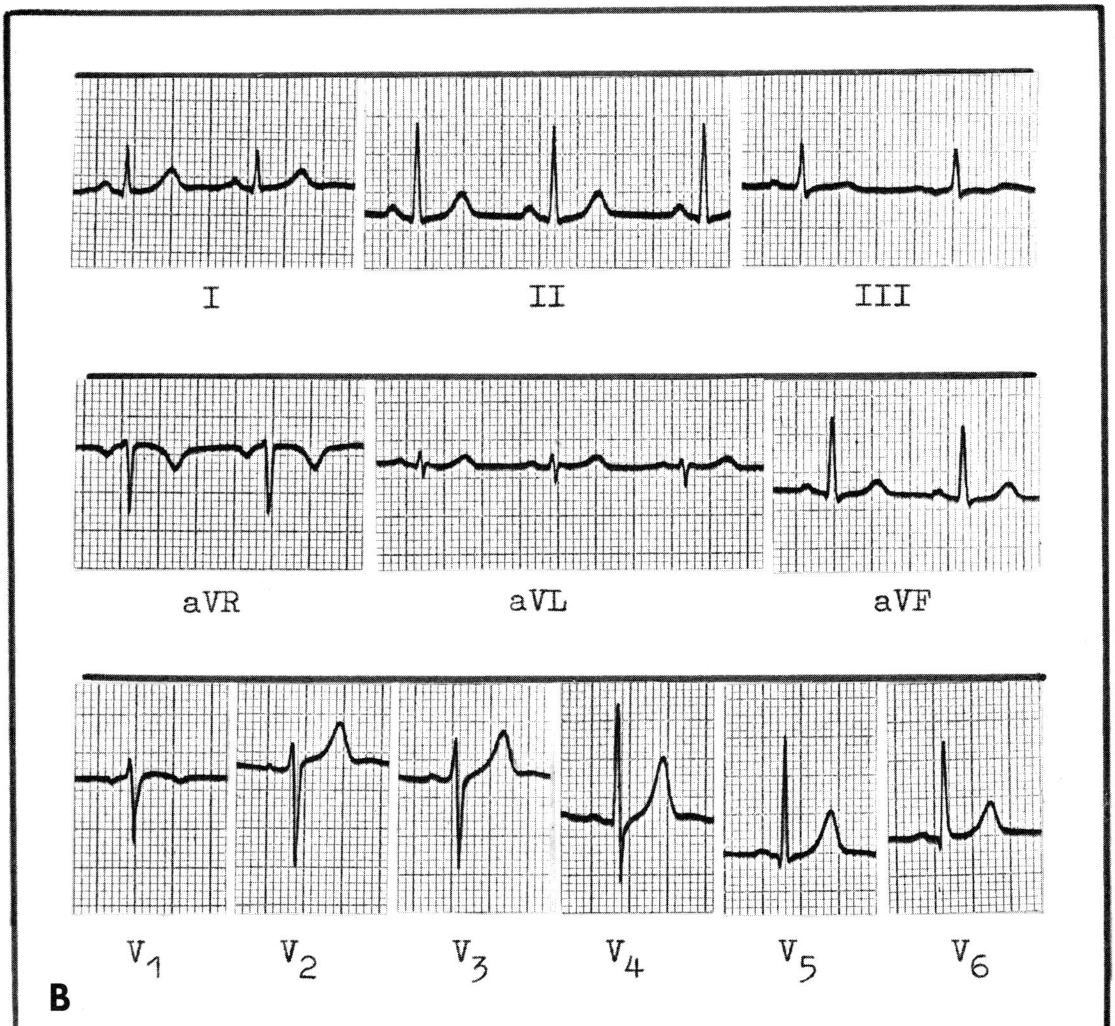

FIGURE 5–47 *Continued.* *B,* Same patient as in Figure 5–47*A*. This electrocardiogram was taken two weeks before the previous one, just before the onset of clinical symptoms of myocardial infarction.

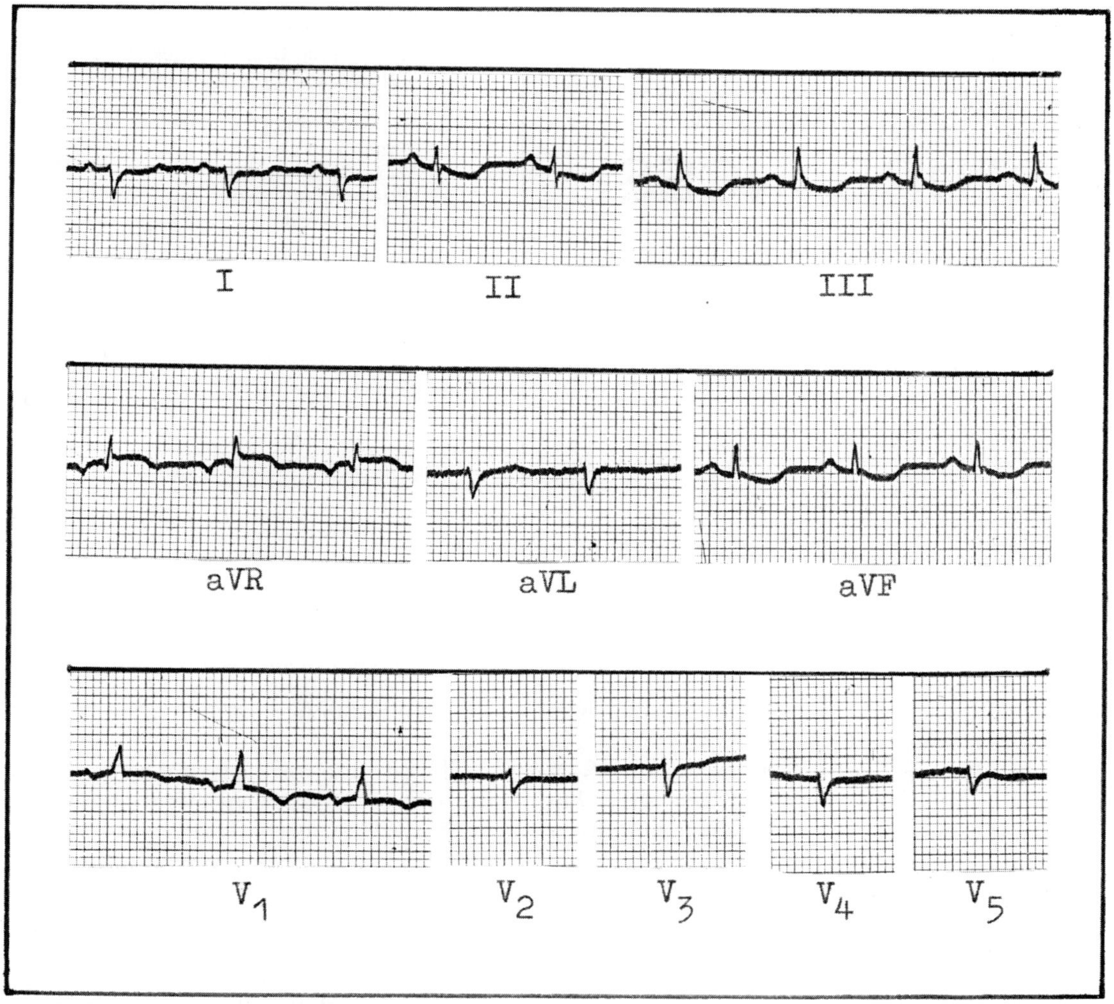

FIGURE 5–48. True posterior myocardial infarction. The right axis deviation will be discussed in the section on hemiblocks in Chapter 6. Without knowing the patient one might reasonably assume this to be right ventricular hypertrophy. Other electrocardiograms of the same patient will be seen in Figure 6–27*A*, *B* and *C*.

6

VENTRICULAR CONDUCTION DISTURBANCES

Cassette Side 15

As noted earlier, the heart possesses its own specialized conduction system. The impulse originates in the sinoatrial (S–A) node and spreads through the atria. The excitation then reaches the atrioventricular (A–V) node, located in the right atrium near the tricuspid valve. Conduction proceeds to the bundle of His, then to the left and right bundle branches (LBB and RBB). The left bundle branch is very short and branches early into an anterior division and a posterior division (Fig. 6–1). The right bundle branch, on the other hand, continues almost to the apex of the right ventricle before branching. The impulse then enters the Purkinje system and ventricular depolarization proceeds from endocardium to epicardium.

The earliest ventricular depolarization is from left to right. This is translated on the clinical electrocardiogram into an initial negative deflection in lead I and in the left precordial leads, and into an initial positive deflection in the right precordial leads.

The conduction system may be likened unto a series of superhighways over which the impulse travels. If there is a block in any of these pathways, if one of the superhighways is obstructed, the impulse may still detour via other available specialized conduction tissue. In so doing there may not be any delay in the depolarization, and the duration of the QRS complex may still be within the limits of normal. If the impulse has to travel through muscle tissue, however, there will be a delay in depolarization and a prolongation of the QRS complex. The "roads" through muscle tissue are small in comparison with the "superhighways" of the specialized conduction system.

Ventricular conduction disturbances will be studied in the following order:

A. Right bundle branch block (RBBB).
B. Left bundle branch block (LBBB).

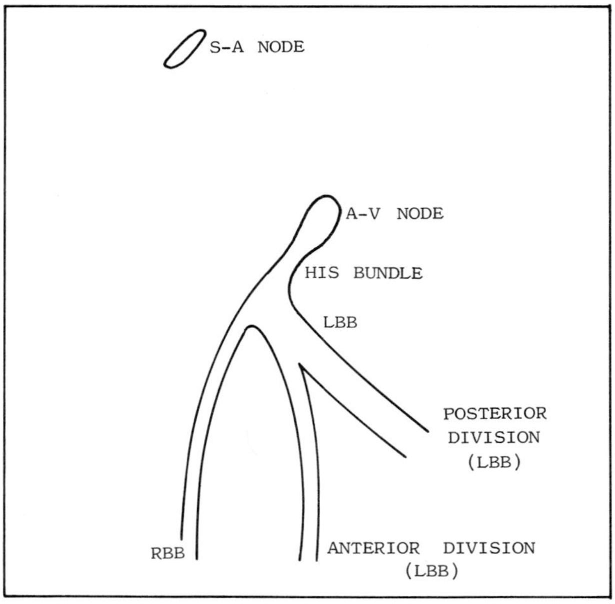

FIGURE 6–1. Atrioventricular (A–V) conduction of the heart. This is a schematic; it does not represent anatomic accuracy.

C. The hemiblocks and the trifascicular system.
D. S_1 S_2 S_3 syndrome.
E. Preexcitation (Wolff-Parkinson-White or W-P-W) syndrome.

A. Right Bundle Branch Block

Right bundle branch block refers to a lesion somewhere along the course of the right bundle branch (Fig. 6–2). In view of the interruption of the normal pathway, the impulses must then reach the remainder of the right ventricular myocardium either via the left side or from the right bundle branch above the block. Since the QRS complex duration is prolonged, there must be at least a partial intramyocardial spread of activation.

Classically, the QRS complex is prolonged to at least 0.12 sec. in "complete" right bundle branch block and up to 0.12 sec. in "incomplete" right bundle branch block. It is questionable as to whether a QRS duration of 0.12 sec. is required if all the other characteristics are present.

Regardless of where the block may be in right bundle branch block, early depolarization will already have occurred from left to right (small Q waves in lead I and left precordial leads). Only the *terminal* QRS vector is affected by right bundle branch block. This is of importance since the electrocardiographic manifestations of initial QRS vector abnormalities, such as Q waves in myocardial infarction, are not obscured. This *terminal delay* is to the *right* (S wave in lead I) and *anterior* (R′ in lead V_1). Right bundle branch block is easily recognized by the following:

a. Widened QRS complex (beyond 0.10 sec.).
b. S wave in lead I.
c. R′ in lead V_1.

Right bundle branch block may be found congenitally without any clinical evidence of heart disease. It may also be

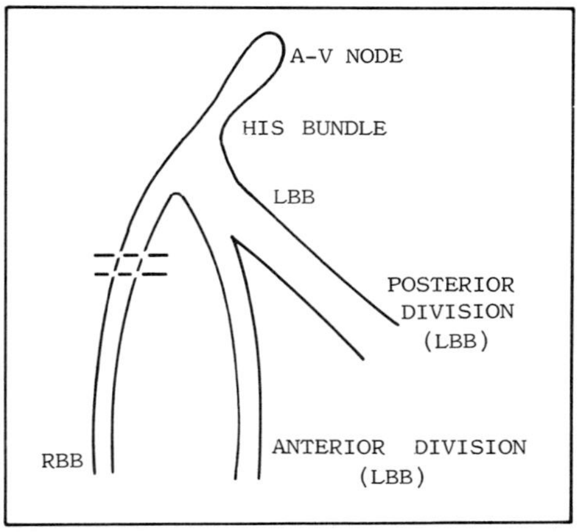

FIGURE 6–2. Block along the course of the right bundle branch.

found in association with an enlarged right ventricle, myocardial infarction and hypertensive cardiovascular disease.

Figures 6–3 and 6–4 are examples of right bundle branch block. Analyze these on the basis of the above three criteria (*a*, *b* and *c*).

The next three figures, Figures 6–5 *A* and *B*, 6–6 *A* and *B* and 6–7 *A* and *B*, are electrocardiograms before and after the development of right bundle branch block. In each right bundle branch block (*B* part) you will find that:

a. The QRS has widened.

b. There is an S wave in lead I. If an S wave was present before the onset of right bundle branch block, it becomes wider and possibly more slurred.

c. There is an R′ in lead V_1.

The initial QRS vector is not affected.

Text continued on page 271.

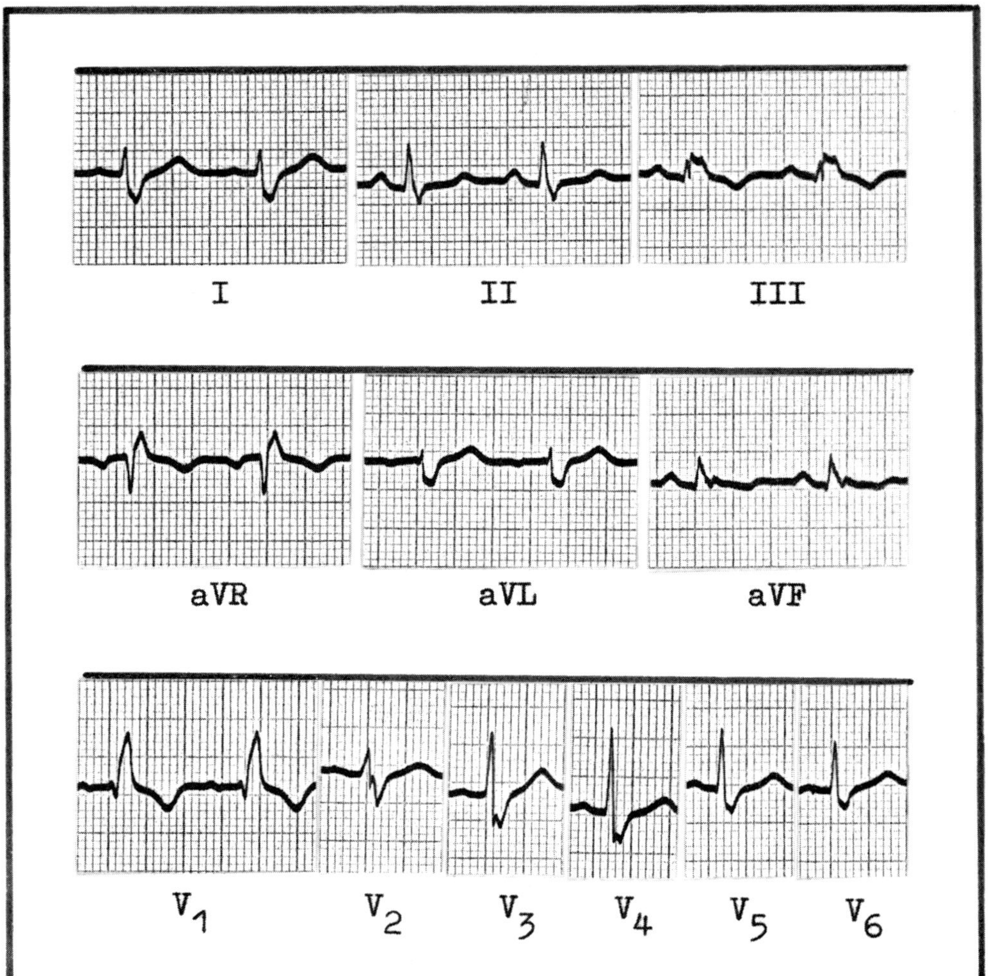

FIGURE 6–3. Right bundle branch block (RBBB). How many of the characteristic criteria of RBBB do you see here?

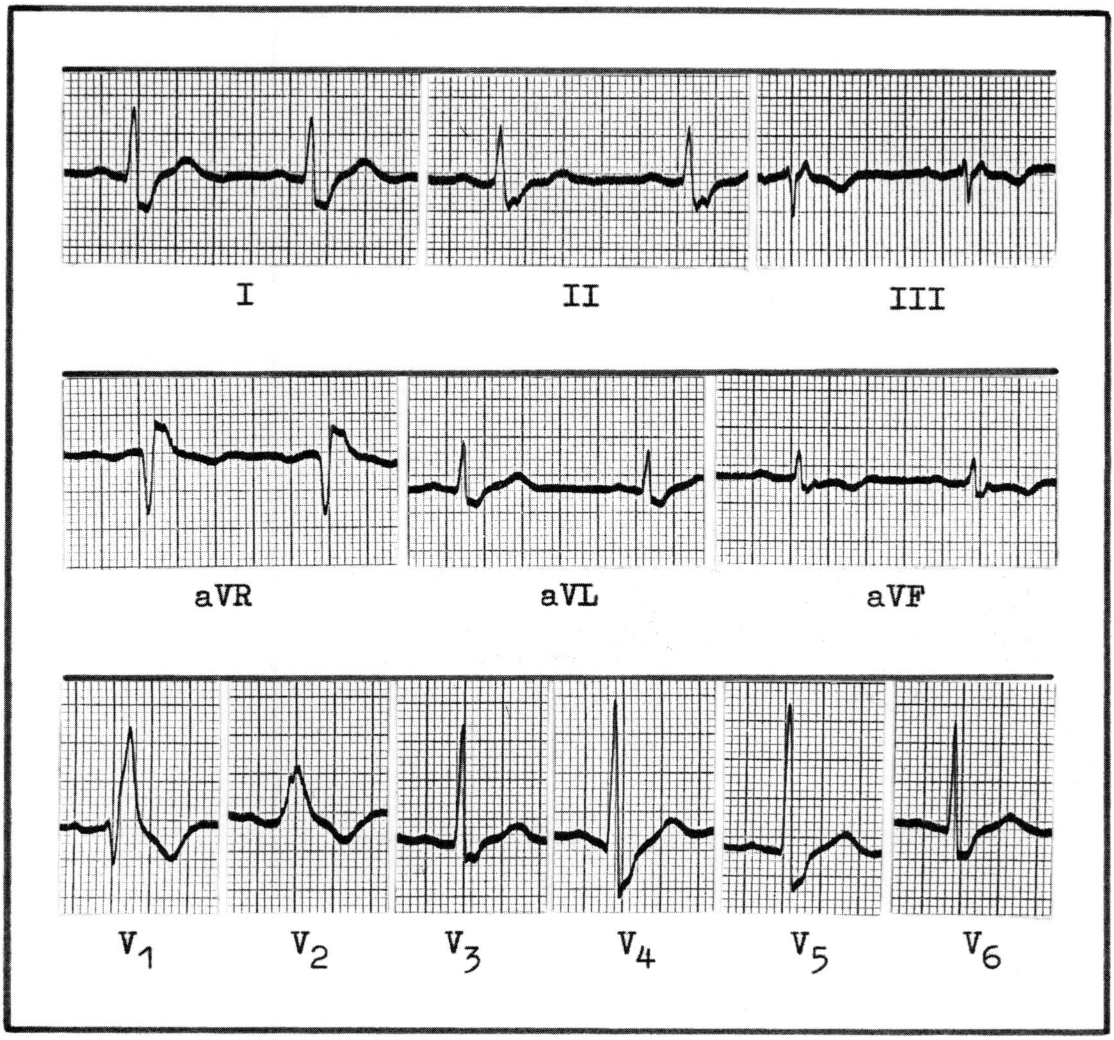

FIGURE 6–4. Right bundle branch block. Review all the criteria for RBBB.

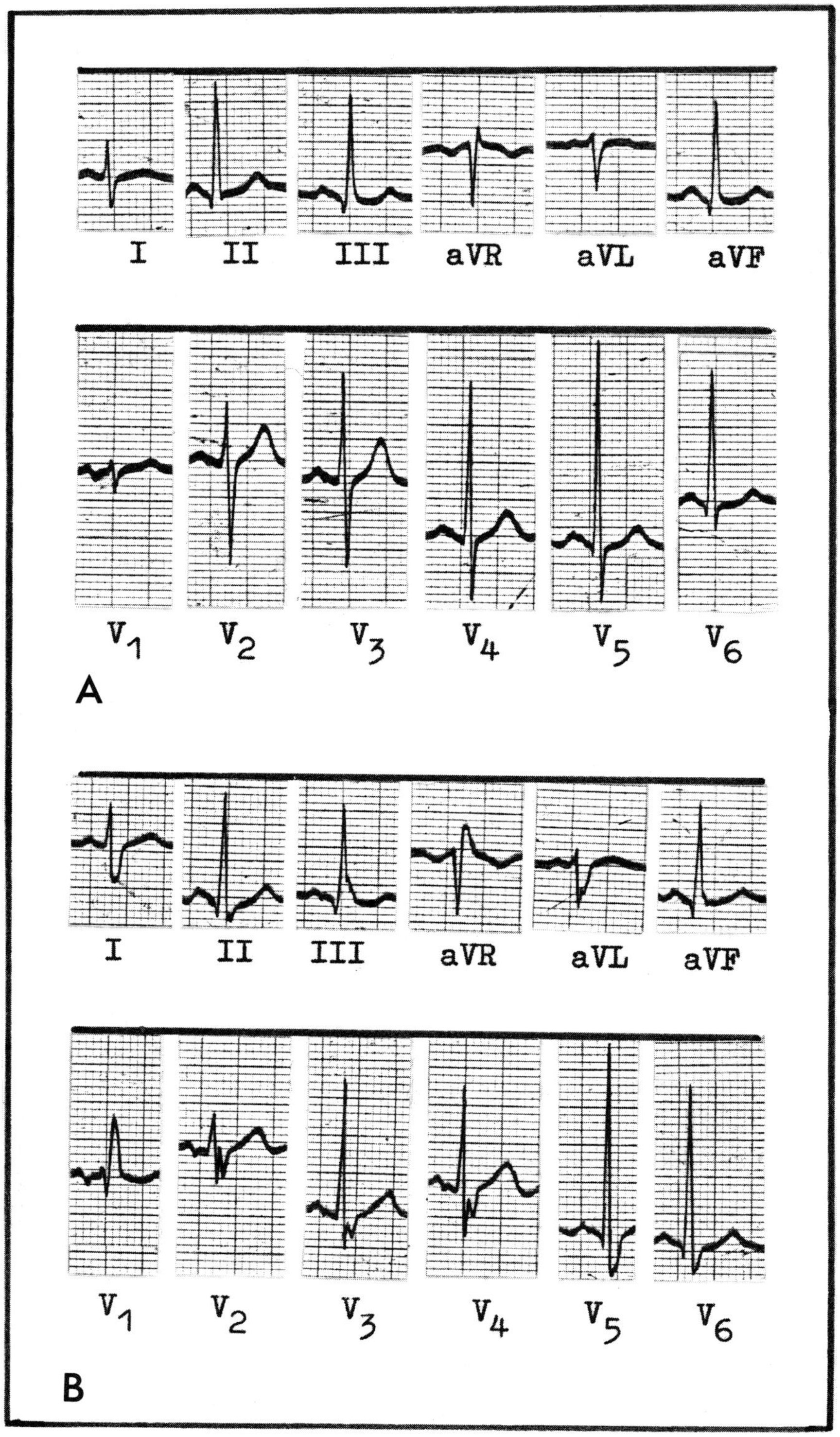

FIGURE 6–5. Before and after development of right bundle branch block. *A*, Baseline; *B*, following onset of RBBB.

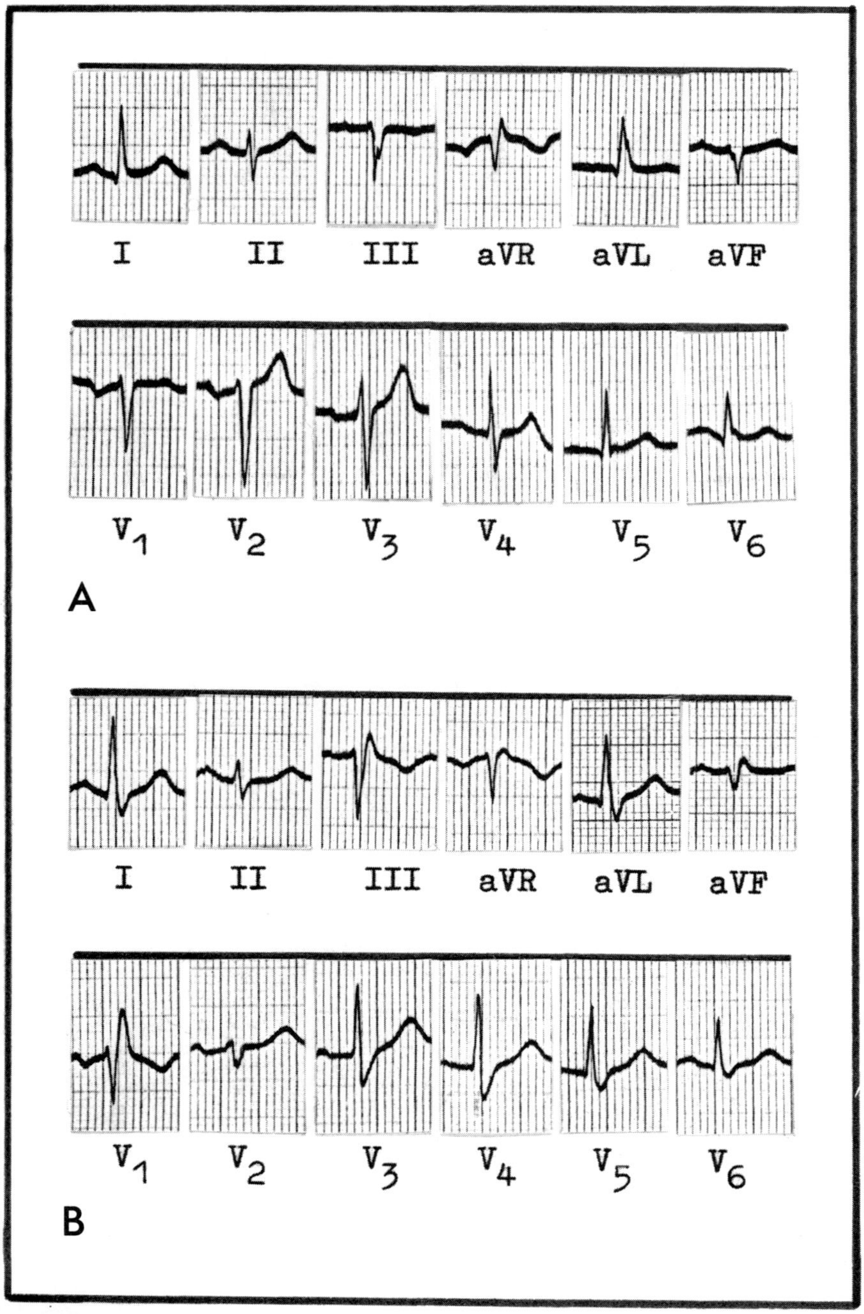

FIGURE 6–6. Before and after development of right bundle branch block. *A,* Baseline; *B,* following onset of RBBB.

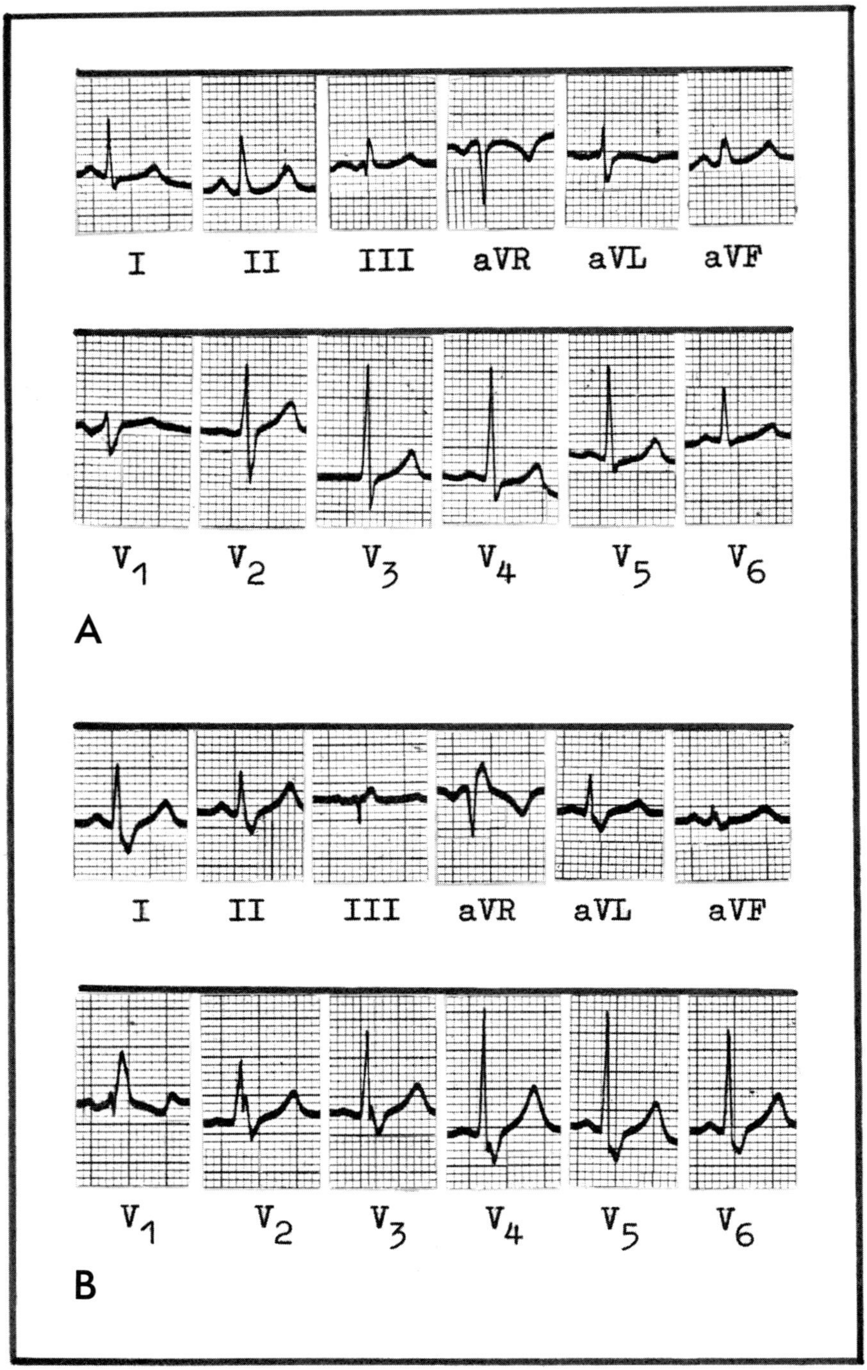

FIGURE 6–7. Before and after development of right bundle branch block. *A,* Baseline; *B,* following onset of RBBB.

Right Bundle Branch Block and Myocardial Infarction

Figures 6–8*A* and *B* are from a patient with diaphragmatic myocardial infarction, before and after development of right bundle branch block. That the initial QRS vectorial forces are *not* affected by the right bundle branch block is of the utmost importance. The Q waves of myocardial infarction are *not* obscured by right bundle branch block. Figure 6–8*A* reveals a diaphragmatic myocardial infarction prior to the development of right bundle branch block. In Figure 6–8*B* the findings of diaphragmatic myocardial infarction remain in the presence of right bundle branch block.

Figures 6–9 and 6–10 are from patients with diaphragmatic myocardial infarction in the presence of right bundle branch block.

The electrocardiographic manifestations of right bundle branch block in the presence of *anterior* myocardial infarction are of special interest. The initial Q wave in lead V_1 is preserved with a resulting *QR* rather than an *RSR′* pattern. This should not detract from the diagnosis of right bundle branch block if the other criteria are present; an illustration is presented in Figure 6–11. In Figure 6–12 right bundle branch block is seen in the presence of both anterior and inferior myocardial infarction.

Text continued on page 277.

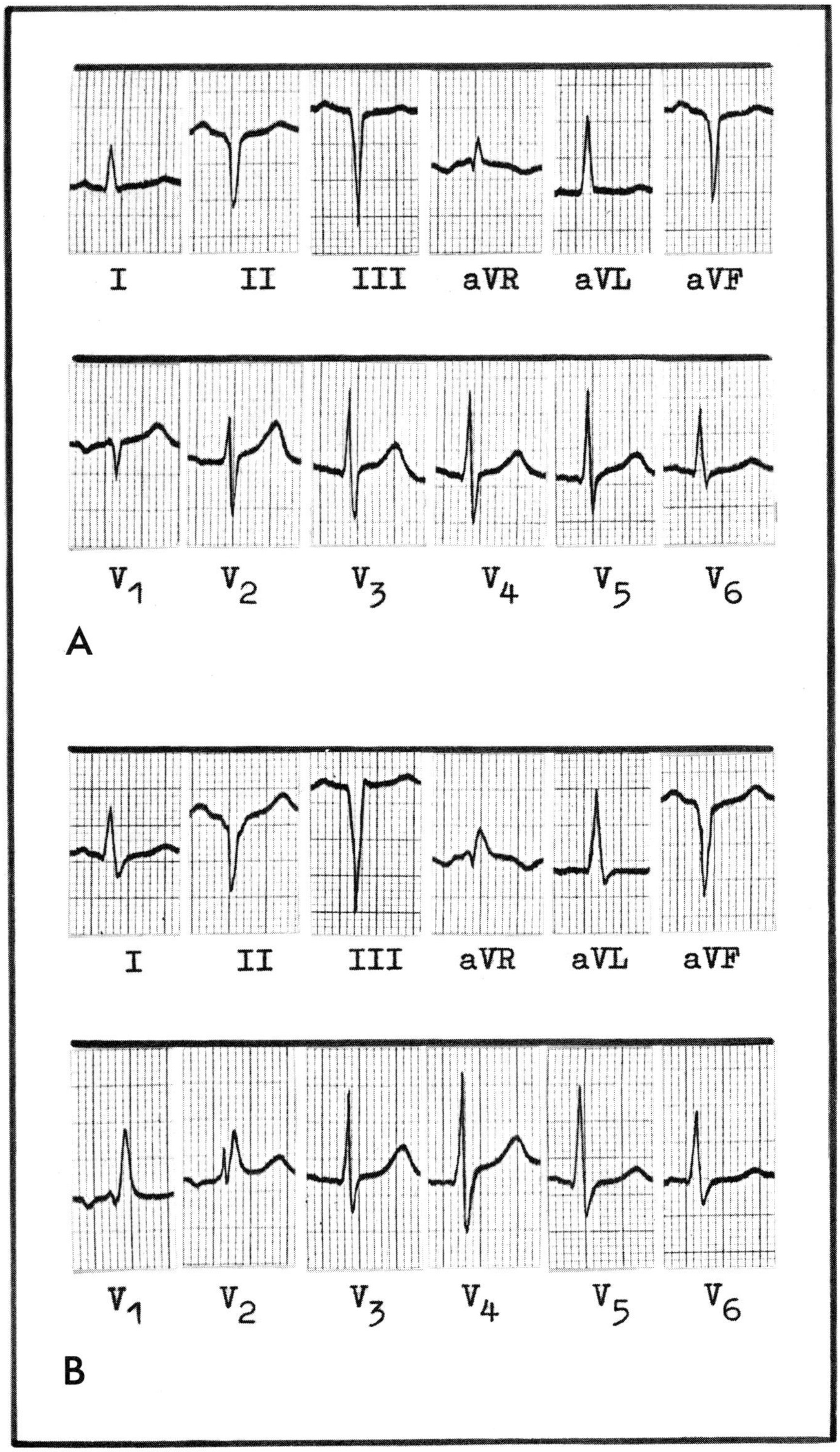

FIGURE 6–8. Before and after development of right bundle branch block in a patient with diaphragmatic myocardial infarction. *A,* Baseline, with diaphragmatic myocardial infarction; *B,* following onset of RBBB.

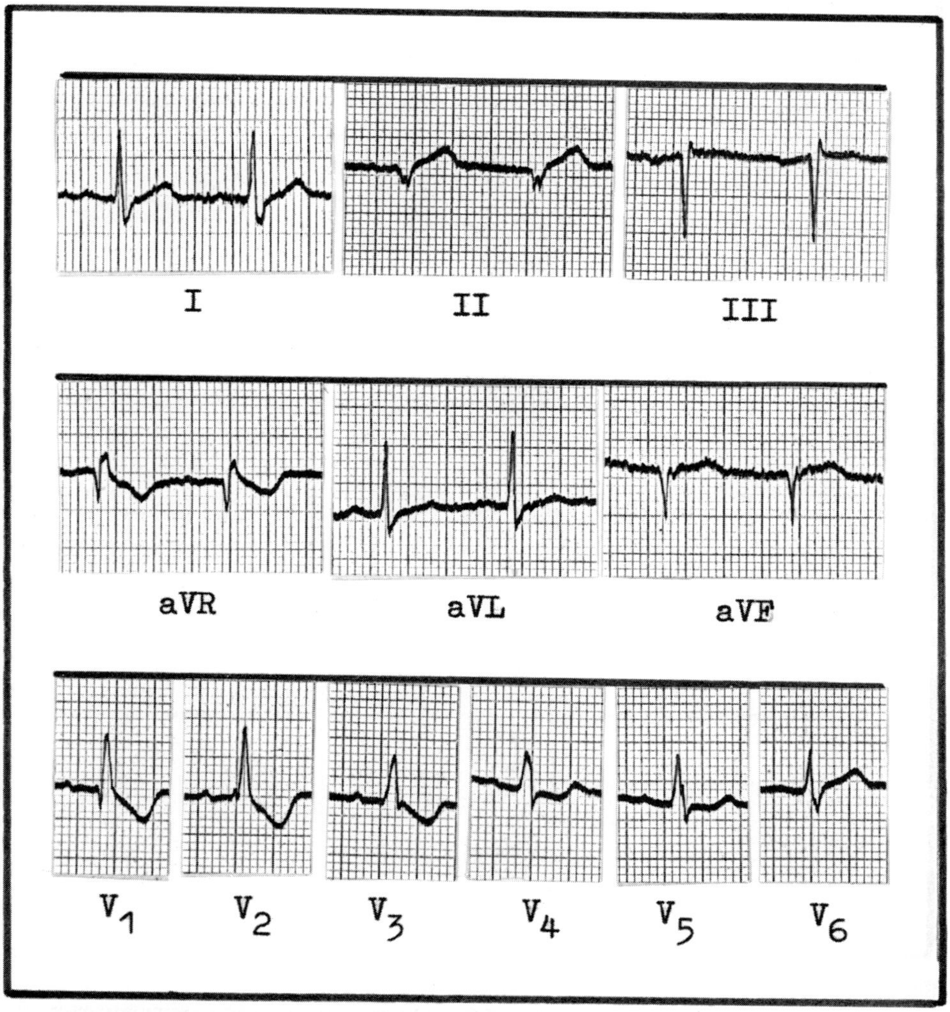

FIGURE 6–9. Diaphragmatic myocardial infarction in the presence of right bundle branch block.

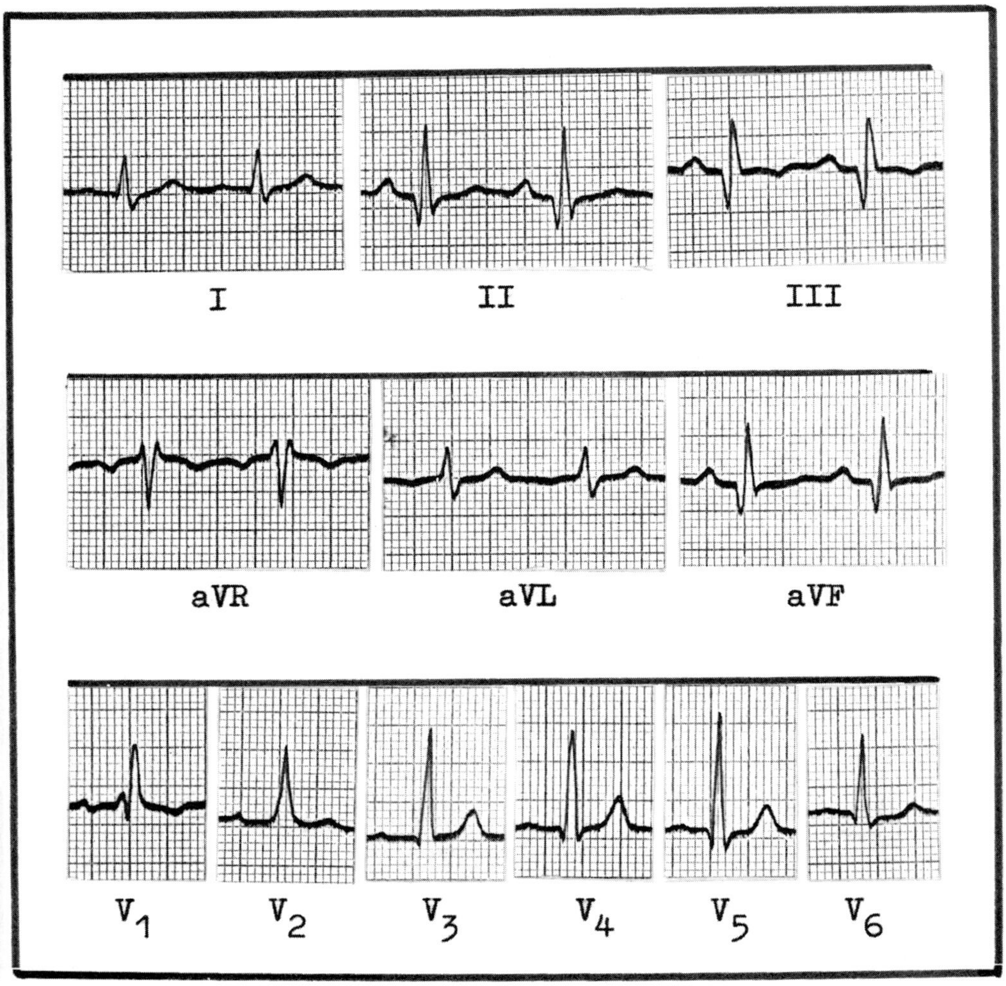

FIGURE 6–10. Diaphragmatic myocardial infarction in the presence of right bundle branch block.

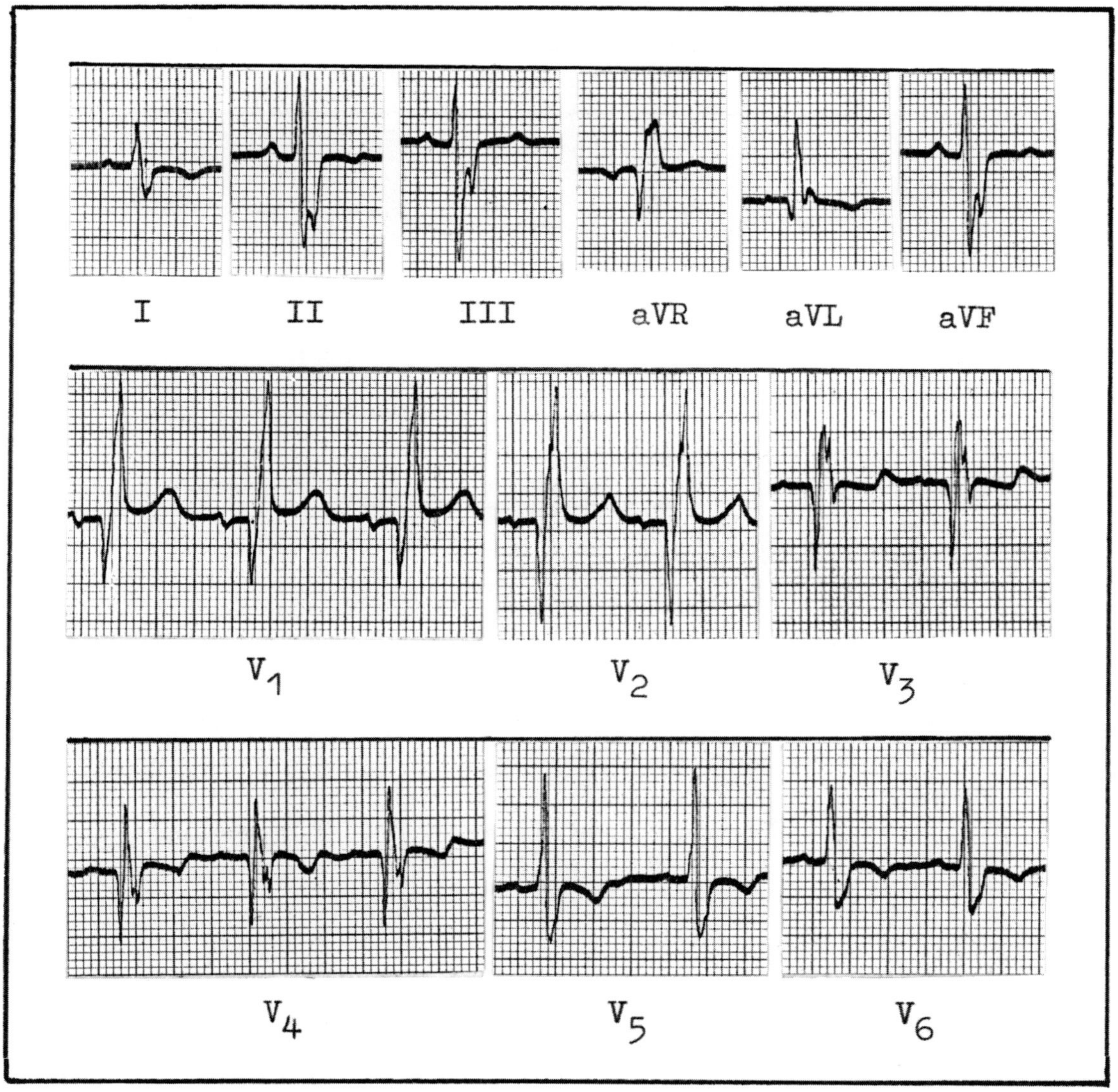

FIGURE 6–11. Anterior myocardial infarction in the presence of right bundle branch block. Note the QR pattern in leads V_1, V_2, V_3 and V_4; the QR replaces the RSR′ in lead V_1.

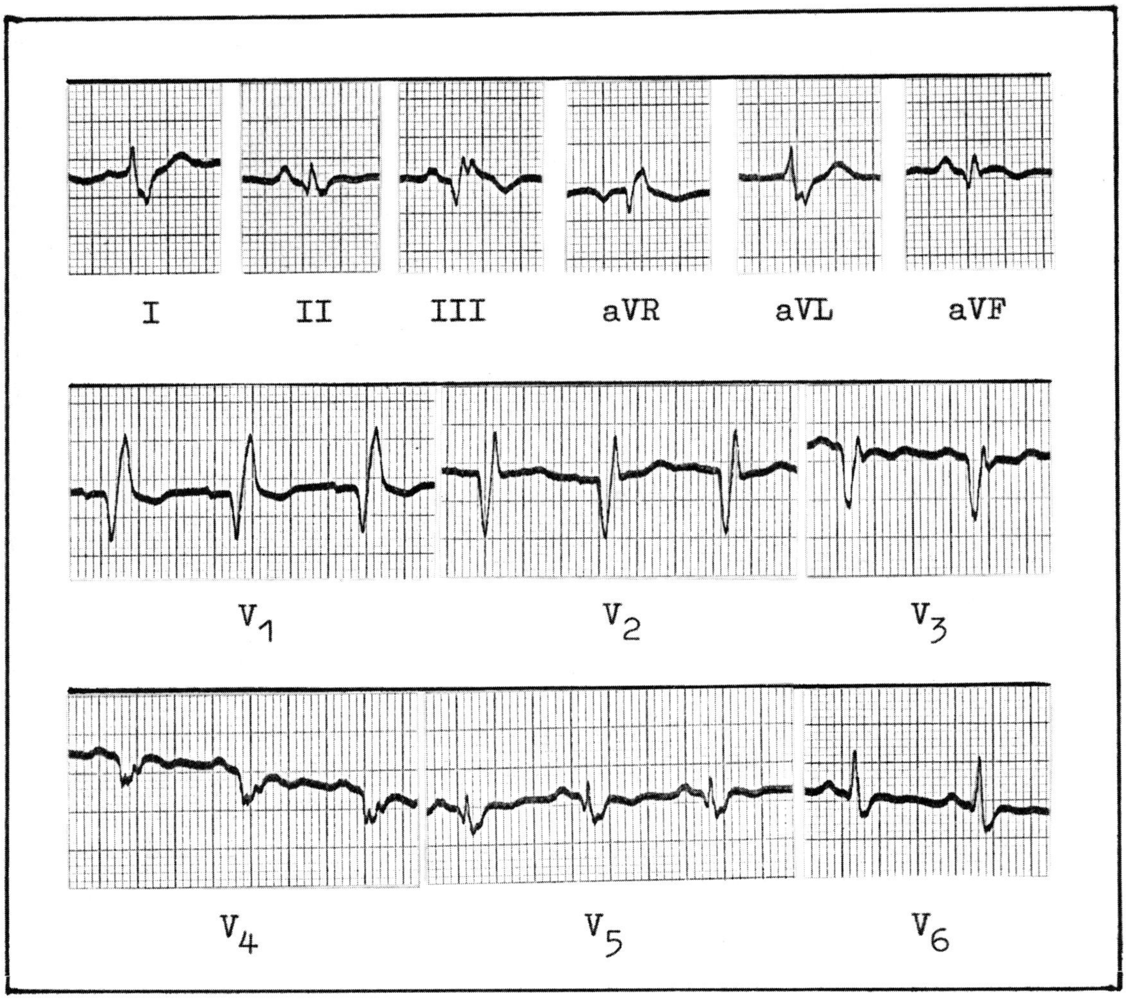

FIGURE 6–12. Anterior and inferior myocardial infarction in the presence of right bundle branch block.

B. Left Bundle Branch Block

In left bundle branch block (Fig. 6–13), in contrast to right bundle branch block, the entire sequence of ventricular depolarization is altered. Both the initial and the terminal QRS vectorial forces point more leftward and posteriorly in comparison with normal conduction. Left bundle branch block, again in contrast to right bundle branch block, is not often found without organic disease of the left ventricle. The characteristics of left bundle branch block follow.

a. The QRS interval is prolonged to greater than 0.12 sec. (if the QRS duration is 0.10 to 0.12 sec. it is labelled "incomplete").
b. The initial QRS vector is changed in orientation to have a more leftward and posterior orientation, so that:
   1. The initial Q waves disappear in leads I and V_6.
   2. The initial R waves seen in the normal electrocardiogram in leads V_1, V_2 and V_3 are much smaller and have often disappeared in leads V_1 and V_2.

      Note: Do not make the diagnosis of myocardial infarction from the lack of R waves in the right precordial leads in the presence of left bundle branch block.
c. The terminal vector has changed in orientation pointing more leftward, so that:
   1. The small S waves in lead aVL, during normal conduction, disappear during left bundle branch block.
   2. Lead III has a terminal R wave during normal conduction and a terminal S wave with left bundle branch block.
   3. Lead aVR has a terminal S wave with left bundle branch block.

These criteria are not invariable and may not be found in every case. They do, however, provide important guideposts.

In examining the electrocardiographic manifestations of left bundle branch block the repolarization (S–T segment and T wave) alterations must be given careful attention. Review primary and secondary repolarization alterations in Chapter 4.

Always consider left bundle branch block when the QRS complex is prolonged and both the initial and terminal QRS vectorial forces are altered. Figures 6–14*A* and *B* are from a patient with intermittent left bundle branch block. Compare each lead using the above listed criteria: there must be QRS widening and initial and terminal QRS vectorial alterations in addition to repolarization alterations. Are these latter changes primary or secondary?

Figure 6–15*B* represents "incomplete" left bundle branch block and Figure 6–15*A* is the baseline; the left branch block criteria are present but the QRS interval is less than 0.12 sec. Figures 6–16, 6–17 and 6–18 are examples of left bundle branch block; analyze each one carefully.

Text continued on page 283.

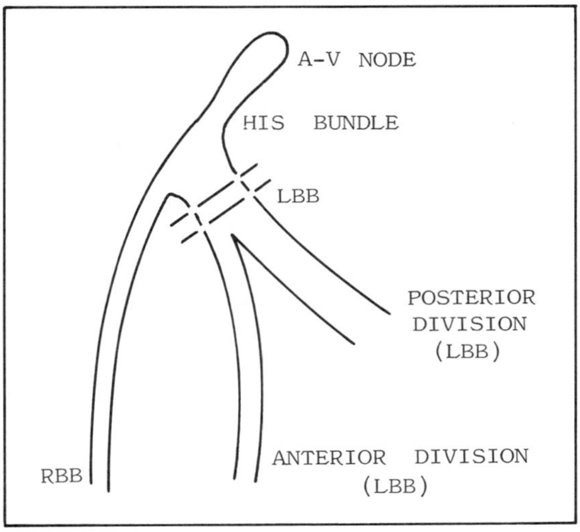

FIGURE 6–13. Left bundle branch block (LBBB).

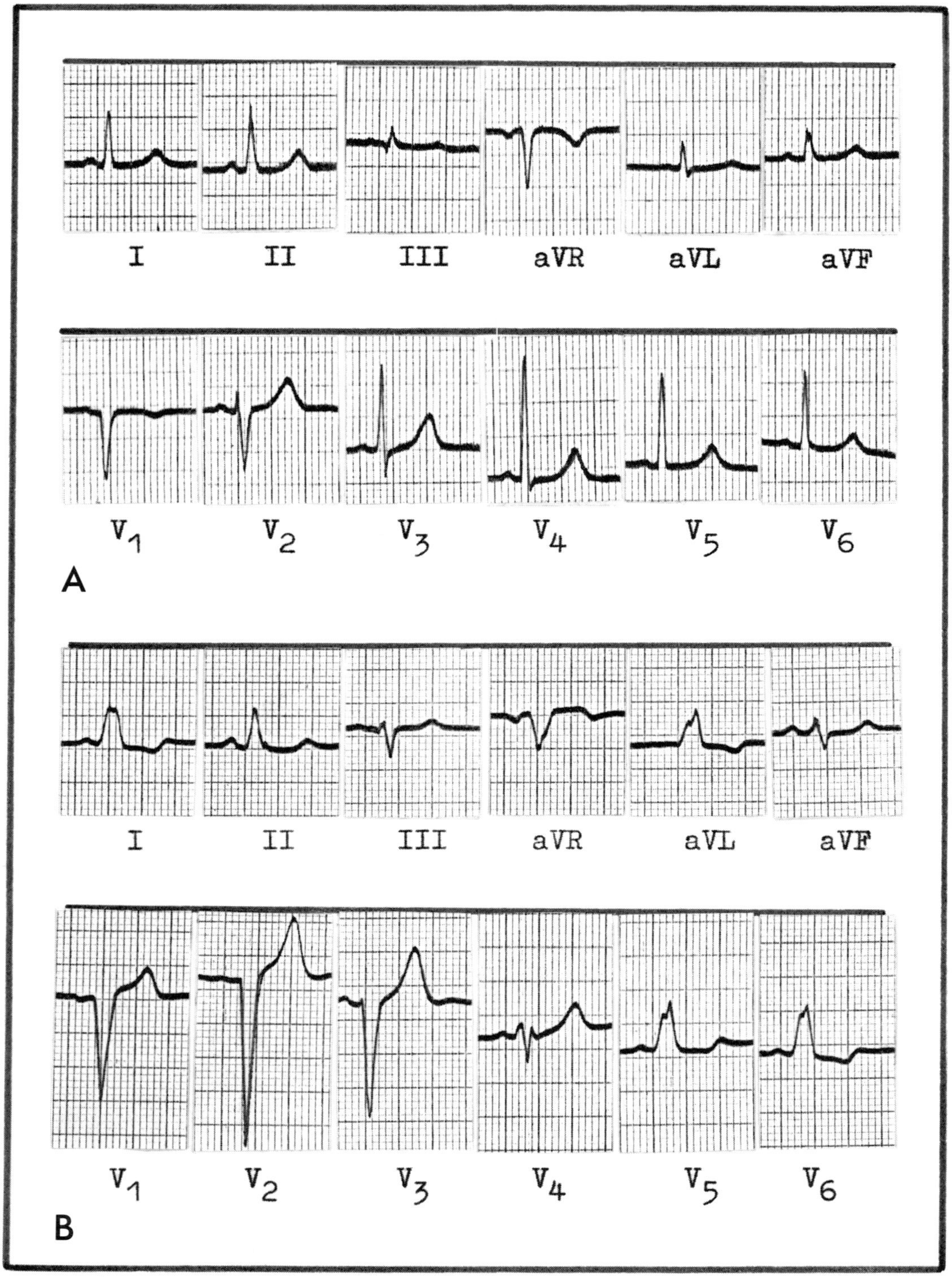

FIGURE 6–14. Before and after development of left bundle branch block. In this patient it was intermittent. How many characteristics of left bundle branch block do you see? *A*, Baseline; *B*, following onset of LBBB.

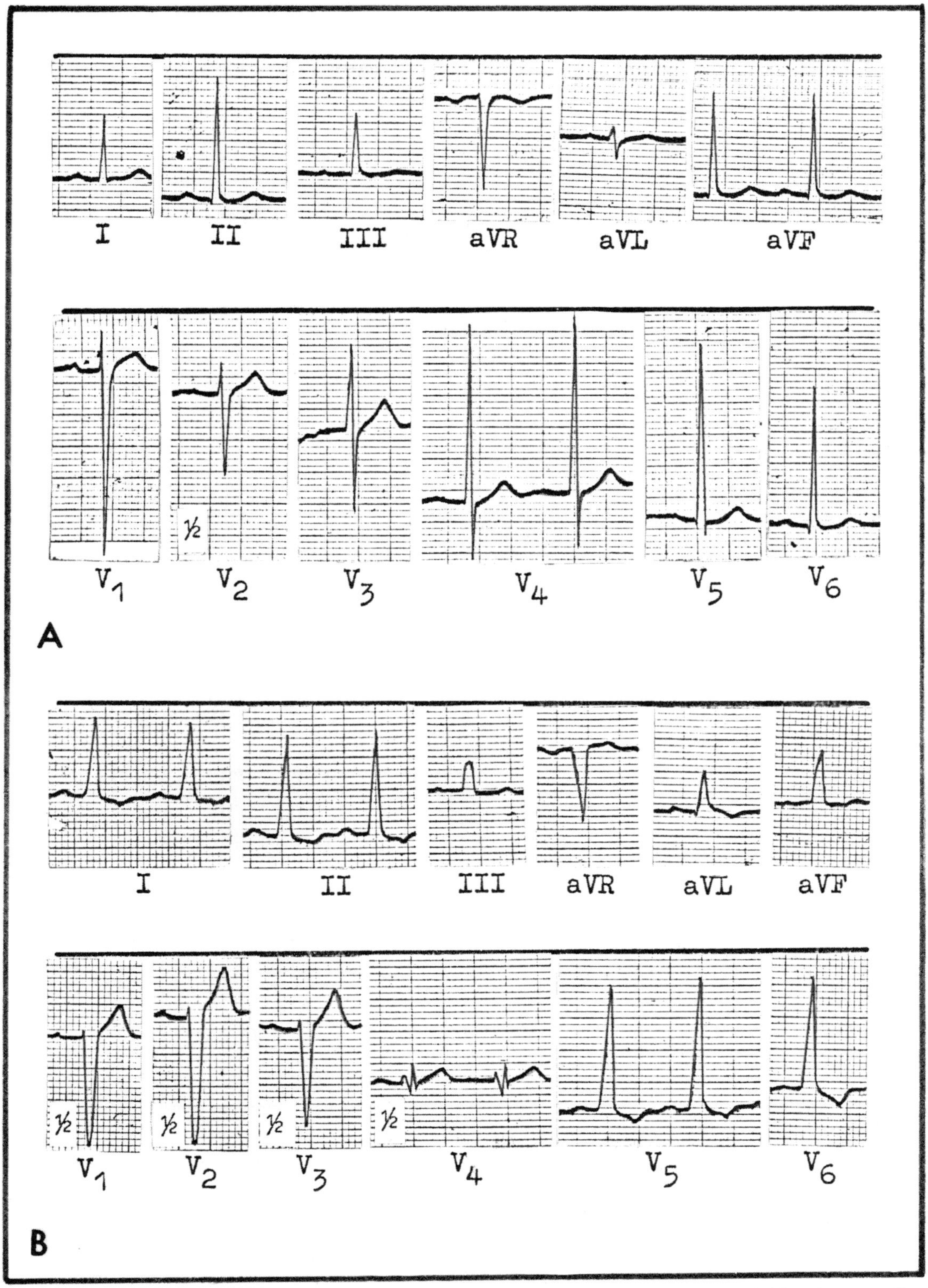

FIGURE 6–15. Before and after the development of "incomplete" left bundle branch block. The electrocardiogram in *B* would be listed classically as "incomplete" left bundle branch block, since the above described changes are present, but the QRS interval is less than 0.12 sec. *A,* Baseline; *B,* following onset of "incomplete" LBBB.

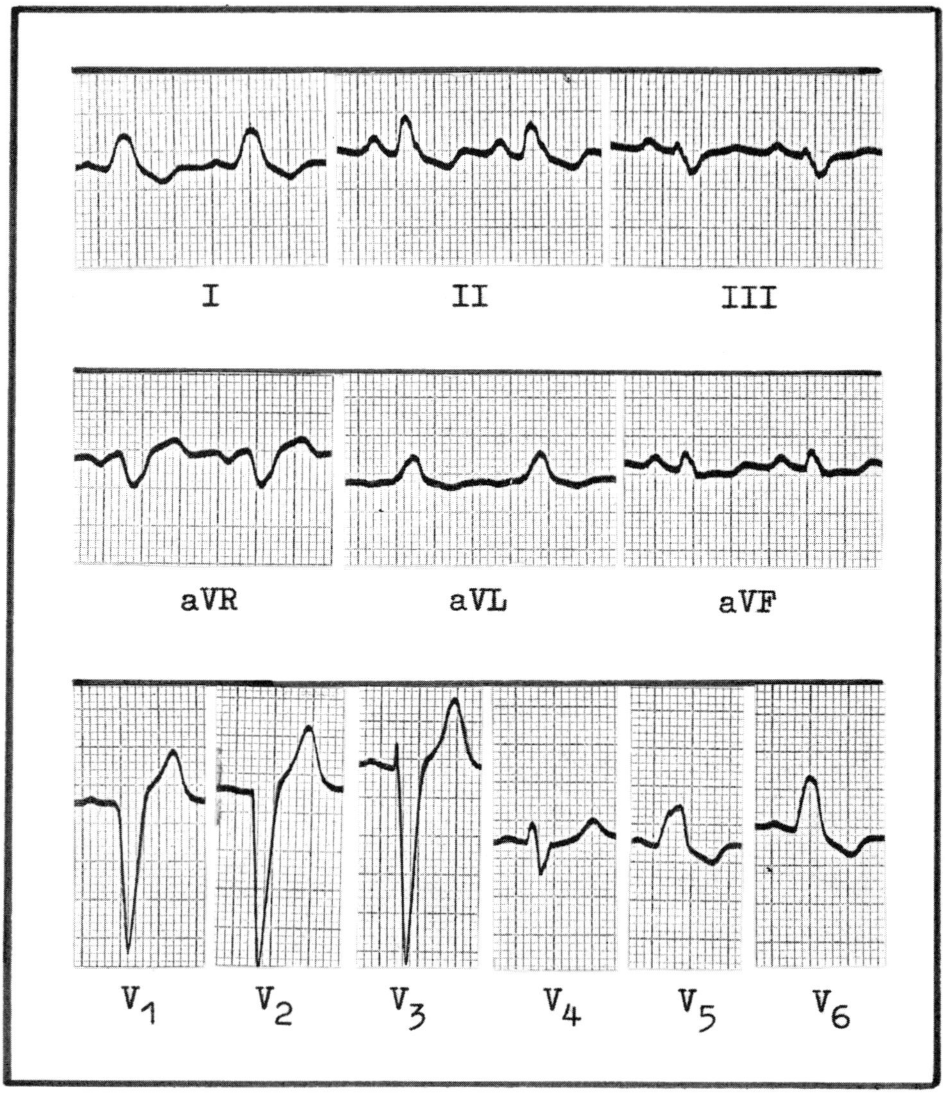

FIGURE 6–16. Left bundle branch block.

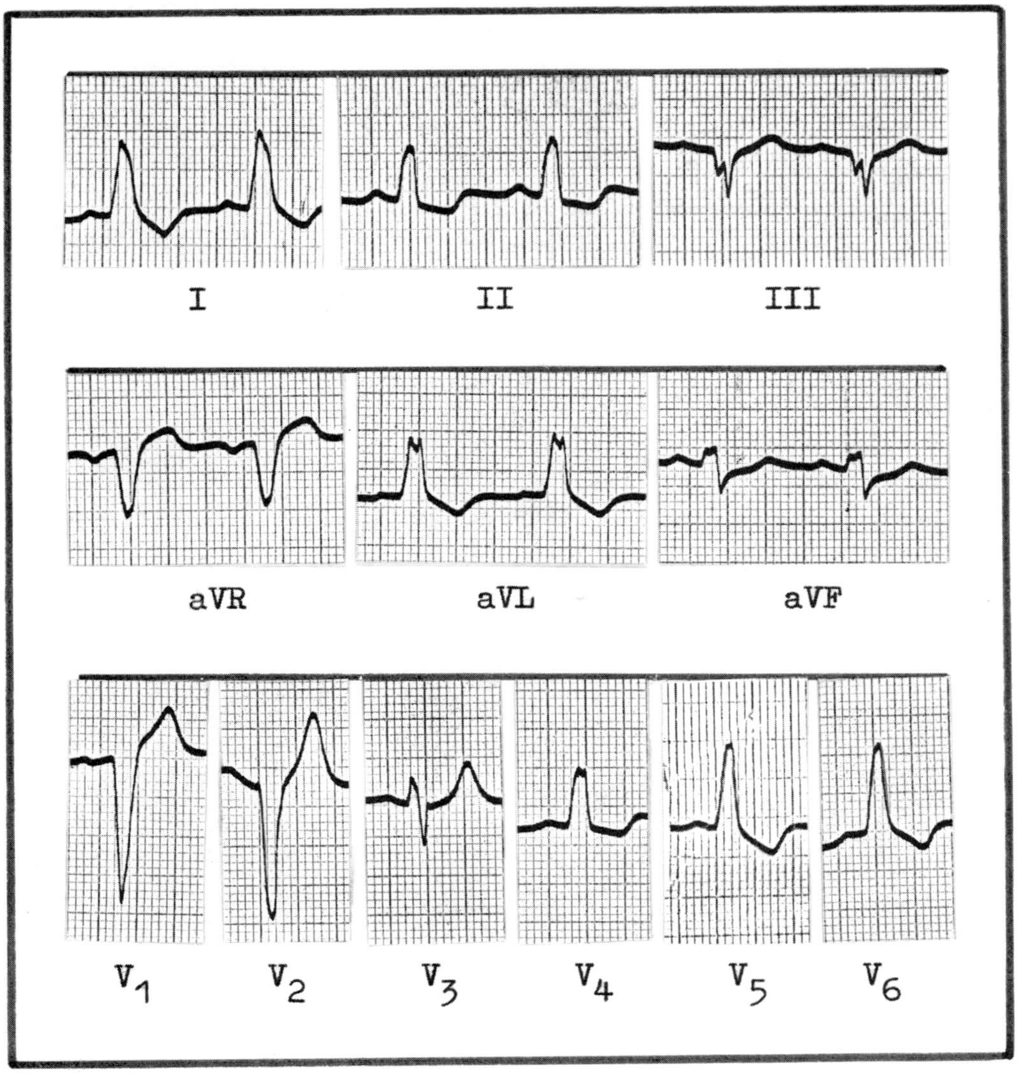

FIGURE 6–17. Left bundle branch block.

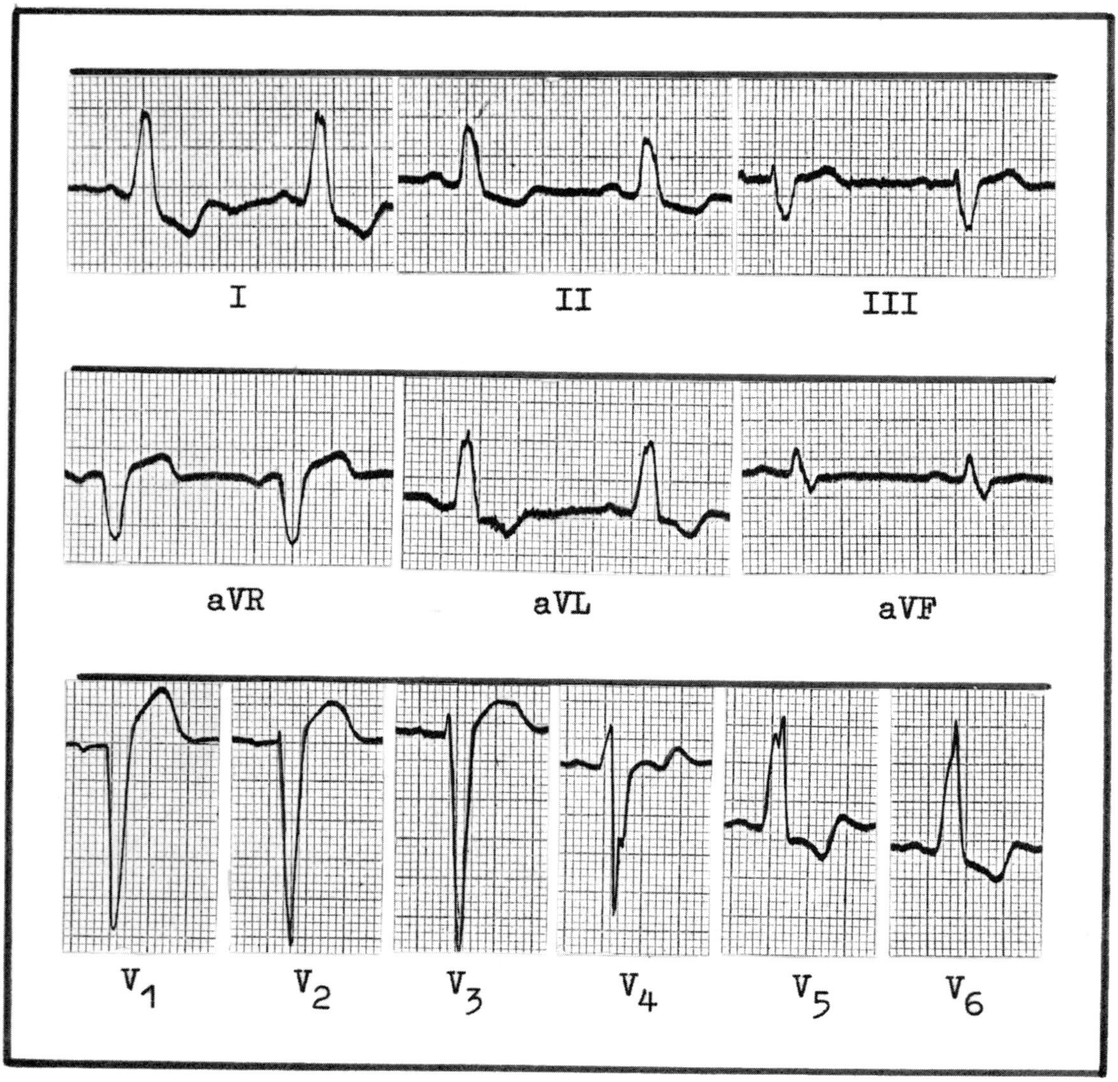

FIGURE 6–18. Left bundle branch block.

Left Bundle Branch Block and Myocardial Infarction

Due to the alterations in the initial QRS vectorial forces in left bundle branch block:

a. Myocardial infarction may be simulated.

b. Myocardial infarction may be masked.

a. In Figure 6–14*B*, during intermittent left bundle branch block, the small R wave in lead V_1 and the larger R wave in V_2 disappeared entirely. The predominant R wave in V_3 became a predominant S wave. The erroneous diagnosis of anteroseptal myocardial infarction should not be made.

b. Figures 6–19*A* and *B* are from a patient with known diaphragmatic myocardial infarction (*A*) who developed left bundle branch block (*B*). Following development of left bundle branch block the Q waves in lead II are no longer present and the Q waves in leads III and aVF have become extremely small.

The electrocardiographic diagnosis of myocardial infarction *should not* be made in the presence of left bundle branch block.

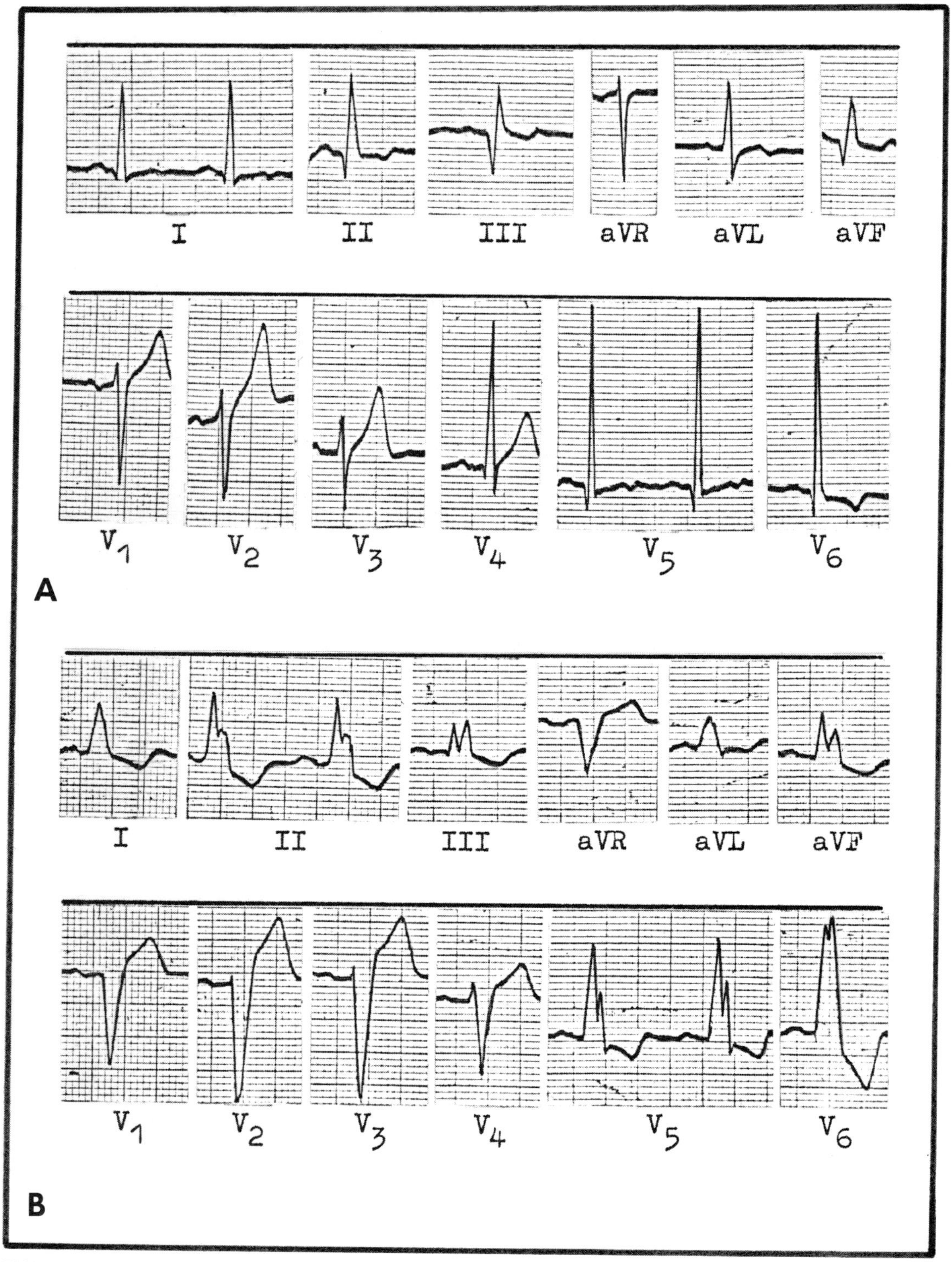

FIGURE 6–19. Development of left bundle branch block in a patient with known diaphragmatic myocardial infarction. *A,* Baseline, with diaphragmatic or inferior myocardial infarction; *B,* following development of LBBB.

TABLE 6–1. HEMIBLOCK CRITERIA

A. Left Anterior Hemiblock
1. FRONTAL PLANE
   a. Mean QRS vector usually −45° to −75° (often > −60°).
   b. Small Q wave in lead I, small R wave in lead III.
   c. QRS interval up to 0.1 sec.
2. HORIZONTAL PLANE (Criteria not constant)
   a. S waves in leads V_5 and V_6 with absence of Q waves.
   b. In right precordial leads there may be a small Q wave or R′.

B. Left Posterior Hemiblock
1. FRONTAL PLANE
   a. Mean QRS vector usually at +120° and beyond (right axis deviation).
   b. Small R wave in lead I and small Q wave in lead III.
   c. QRS interval up to 0.1 sec.
   d. No evidence of right ventricular hypertrophy.
2. HORIZONTAL PLANE (Criteria not constant)
   a. R wave or R with small S wave in leads V_5 and V_6 with absence of Q waves.

C. The "Hemiblocks" and the "Trifascicular" System

Left axis deviation of the mean QRS vector had, for many years, been considered a major criterion for left ventricular hypertrophy. It has been shown, quite conclusively, that left ventricular hypertrophy, even to a marked degree, is not necessarily accompanied by left axis deviation. Left axis deviation, or perhaps a better term, superiorly oriented QRS vector (in the frontal plane), may be caused by a conduction disturbance in the anterior division of the left bundle branch. Since the left bundle branch comprises two major divisions, the anterior and the posterior division, Rosenbaum, who has helped clarify the subject of intraventricular conduction, recommended the use of the term "hemiblock" to describe a disturbance in either of the divisions. *Left anterior hemiblock (LAH)*, therefore, describes a conduction disturbance in the anterior division, and *left posterior hemiblock (LPH)*, a disturbance in the posterior division of the left bundle branch. In left anterior hemiblock the mean QRS vector, in the frontal plane, is leftward and superior, or simply superior, and in left posterior hemiblock the mean QRS vector, in the frontal plane, is rightward or frank right axis deviation.

Figure 6–20 is a schematic illustration of the hemiblocks.

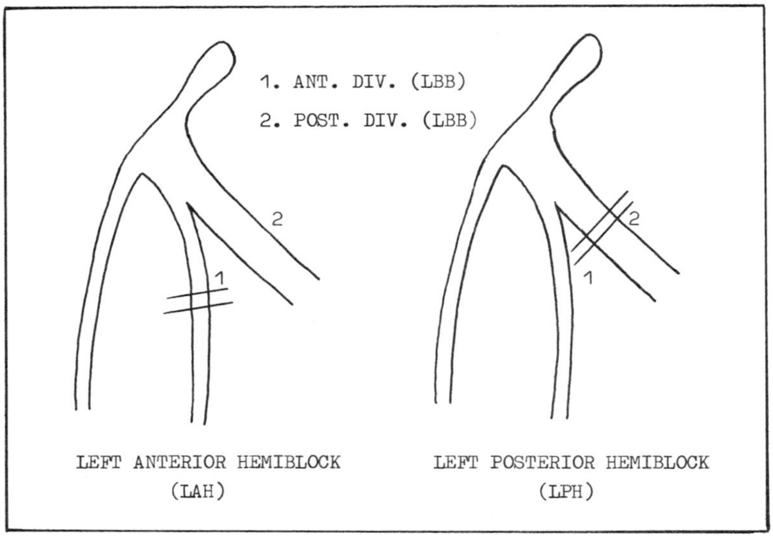

FIGURE 6–20. The "hemiblocks."

Cassette 16

Left anterior hemiblock is a much more common finding than left posterior hemiblock.

1. *Left Anterior Hemiblock Associated with Anterior Myocardial Infarction*

In the study of myocardial infarction it was noted that the *terminal* portion of the QRS complex may *also* be altered by infarction, with no, or almost no, prolongation of the QRS complex itself (Chapter 5, Figure 5–22). This is not an infrequent finding in clinical electrocardiography and deserves careful scrutiny. A major cause of *left axis deviation* of the mean QRS vector is an abnormal sequence of depolarization of the left ventricle due to a conduction disturbance in the anterior division of the left bundle branch. Terminal activation must then spread leftward and superiorly from the posterior division, resulting in a leftward and superior orientation of the terminal QRS vector. Before stating that the left anterior hemiblock is due to myocardial infarction, serial electrocardiograms should show that it did not antedate the infarction. Figure 6–21*A* is from a patient with an acute myocardial infarction. During the

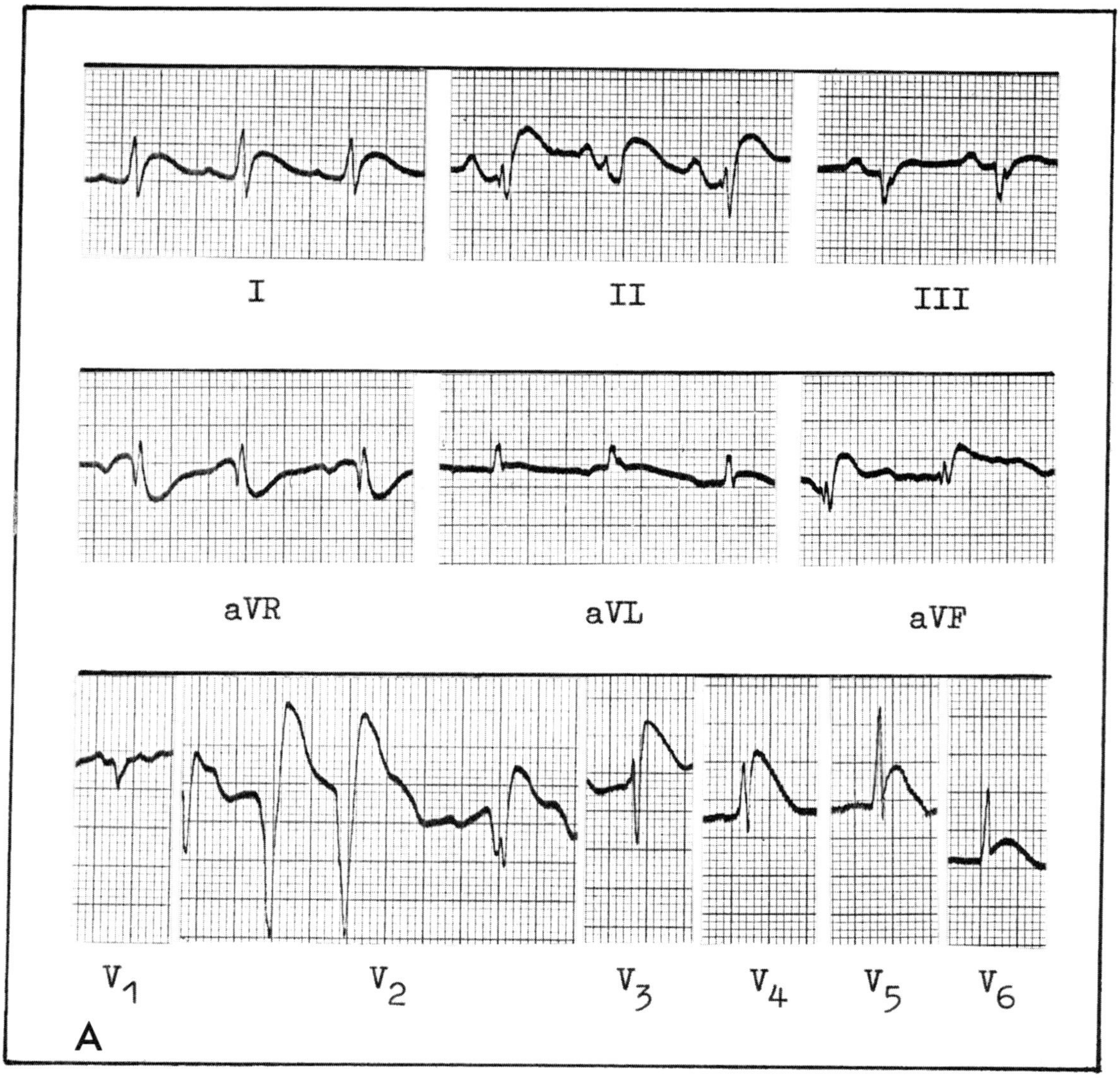

FIGURE 6–21. *A,* Left anterior hemiblock occurring in a patient with acute myocardial infarction.
Illustration continued on opposite page.

recovery phase the mean QRS vector remains oriented abnormally to the left, as seen in Figure 6–21*B*. Figure 6–21*C* is the baseline tracing. Eventually, the patient's mean QRS vector returned to the prior state, demonstrating that this disturbance need not be anatomic nor permanent.

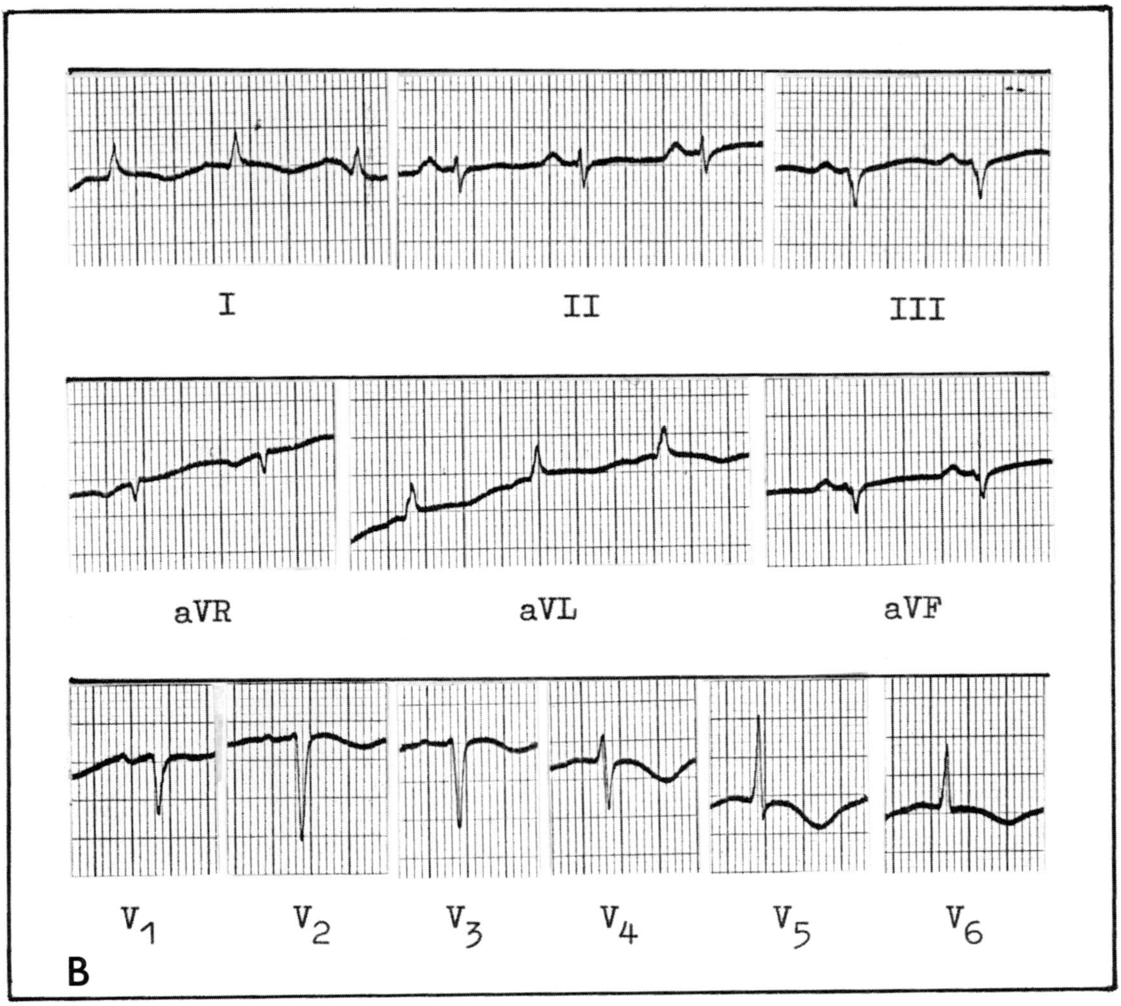

FIGURE 6–21 *Continued.* *B,* Evolutionary changes after myocardial infarction. The mean QRS vector still oriented abnormally to the left.

Illustration continued on following page.

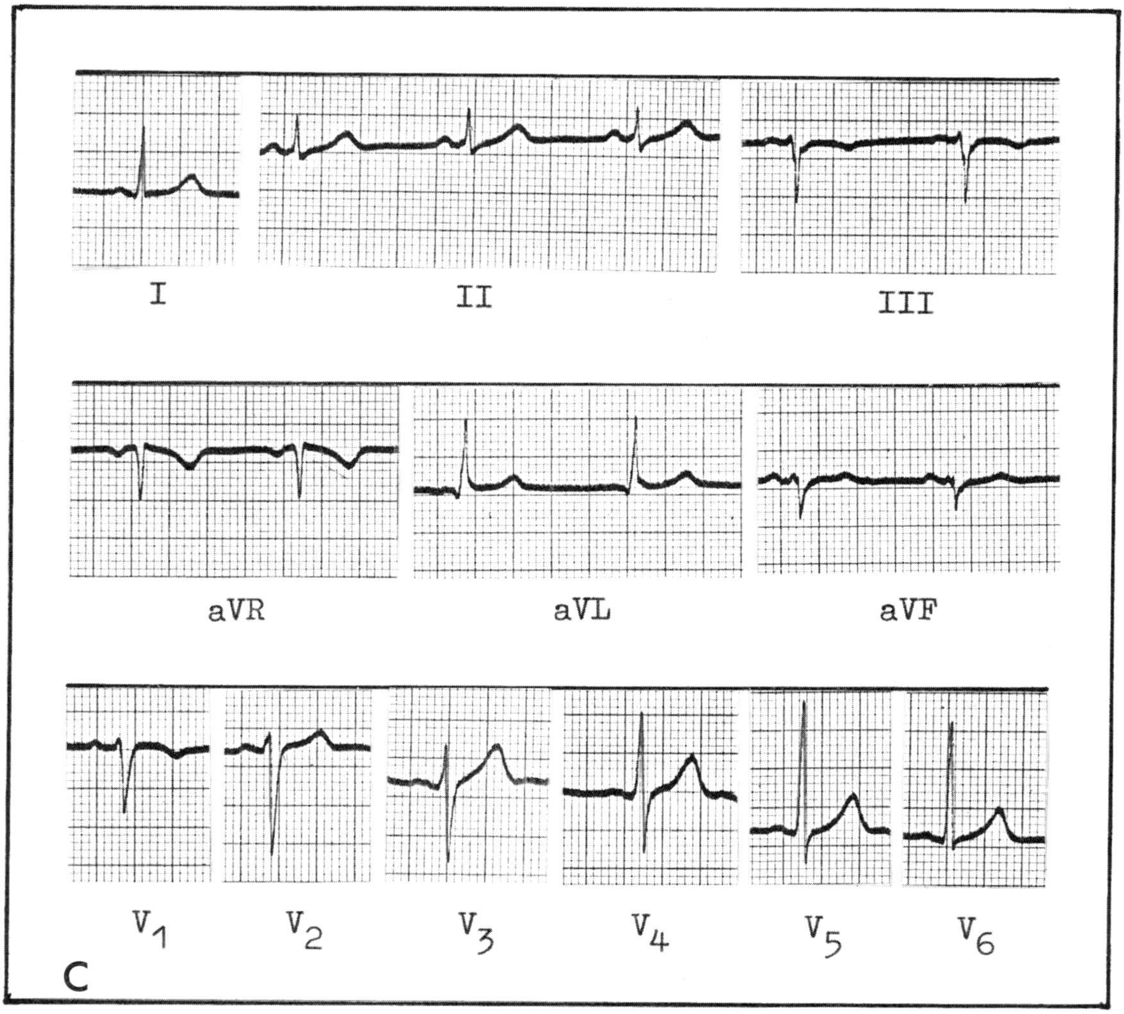

FIGURE 6–21 *Continued.* *C*, Baseline electrocardiogram of same patient as in Figures 6–21*A* and 6–21*B*. Eventually the patient's mean QRS vector returned to the prior state, demonstrating that this disturbance need not be anatomic or permanent.

2. *Left Anterior Hemiblock Associated with Chronic Coronary Artery Disease*

Frequently, in the absence of myocardial infarction, left anterior hemiblock is present in patients with chronic coronary artery disease. Figure 6–22 is from an elderly patient with angina pectoris and diabetes mellitus. There is no electrocardiographic evidence of myocardial infarction or an enlarged left ventricle. There may, or may not, be repolarization (S–T segment and T wave) abnormalities. It is postulated that the left anterior hemiblock is due to *fibrosis* in the anterior division of the left bundle branch.

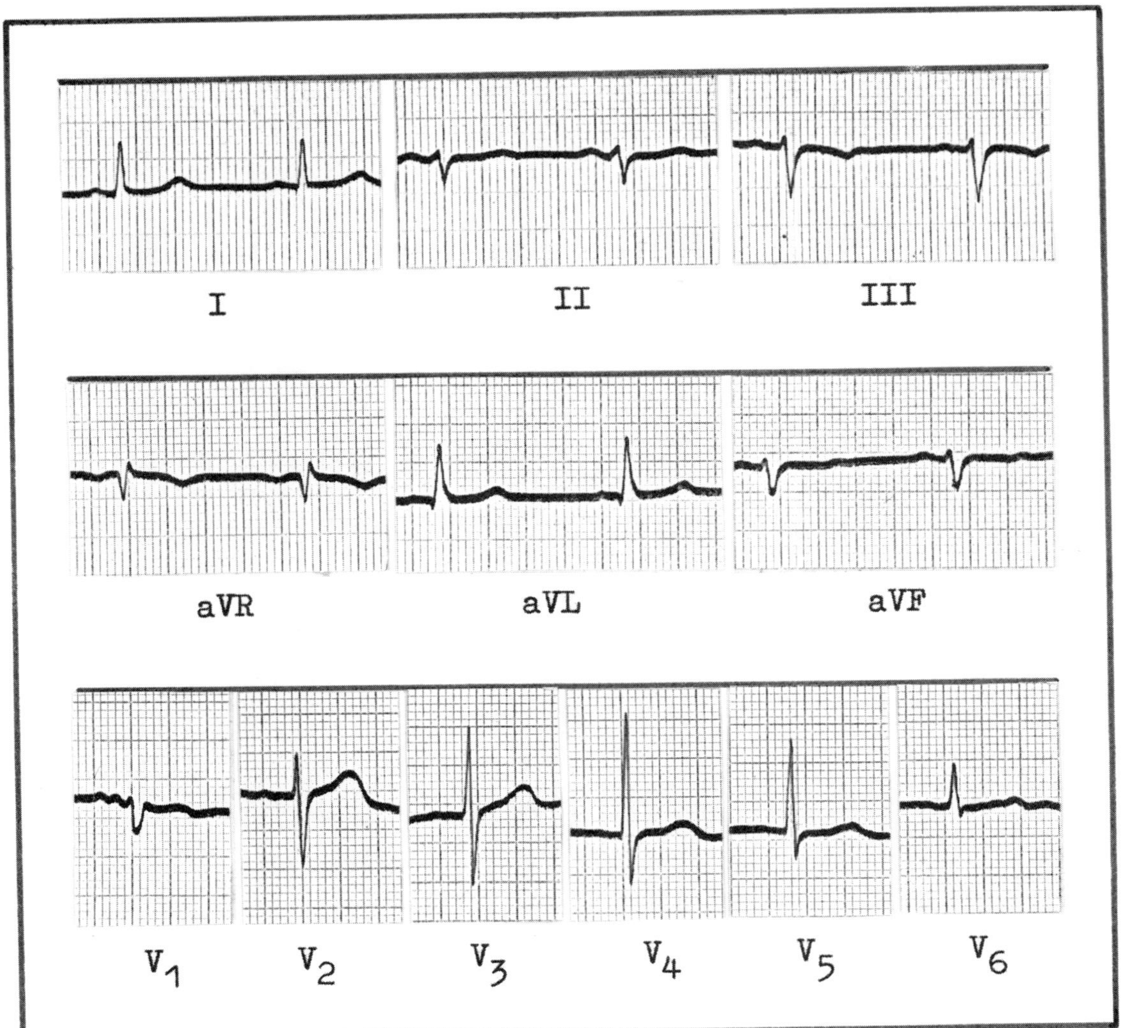

FIGURE 6–22. Left anterior hemiblock in an elderly patient with chronic coronary artery disease and diabetes mellitus.

3. *Left Anterior Hemiblock Associated with Left Ventricular Hypertrophy*

Left axis deviation had for many years been considered a major criterion of left ventricular hypertrophy. It is now considered to be a conduction disturbance (left anterior hemiblock) which may or may not accompany left ventricular hypertrophy. In the presence of fibrosis involving the conduction system the two may be found together. Review all the criteria of left ventricular hypertrophy in Figure 6–23.

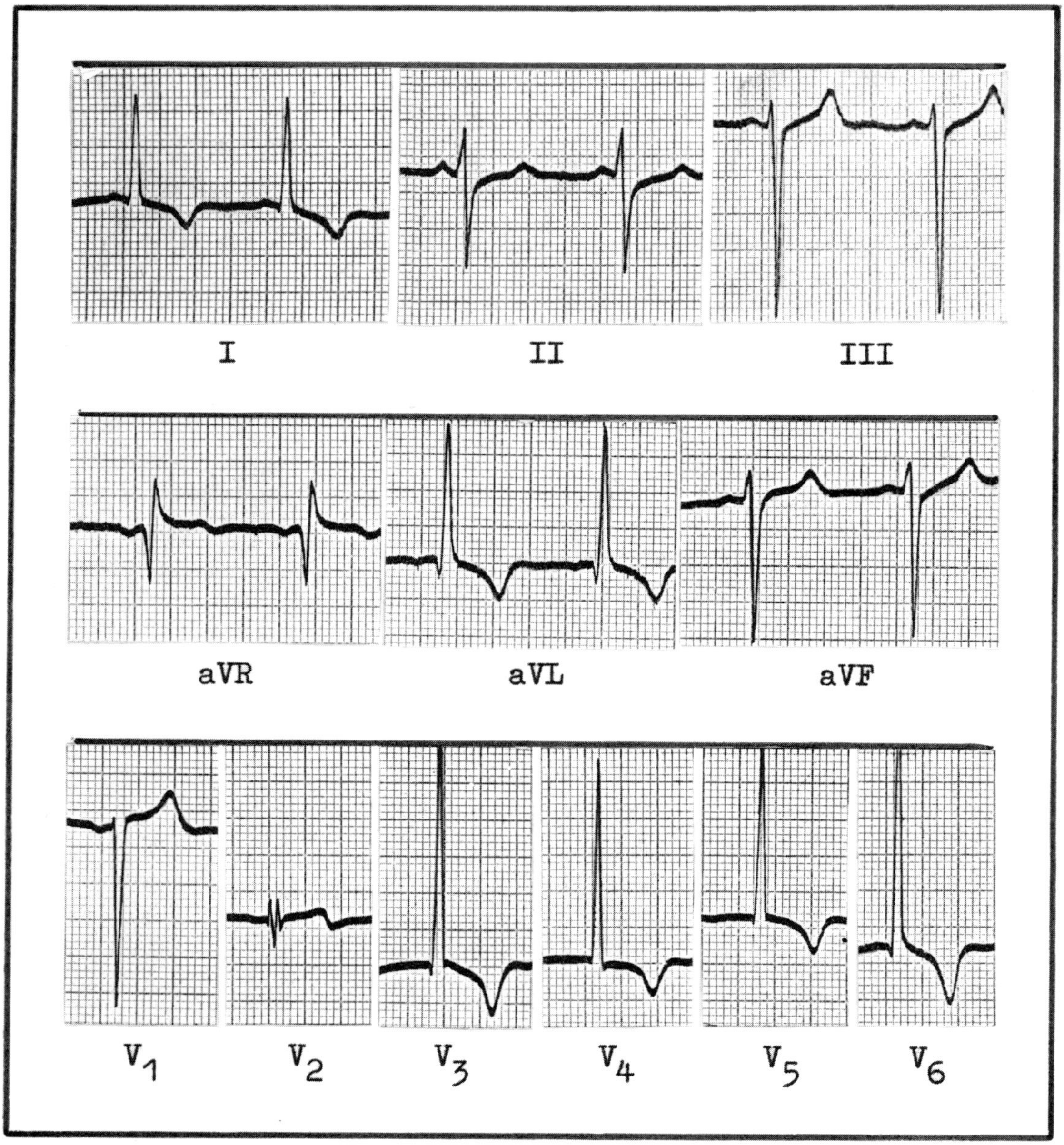

FIGURE 6–23. Left anterior hemiblock in a patient with left ventricular hypertrophy.

Not every abnormal left axis deviation of the mean QRS vector represents left anterior hemiblock.

1. *Left Axis Deviation Associated with Diaphragmatic Myocardial Infarction*

The abnormal leftward axis of the mean QRS vector in Figure 6–24 is due to the Q waves or QS complexes in leads II, III and aVF, representing the inferior wall myocardial infarction, rather than to large terminal S waves preceded by smaller initial R waves. Review the criteria for left anterior hemiblock.

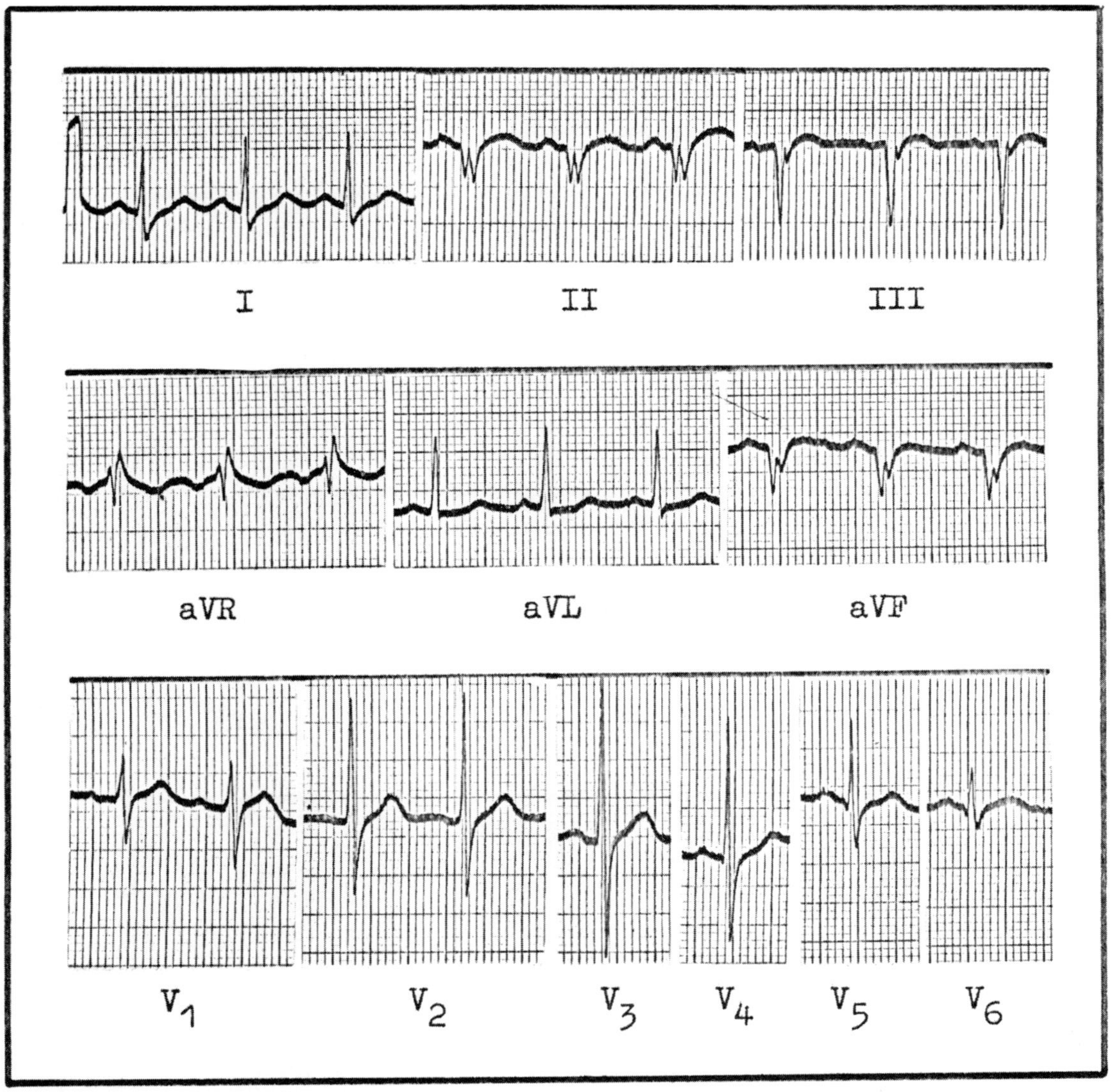

FIGURE 6–24. Diaphragmatic-posterior myocardial infarction. The left axis deviation is *not* left anterior hemiblock.

2. Left Axis Deviation Associated with Pulmonary Emphysema

Left axis deviation is found in a small percentage of patients with pulmonary emphysema. *The mechanism is not clear* since, in the majority of patients with emphysema, who have similar deformity of the chest and hyperinflation of the lungs, the mean QRS vector is normal, vertical or even rightward. Figure 6–25 is from a patient with severe, chronic obstructive lung disease. Recognized authorities have argued that the left axis deviation associated with pulmonary emphysema is really left anterior hemiblock and may be the only indication of disease of the left ventricle. Research in this area is in progress. Low QRS complex amplitude is common in patients with emphysema.

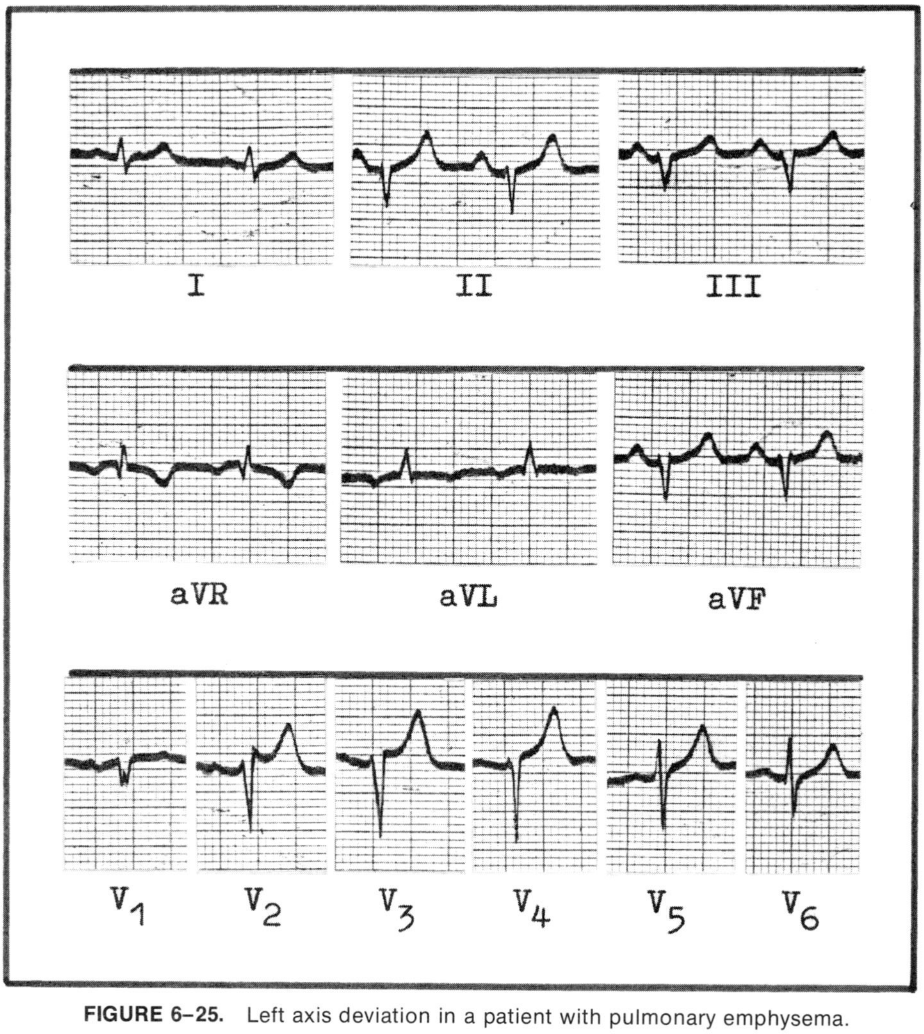

FIGURE 6–25. Left axis deviation in a patient with pulmonary emphysema.

Left axis deviation is sometimes found in a young "otherwise normal" patient. Figure 6–26 is from a 30 year old "healthy" man. Laboratory studies and chest x-ray were within normal limits. Although the left axis deviation is abnormal, the criteria for left anterior hemiblock are not clearly met. Still, the possibility of a congenital block in the anterior division of the left bundle branch must be considered. Thorough follow-up of these patients for many years is needed for evaluation of this entity.

Although discussion of these is beyond the scope of our present study, left axis deviation has also been associated with various congenital heart lesions.

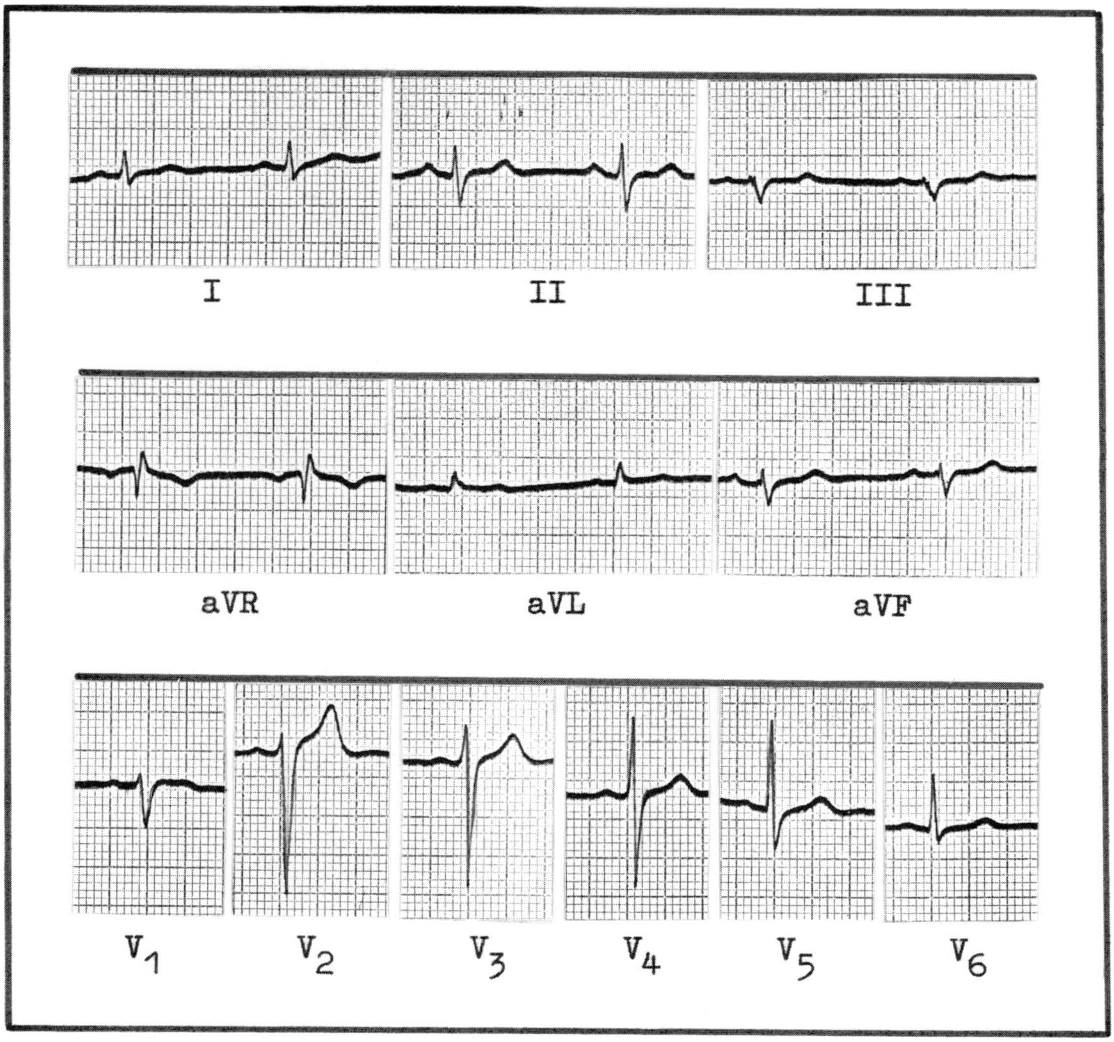

FIGURE 6–26. Left axis deviation in an "otherwise normal" patient.

Left posterior hemiblock is less common than left anterior hemiblock due to the more secure blood supply to the posterior division of the left bundle branch. Figure 6–27*A* is from a patient with true posterior myocardial infarction who developed left posterior hemiblock. Review the criteria for left posterior hemiblock at this point. The criteria for left posterior hemiblock, especially in the precordial leads, are not strictly met on this electrocardiogram. However, a major change in the orientation of the mean QRS vector took place which cannot be explained on the basis of the myocardial infarction alone. There was no right ventricular hypertrophy nor increased pressure in the right atrium, right ventricle and pulmonary artery. The left posterior hemiblock is presumed here. As clearly stated by Rosenbaum, LPH cannot be a pure electrocardiographic diagnosis; it must necessarily be a clinical-electrocardiographic diagnosis. Figure 6–27*B* is the baseline electrocardiogram.

At the time of the myocardial infarction the patient also had an atrioventricular conduction disturbance known as Mobitz I block or the classical Wenckebach block. This is illustrated in Figure 6–27*C* and will be seen again in Chapter 7 (Fig. 7–42).

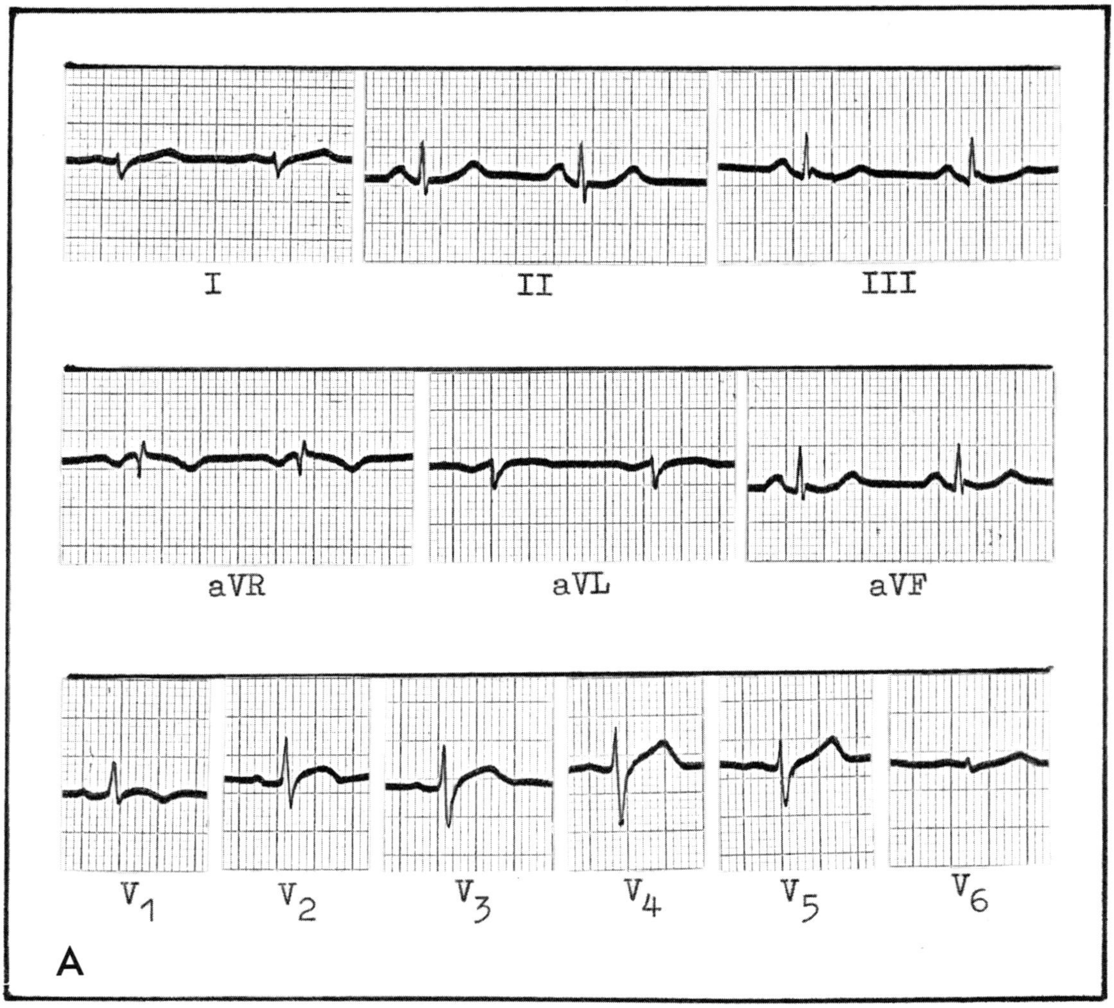

FIGURE 6–27. *A,* Right axis deviation in a patient with true posterior myocardial infarction, presumed left posterior hemiblock. Although the criteria for left posterior hemiblock are not strictly met, there was no right ventricular hypertrophy nor increased pressure in the right atrium, right ventricle and pulmonary artery. See also Figure 5–48, which is another electrocardiogram of the same patient.

Illustration continued on opposite page.

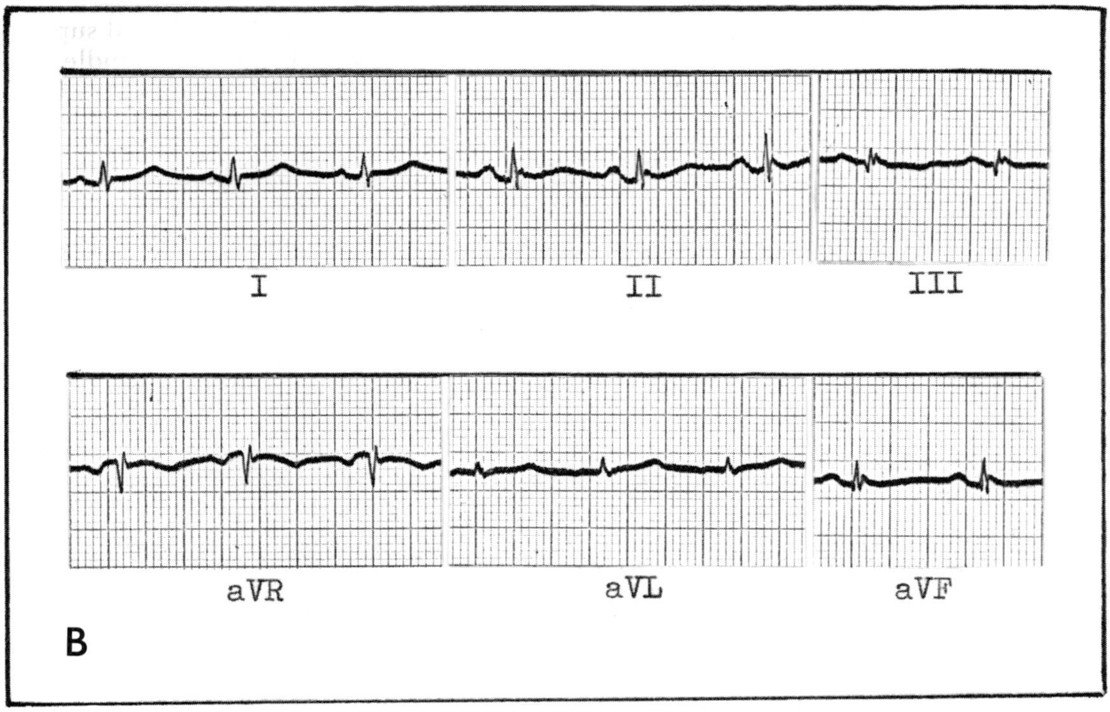

FIGURE 6–27 *Continued.* *B,* Same patient as in Figure 6–27*A,* prior to development of right axis deviation.

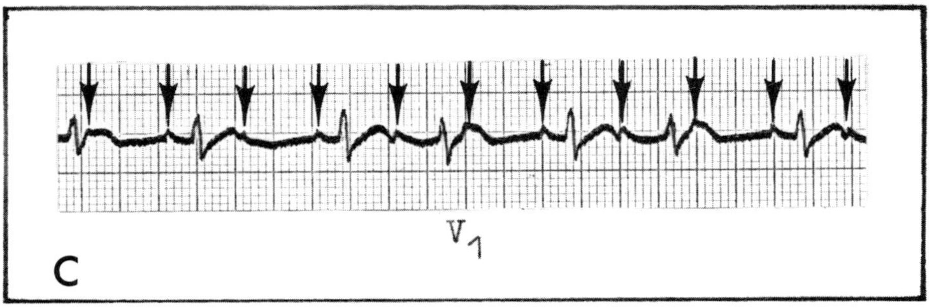

FIGURE 6–27 *Continued.* *C,* Same patient as in Figures 6–27*A* and 6–27*B.* Atrioventricular conduction disturbance at time of true posterior myocardial infarction. See text. The arrows point to the P waves.

The "Trifascicular" System

Both divisions of the left bundle branch (*1* and *2* in Fig. 6–28) plus the right bundle branch (*3*) have been termed the "trifascicular" system of intraventricular conduction. Each of the three component parts is called a fascicle. For example, right bundle branch block plus left anterior hemiblock or right bundle branch block plus left posterior hemiblock could be called *bifascicular* block. Examples and diagrams will be seen in the figures to follow. Block in all three fascicles would result in complete atrioventricular (A–V) block.

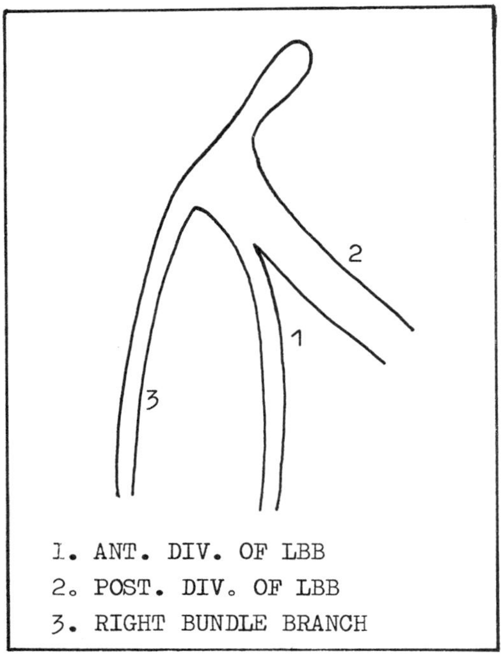

FIGURE 6–28. The "trifascicular" system.

Left anterior hemiblock is much more common than left posterior hemiblock, as already noted, since the anterior division of the left bundle branch is longer, thinner and has a more tenuous blood supply.

The combination of right bundle branch block (RBBB) plus left anterior hemiblock (LAH) is seen in Figures 6–29*A*, 6–30 and 6–31. Right bundle branch block plus left posterior hemiblock (LPH) is seen in Figures 6–29*B* and 6–32*B*. This combination may augur ill for the patient since the atrioventricular (A–V) conduction system depends on only one of the three "fascicles" functioning. These patients must be closely followed; pacemaker therapy must be considered with progression of disease to the third fascicle.

Text continued on page 300.

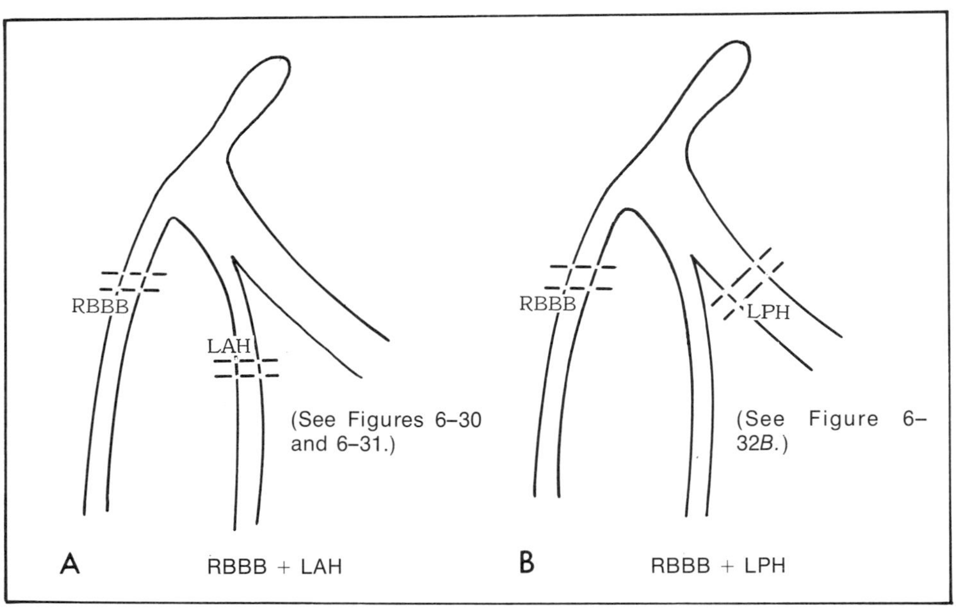

FIGURE 6–29. Types of "bifascicular" block.

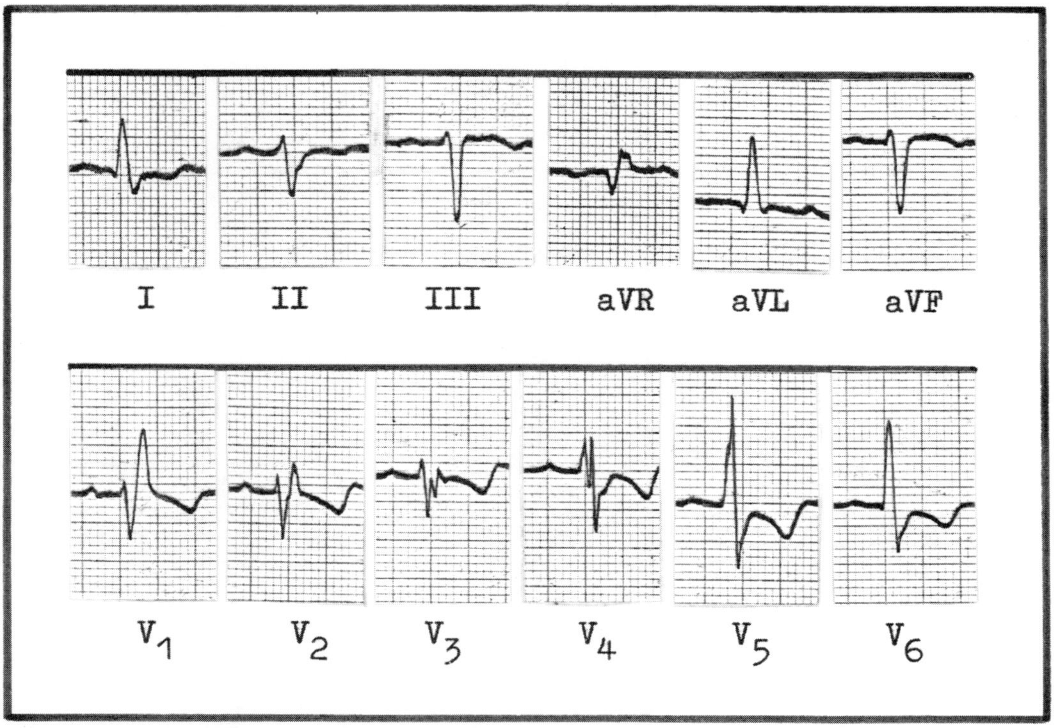

FIGURE 6–30. Bifascicular block. Right bundle branch block plus left anterior hemiblock is a not infrequent association. What may follow this stage?

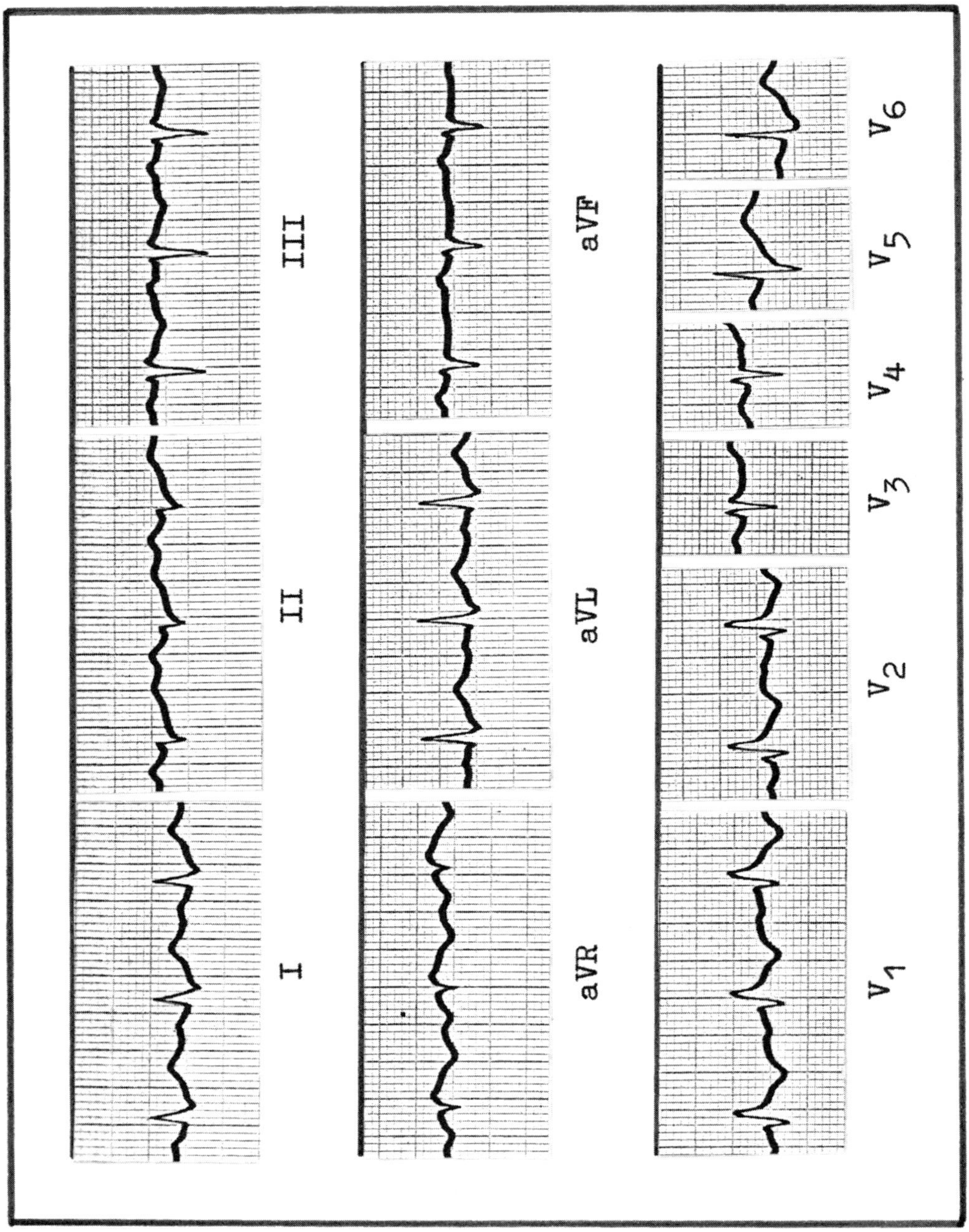

FIGURE 6–31. Right bundle branch block plus left anterior hemiblock. In this combination of conduction disturbances the S wave in lead I is often quite small and the QRS complex might resemble that of a left bundle branch block. The RSR′ in lead V_1, however, remains the key to the correct diagnosis.

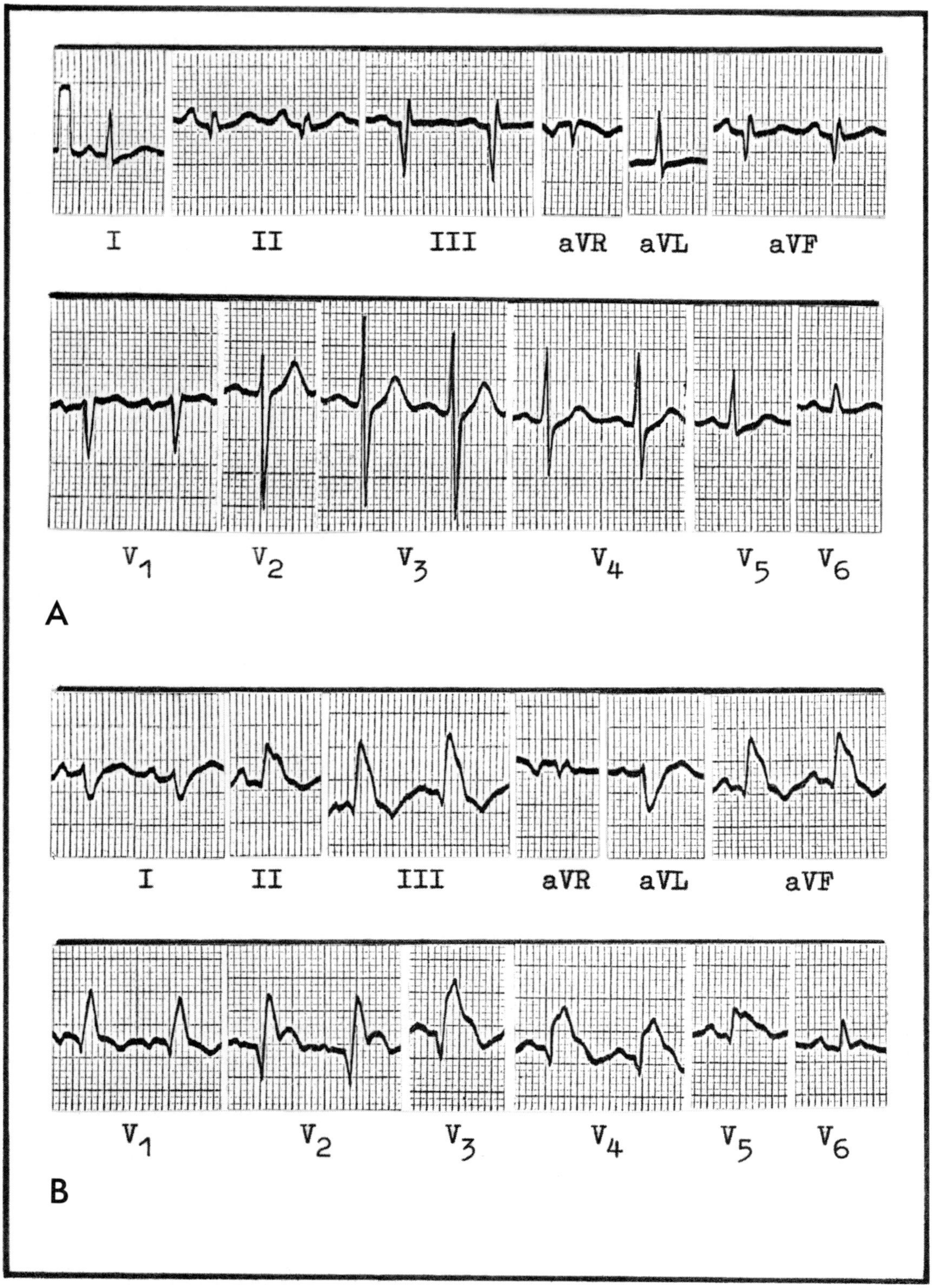

FIGURE 6–32. Development of *right bundle branch block* plus *left posterior hemiblock* with acute anterior myocardial infarction in a patient with a history of old diaphragmatic myocardial infarction. Note the marked shift of the mean QRS axis to the right in *B*. *A*, Baseline, with diaphragmatic or inferior myocardial infarction; *B*, following acute onset of anterior myocardial infarction, RBBB with right axis deviation.

The electrocardiograms in Figure 6–33 (*A* to *E*) are from a patient who in the course of an anterior myocardial infarction (*B*) developed right bundle branch block plus left anterior hemiblock (*C*). Cardiac pacing was required with the development of atrioventricular block (*D*). When the patient's sinus rhythm returned spontaneously he no longer had left anterior hemiblock but left posterior hemiblock plus right bundle branch block (*E*).

Text continued on page 305.

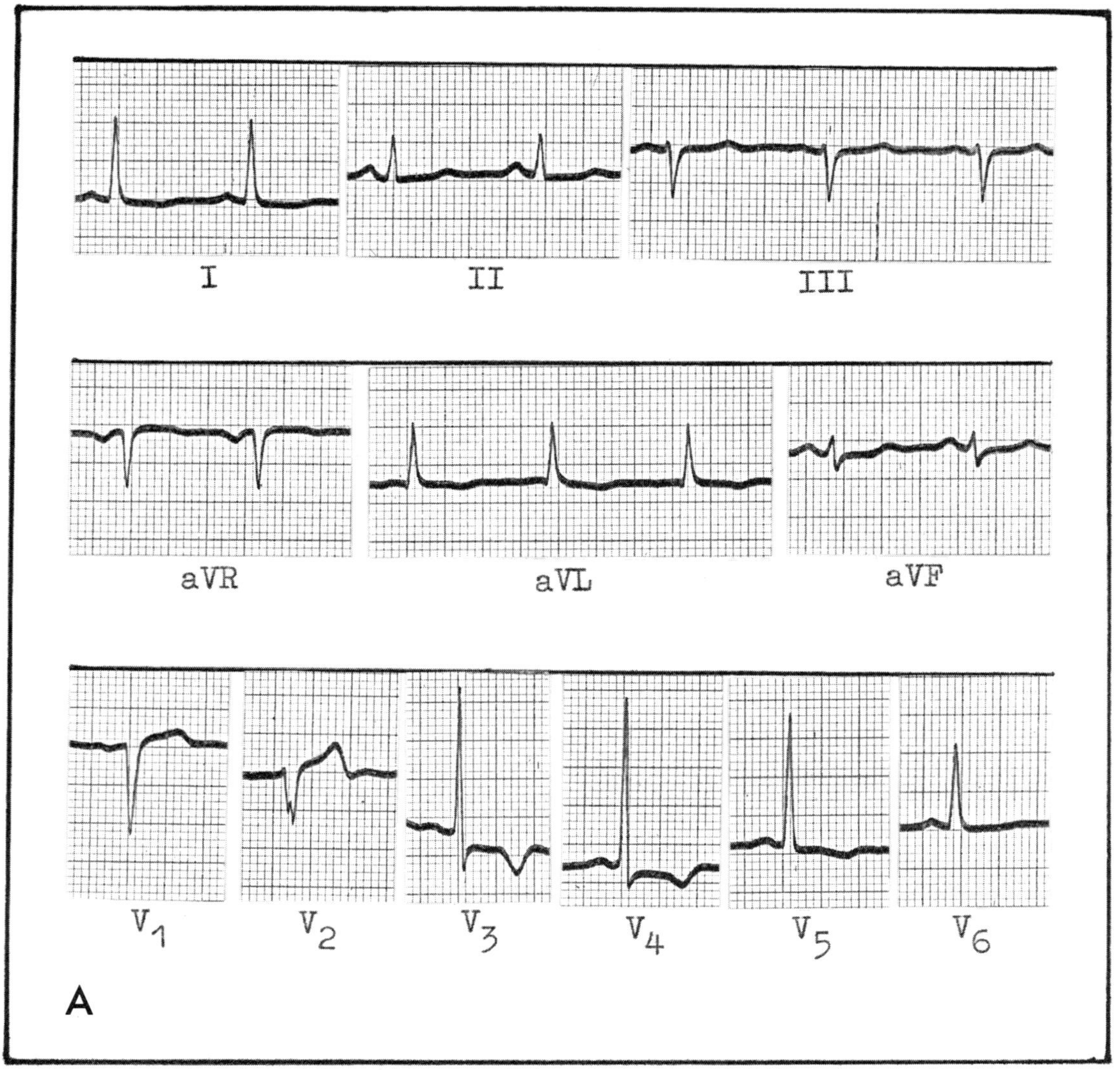

FIGURE 6–33. *A*, Baseline. Figures 6–33*B* to 6–33*E* are from the same patient during an anterior wall myocardial infarction.

Illustration continued on opposite page.

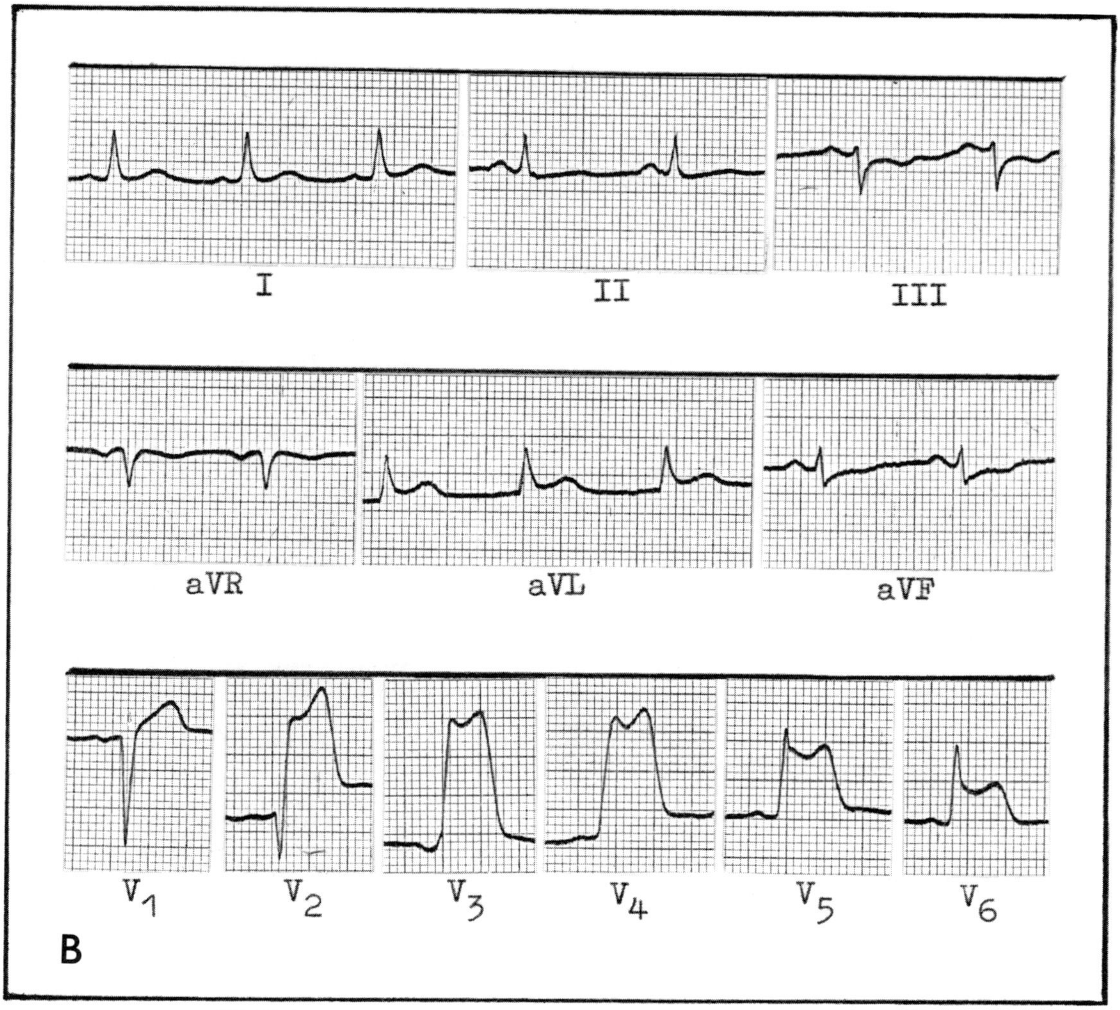

FIGURE 6–33 *Continued.* *B,* Acute anterior myocardial infarction.

Illustration continued on following page.

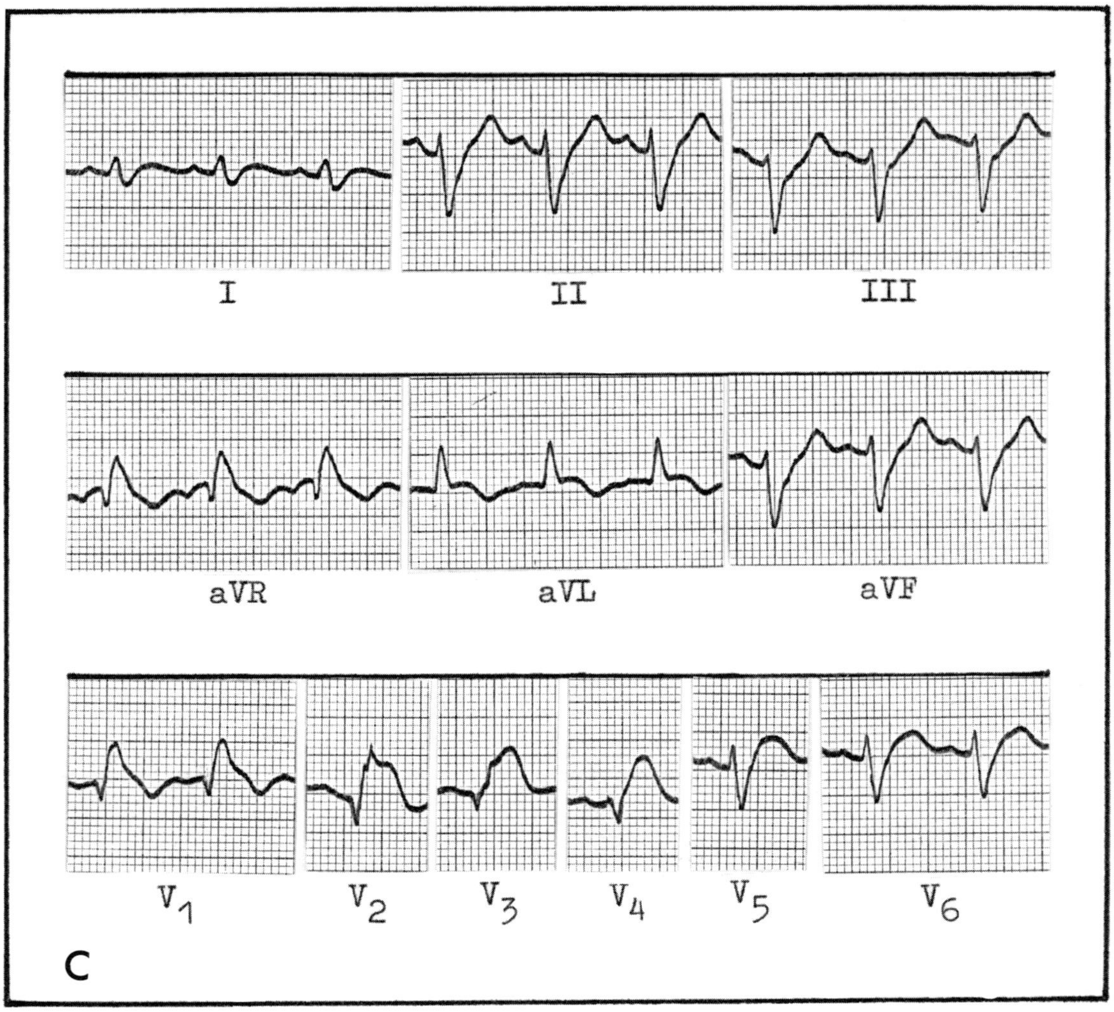

FIGURE 6–33 *Continued.* *C,* Bifascicular block (right bundle branch block plus left anterior hemiblock) one day after electrocardiogram in Figure 6–33*B*.

Illustration continued on opposite page.

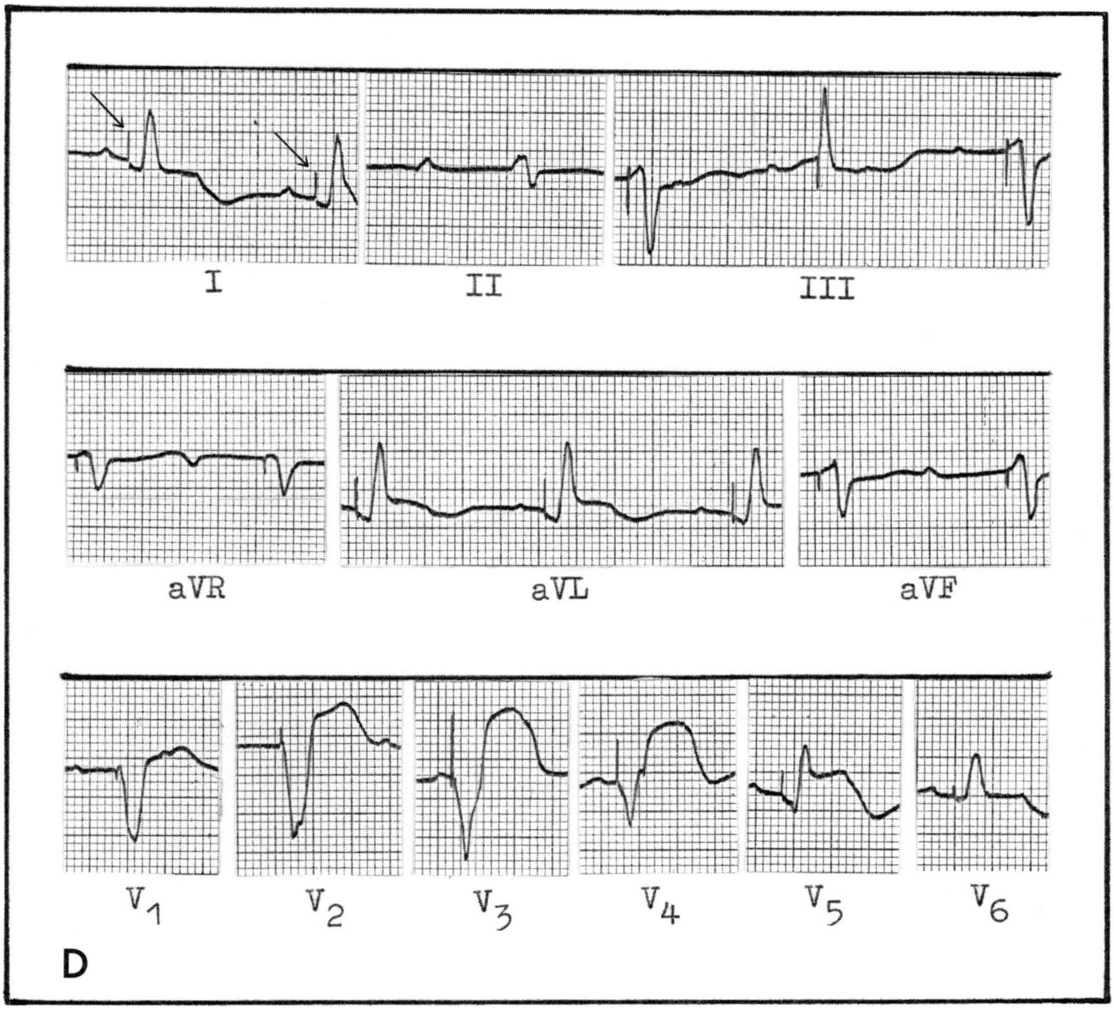

FIGURE 6–33 *Continued.* *D,* Cardiac pacing due to A–V block. The arrows in lead I point to the pacemaker impulses. The middle beat in lead III is conducted, with a prolonged P–R interval. Same evening as electrocardiogram in Figure 6–33*C*.

Illustration continued on following page.

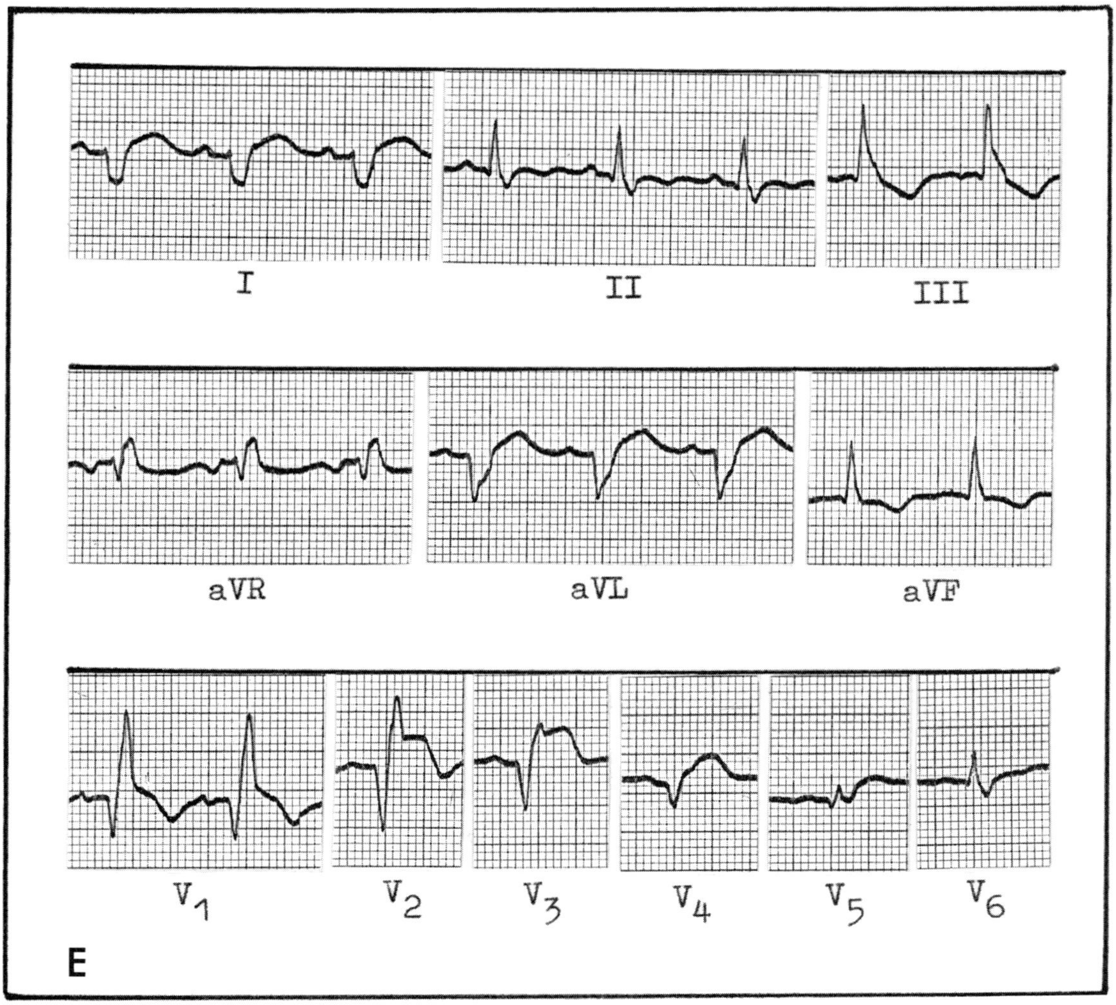

FIGURE 6–33 *Continued.* *E,* Bifascicular block (right bundle branch block plus *left posterior hemiblock*) one week after electrocardiogram in Figure 6–33*D.*

In studying left bundle block, in contrast to left anterior or left posterior hemiblock we note no significant mean QRS vectorial shifts. Following onset of left bundle branch block there is *neither* left nor right axis deviation, as seen in Figures 6–14 (*A* and *B*), 6–15 (*A* and *B*) and 6–19 (*A* and *B*). Where we did find a combination of left bundle branch block plus left axis deviation, the left axis deviation antedated the left bundle branch block. The location of the lesion or lesions is the subject of investigation today. This combination is seen in Figures 6–34 to 6–36.

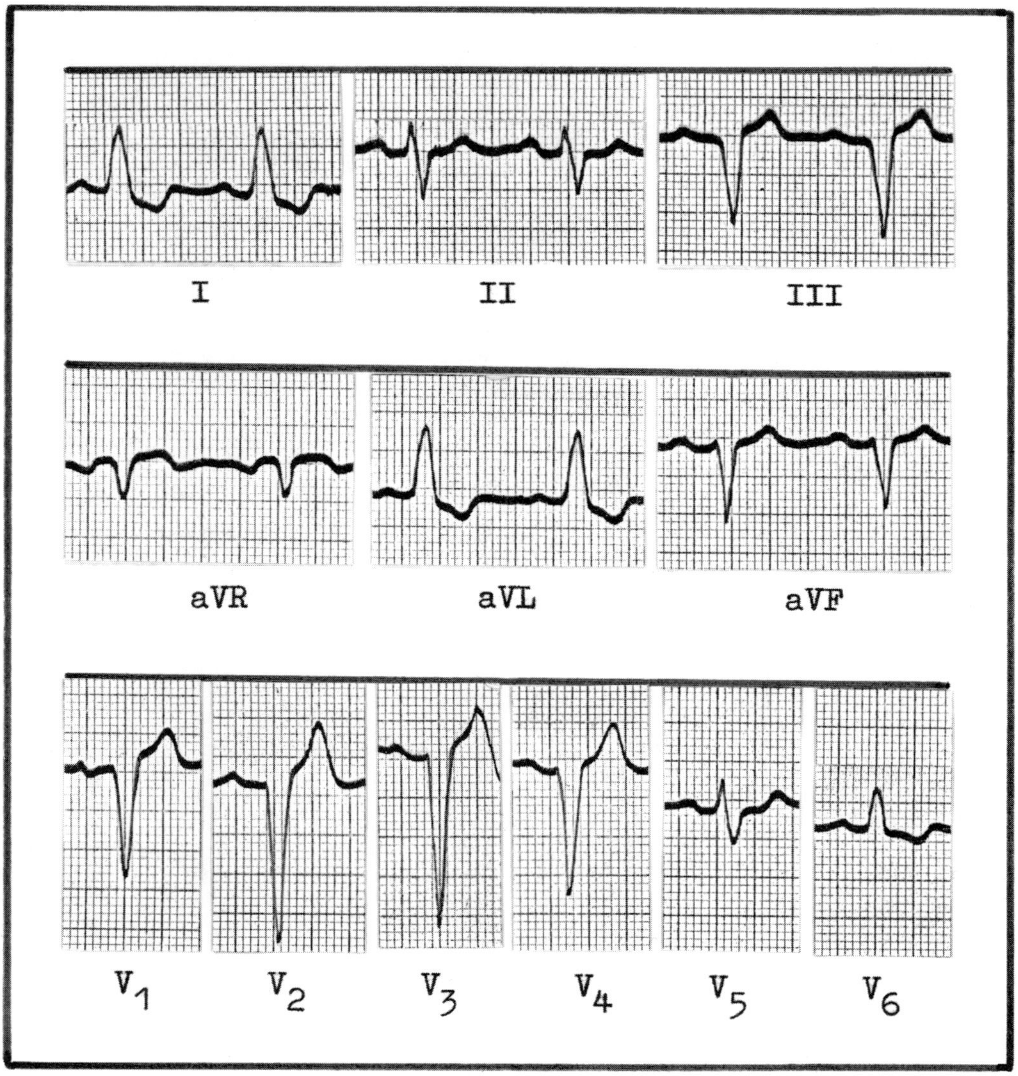

FIGURE 6–34. Left bundle branch block associated with left axis deviation. In this patient and in the next two (Figures 6–35 and 6–36) the left axis deviation antedated the left bundle branch block. This has been the case in most of our patients. In general, the mean QRS vector is not changed to any significant degree by left bundle branch block so that left axis deviation may be diagnosed in the presence of left bundle branch block. The location of the lesion or lesions in this combination is the subject of much study today. Be ready to revise your present concepts with the accumulation of new data.

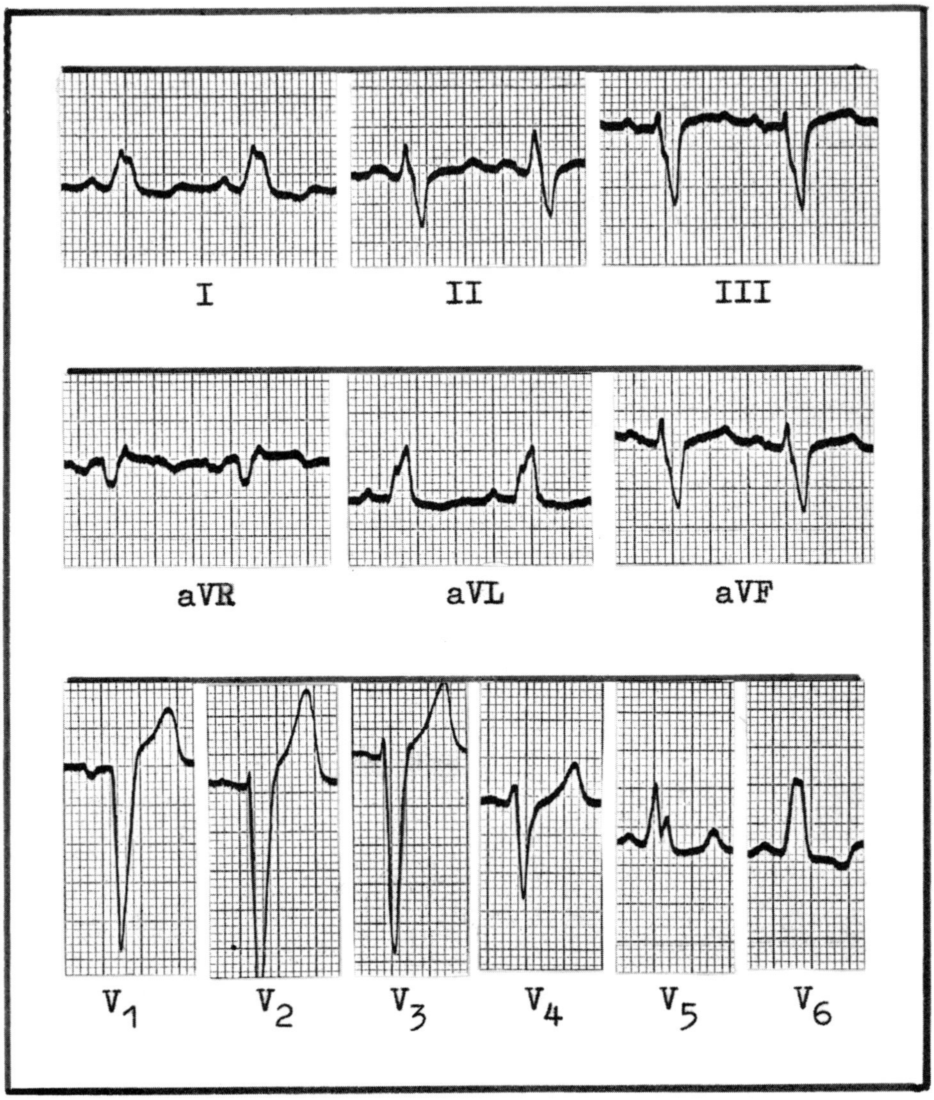

FIGURE 6–35. Left bundle branch block associated with left axis deviation (see Figure 6–34).

The hemiblocks differ from left bundle branch block in that in the hemiblocks there is no significantly prolonged QRS interval (up to 0.1 sec.). In left anterior hemiblock the mean QRS vector is usually at least −45° and in left posterior hemiblock the mean QRS vector is usually at +120° or beyond. In left bundle branch block there *is* prolongation of the QRS complex and no mean QRS vectorial shift. In left posterior hemiblock, with shift of the mean QRS vector to the right, right ventricular hypertrophy must be ruled out.

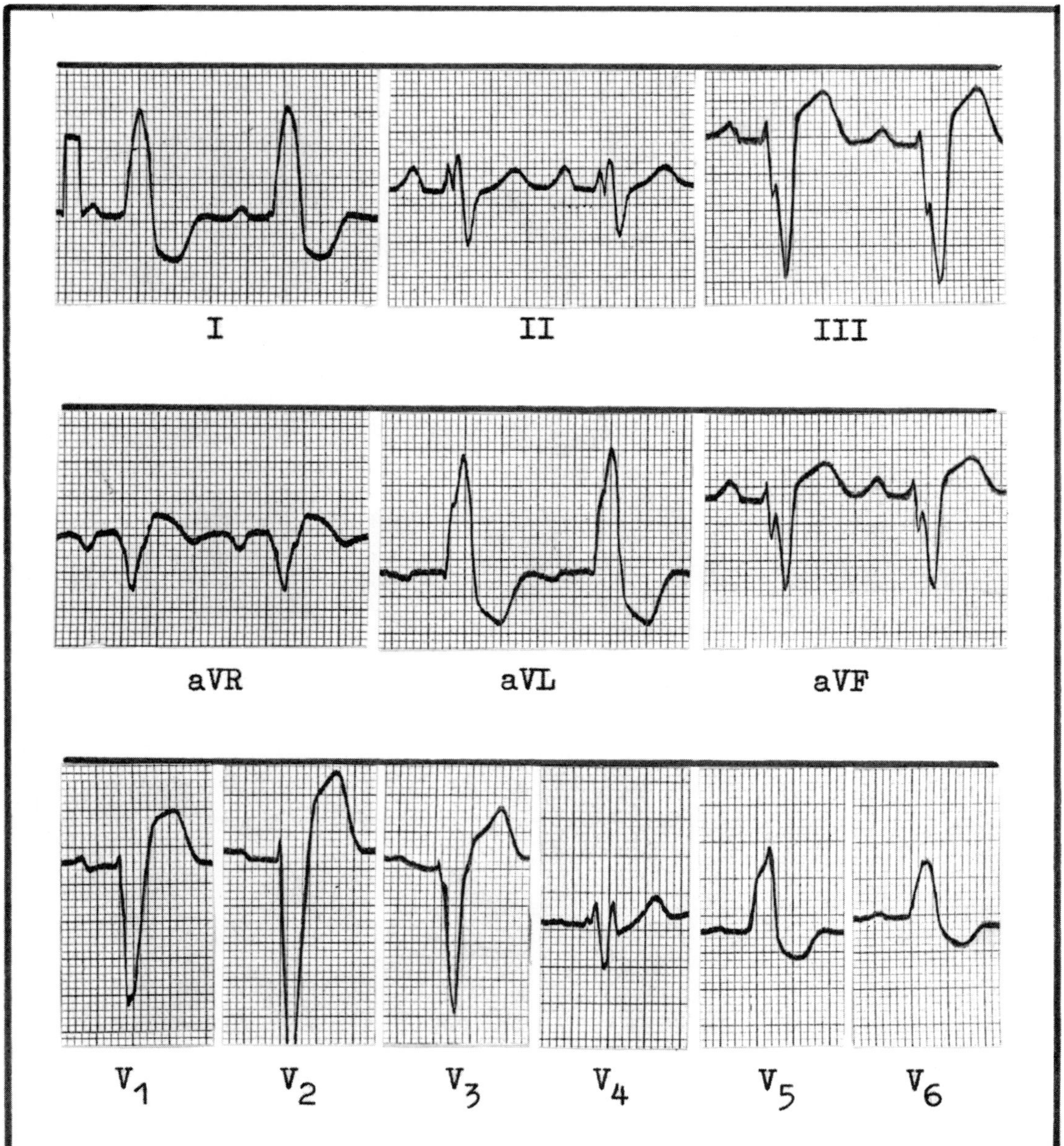

FIGURE 6–36. Left bundle branch block associated with left axis deviation (see Figure 6–34).

D. S_1 S_2 S_3 Syndrome

The S_1 S_2 S_3 syndrome, in which there are prominent S waves in the three standard leads with no prolongation of the QRS interval and, at times, with an R′ in lead V_1 (terminal QRS vector which is to the right, superior and sometimes anterior) has been found:

1. In normal patients.
2. In patients with right ventricular hypertrophy, both congenital and acquired (such as cor pulmonale).
3. In patients with acute myocardial infarction without complicating cor pulmonale.

Figure 6–37 is from a "normal" patient with the S_1 S_2 S_3 syndrome. The patient was normotensive with no evidence of heart disease by history, on physical examination, chest x-ray and laboratory studies.

Figure 6–38 is from a patient with severe chronic obstructive lung disease and cor pulmonale and Figures 6–39 *A* and *B* are from a patient who developed the S_1 S_2 S_3 syndrome with acute anterior myocardial infarction.

Text continued on page 312.

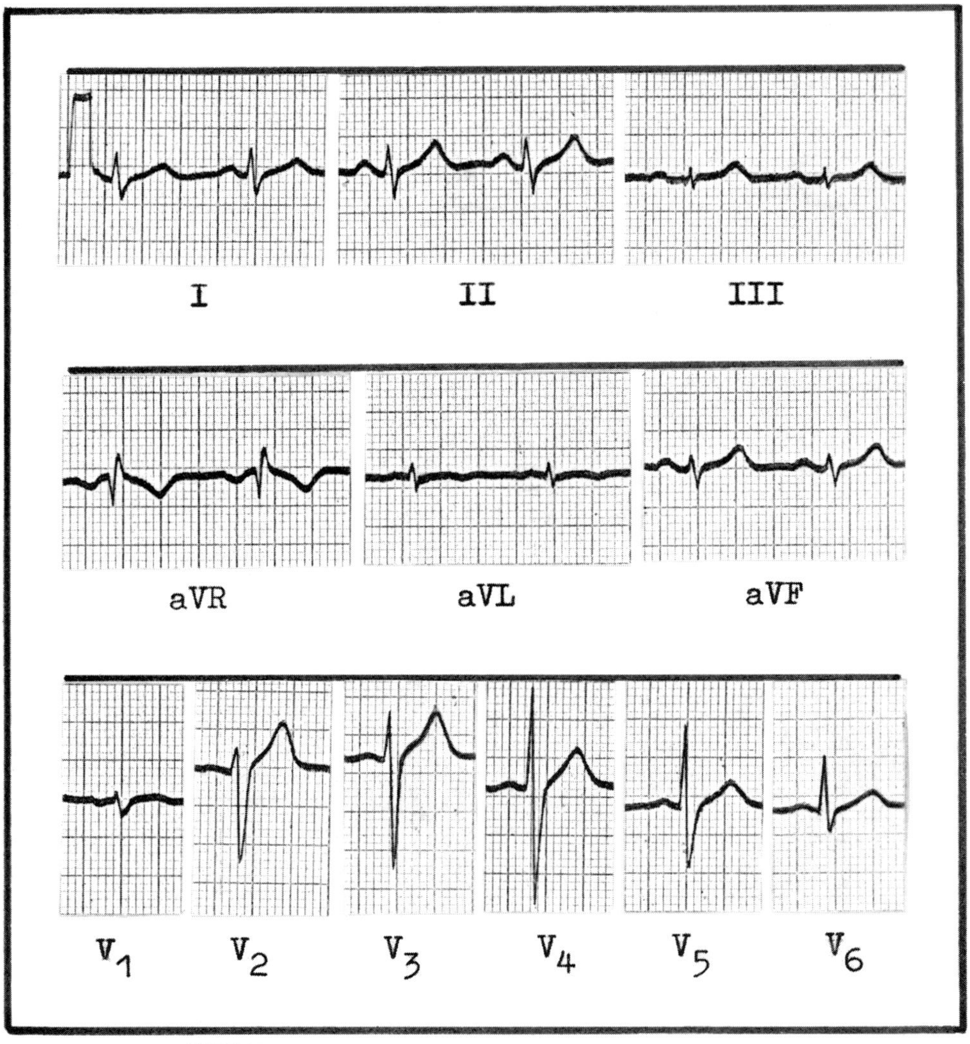

FIGURE 6–37. The S_1 S_2 S_3 syndrome in a normal patient.

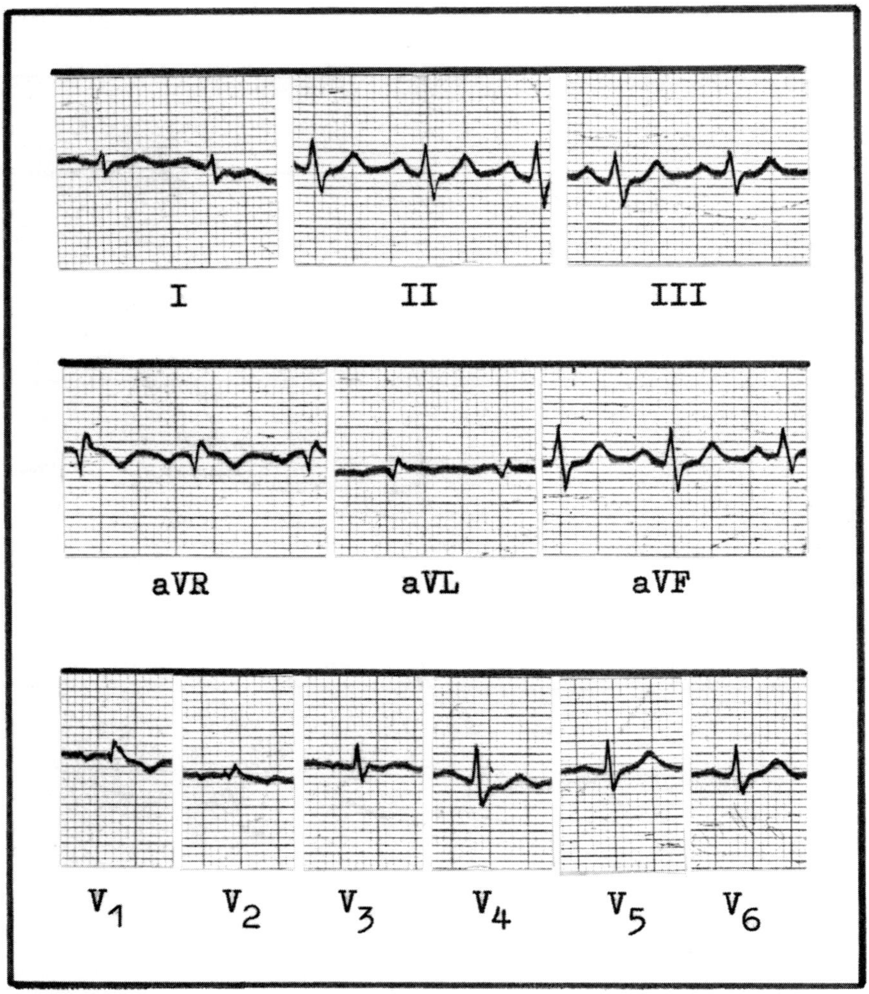

FIGURE 6–38. The S_1 S_2 S_3 syndrome in a patient with severe chronic obstructive lung disease and cor pulmonale. Note the small QRS deflections in all the leads, not uncommon in patients with severe hyperinflation of the lungs (pulmonary emphysema).

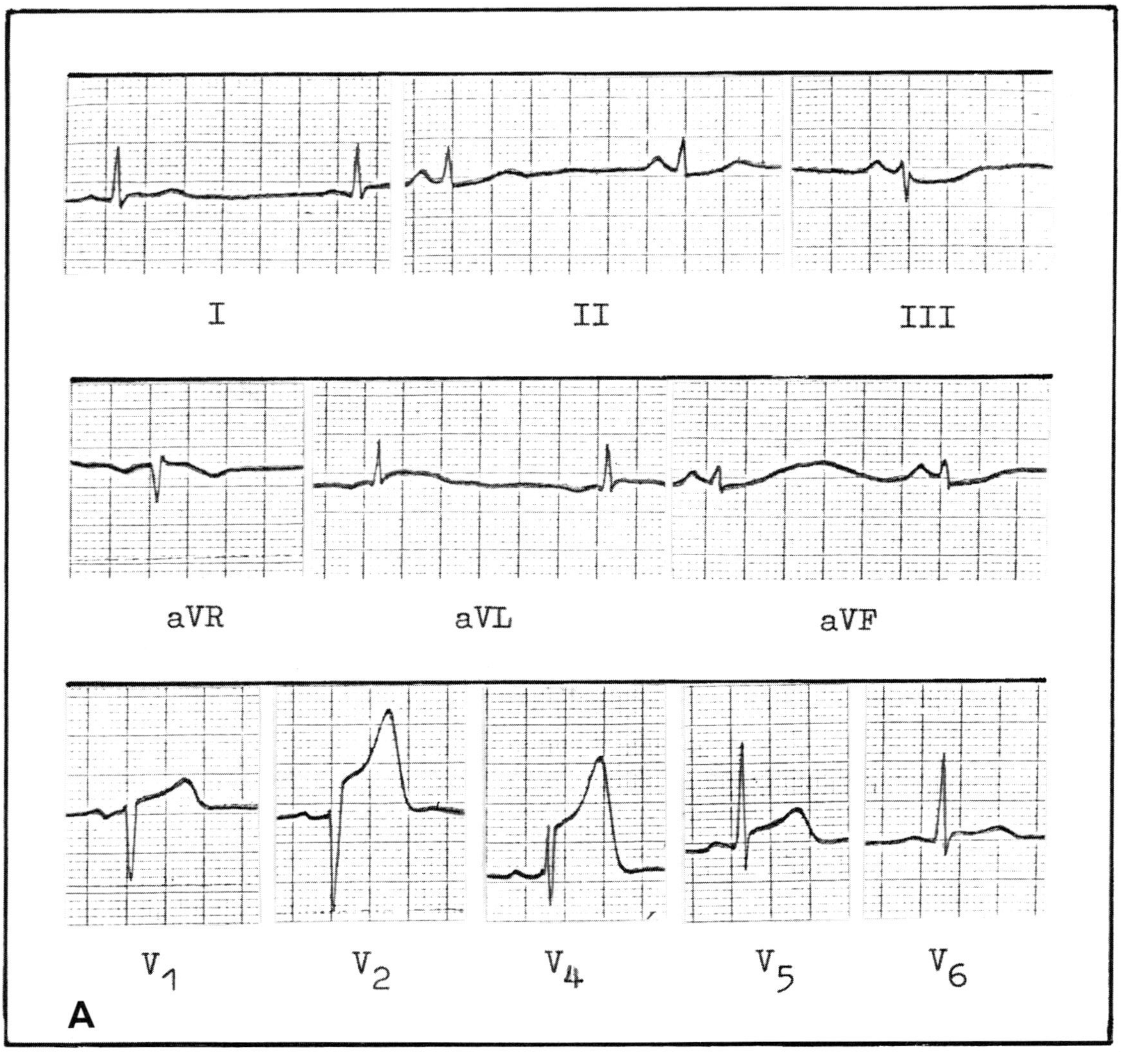

FIGURE 6–39. *A,* Patient with acute anterior myocardial infarction. Note the mean QRS vector.

Illustration continued on opposite page.

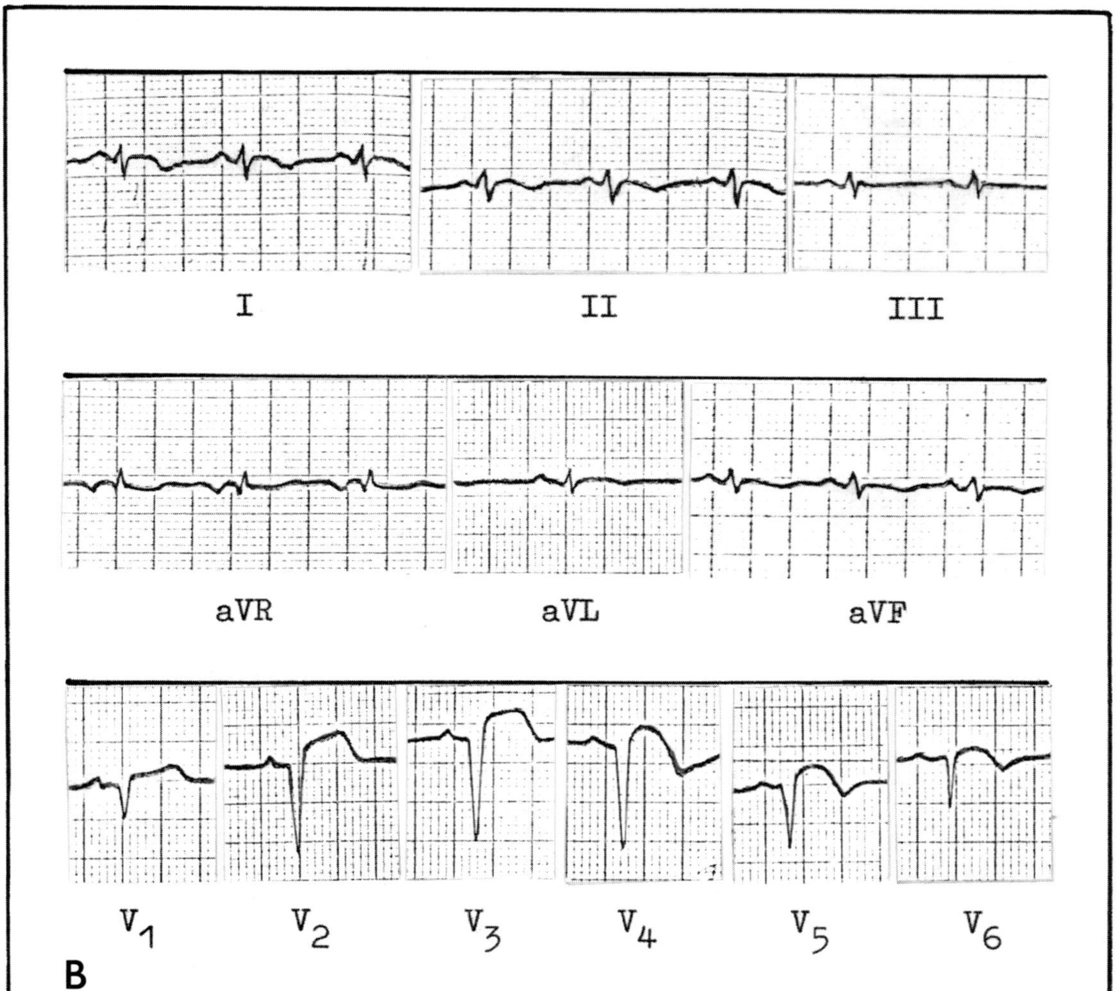

FIGURE 6–39 *Continued.* *B,* Same patient as in Figure 6–39 *A,* with onset of S_1 S_2 S_3 syndrome during the acute myocardial infarction.

In Figures 6–37, 6–38 and 6–39*B* it is not possible to plot a mean QRS vector in the frontal plane using the entire QRS complex, since in every lead of the frontal plane the QRS complex is biphasic. To properly plot the QRS vectorial forces, the QRS complexes must be divided into initial and terminal vectors. In Figure 6–40 it is seen that the initial QRS vectorial forces are approximately along the axis of +lead II and the terminal QRS vectorial forces are along the axis of −lead II, in the opposite direction. In summary, in the S_1 S_2 S_3 syndrome the initial QRS is to the left and inferior, and the terminal QRS vector is to the right and superior in the frontal plane.

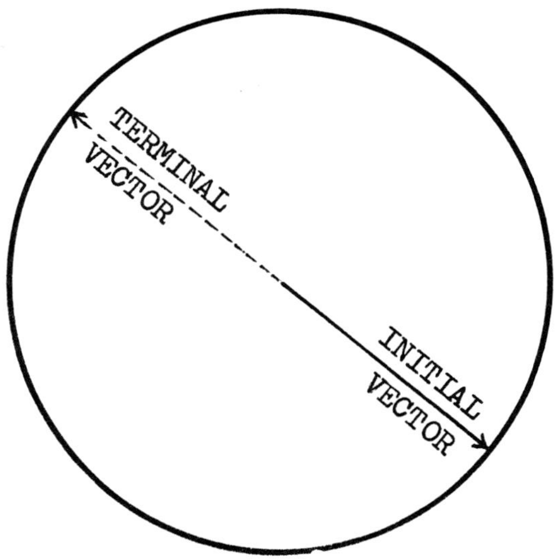

FIGURE 6–40. Initial and terminal vectorial forces of the QRS in the S_1 S_2 S_3 syndrome.

E. Preexcitation (Wolff-Parkinson-White or W-P-W) Syndrome

A very distinctive electrocardiogram was reported in patients subject to attacks of paroxysmal tachycardia. The electrocardiographic pattern is characterized by a:

a. Short P–R interval (0.12 sec. or less).

b. Prolonged QRS interval (greater than 0.1 sec.).

c. Slurring of the upstroke by a *delta* wave.

The short P–R interval may be more apparent than real since the measurement from the beginning of the P wave to the end of the QRS complex may be normal. A typical electrocardiographic cycle is diagrammed in Figure 6–41.

The mechanism responsible for this syndrome is under intensive investigation in numerous laboratories. The theories will not be discussed here, but the entity is not a mere curiosity, and certain features must be emphasized.

1. There is a frequent association of the W-P-W syndrome with paroxysmal supraventricular tachycardia—namely, paroxysmal atrial tachycardia, atrial fibrillation and atrial flutter. A typical case history is of an older patient stating that he has had bouts of rapid heart action throughout his life, but only in recent years, with increasing age and coronary disease, have these episodes caused him chest pain.

2. The alternation of normal conduction with the W-P-W syndrome is frequent and can make the search for the etiology of a supraventricular tachycardia a difficult one.

3. The electrocardiogram must be carefully scrutinized, and at times, the patient must be evaluated in a sophisticated cardiac laboratory since:

a. The delta waves may cause Q waves and QS complexes resembling myocardial infarction (Fig. 6–43:QS complexes are seen in leads III and V_1).

b. The delta waves may obscure the electrocardiographic evidence of myocardial infarction.

c. The tall R waves in lead V_1 in the W-P-W syndrome, type A (Fig. 6–42), may cause the diagnosis of posterior myocardial infarction or right ventricular hypertrophy to be made.

d. Secondary S–T segment and T wave abnormalities occur and may obscure primary abnormalities.

Text continued on page 318.

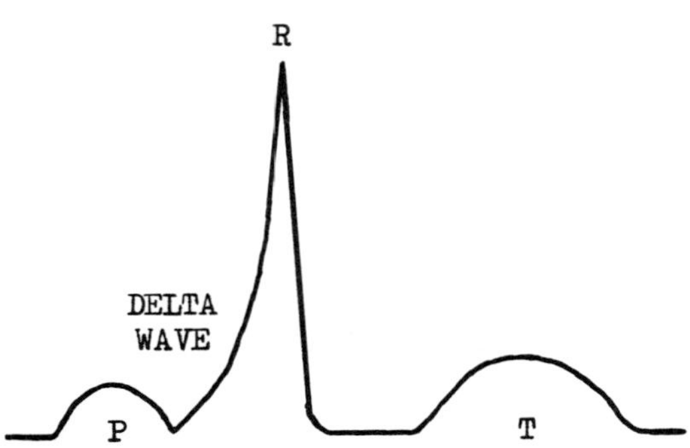

FIGURE 6–41. Preexcitation (Wolff-Parkinson-White or W-P-W) syndrome.

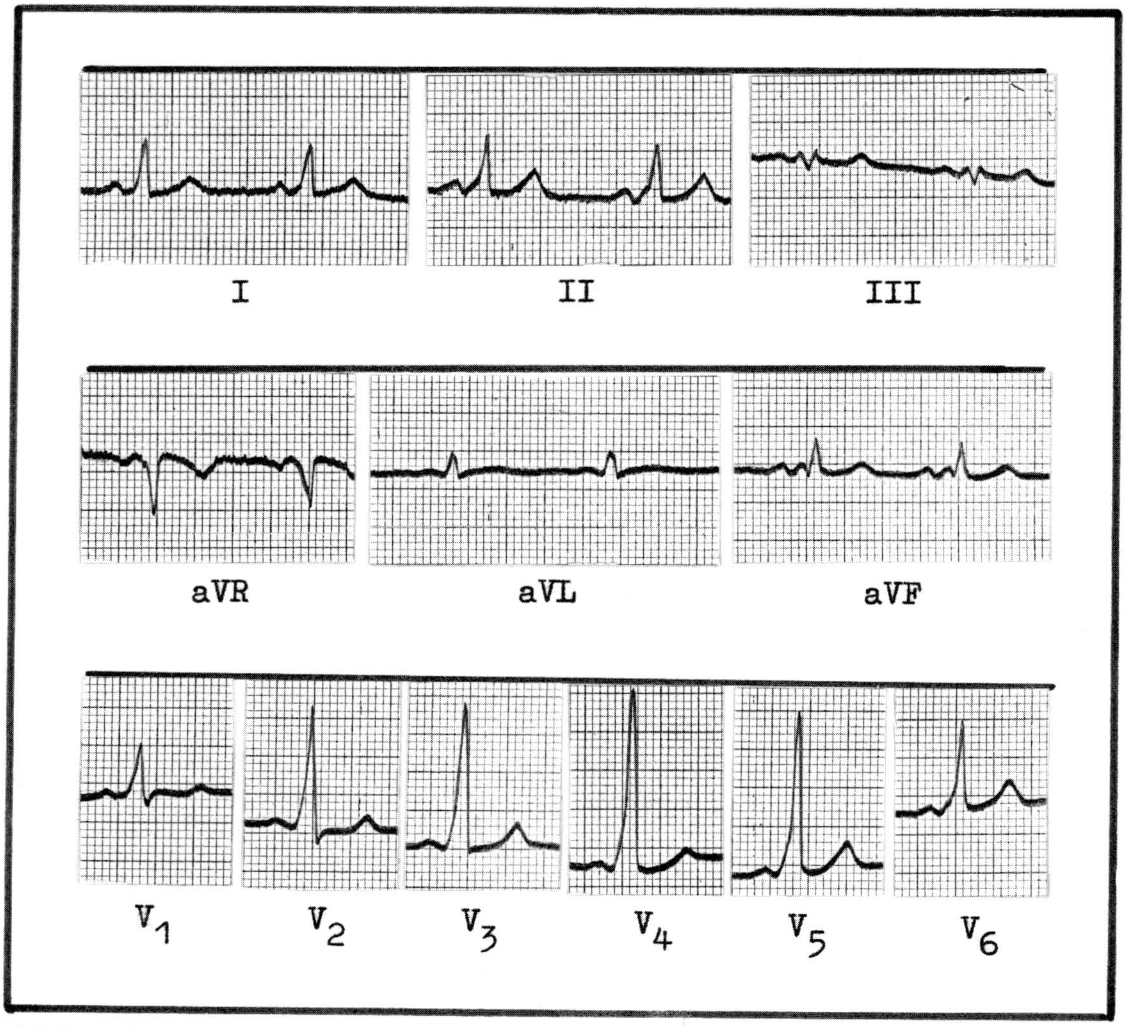

FIGURE 6–42. Wolff-Parkinson-White syndrome, type A. Note that all the precordial complexes are upright. Describe the typical findings in this syndrome.

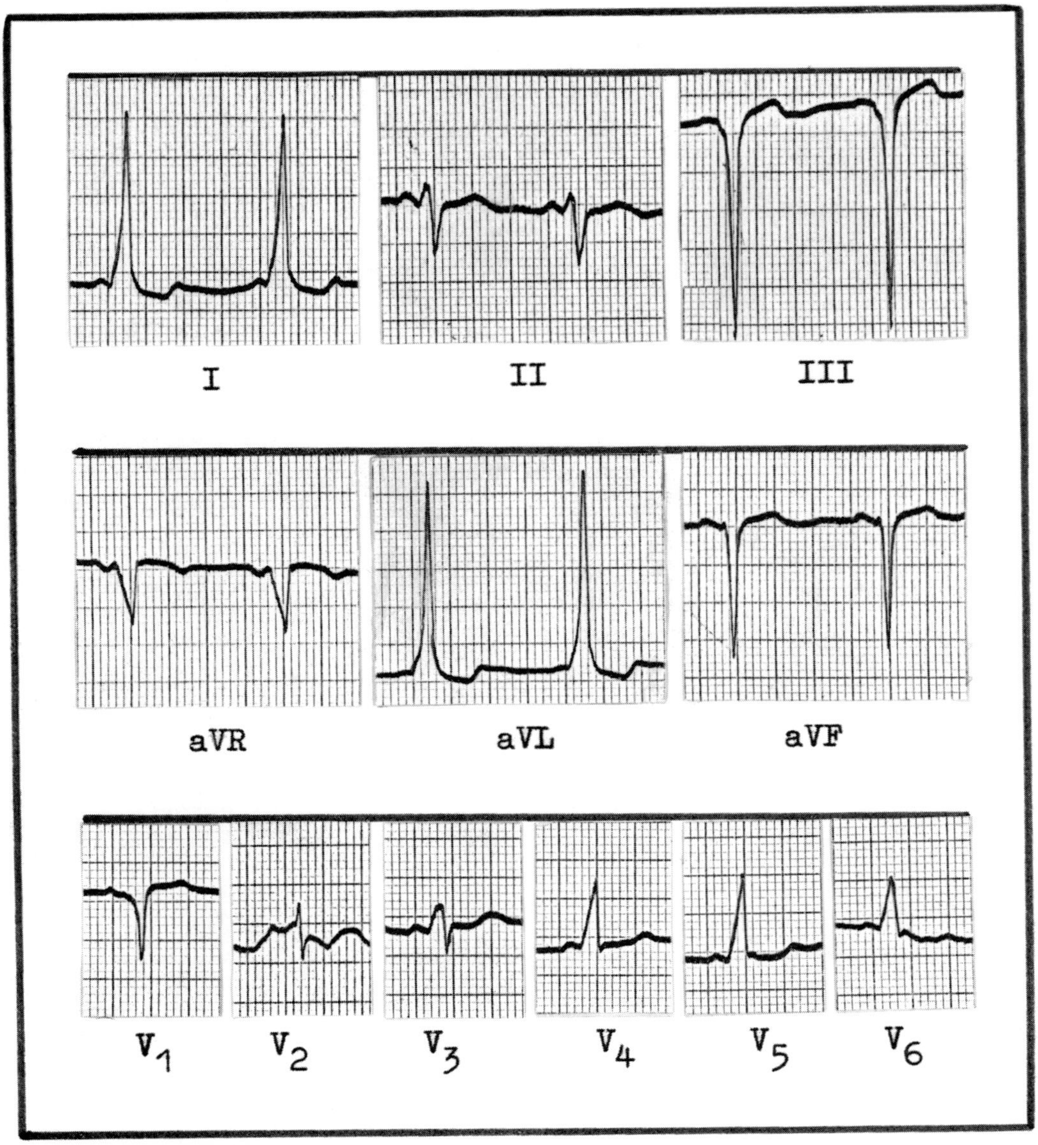

FIGURE 6–43. Wolff-Parkinson-White syndrome, type B. Note that the QRS complex in lead V_1 is negative, in contrast to the electrocardiogram in Figure 6–42.

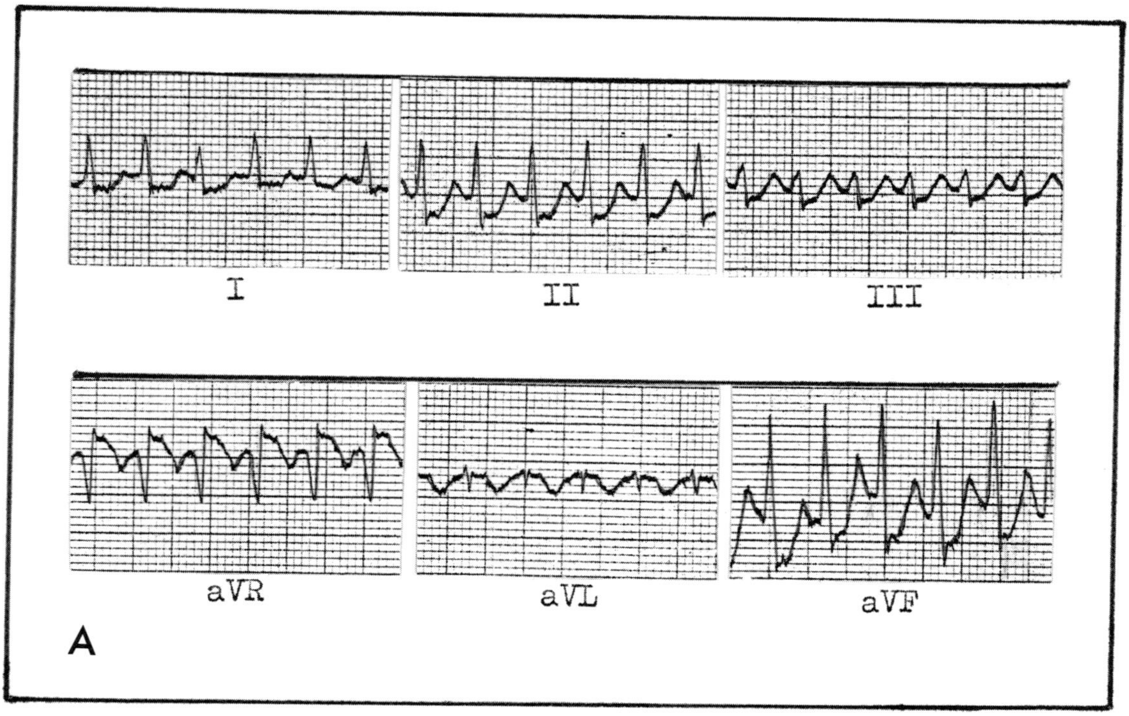

FIGURE 6–44. *A,* Electrocardiogram of an 18 year old patient who came to emergency room because of rapid heart action. Diagnosis?

Illustration continued on opposite page.

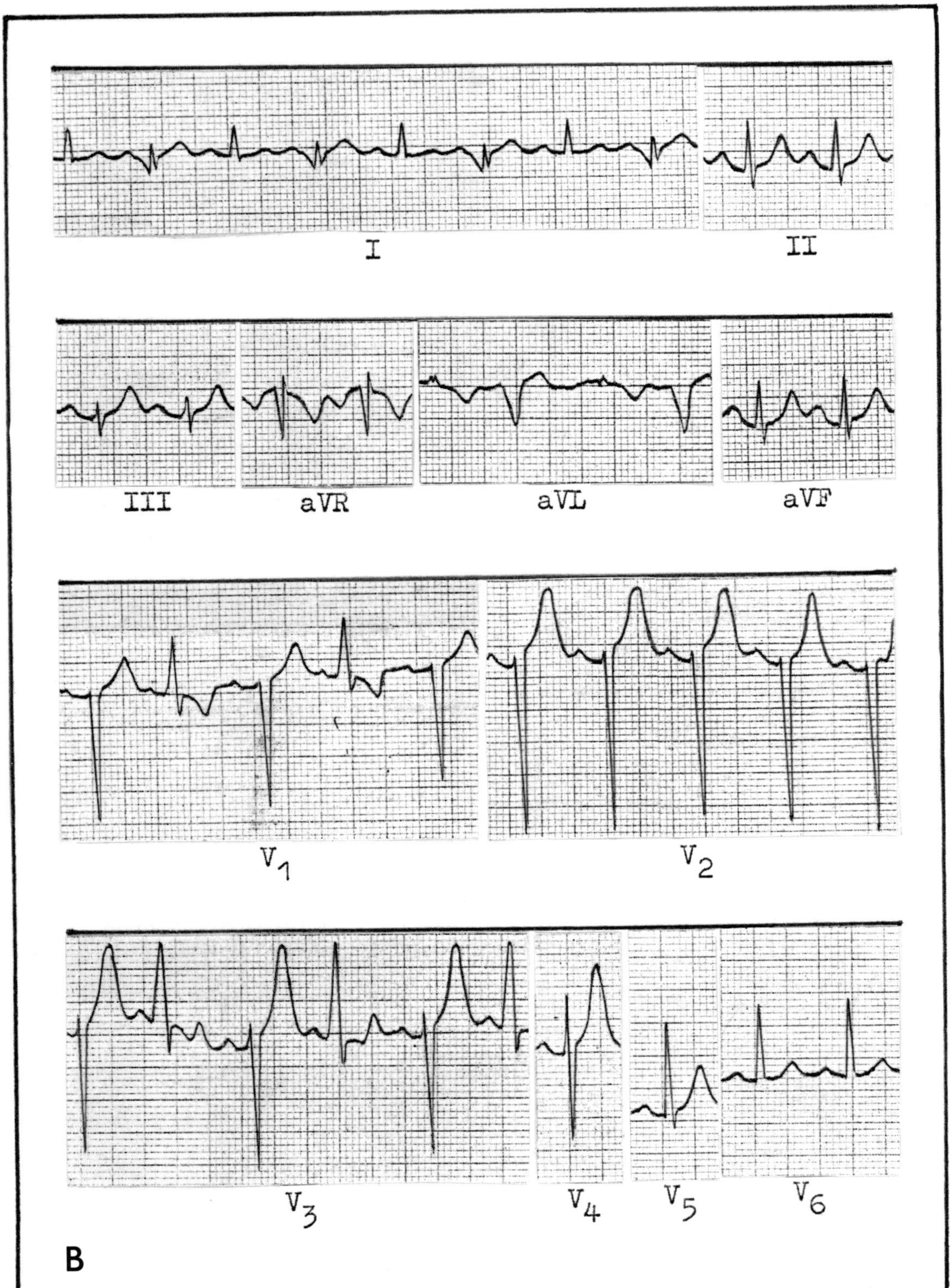

FIGURE 6–44 *Continued.* *B,* After cardioversion: same patient as in Figure 6–44*A*. What are the "aberrant" beats? premature atrial contractions? premature ventricular contractions?

Illustration continued on following page.

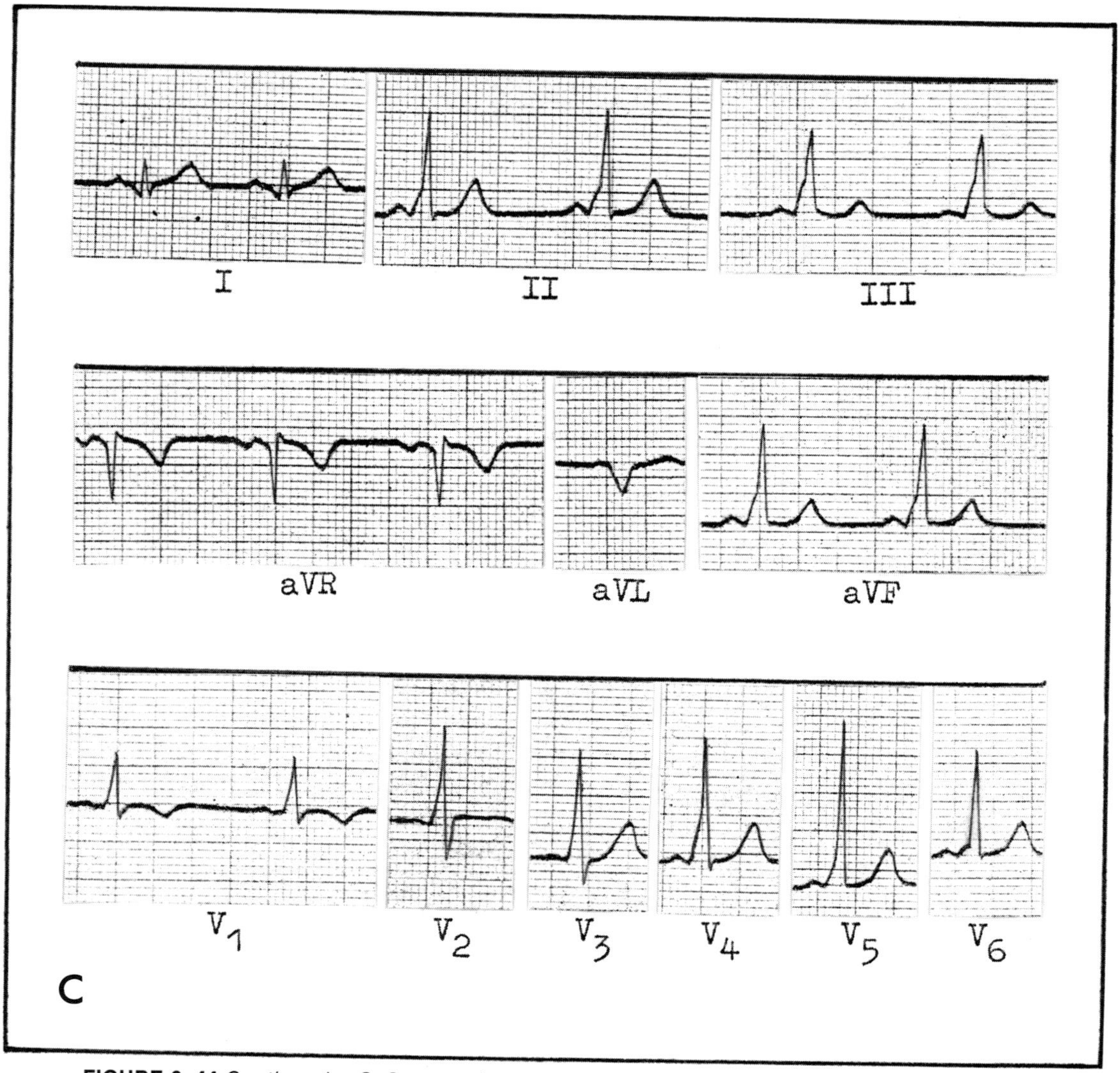

FIGURE 6–44 *Continued.* *C,* Same patient as in Figure 6–44*A* and 6–44*B* (W-P-W, Type A).

The patient presented with a heart rate of 200 beats per minute (Fig. 6–44 *A*). Even an 18 year old patient may be quite symptomatic at this heart rate. Following cardioversion the W-P-W syndrome became apparent intermittently (Fig. 6–44*B*). On the following day (Fig. 6–44*C*) we see W-P-W syndrome, type A.

Did you correctly diagnose electrocardiograms in Figure 6–44 *A* and *B*?

As you continue with electrocardiography you will encounter additional ventricular conduction disturbances. This is also an area of active research, both anatomically and physiologically. Additional fascicular components and derangements will surely be brought to light.

7
ARRHYTHMIAS

Cassette Side 17

ARRHYTHMIAS

A. Sinoatrial (S–A) Node and Atria: Normal Sinus Rhythm
   1. Sinus Arrhythmia
   2. Sinus Tachycardia
   3. Sinus Bradycardia
   4. Wandering Pacemaker
   5. Sinoatrial (S–A) Block
   6. Sinus Arrest
   7. Escape Beats and Escape Rhythms
   8. The Short P–R Interval and W–P–W Syndromes
   9. Coronary Sinus Rhythm
   10. Premature Atrial Contractions
   11. Paroxysmal Atrial Tachycardia (PAT)
   12. Atrial Flutter
   13. Atrial Fibrillation

B. Atrioventricular (A–V) Node
   1. Upper Nodal Rhythm
   2. Middle Nodal Rhythm
   3. Lower Nodal Rhythm

   His Bundle Studies

C. Ventricles
   1. Idioventricular Rhythm
   2. Premature Beats of the Ventricle
   3. Ventricular Tachycardia
   4. Ventricular Flutter
   5. Ventricular Fibrillation

D. Atrioventricular (A–V) Conduction Disturbances
   1. First Degree A–V Block
   2. Second Degree A–V Block
   3. Third Degree (Complete) A–V Block

   Pacemaker Therapy

ARRHYTHMIAS

The study of arrhythmias has been of special interest to me and I have always considered this a subject of major importance. All the heartbeat disorders have been under intensive investigation. Proliferation of coronary care units has given great impetus to this study; many arrhythmias arising in the patient with a myocardial infarction may be stopped or prevented entirely. New methods have been developed which help in the interpretation of arrhythmias and facilitate understanding of the underlying electrophysiological principles. Foremost among these has been the technique of His bundle recording for clinical use, which was developed in our laboratory and which represents one of the great advances of the past decade.

It was hard to keep this as one chapter among others in an introductory course of electrocardiography; it would have been much easier to prepare a monograph on arrhythmias. Fully half of the material in the original course was devoted to arrhythmias. I am certain that a cardiologist reviewing this section, as well as others, could recommend a number of additions, especially in the areas of his own research. It was a difficult task to remove this material but it is sincerely hoped that this brief review will stimulate you to study further this most dynamic field. Once the basics in this chapter are known, the other concepts may be easily acquired from works devoted specifically to arrhythmias and by keeping abreast of the current literature.

The arrhythmias will be described in the classical manner. Be ready, however, to revise these concepts as knowledge which may nullify time-honored ideas accumulates. New thoughts have been incorporated where applicable.

The atrioventricular (A–V) conduction system of the heart had been discussed earlier. The impulse originates in the

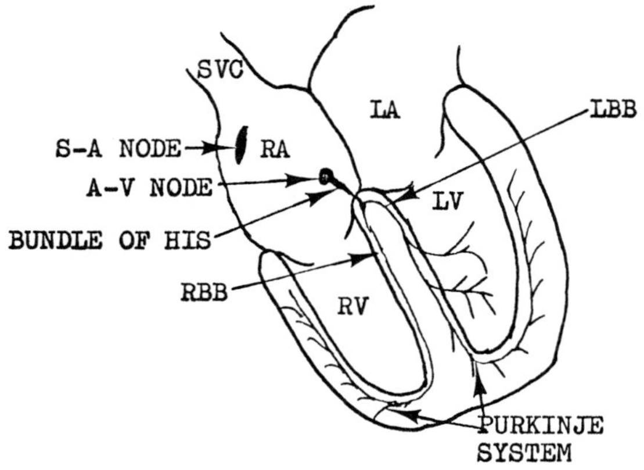

FIGURE 7–1. Conduction system of the heart. Abbreviations are as follows:

SVC	Superior vena cava
RA	Right atrium
LA	Left atrium
RV	Right ventricle
LV	Left ventricle
S–A	Sinoatrial (node)
A–V	Atrioventricular (node)
RBB	Right bundle branch
LBB	Left bundle branch

sinoatrial (S–A) node, spreads to the atria, then to the atrioventricular (A–V) node, and on to the bundle of His, bundle branches and Purkinje network of the ventricles. In Figure 7–1 the conduction of the heart is diagrammed. Once again emphasis is placed on ease of understanding rather than on absolute anatomic accuracy.

The structure of our study of arrhythmias will be as follows:

A. Sinoatrial (S–A) node and atria.
B. Atrioventricular (A–V) node.
C. Ventricles.
D. Atrioventricular conduction disturbances.

When we order our chapter according to the structure listed in *A, B* and *C,* we are starting from above and working down. Normally the S–A node is the dominant pacemaker, but if anything occurs to the S–A node a lower pacemaker may take over. If anything happens to that pacemaker, a still lower pacemaker may take over, and so on. Although the dominant pacemaker of the heart is the S–A node, under various circumstances and stimuli any part of the specialized conduction system or myocardial tissue may become the dominant pacemaker. There may even be two or more pacemakers propagating impulses at the same time. The S–A node emits from 60 to 100 impulses per minute, the A–V node from 40 to 60 per minute and the lower pacemakers, such as an idioventricular pacemaker, less than 40 per minute.

Text continued on page 343.

A. Sinoatrial (S–A) Node and Atria: Normal Sinus Rhythm

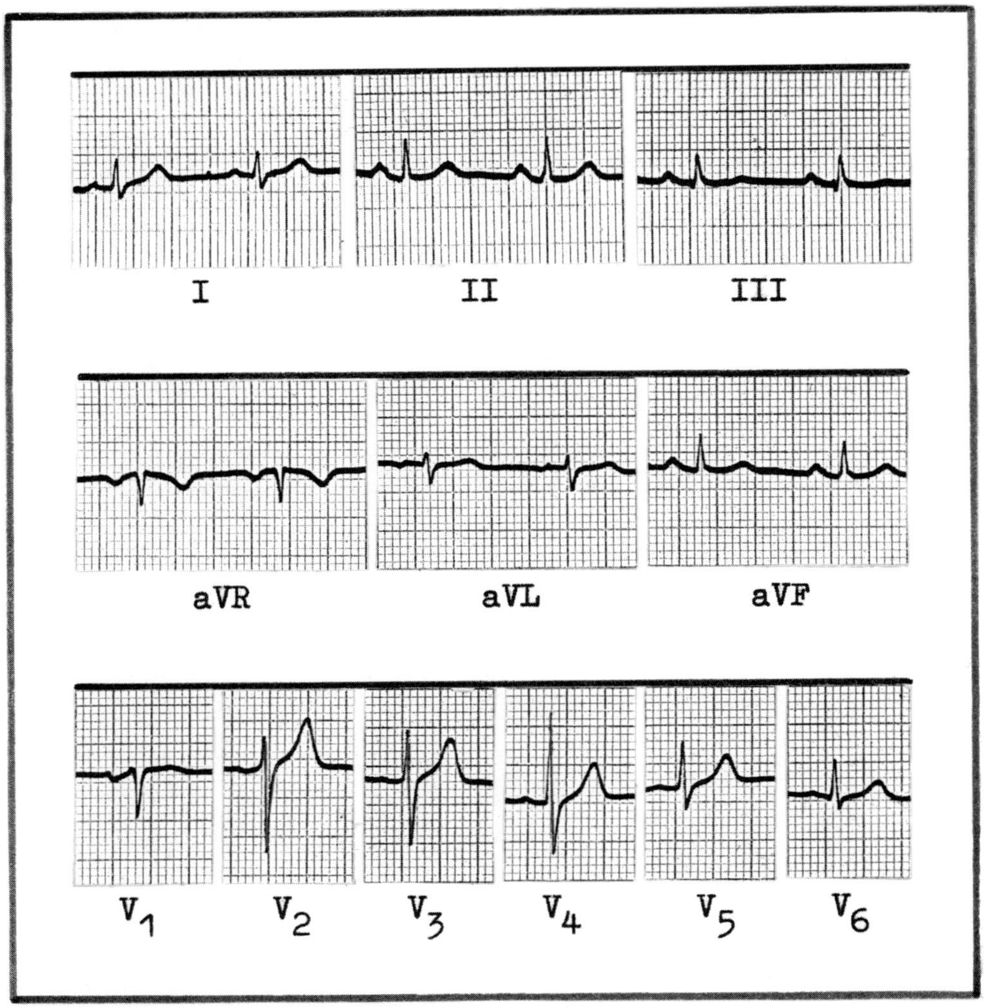

FIGURE 7–2. Normal sinus rhythm. The impulse starts in the S–A node and is propagated normally. The rate is regular, between 60 and 100 beats per minute. The P waves are constant and upright in at least leads I and aVF or I and II. Each P wave is followed by a QRS complex, and each QRS complex is preceded by a P wave. The P–R interval is from 0.12 to 0.2 sec. (3 to 5 small boxes), and constant from beat to beat.

When the word "nodal" is used to describe a rhythm it refers to the A–V node and *not* to the S–A node; "nodal" is never an abbreviation for the S–A node.

Any beat or rhythm originating outside the S–A node is an ectopic beat or rhythm, ectopic in that it does not originate in the normal site.

1. *Sinus Arrhythmia*

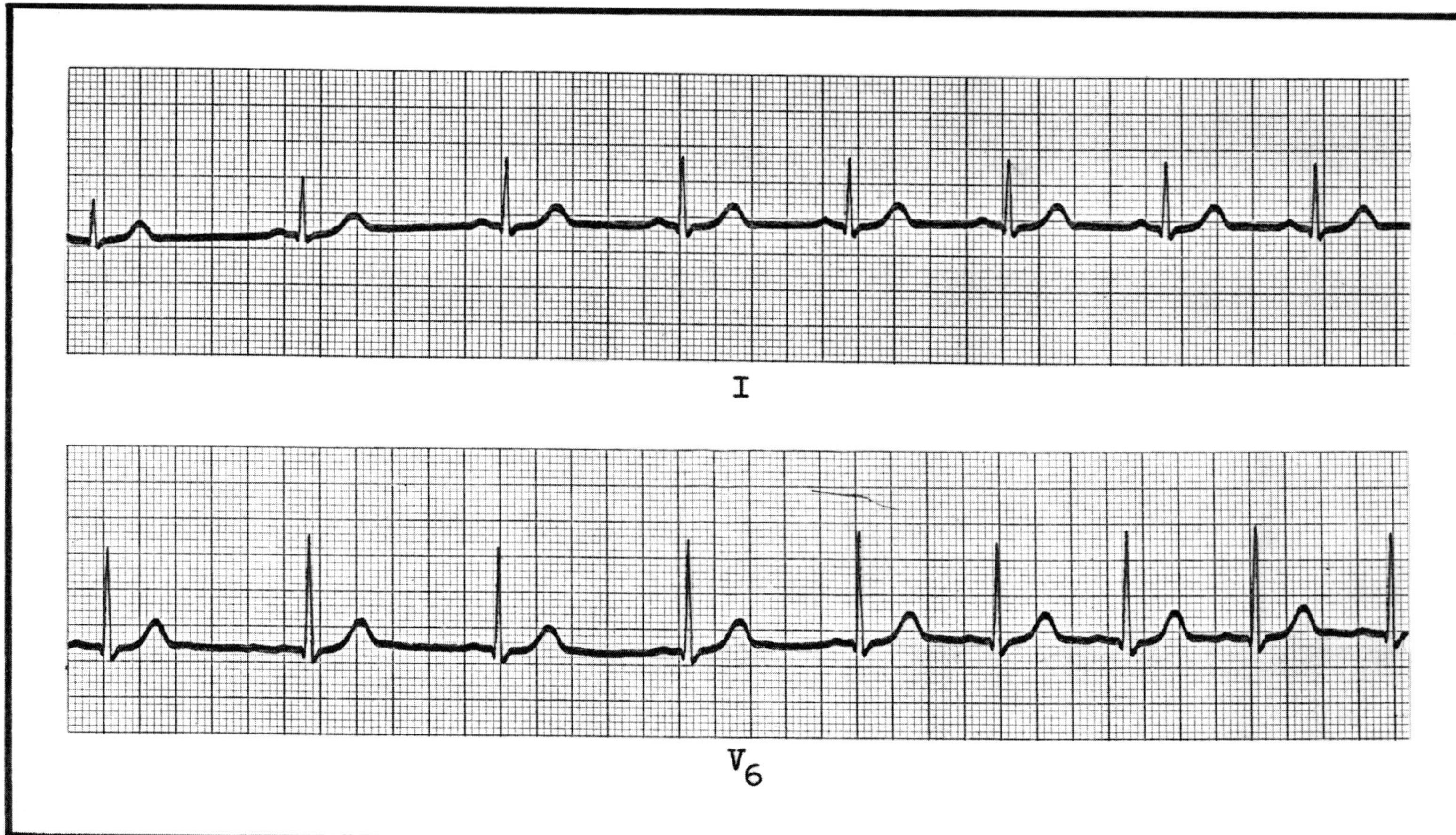

FIGURE 7–3. Sinus arrhythmia. The same characteristics as described under normal sinus rhythm apply, except that there may be marked variation in rate that is often, but not always, associated with the respiratory cycles. It is commonly seen in the young. The P–R intervals are constant but the R–R intervals are continually changing.

2. *Sinus Tachycardia*

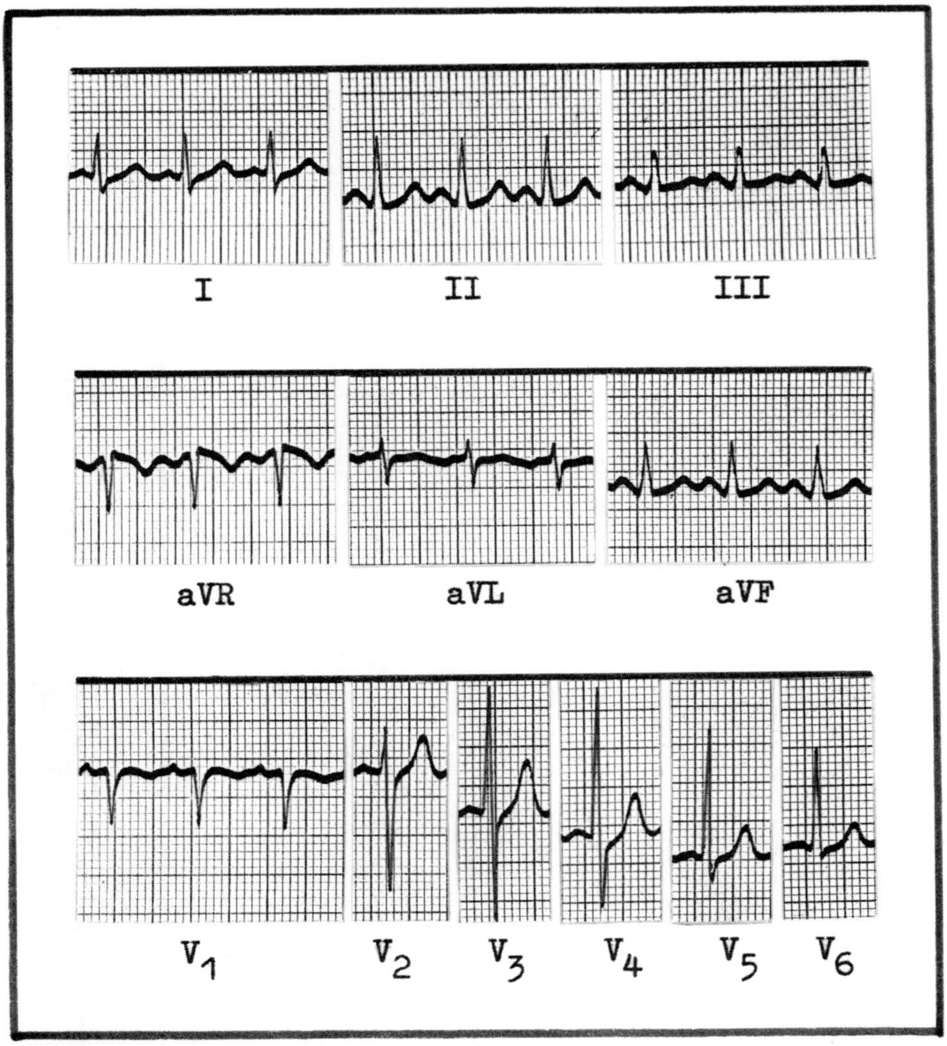

FIGURE 7–4. Sinus tachycardia. As in normal sinus rhythm, except that the rate is greater than 100 beats per minute, usually 100 to 160 beats per minute.

3. *Sinus Bradycardia*

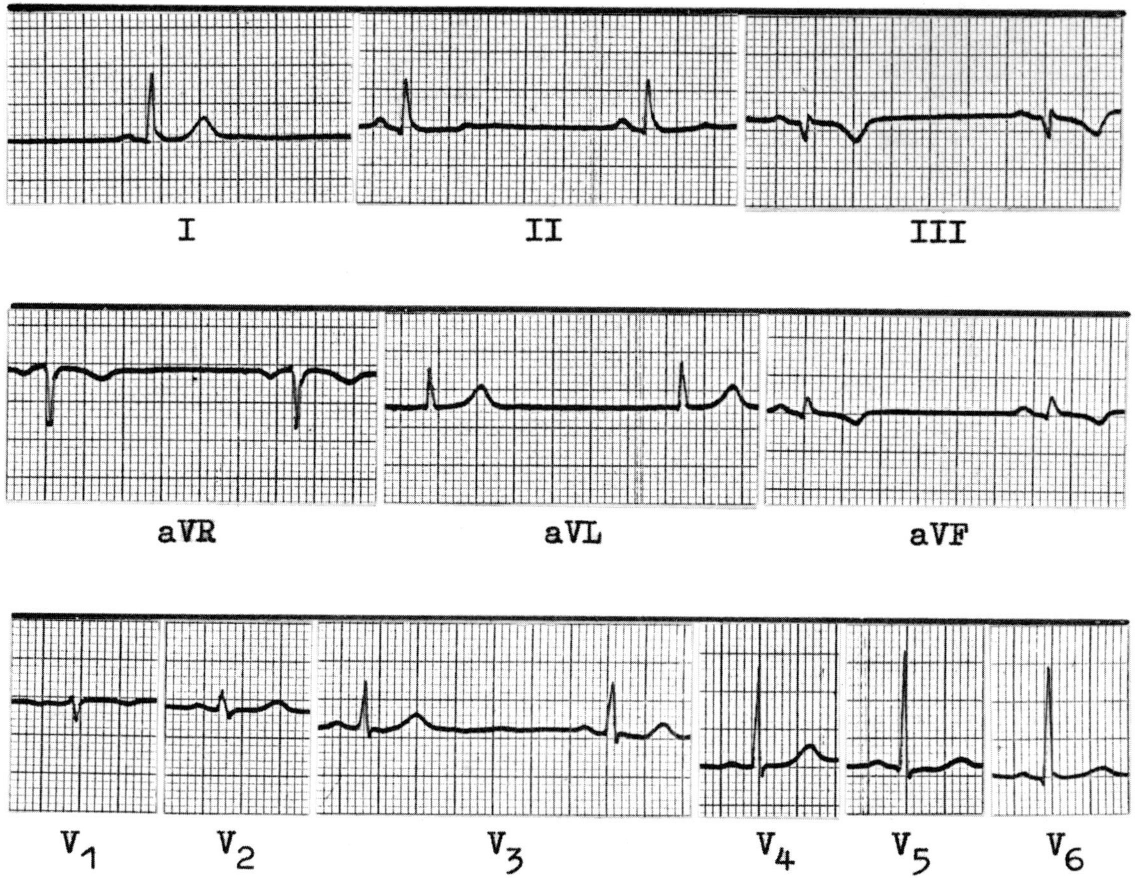

FIGURE 7–5. Sinus bradycardia. As in normal sinus rhythm, except for a rate under 60 beats per minute.

4. *Wandering Pacemaker*

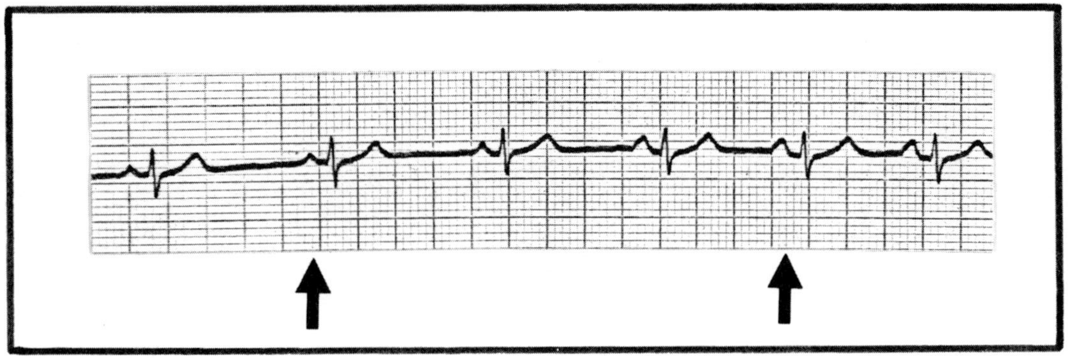

FIGURE 7–6. Wandering pacemaker (S–A node). As under normal sinus rhythm, except for variations in the contour of the P waves (arrows). This may represent a varying origin of the impulse within the S–A node (lead II).

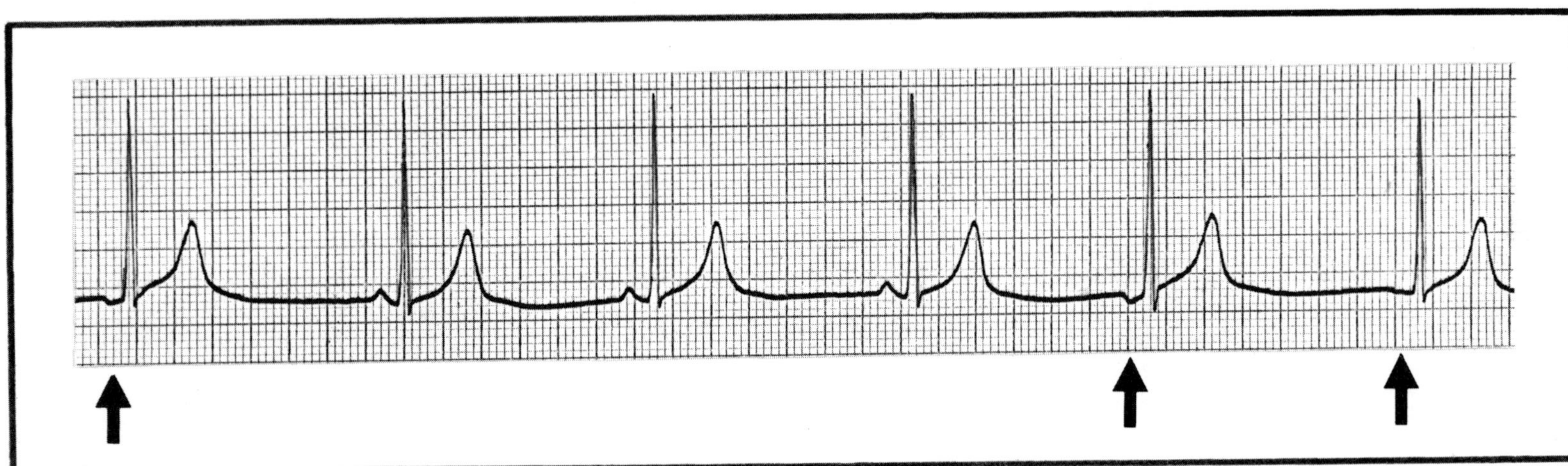

FIGURE 7–7. Wandering pacemaker. Wandering pacemaker is not limited to the S–A node, and may also occur within the A–V node or from the S–A to the A–V node. Note the variation in P wave polarity. The arrows point to the P waves from a *lower* pacemaker.

5. *Sinoatrial (S–A) Block*

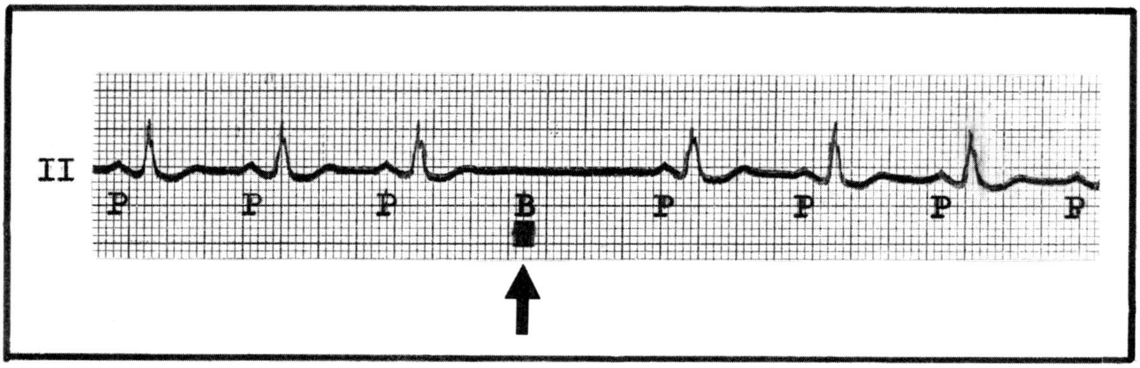

FIGURE 7–8. Sinoatrial (S–A) block. The S–A node is believed to initiate the impulse but the *propagation* is blocked, so that the atria are not depolarized and hence there is no P wave. The pause is a multiple of the regular cycle length. The block, represented by the letter *B* above, is seen where the P wave should normally be. This will again be seen in the study of digitalis.

6. *Sinus Arrest*

7. *Escape Beats and Escape Rhythms*

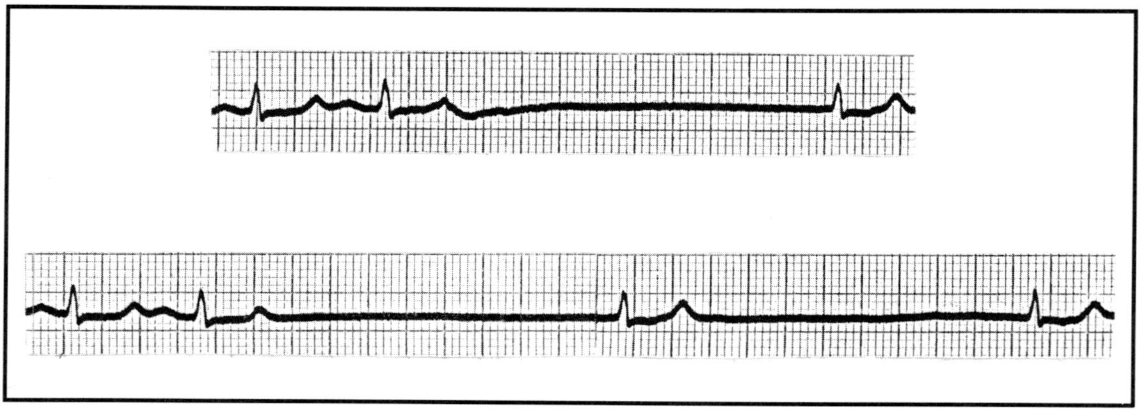

FIGURE 7–9. Sinus arrest with "escape" of lower pacemaker. Sinus arrest is a sudden failure of the S–A node to initiate an expected impulse; it is a failure of impulse *formation,* rather than a failure of impulse *propagation.* If no other pacemaker becomes dominant at this point, death follows quickly. The "escape" beat is usually from a lower pacemaker, as above. When the S–A node fails to initiate an impulse, a lower pacemaker may become dominant. The beat that follows the "arrest" is then called an "escape" beat. If the pacemaker originating the escape beat remains the dominant one, the rhythm may then be called an escape rhythm.

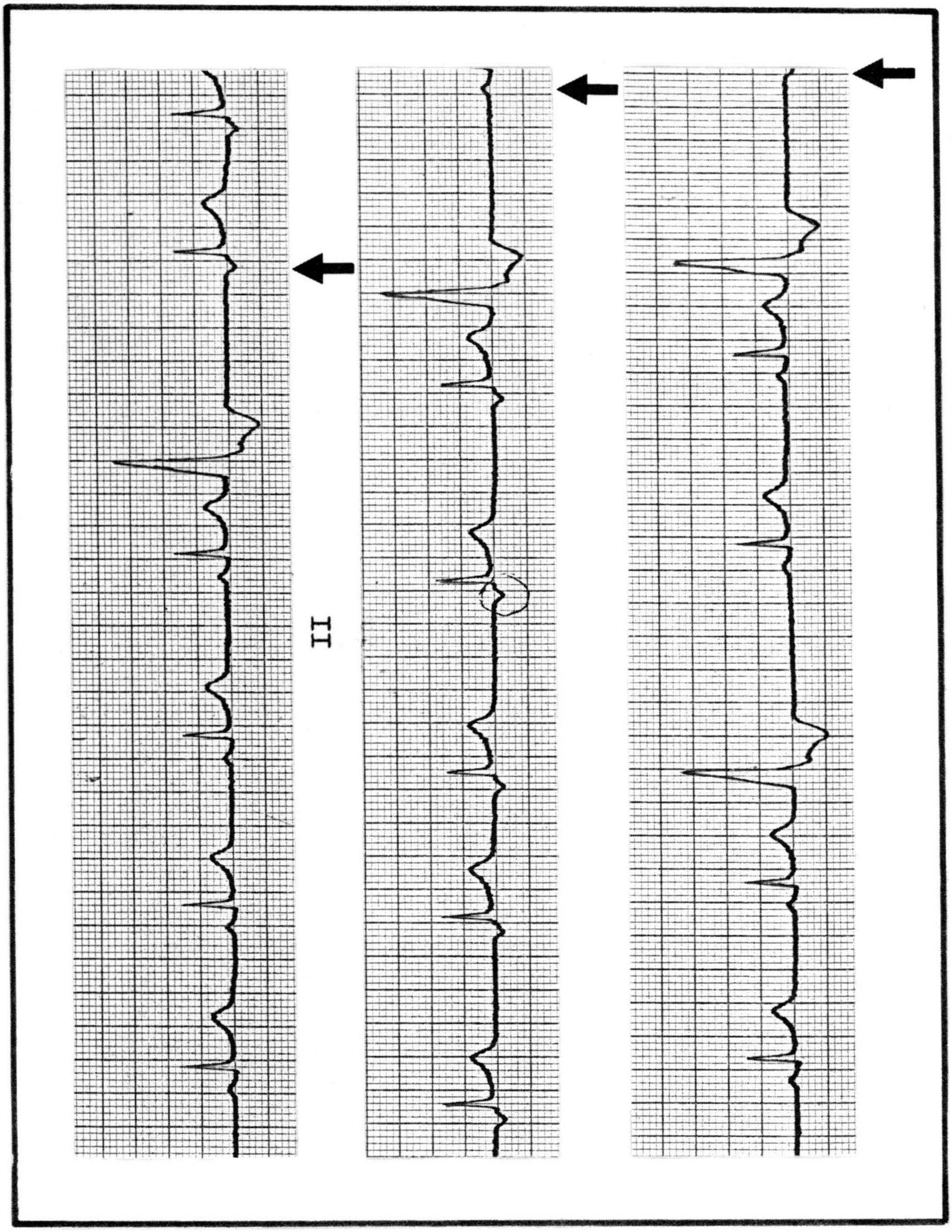

FIGURE 7–10. Note the change in rhythm following interruption of the basic rhythm by premature ventricular contractions (lead II).

8. The Short P–R Interval and W–P–W Syndromes

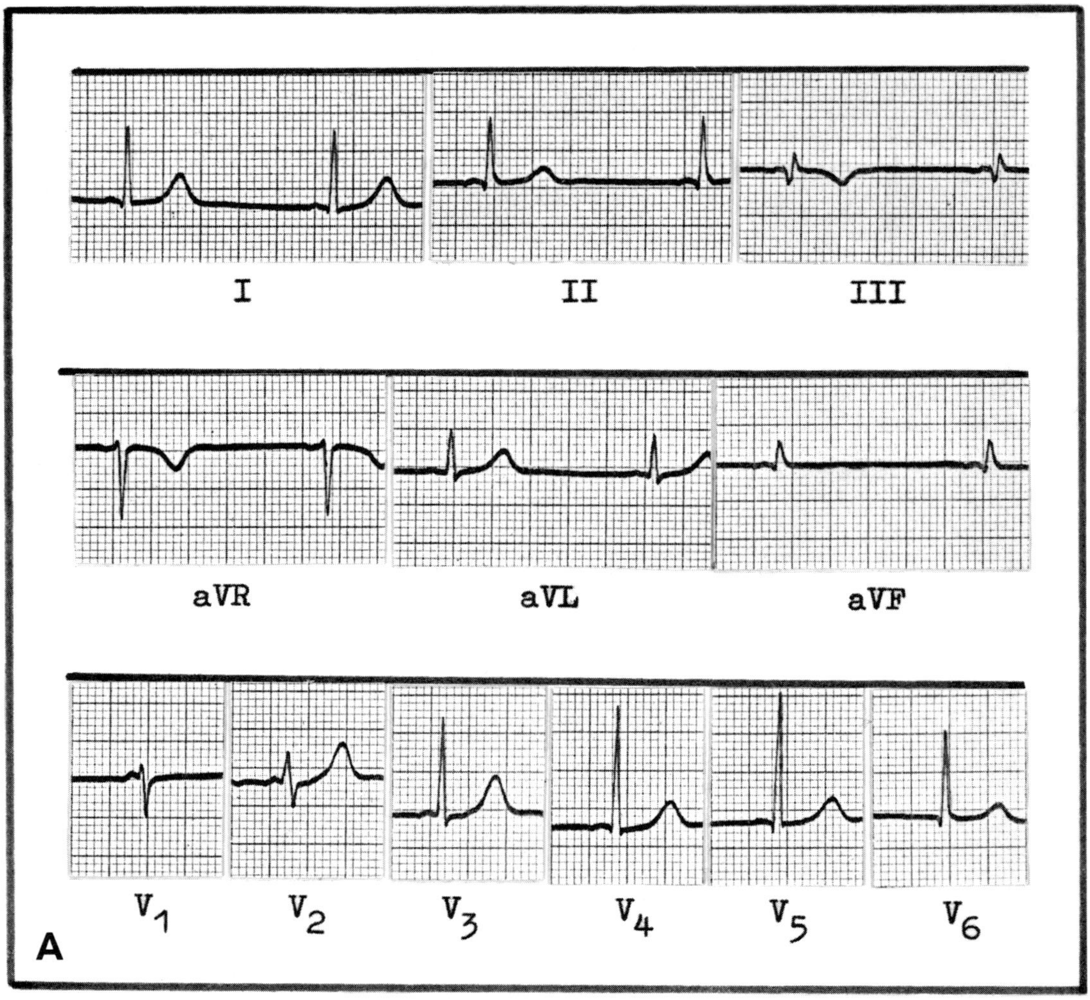

FIGURE 7–11. *A,* The short P–R interval syndrome. The syndrome of the short P–R interval with the normal QRS complex has characteristics of normal sinus rhythm except for the short P–R interval (usually 0.10 sec. or less). The vectorial forces of the P wave are normal, with the P wave upright in leads I, II and aVF. There is no delta wave, as in the W-P-W syndrome (Figure 7–11*B*). Other eponyms have been associated with this syndrome and it is under study today. There may be a complete or incomplete bypass of the A–V node, or rapid conduction through a small A–V node. Some investigators postulate that the impulse originates near the tail of the S–A node, which accounts for the normal mean P vector. Many patients with this type of conduction have experienced paroxysmal tachycardias, hence the inclusion of this syndrome in the arrhythmia chapter.

Illustration continued on opposite page.

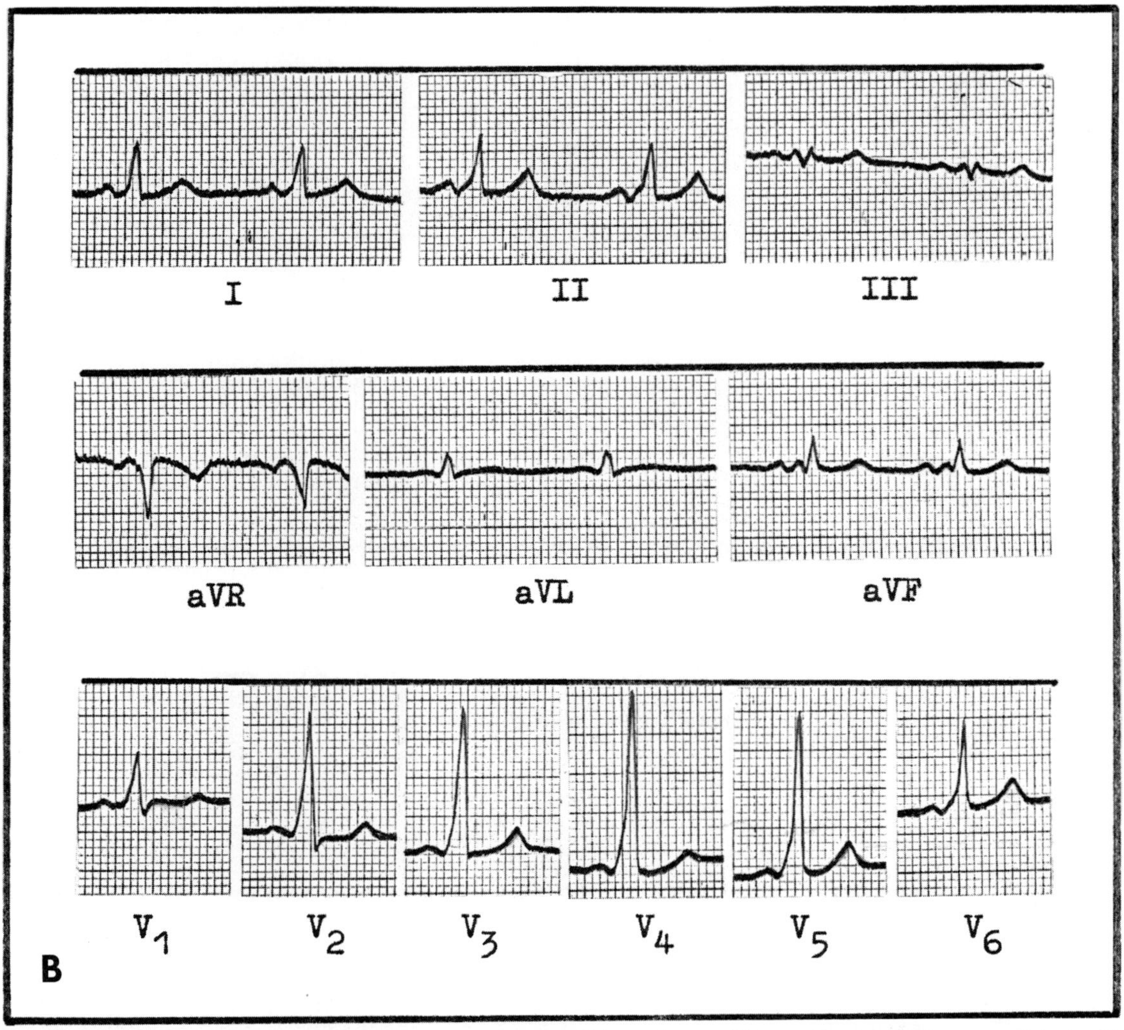

FIGURE 7–11 *Continued.* *B,* Wolff-Parkinson-White (W-P-W) syndrome. This syndrome is often associated with paroxysmal tachycardias (paroxysmal atrial tachycardia, atrial fibrillation and atrial flutter) and should be mentioned in any discussion of arrhythmias. Refer to the chapter on conduction disturbances (Chapter 6) for a fuller discussion of this entity. Is this W-P-W type A or type B?

9. *Coronary Sinus Rhythm*

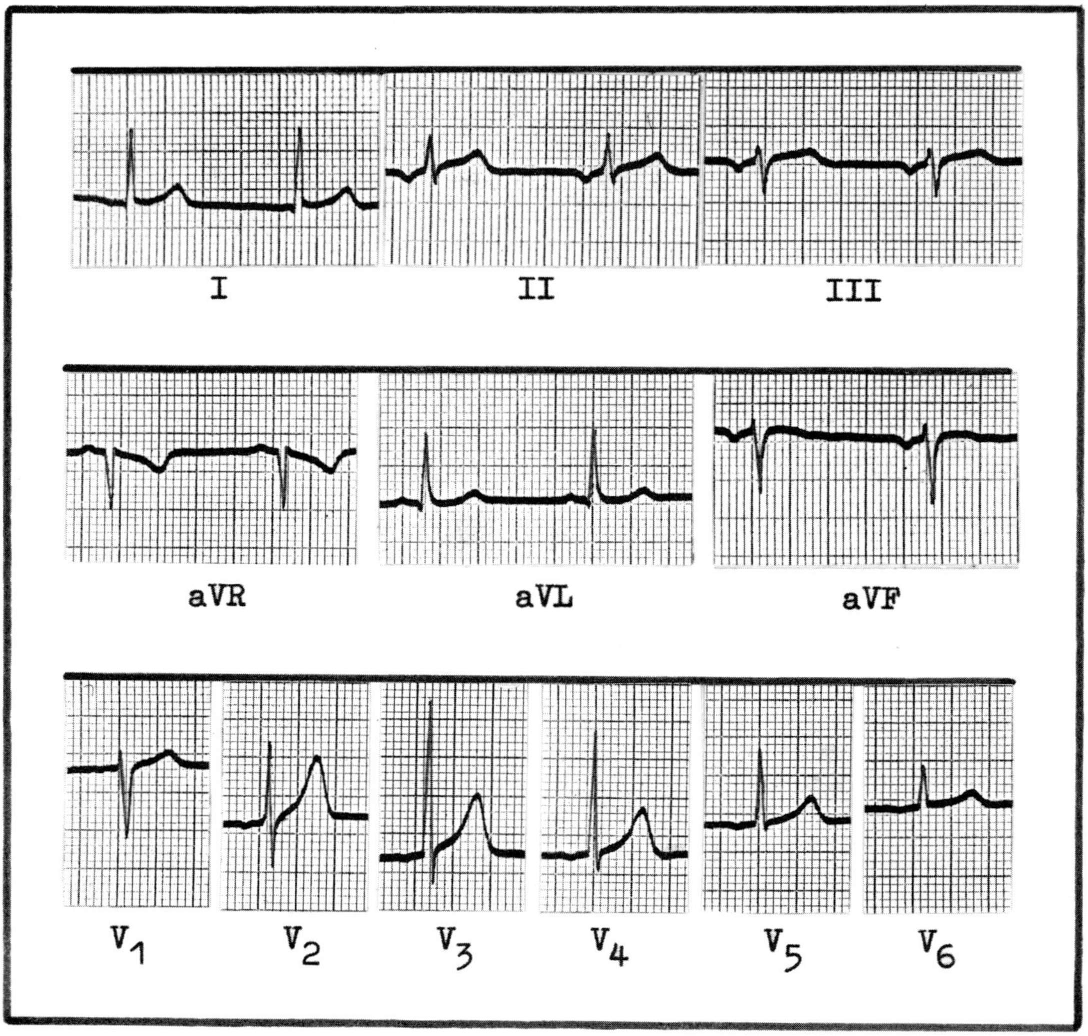

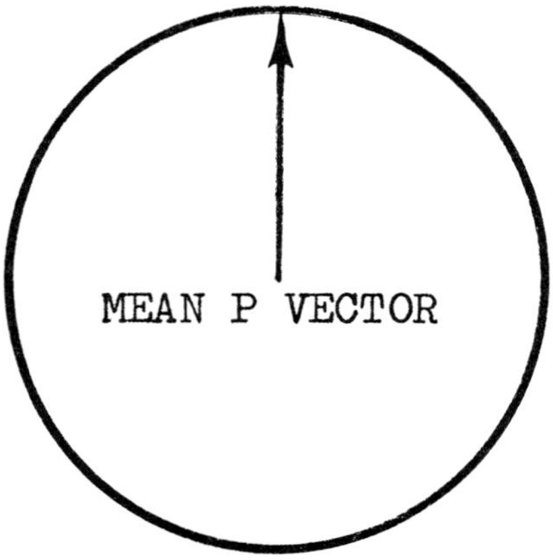

FIGURE 7–12. Coronary sinus rhythm. When the impulse arises from the area of the coronary sinus the atria are activated *retrogradely* and the P waves are usually inverted in leads II and III, with a P–R interval of at least 0.12 sec.

The mean P vector is superiorly oriented.

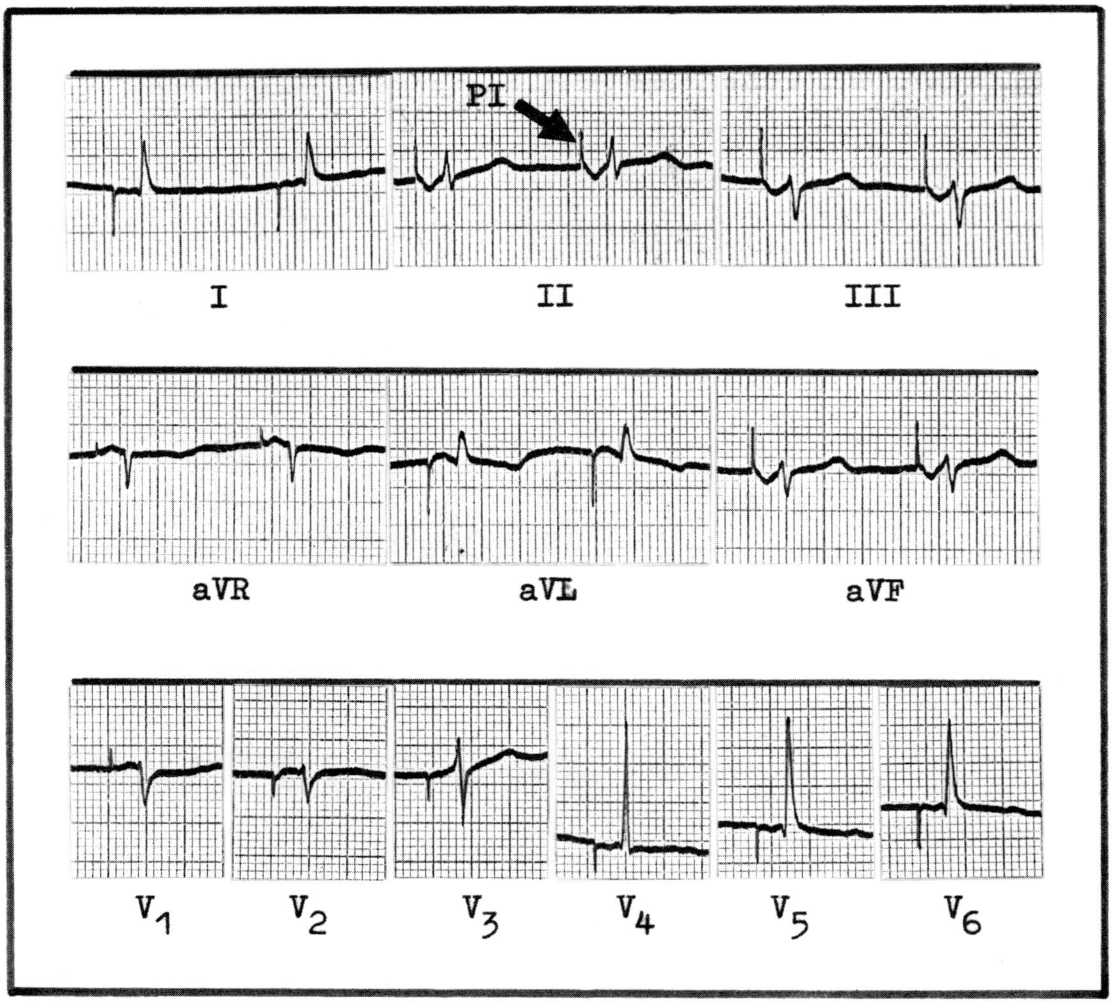

FIGURE 7–13. This electrocardiogram is from a patient who was treated with electrical pacing of the coronary sinus. Note the characteristic mean P vector of coronary sinus rhythm. The narrow deflection preceding each P wave is the pacemaker impulse (labeled PI in lead II).

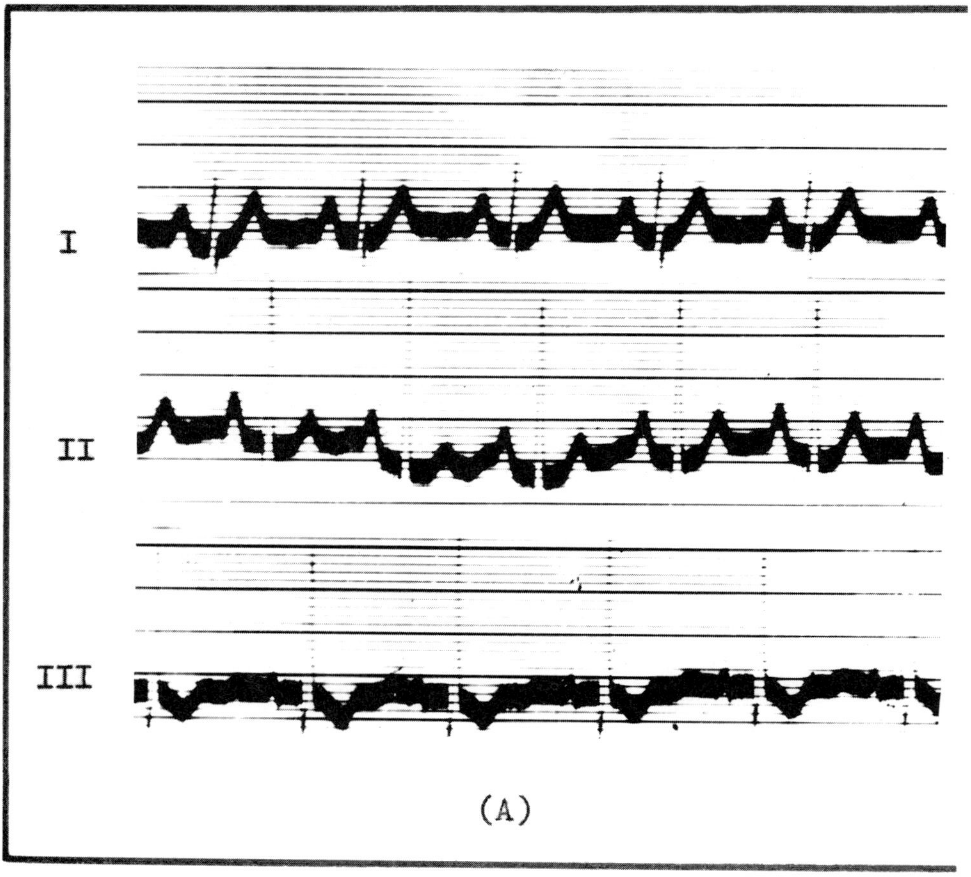

FIGURE 7–14. Onset of *coronary sinus rhythm (B)* in a patient taking digitalis; there is no significant change in heart rate.
(Electrocardiogram enlarged for clarity.)

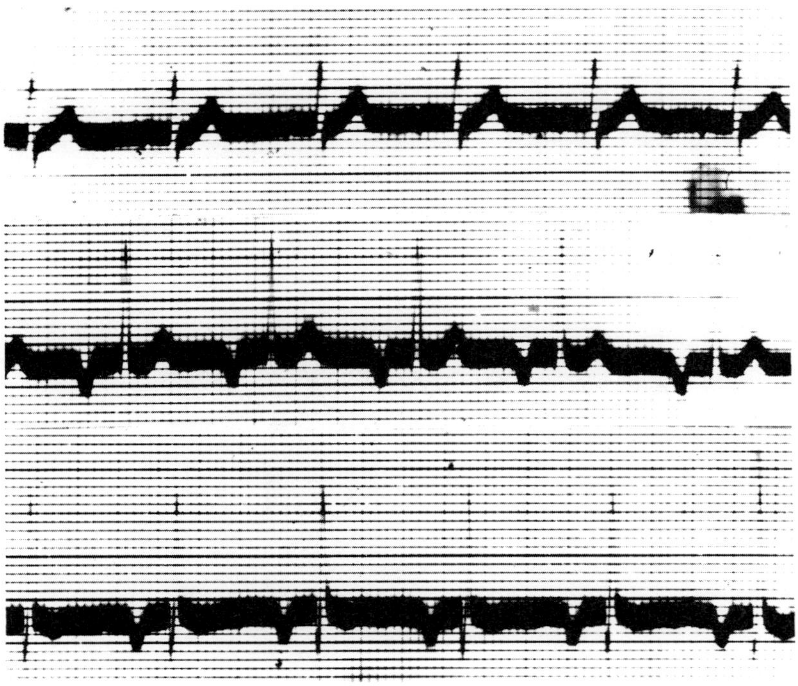

(B)

10. Premature Atrial Contractions

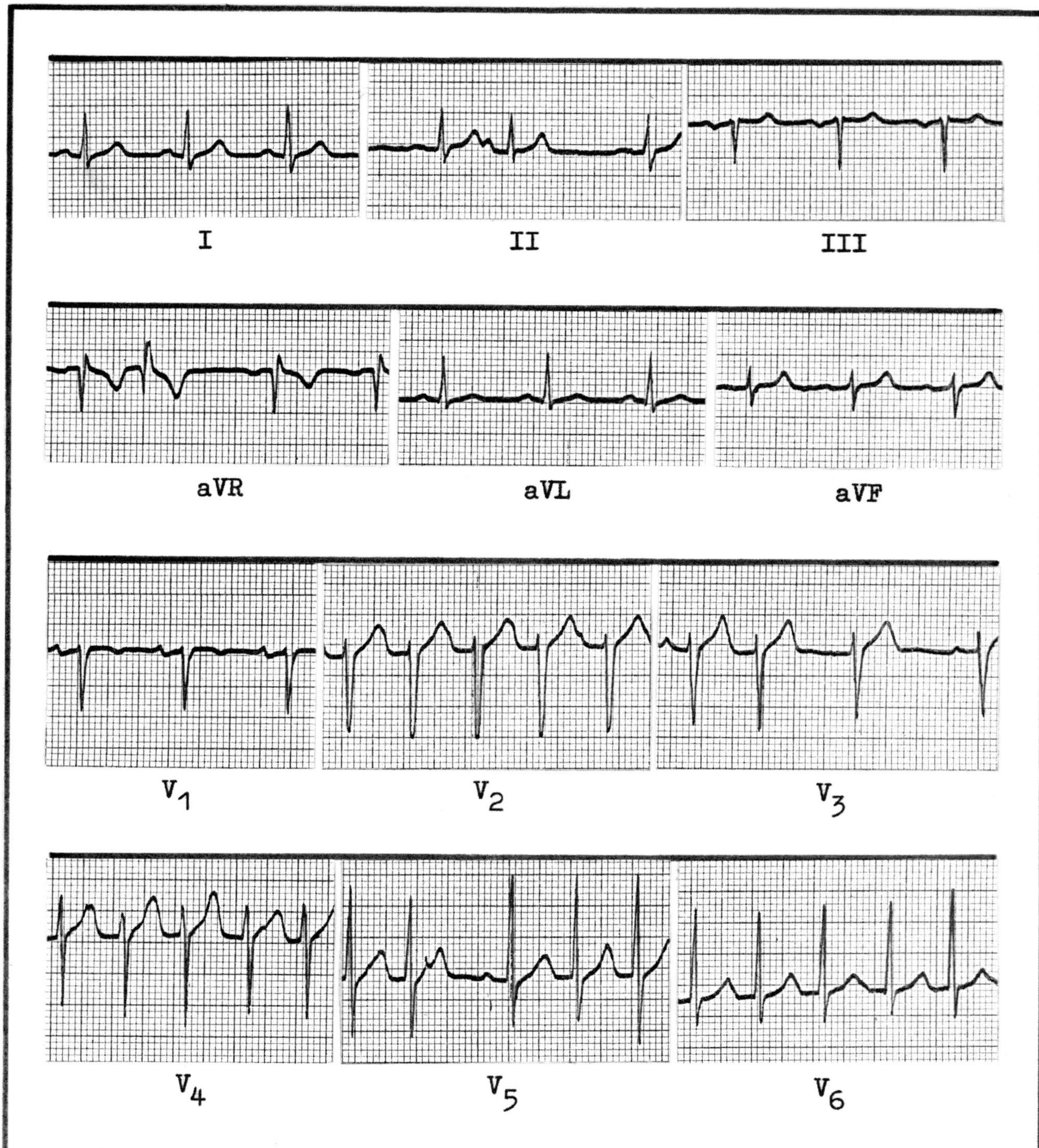

FIGURE 7–15. Premature atrial contractions. Premature beats of the atria are seen when an ectopic atrial pacemaker propagates an impulse before the next normal beat is due. The premature beat may be conducted to the ventricles, as seen in leads II and aVR. The P waves of the premature beat differ from the sinus P waves in contour and probably come from an ectopic atrial pacemaker. In general, following atrial premature beats, the P–R interval may be normal or prolonged, and the QRS complexes may be of normal contour and duration or of changed configuration and prolonged, depending upon the state of refractoriness of the conduction tissue. The premature beats of the atria may herald paroxysms of atrial tachycardia (leads V_2, V_4, V_5 and V_6).

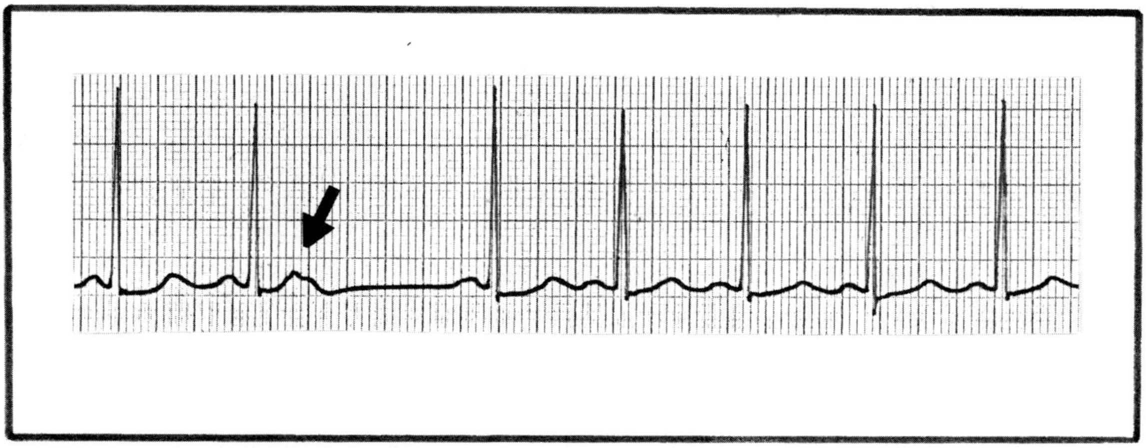

FIGURE 7–16. Blocked atrial premature beats. If the premature beat of the atria does not conduct to the ventricles, it is said to be blocked, and is not followed by a QRS complex. The arrow above points to the blocked atrial premature beat.

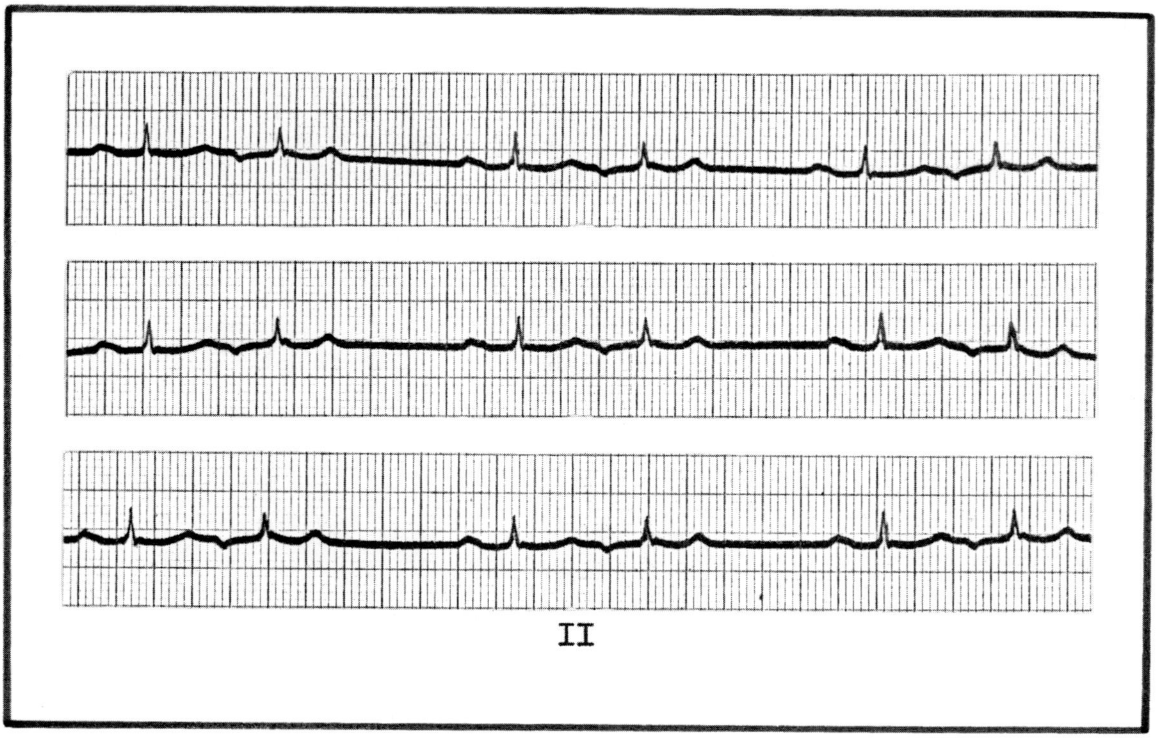

FIGURE 7–17. Bigeminy. Bigeminy refers to heart beats in groups of two. In this case the second beat in each pair is of coronary sinus origin. You must describe what you see since the word "bigeminy" does not give you any clue as to the component parts of each pair.

11. *Paroxysmal Atrial Tachycardia (PAT)*

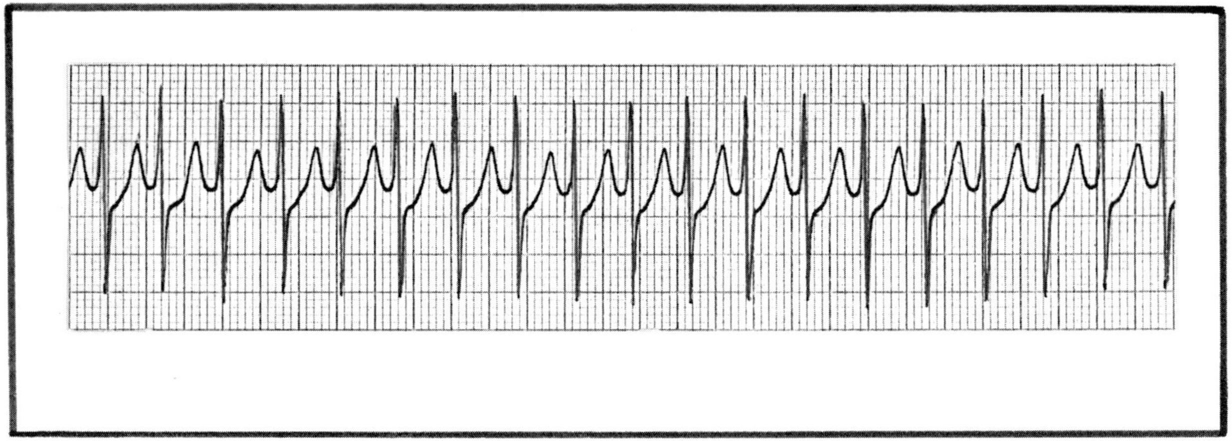

FIGURE 7–18. Paroxysmal atrial tachycardia (PAT). The pacemaker responsible for the premature beats of the atria is capable of becoming the dominant pacemaker, superseding the S–A node and setting up paroxysms of atrial tachycardia. These are usually characterized by a rapid (160 to 250 beats per minute) rate and regular rhythm, sudden in onset, terminating abruptly, and may be followed by a pause. The P waves, when seen, differ from the sinus P waves in contour but are usually upright in leads I and II. When each P wave is followed by a QRS complex (the P waves often are not seen without an esophageal lead or intra-atrial recording) the arrhythmia is called paroxysmal atrial tachycardia with 1:1 conduction (above).

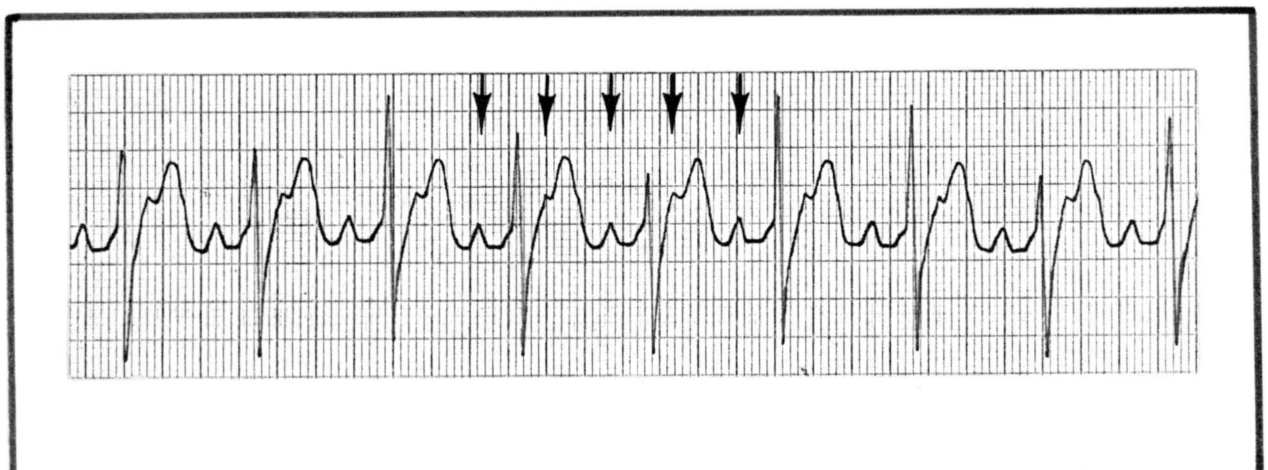

FIGURE 7–19. Paroxysmal atrial tachycardia with 2:1 A–V block is seen with alternate blocked P waves. Arrows point to the P waves.

12. Atrial Flutter

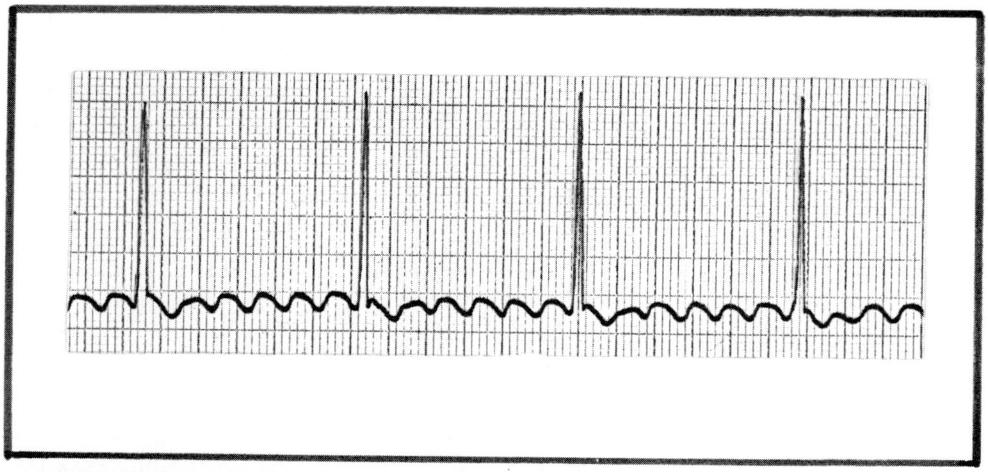

FIGURE 7–20. Atrial flutter. The fluttering atria are represented by the undulating waves, rising and falling to the baseline. There are 6 atrial waves (F or flutter waves) for each QRS complex; hence 6:1 atrial flutter. In each case determine, in the usual manner, the atrial rate and the ventricular rate to set up the ratio. In the present case the atrial rate is 312 per minute and the ventricular rate is approximately 52 per minute. The atrial rate in flutter is frequently 250 to 350 per minute.

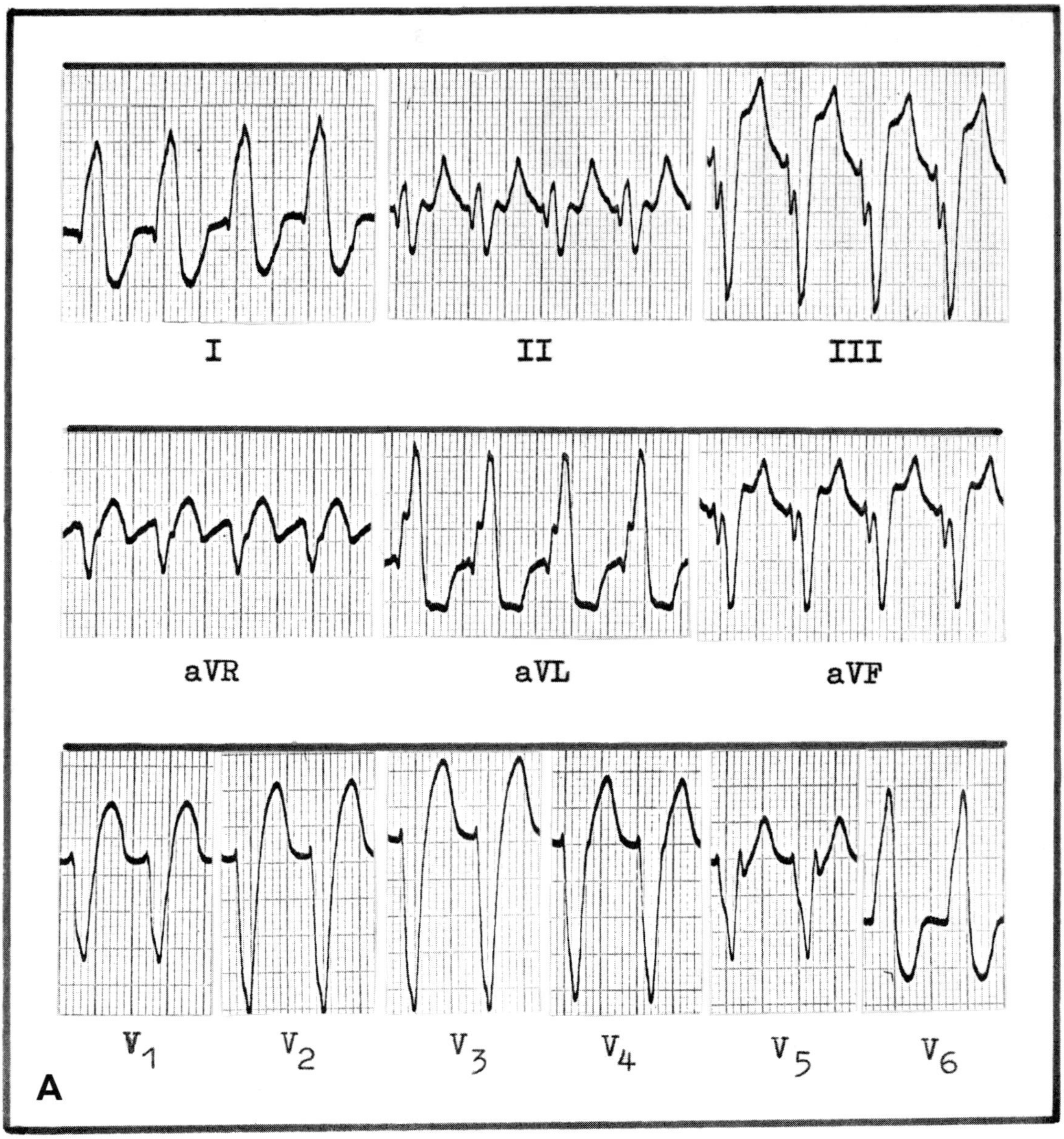

FIGURE 7–21. *A,* The elaboration on the following patient will serve as an example of how difficult an arrhythmia problem may be. A 67 year old man with hypertensive, atherosclerotic heart disease presented with a heart rate of 145 beats per minute and the electrocardiogram above. The ventricular rate was rapid and the QRS complexes wide. What was the underlying rhythm? Was this a ventricular tachycardia or a supraventricular tachycardia with a conduction disturbance? Try to answer these questions before proceeding.

Illustration continued on opposite page.

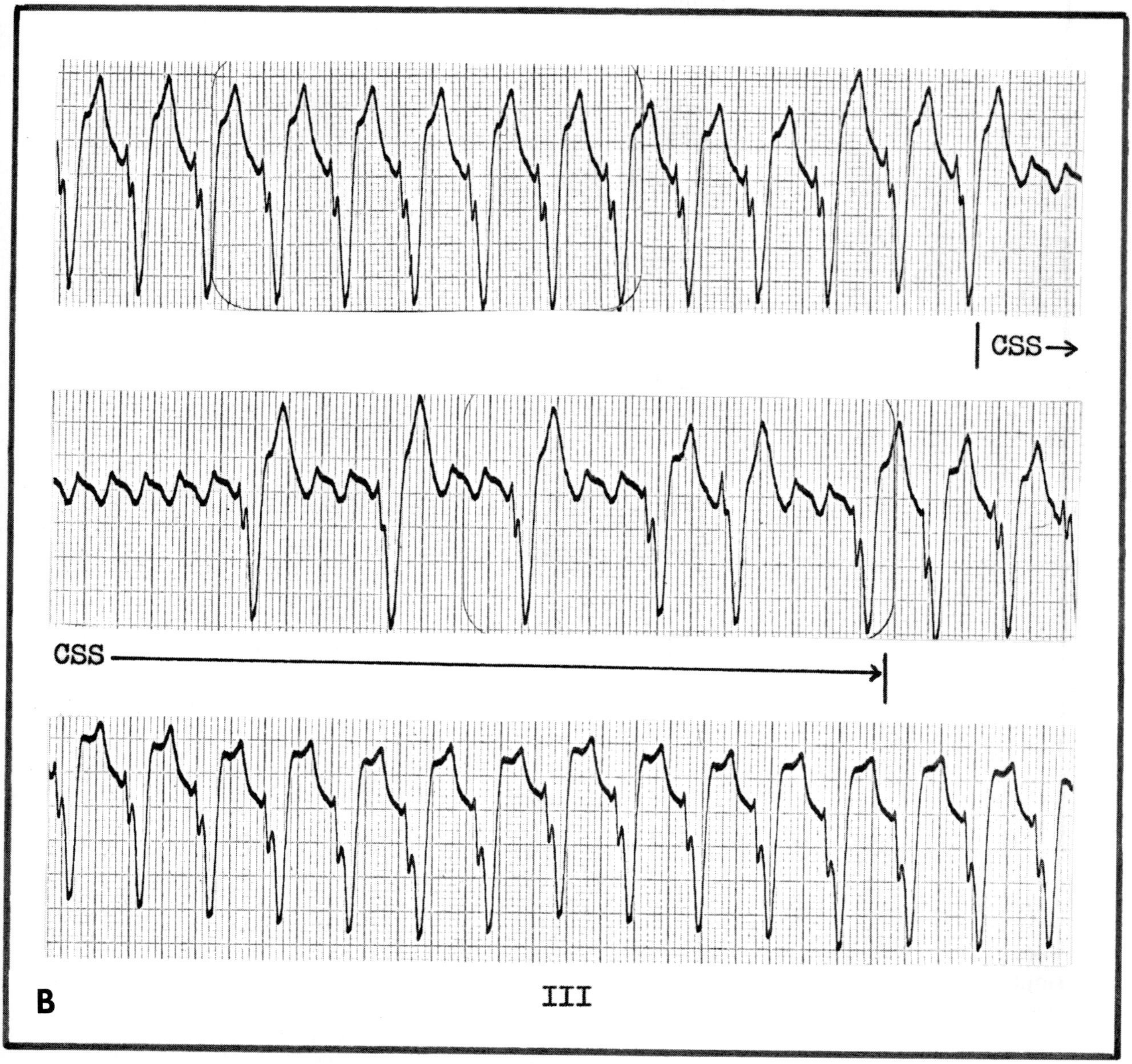

FIGURE 7–21 *Continued.* *B,* Carotid sinus stimulation (CSS above) was used, with caution, and the atrial flutter became evident. The flutter waves have the often described "saw-tooth" appearance.

Illustration continued on following page.

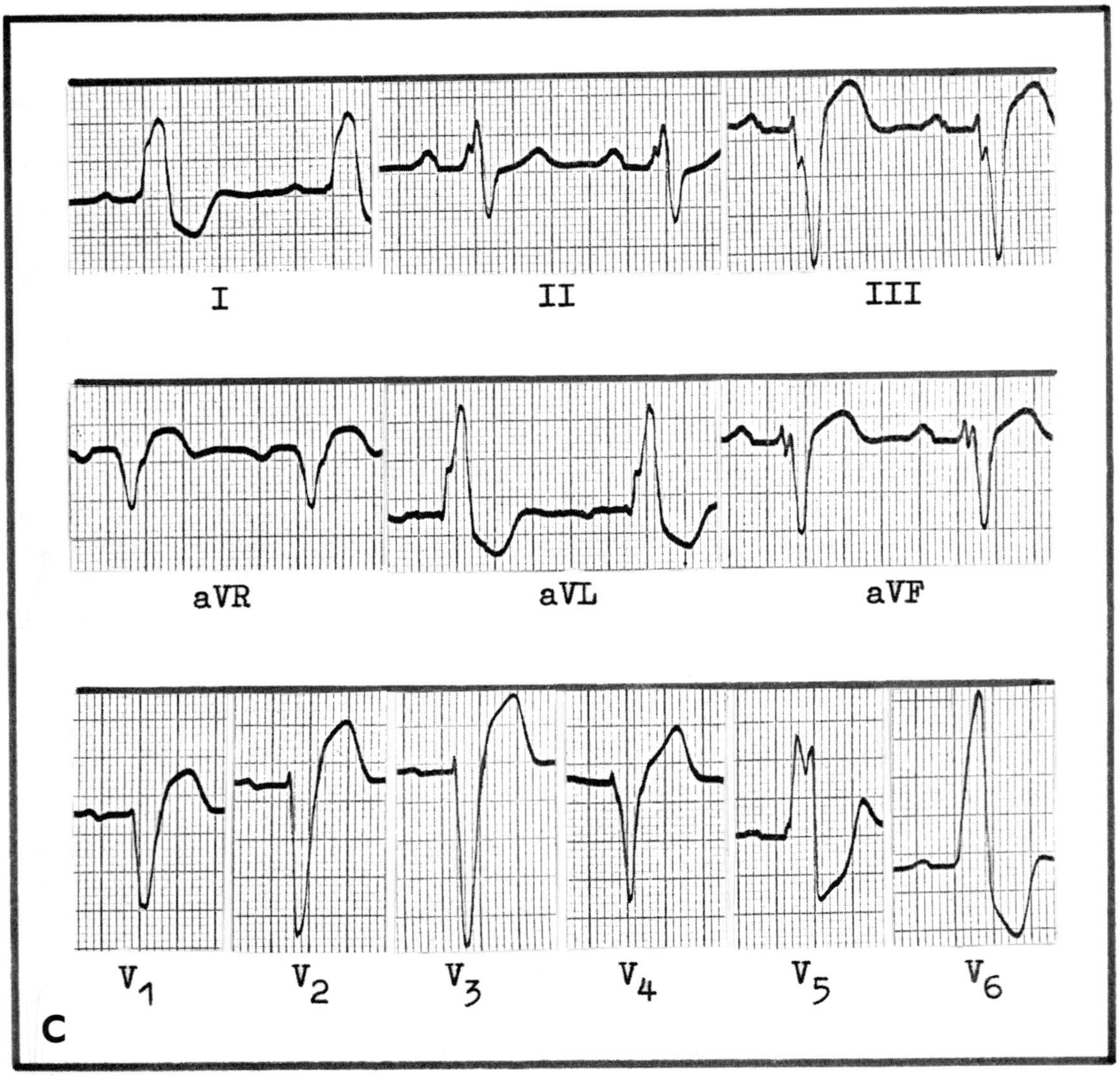

FIGURE 7–21 *Continued.* *C,* After resumption of his previous rhythm it became clear that left bundle branch block was responsible for the wide QRS complexes. Did you answer the questions (in Figure 7–21*A*) correctly?

13. Atrial Fibrillation

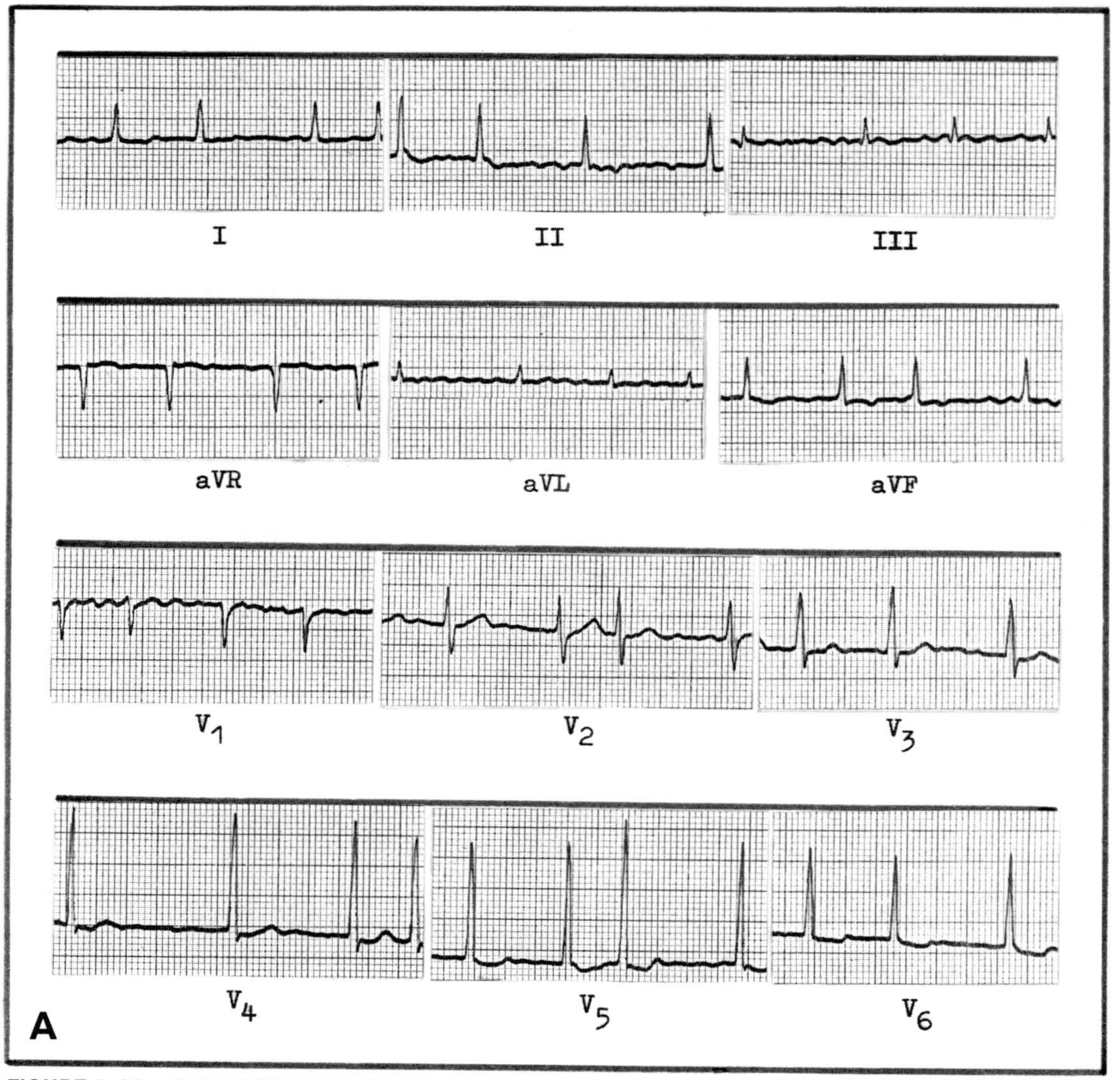

FIGURE 7–22. *A,* Atrial fibrillation. Disorganized, ineffective contractions of the atria (350 to 600 per minute) characterize atrial fibrillation. No P waves are seen, and the ventricular response is irregular depending on how many of the 350 to 600 impulses are conducted to the ventricles. If the atrial rate is 500 per minute and the ventricular rate is 125 per minute, it means that one in every four atrial impulses is conducted, irregularly, to the ventricles.

The discussion from sinus tachycardia (up to 160/minute) to atrial tachycardia (160 to 250/minute) to atrial flutter (250 to 350/minute), to atrial fibrillation (350 to 600/minute) has included rate as a criterion. These classical figures should be considered as guideposts rather than as rigid absolutes, for there is much overlap. It is beyond our scope to discuss the interesting theories as to mechanisms behind these entities, but again it is hoped that your interest will be stimulated to continue your study.

(Electrocardiogram reduced in size.)

Illustration continued on following page.

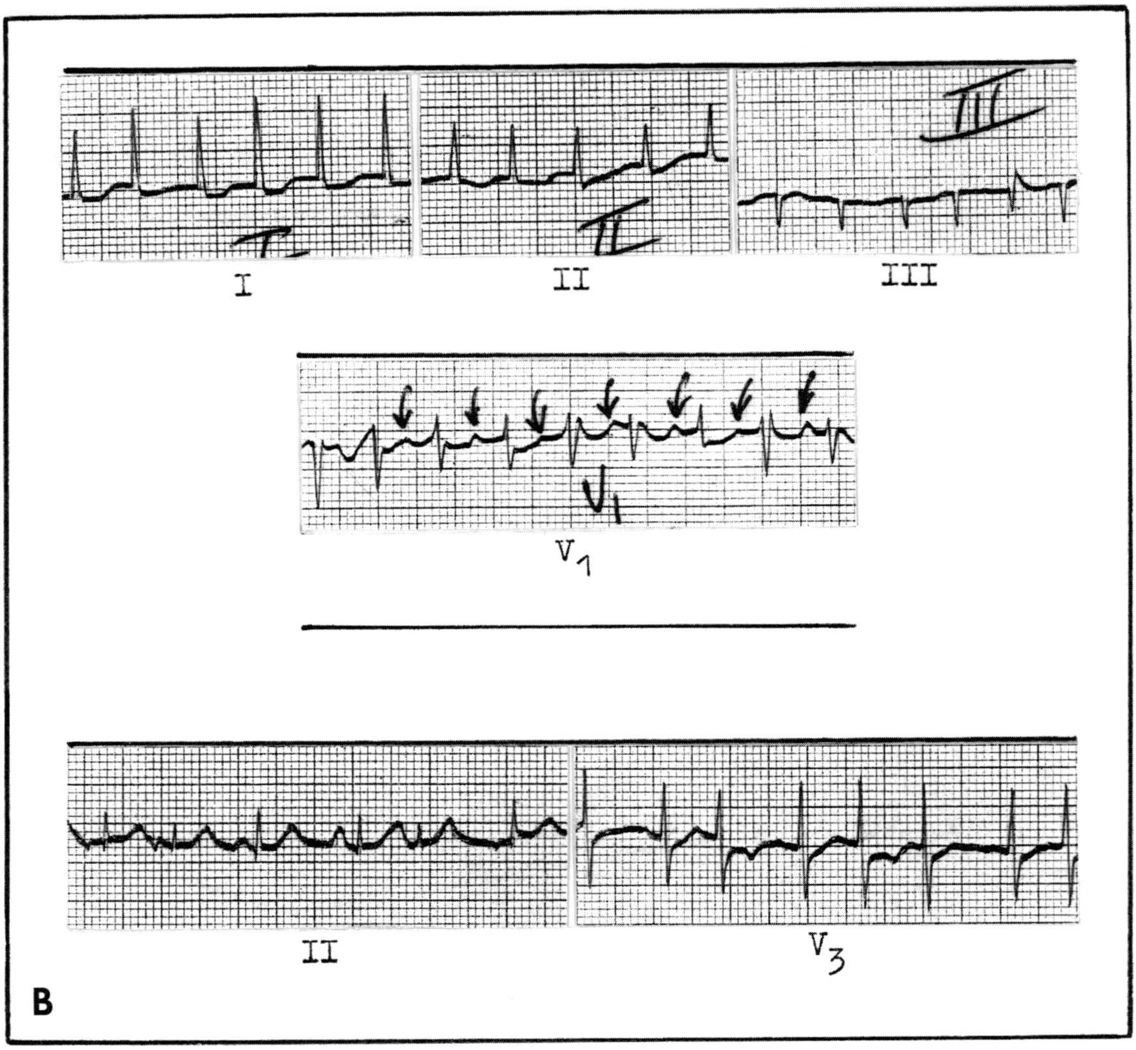

FIGURE 7–22 *Continued.* *B,* Two patients with multifocal (chaotic) atrial tachycardia. Leads I, II and III in the first patient and lead V_3 in the second patient, at a quick glance, might appear to be examples of atrial fibrillation. Leads V_1 and II, respectively, show that the rhythm is *not* atrial fibrillation. This rhythm is frequently found in patients with chronic obstructive pulmonary disease with hypoxia.
(Electrocardiogram reduced in size.)

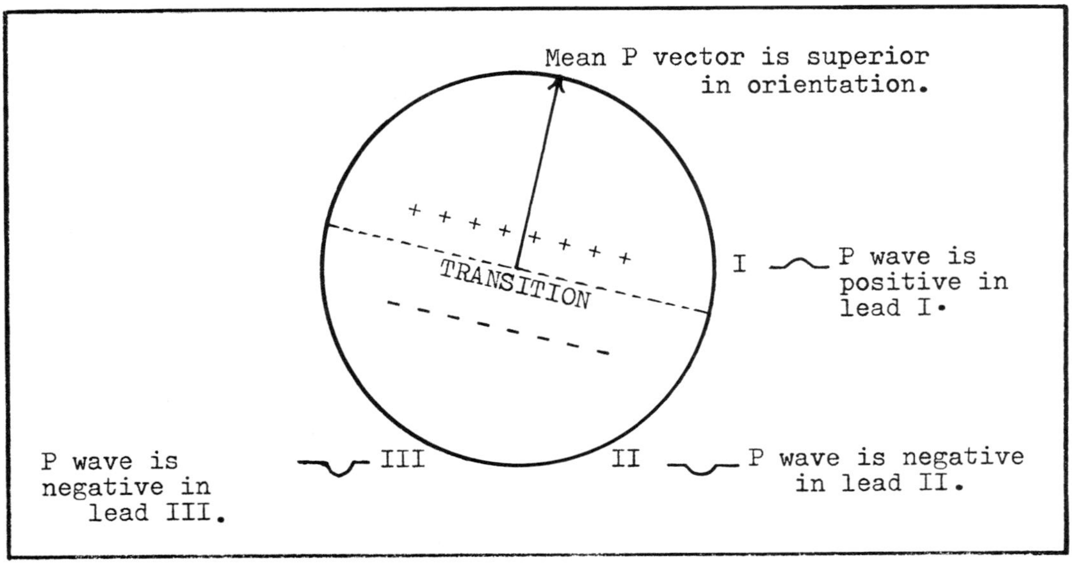

FIGURE 7–23. Mean P vector in "A–V nodal" rhythm.

B. Atrioventricular (A–V) Node (The A–V Node Will Be Described in the "Classical" Manner for Historical Interest Followed by a Discussion of Newer Concepts)

The atrioventricular (A–V) node is a lower center of excitation and may become the dominant pacemaker when the S–A node is depressed. The A–V node may be the dominant pacemaker congenitally, or may share dominance with the S–A node throughout life. The heart rate, with the A–V node as the pacemaker, is regular and from 40 to 60 beats per minute. However, the rate may be equivalent to the sinus rate or even quite rapid (A–V nodal tachycardia). The P waves are usually upright in lead I, but may be transitional, inverted in leads II and III (Fig. 7–23), and may come before, during or after the QRS complex.

As noted, A–V nodal rhythms will be described in the "classical" manner, followed by a discussion of newer concepts. These rhythms have been divided into upper, middle and lower, with characteristics as follows:

1. Upper nodal rhythm: The P wave precedes the QRS complex, with a P–R interval up to 0.12 sec.
2. Middle nodal rhythm: The P wave is within the QRS complex.
3. Lower nodal rhythm: The P wave follows the QRS complex, with an R–P interval up to 0.2 sec.

As noted earlier, when the word "nodal" is used to describe a rhythm it refers to the A–V node and *not* to the S–A node.

Since the "normal" rate in nodal rhythm is 40 to 60 beats per minute, a rate above 60 is really a "nodal tachycardia" although many electrocardiographers will not label a rhythm a tachycardia unless the rate is greater than 100 beats per minute.

A way to understand the "classical" concept of A–V nodal rhythms, although it may not be anatomically accurate, is diagrammed in Figures 7–24, *A*, *B* and *C*.

Text continued on page 350.

1. Upper Nodal Rhythm

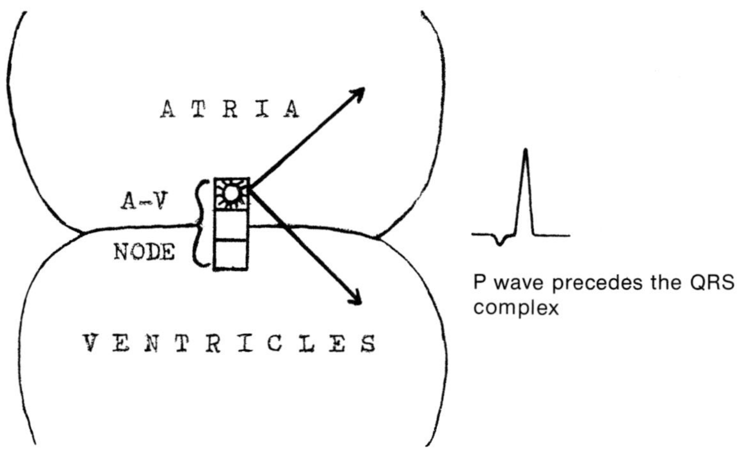

A

FIGURE 7–24. *A,* Upper nodal rhythm. The upper part of the A–V node initiates the impulse. Since it is closer to the atria (see above), the atria are first depolarized retrogradely, followed by the antegrade depolarization of the ventricles. The P wave precedes the QRS complex.

Illustration continued on opposite page.

2. *Middle Nodal Rhythm*

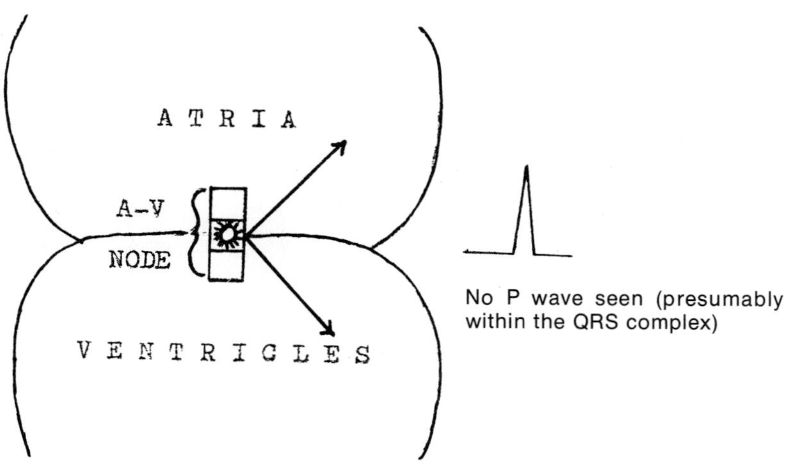

B

FIGURE 7–24 *Continued. B,* Middle nodal rhythm. The atria and ventricles are depolarized at the same time, the atria in a retrograde and the ventricles in an antegrade manner. The P wave is not seen and is presumed to be within the QRS complex.

Illustration continued on following page.

3. *Lower Nodal Rhythm*

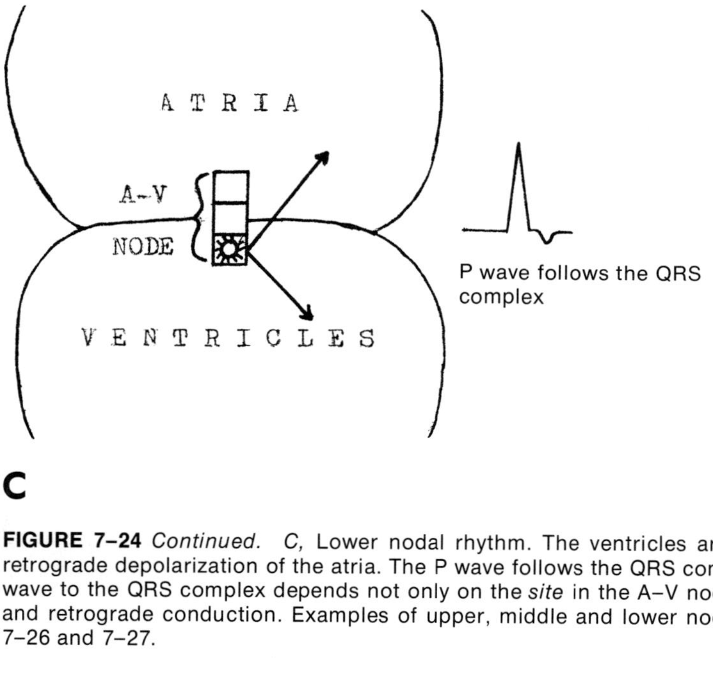

C

FIGURE 7–24 *Continued.* *C,* Lower nodal rhythm. The ventricles are depolarized antegradely before the retrograde depolarization of the atria. The P wave follows the QRS complex. The relation of the retrograde P wave to the QRS complex depends not only on the *site* in the A–V node but also on the *speed* of antegrade and retrograde conduction. Examples of upper, middle and lower nodal rhythms are seen in Figures 7–25, 7–26 and 7–27.

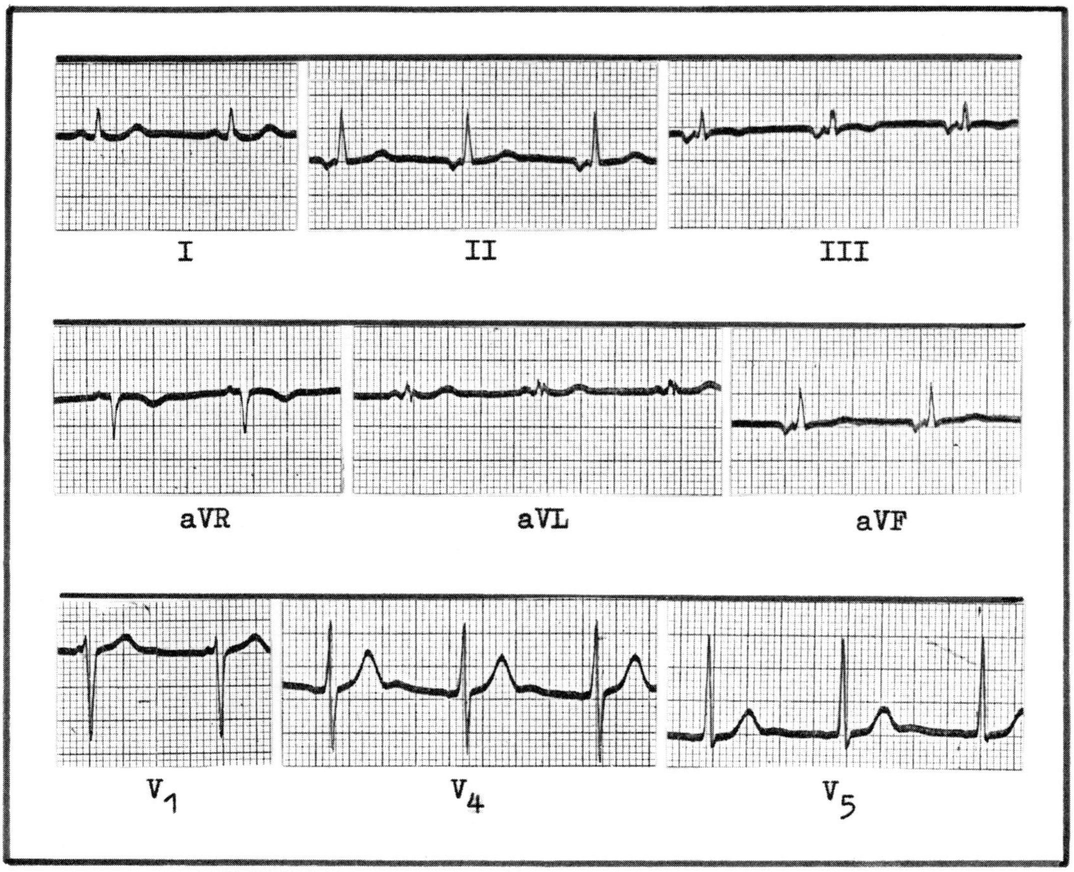

FIGURE 7–25. Upper nodal rhythm. Describe the mean P vector. (Electrocardiogram reduced in size.)

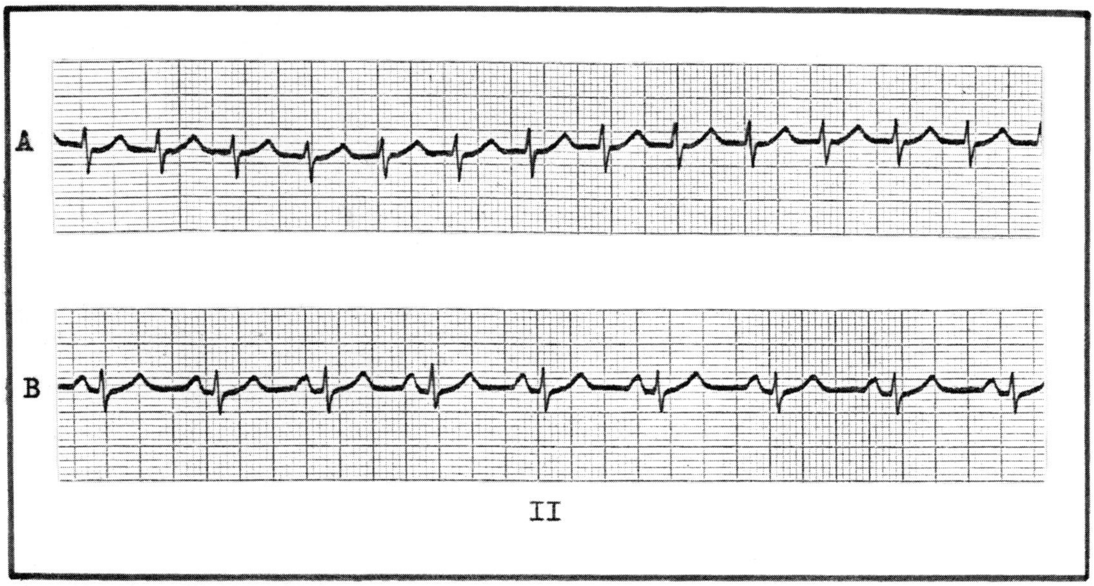

FIGURE 7–26. *A,* Paroxysmal middle nodal tachycardia. Where are the P waves? Are you sure? *B,* Restoration of sinus rhythm following the paroxysm.
(Electrocardiogram reduced in size.)

Cassette Side 18

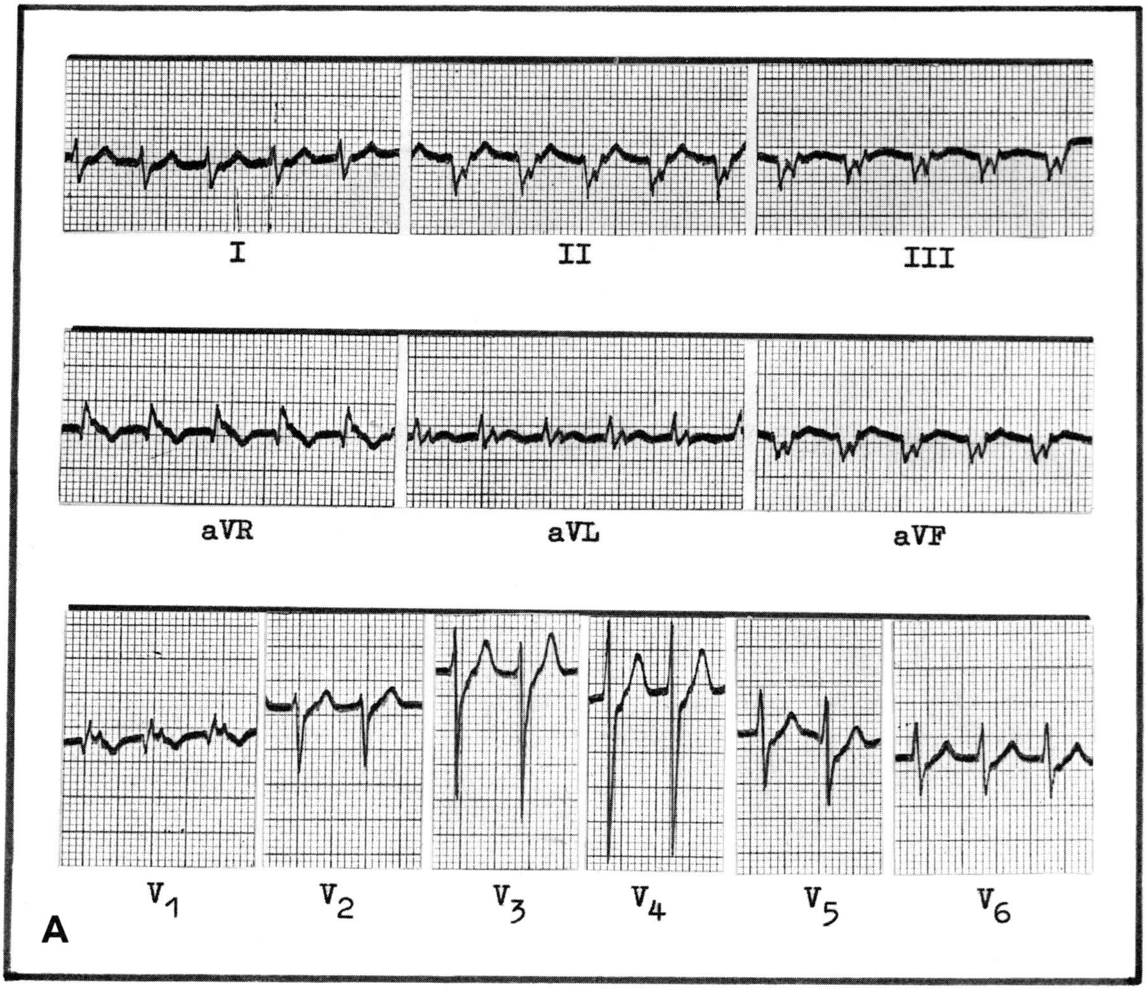

FIGURE 7–27. *A,* A patient presented with a heart rate of approximately 155 beats per minute. The QRS complexes appear wide and P waves may not be obvious. Is this a ventricular tachycardia or supraventricular tachycardia? Diagnosis? On what basis? Try to answer these questions before proceeding.
(Electrocardiogram reduced in size.)

Illustration continued on opposite page.

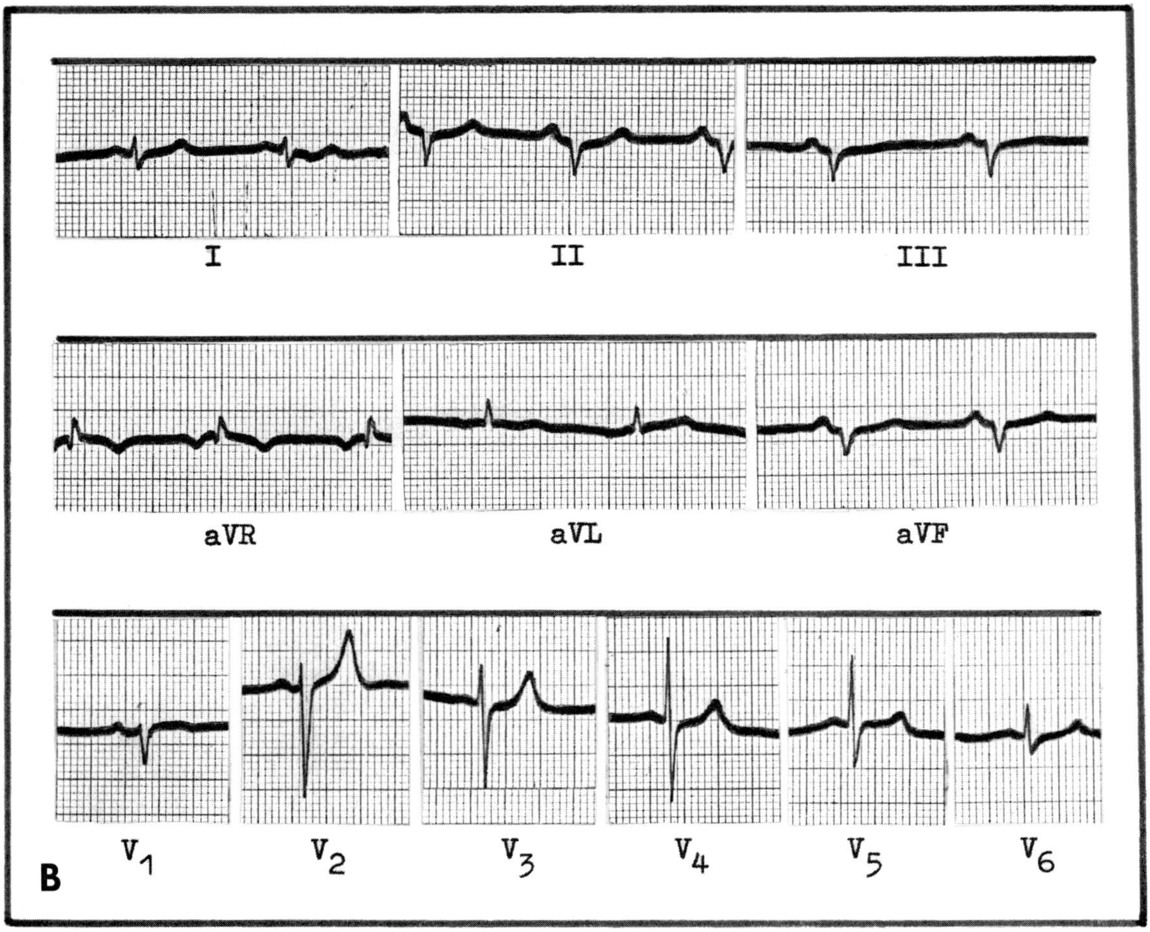

FIGURE 7–27 *Continued.* *B,* Following reversion to normal sinus rhythm, it became clear that the QRS complexes during the tachycardia were not actually widened, but were closely followed by retrograde P waves. The classical diagnosis would be lower nodal tachycardia. Was your diagnosis correct?
(Electrocardiogram reduced in size.)

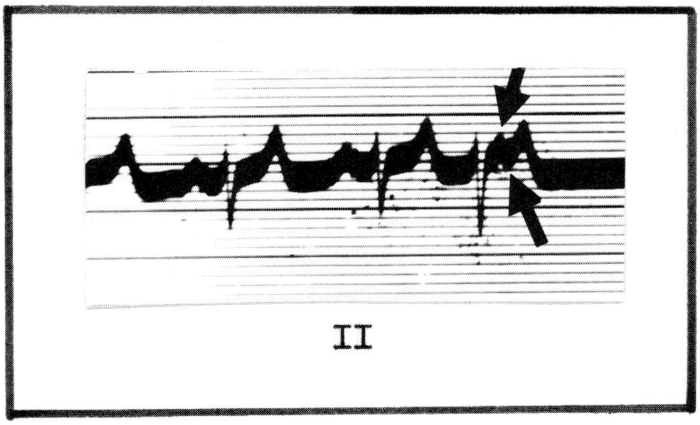

FIGURE 7–28. A "lower nodal" premature beat is seen followed by a retrograde P wave (lower arrow). An alternate interpretation, since the strip is very short and no esophageal or intra-atrial recordings are available, is that the premature beat is really a "middle nodal" premature beat followed by an upright "sinus" P wave (upper arrow), which is blocked due to the refractory state of the ventricular myocardium. A third alternative will be discussed in Figure 7–31 using His bundle recordings.

His Bundle Studies

Evidence is accumulating to show that the A–V node itself may not be the actual site of impulse formation in rhythms attributed to the A–V node. "Junctional," referring to the A–V junction, may be a better term.

I would like to illustrate examples from His bundle studies so that you may keep your minds open until the evidence is conclusive. Concepts will continually change and new ones will evolve as new information emerges. The His bundle study is a technique whereby an electrode catheter is placed near the tricuspid valve via the femoral vein or an arm vein, and recordings made from the area of the His bundle. The recordings reveals a sharp deflection, labeled *H* in Figure 7–29, between the atrial and ventricular deflections. The next two illustrations, Figures 7–30 and 7–31, are from His bundle studies.

His bundle recordings have terminated the "silence" of the P–R segment and have added an important tool to the understanding of arrhythmias.

Text continued on page 371.

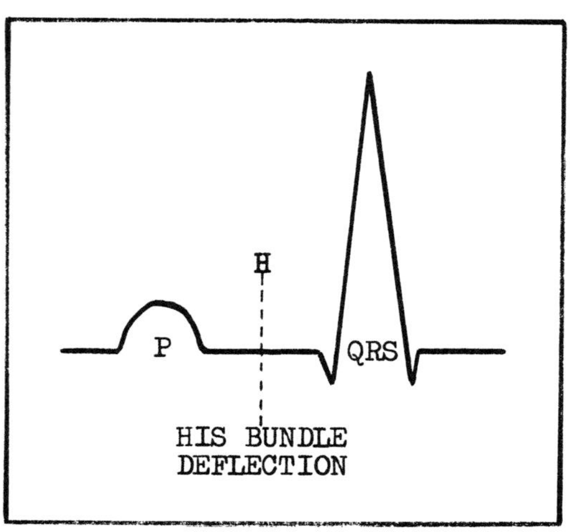

FIGURE 7–29. Diagram showing location of His bundle deflection.

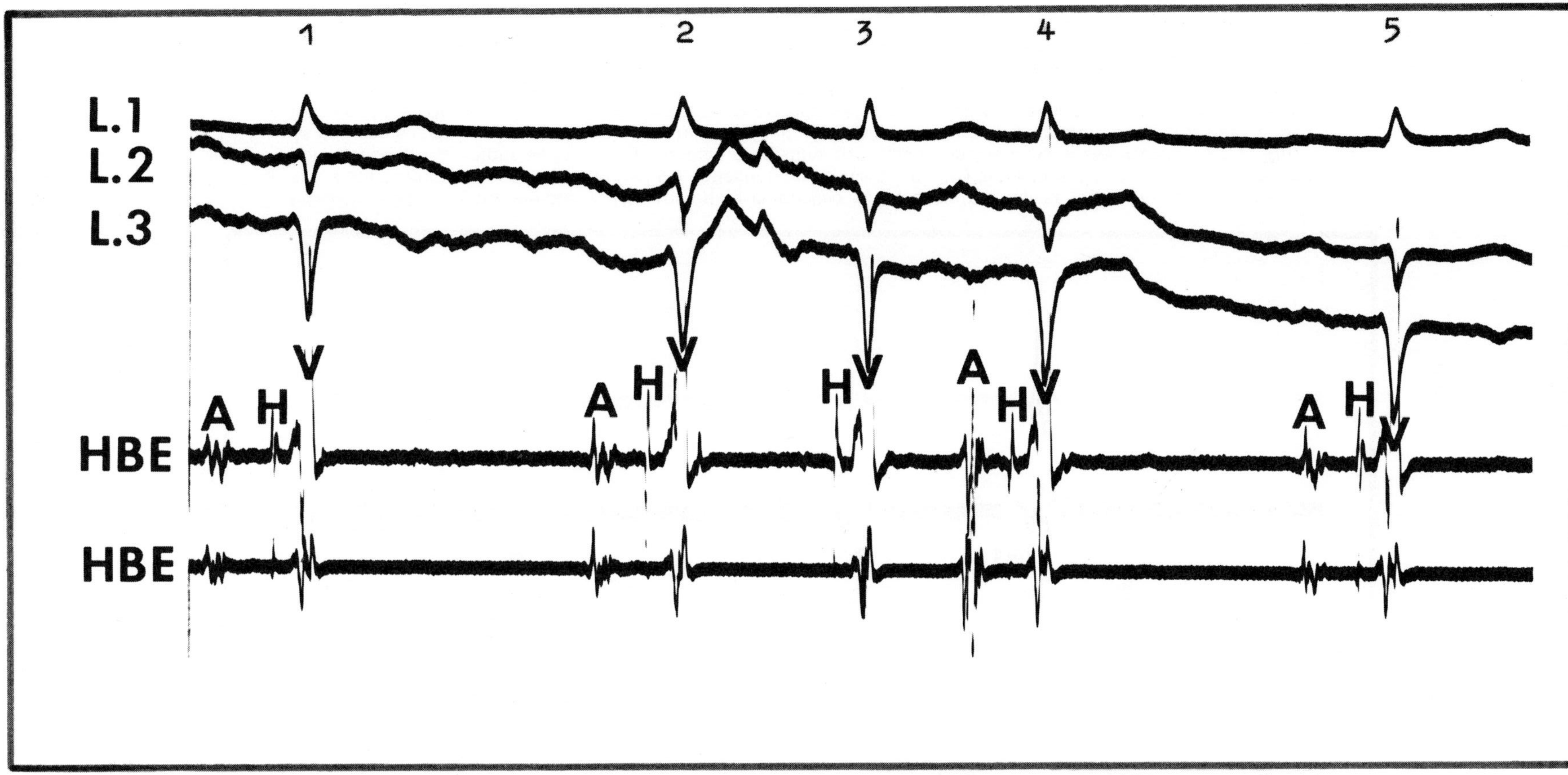

FIGURE 7–30. His bundle study. From above down are seen standard leads I, II and III, in addition to recordings from within the heart. *HBE* is the His bundle electrogram; *A,* atrial deflection; *H,* His deflection; *V,* ventricular deflection. The five ventricular complexes are labelled 1, 2, 3, 4 and 5. Ventricular complexes (V 1, 2, 4 and 5) are preceded by an atrial deflection (A), lining up with the P wave on the clinical electrocardiogram, and a His deflection (H), representing normal A–V conduction. Complex number 3, on the other hand, might be called a "middle nodal" extra beat if we had only the clinical electrocardiogram at our disposal, since it is not preceded or followed by a P wave. The His bundle electrogram shows us, however, that complex number 3 is preceded only by a His bundle (H) deflection—it is a His bundle (or above) beat and *not* a "middle nodal" beat. There is no "hidden" P wave within the QRS complex.

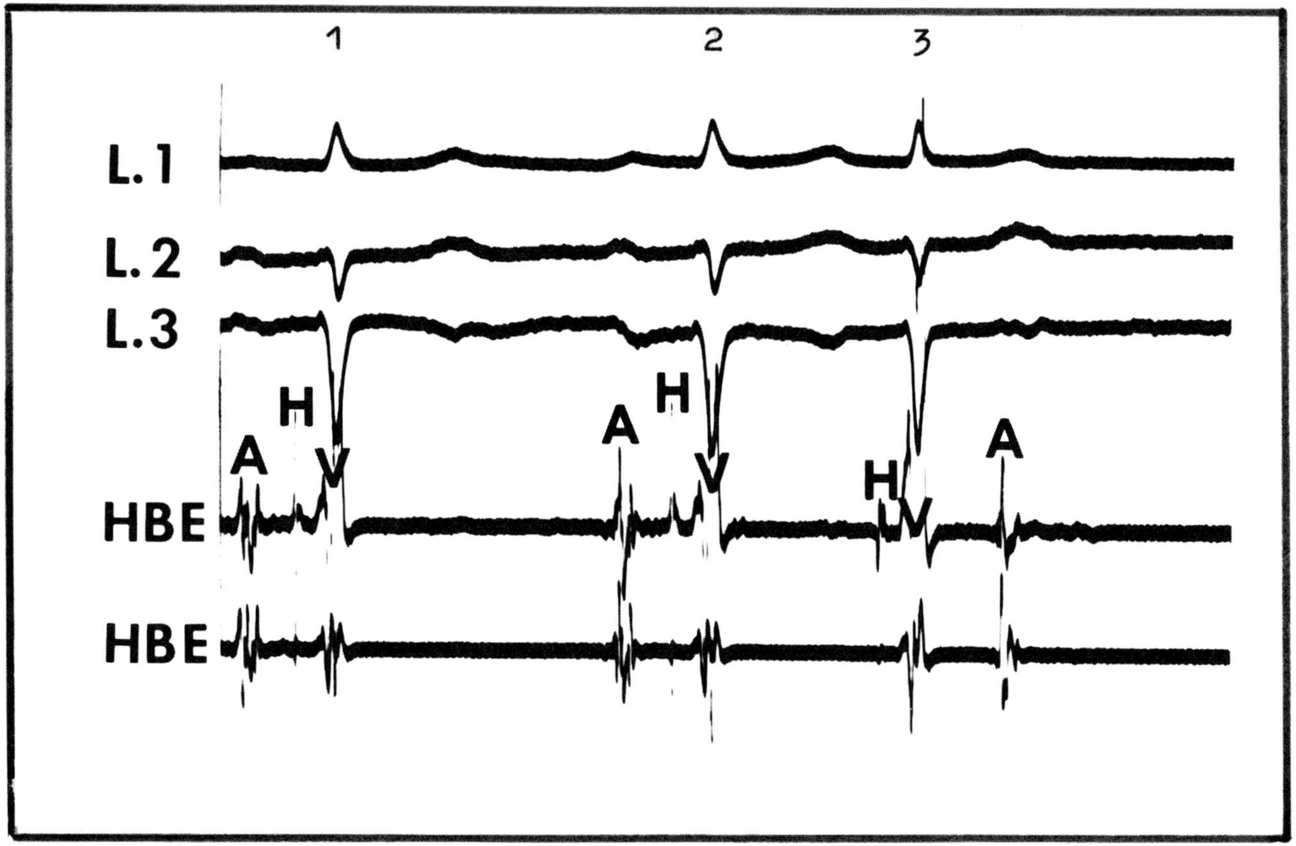

FIGURE 7–31. His bundle study. This recording is labelled in the same manner as Figure 7–30. Complexes 1 and 2 are normal, preceded by an atrial (*A*) deflection and a His bundle (*H*) deflection. Complex 3 is a premature contraction which might be labelled a "nodal" premature contraction on the clinical electrocardiogram. Why? As you can see on the His bundle electrogram (*HBE*), it is actually a *His bundle* premature beat. This beat is then followed by a normal atrial deflection, which cannot conduct to the ventricles because the ventricular conduction system is in a refractory state due to the premature contraction. Review Figure 7–28. Any similarity? On the basis of similar studies it has been postulated that "lower" and "middle nodal" rhythms are actually His bundle rhythms with or without retrograde depolarization of the atria. "Upper nodal" rhythms may actually be rhythms originating in the area of the coronary sinus or in the left atrium. Notice how a new technique can revolutionize time-honored concepts.

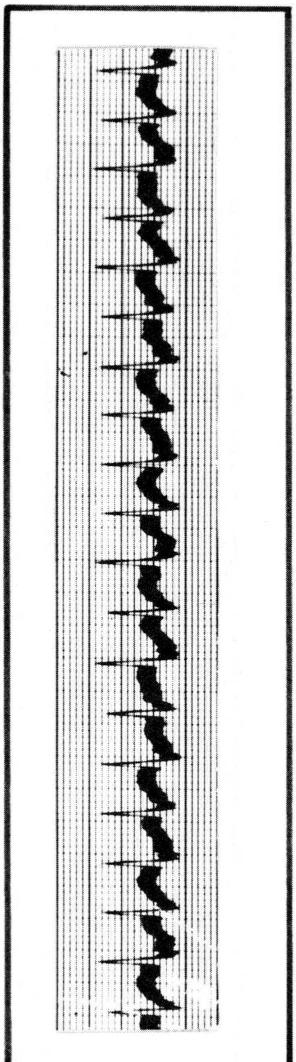

FIGURE 7–32. Supraventricular tachycardia. An arrhythmia is not infrequently encountered where the ventricular rate is so rapid that P waves cannot be readily identified on the standard electrocardiogram. The rate appears fairly regular and the duration of the QRS complexes normal. In the absence of esophageal recordings or of more definitive laboratory studies, the term "supraventricular tachycardia" is often used. (Electrocardiogram reduced in size.)

C. Ventricles

1. *Idioventricular Rhythm*

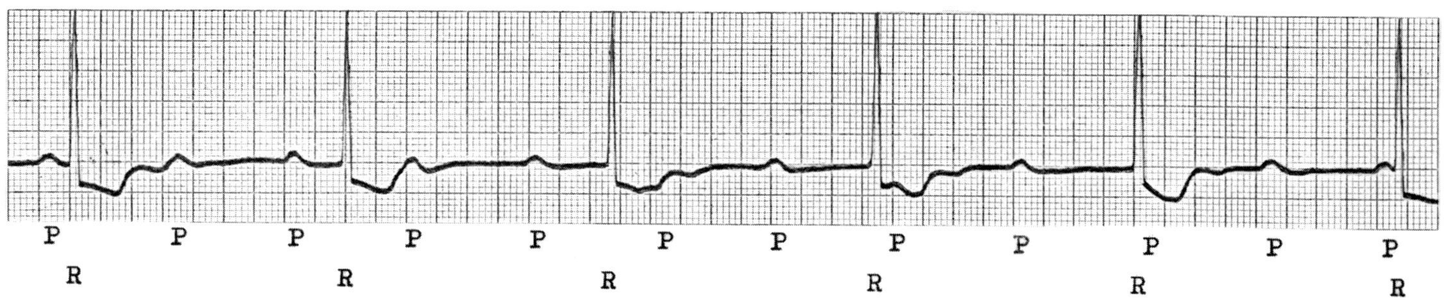

FIGURE 7–33. Idioventricular rhythm. When the dominant pacemaker is within the ventricles, due to drugs such as digitalis or disease of the conduction system, the rate may be quite slow (20 to 40 per minute) and the rhythm is called idioventricular. Depending on the site of impulse formation, the QRS complexes may be very bizarre or almost normal. In the above electrocardiogram, the ventricular rate is 33 per minute and regular. The atria, remaining under control of the S–A node, are beating at 75 per minute and are completely dissociated from the ventricles.
(Electrocardiogram reduced in size.)

2. Premature Beats of the Ventricle

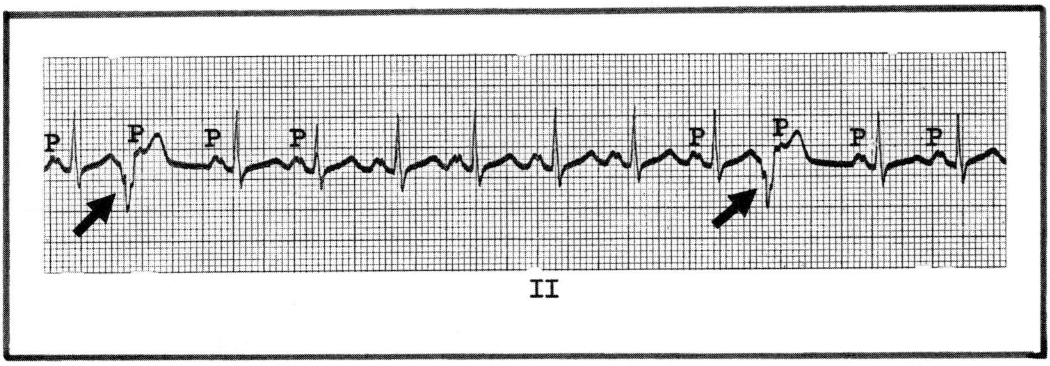

FIGURE 7–34. Premature beats of the ventricle (arrows above) are seen when an impulse is propagated from a ventricular focus before the next normal beat is due. The QRS is commonly widened and not preceded by a P wave. A "compensatory" pause usually follows. There may be retrograde activation of the atria following a premature ventricular contraction or the normal sinus P waves may continue (as in the present case). The sinus P waves following the premature ventricular contractions are blocked because of conduction system refractoriness.
(Electrocardiogram reduced in size.)

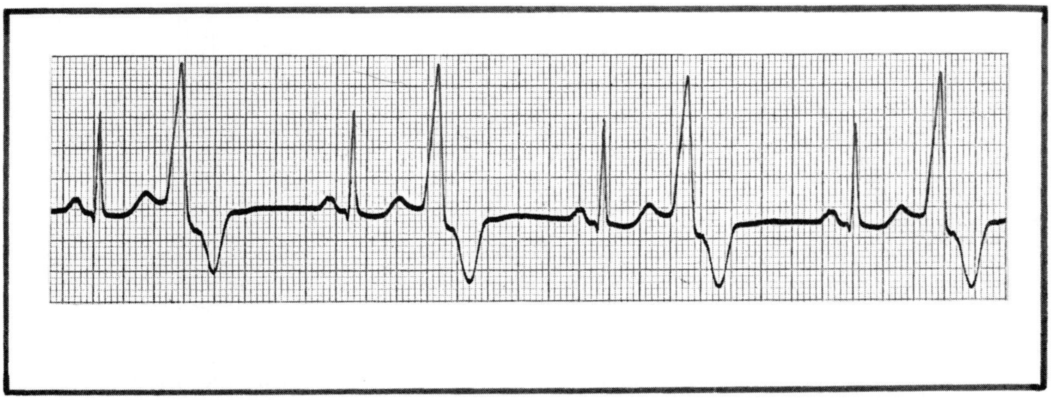

FIGURE 7–35. *Bigeminy* or *coupling* describes the heart beating in groups of two, usually a normal beat followed by a premature ventricular contraction and separated from the next group by a compensatory pause. Beating in groups of three, such as two normal beats followed steadily by a premature ventricular contraction and separated by a compensatory pause, is known as *trigeminy.* The words bigeminy, trigeminy, etc., merely describe group beating; they do not tell you the components of the groups. As seen above, in bigeminy due to a premature ventricular contraction following a normal beat, the *coupling* interval is "fixed"—that is, there is an identical interval between each normal beat and each premature ventricular contraction.
(Electrocardiogram reduced in size.)

3. Ventricular Tachycardia

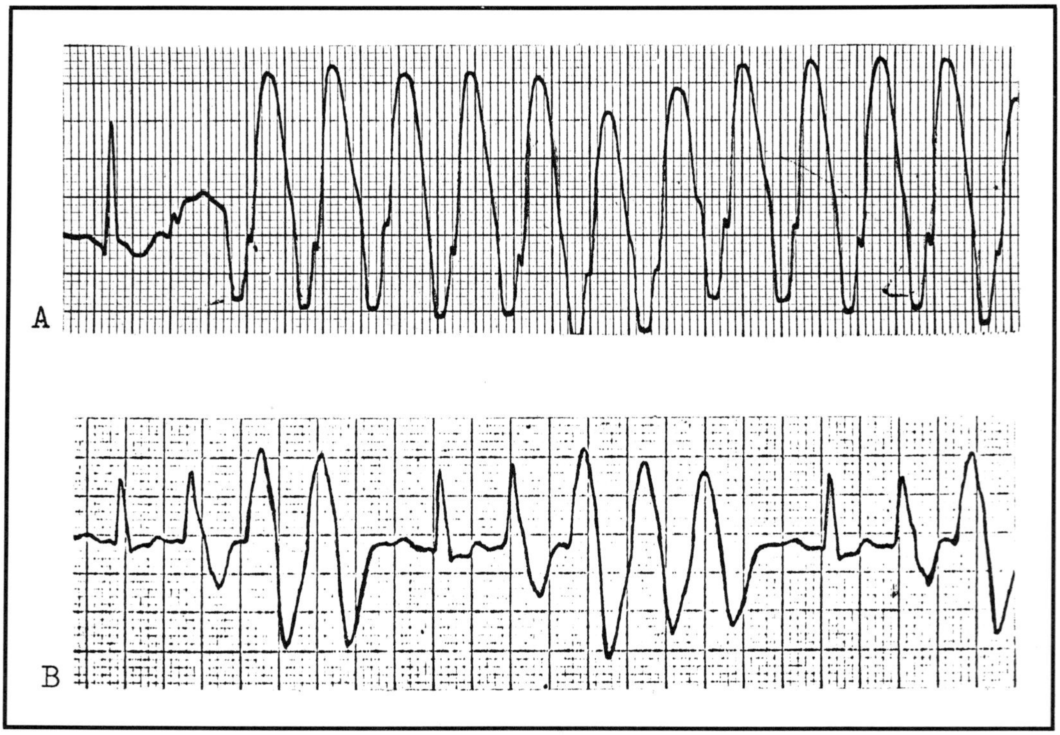

FIGURE 7–36. Ventricular tachycardia. The ectopic pacemaker in the ventricle may produce "runs" of premature contractions under proper circumstances, known as ventricular tachycardia. Once started, ventricular tachycardia may be sustained until terminated spontaneously, by medication or by electrical cardioversion (*A*), or it may be intermittent, with "runs" of premature ventricular contractions (*B*). The QRS complexes are widened and the rate is usually from 150 to 250 per minute. The rhythm may be regular or slightly irregular.

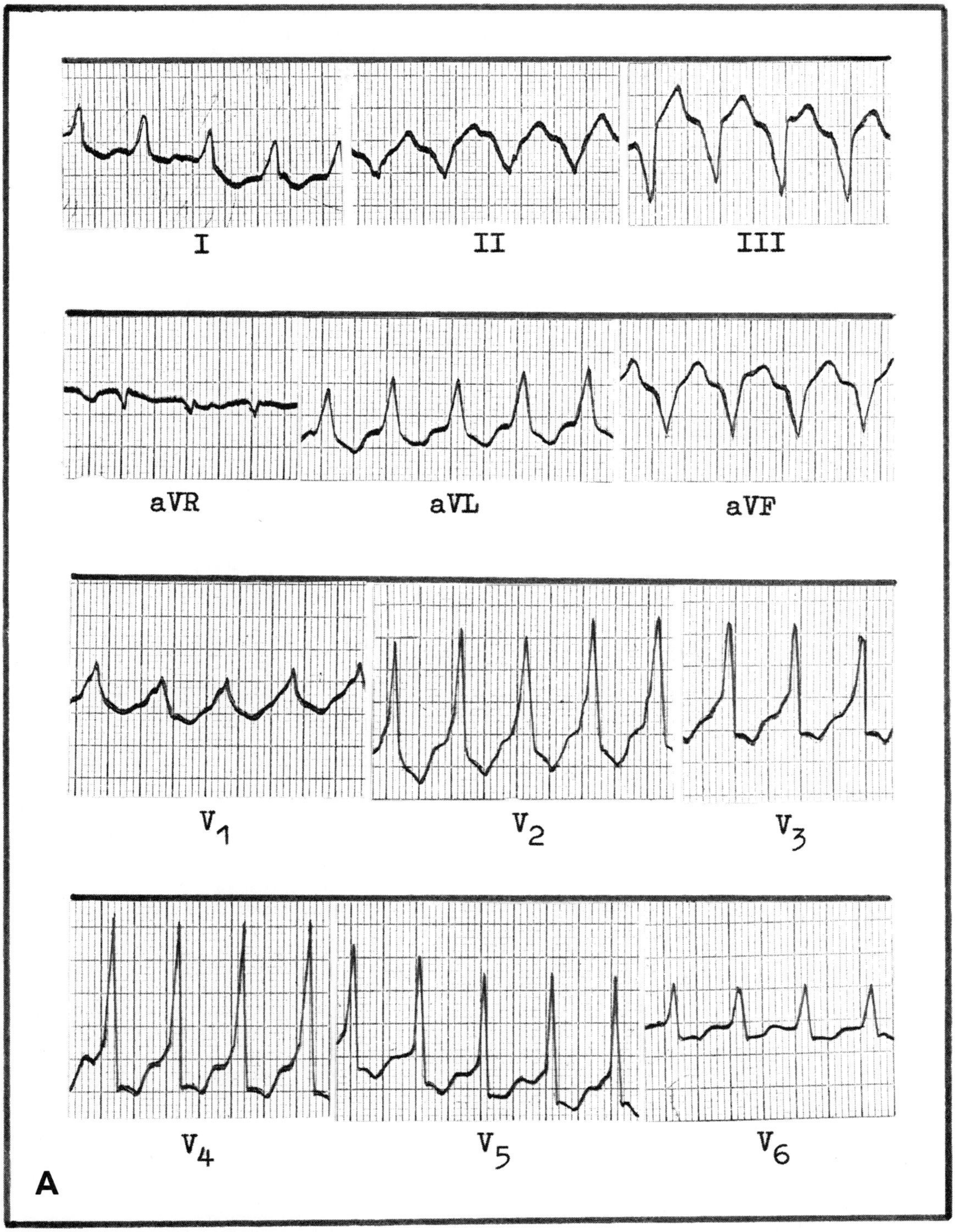

FIGURE 7–37. *A,* Evaluation of this arrhythmia presents an interesting challenge. Review the analyses of the arrhythmias in Figures 7–21 and 7–27. Is this tachycardia, with a ventricular rate of 150 per minute, a ventricular tachycardia or a supraventricular tachycardia with wide QRS complexes (aberration)? Why? Make a decision before proceeding.

Illustration continued on following page.

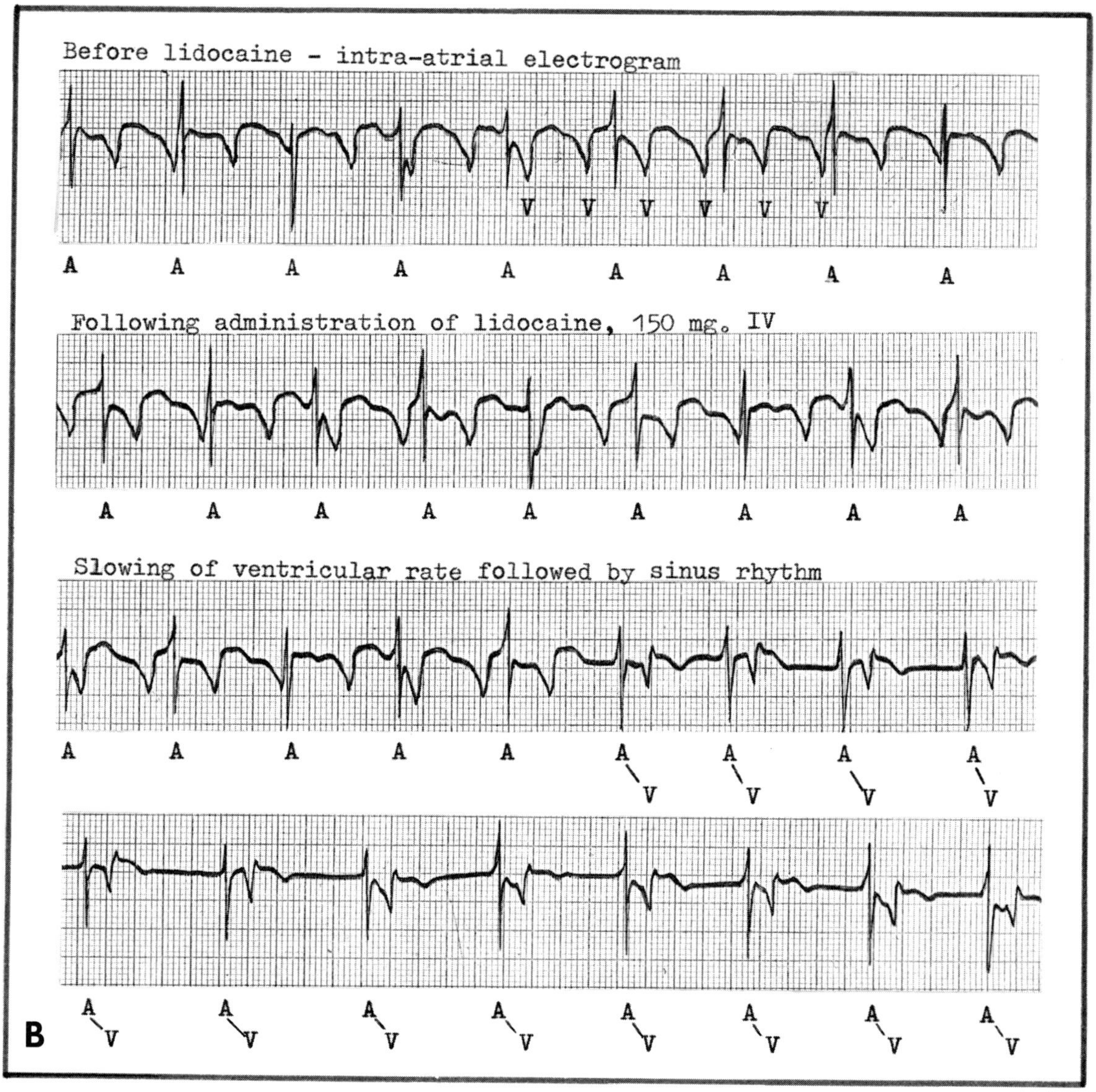

FIGURE 7–37 *Continued.* *B,* Intra-atrial electrogram. During ventricular tachycardia, the ventricles may activate the atria retrogradely. The atria, however, usually remain under sinus control and beat at the normal, slower rate and are dissociated from the ventricles.

Often it is important, in order to make the diagnosis of ventricular tachycardia, to evaluate the atrial activity. Atrial activity may or may not be obvious on the clinical electrocardiogram in the presence of a very rapid ventricular rate. We may not even be dealing with a ventricular tachycardia, as we saw in two cases earlier in this study, one with atrial flutter and left bundle branch block (Fig. 7–21) and the other with "lower nodal" tachycardia (Fig. 7–27). All efforts to identify atrial activity on the clinical electrocardiogram may prove futile. Because of the importance of establishing the diagnosis, in terms of therapy, the cardiology laboratory may be of help. The electrocardiogram in Figure 7–37*A* reveals a tachycardia with a ventricular rate of 150 per minute. Is this a ventricular tachycardia or a supraventricular tachycardia with wide QRS complexes (aberration)? An electrode catheter was inserted into the right atrium and an intra-atrial electrogram recorded an atrial rate of 80 per minute. The demonstration of a slower atrial rate dissociated from the rapid ventricular rate facilitated the diagnosis of ventricular tachycardia and resulted in the initiation of proper therapy. The atrial deflections are marked by the letter *A* and the ventricular deflections by the letter *V* above. Note the slowing of the ventricular rate following the administration of lidocaine, with establishment of normal sinus rhythm, seen in the third panel.

Another aid which may be obtained in the cardiology laboratory is the His bundle recording, as seen earlier in this chapter. If a His bundle deflection does not precede the QRS complex of the tachycardia, the origin of the impulses must be below the His bundle—for example, in the ventricle.

In the absence of a laboratory, esophageal recording can be of great value in locating the atrial deflections or P waves. When P waves are not obvious, and other differentiating features are obscured, it may help, in differentiating supraventricular tachycardia with aberration (e.g., RBBB or LBBB) from ventricular tachycardia, to keep in mind that in *ventricular tachycardia,* the QRS complexes, when examined in all twelve leads, do not resemble classical bundle branch block of either type. In Figure 7–37*A,* lead V_1 suggests RBBB while other leads suggest LBBB. Now go back and analyze Figure 7–21*A* on this basis.
(Electrocardiogram reduced in size.)

4. *Ventricular Flutter*

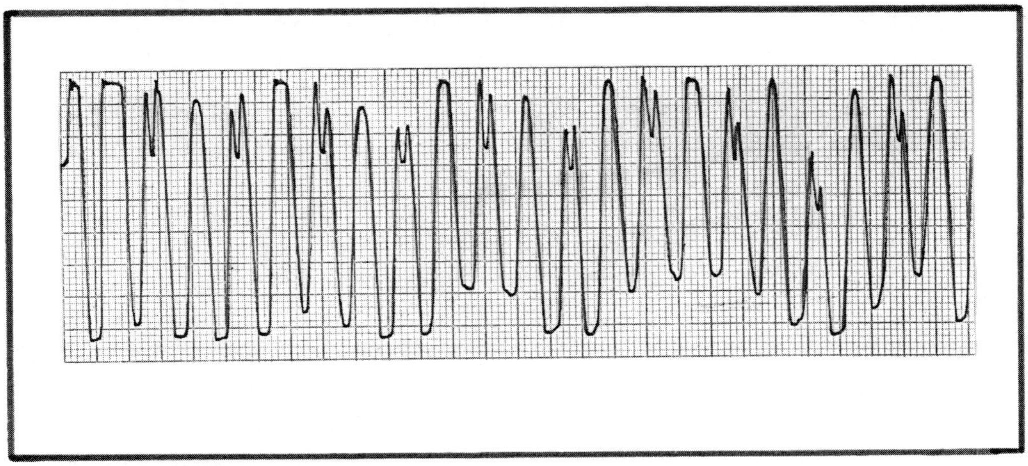

FIGURE 7–38. Ventricular flutter. Undulating waves are seen rising and falling. This rhythm is often an intermediary stage between ventricular tachycardia and ventricular fibrillation. The rate is usually between 250 to 350 beats per minute. When the ventricular rate is at this level, the patient is acutely ill and the pulse may be imperceptible. The differential diagnosis is ventricular flutter versus atrial flutter *in the presence of an aberrant pathway (e.g., W-P-W).* The normal A–V node cannot conduct 1:1 at this rate, and it is too fast for ventricular tachycardia (usually about 160 per min.). (Electrocardiogram reduced in size.)

5. *Ventricular Fibrillation*

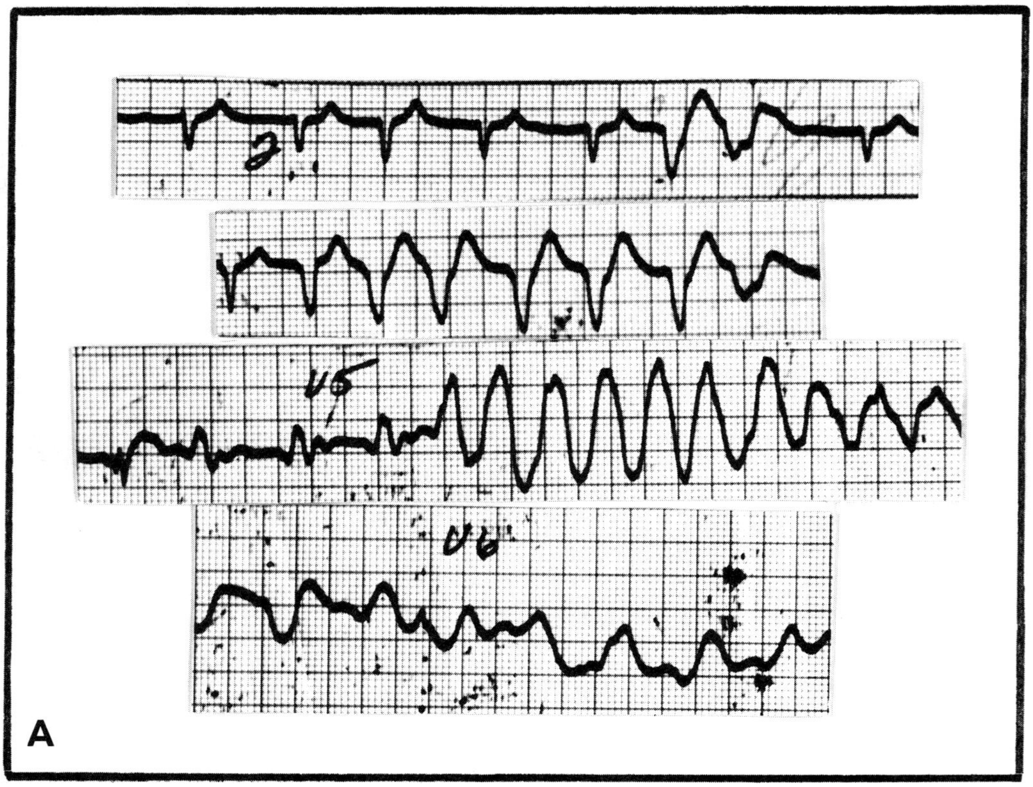

FIGURE 7–39. *A,* Ventricular fibrillation. Very rapid, disorganized contractions of the ventricle characterize ventricular fibrillation and represent cardiac arrest. It may be of sudden onset or may follow ventricular premature contractions and ventricular tachycardia, as seen above. The bottom strip represents chaotic action of the dying heart. This is also seen in Figure 7–39*B.*
(Electrocardiogram reduced in size.)

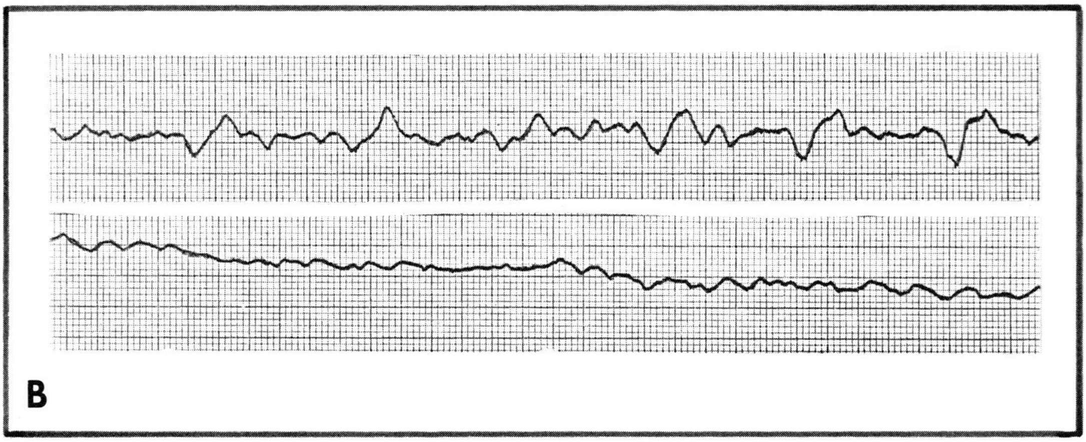

FIGURE 7–39 *Continued. B,* Chaotic action of the dying heart.
(Electrocardiogram reduced in size.)

D. Atrioventricular (A–V) Conduction Disturbances

1. First Degree A–V Block

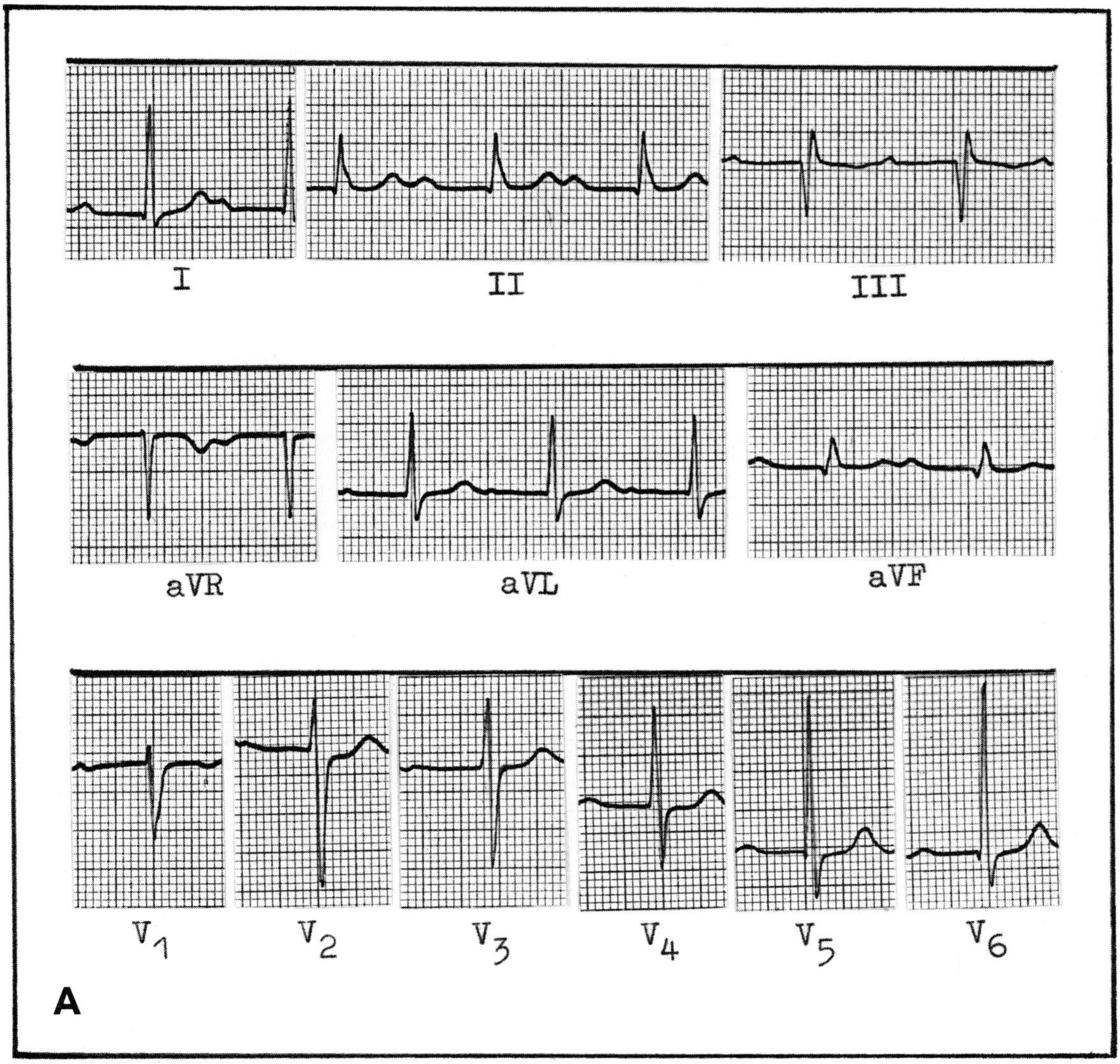

FIGURE 7–40. *A, First degree A–V block* represents a delay in the transmission of impulses from the atria to the ventricles, usually across the A–V node. A prolonged P–R interval (greater than 0.20 sec.) is seen on the electrocardiogram. This patient also had an old diaphragmatic myocardial infarction.

Illustration continued on following page.

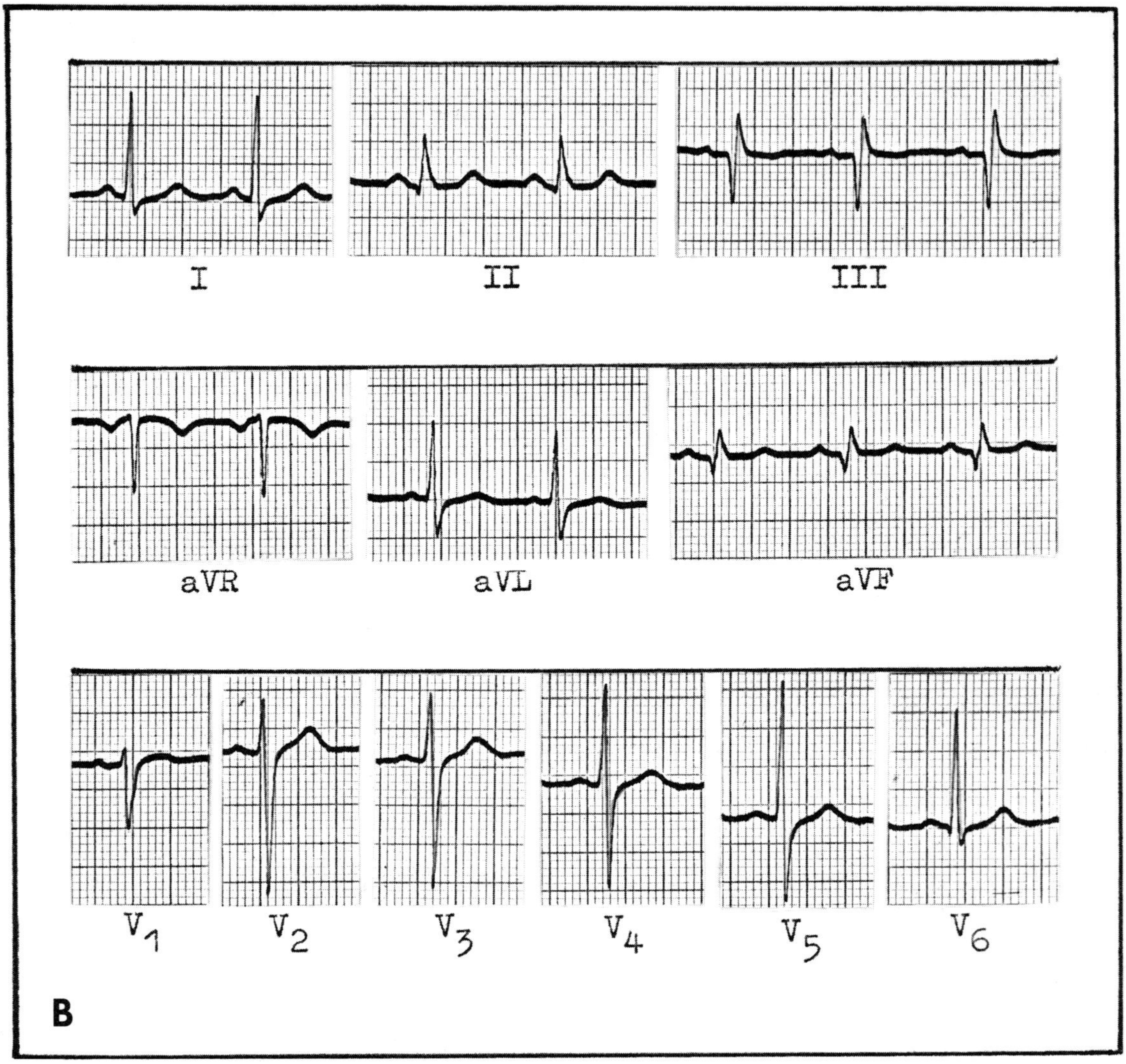

FIGURE 7–40 *Continued. B,* Same patient as in Figure 7–40*A* following the infarct but prior to the development of first degree A–V block.

2. *Second Degree A–V Block*

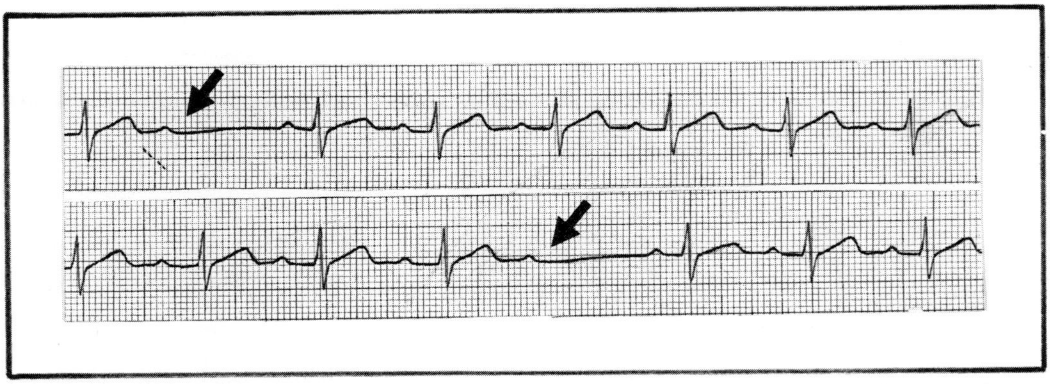

FIGURE 7–41. Second degree A–V block. When the ventricles periodically do not respond to atrial stimuli, the P wave on the electrocardiogram is *not* followed by a QRS complex (arrows). The various grades of second degree A–V block will depend on the frequency and characteristics of the blocked atrial conduction. In the above illustration, a dropped beat occurs periodically with little, if any, change in the other P–R intervals. His bundle studies have shown that the block is frequently below the His bundle and may be a warning of future development of complete A–V block and Adams-Stokes syndrome. This is called Mobitz II block.
(Electrocardiogram reduced in size.)

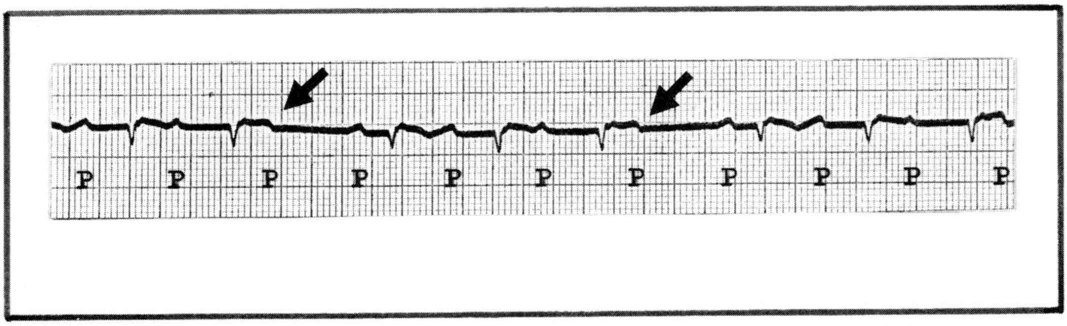

FIGURE 7–42. Another form of second degree A–V block is what is known as Mobitz I block or the classical Wenckebach block. Ventricular beats are "dropped" in a cyclic manner. The P–R interval is less prolonged at first but becomes progressively longer until an atrial contraction no longer initiates a ventricular response. The cycle is then resumed. In the above electrocardiogram, the first P–R interval is shorter than the second and the third P wave does not conduct (first arrow). The fourth P wave starts the cycle again. The seventh P wave does not conduct (second arrow), and the cycle starts again with the eighth P wave. The block in Wenckebach periods has frequently been shown to be above the bundle of His (in contrast to Mobitz II, seen in Fig. 7–41), presumably in the A–V node. However, to be absolutely sure, a His bundle recording is needed.
(Electrocardiogram reduced in size.)

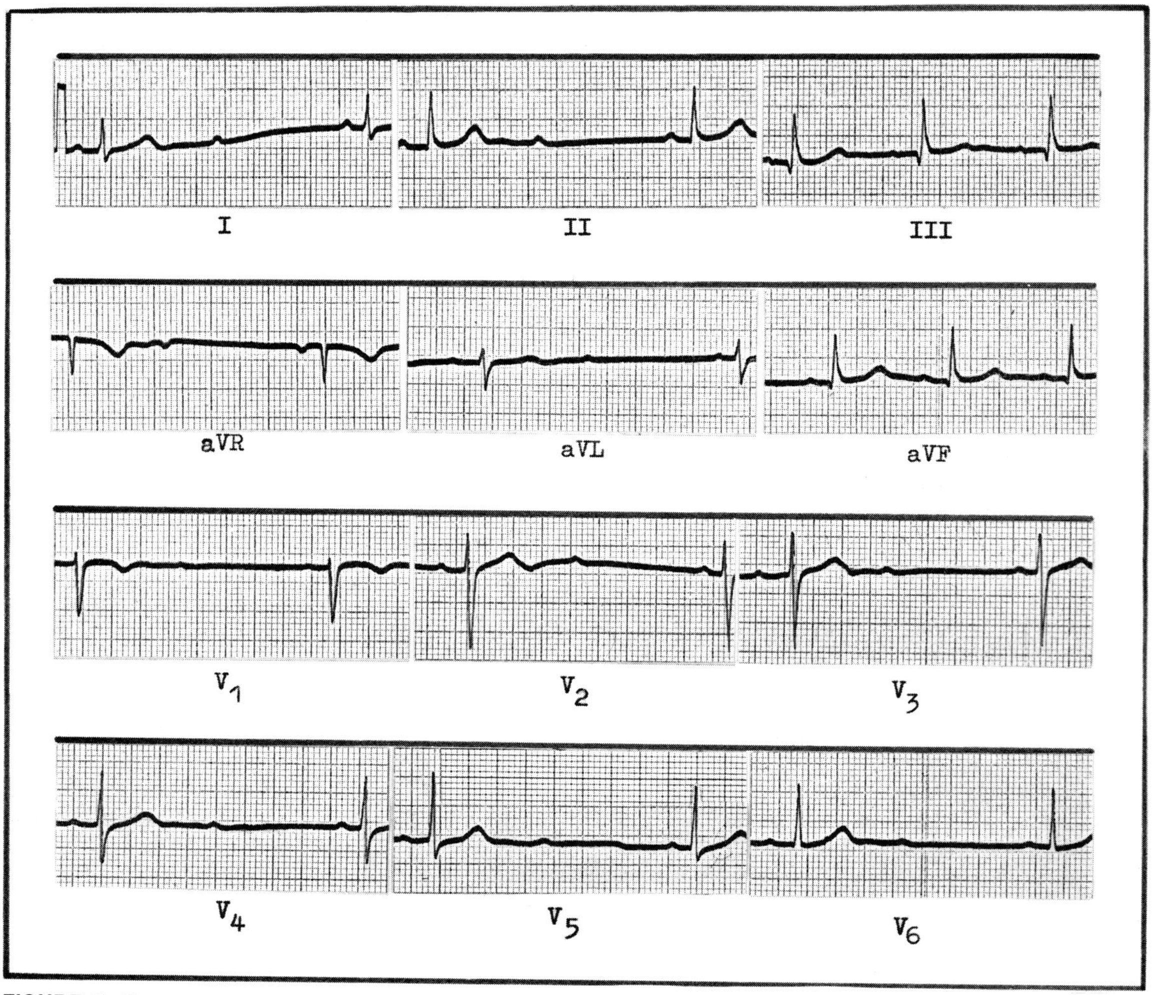

FIGURE 7–43. In more severe forms of second degree A–V block, the ventricles are able to respond only to every second, third, fourth or fifth beat. In the above electrocardiogram, every other P wave (except in leads III and aVF) is not followed by a QRS complex. This is known as 2:1 A–V block (two atrial beats for every ventricular beat).
(Electrocardiogram reduced in size.)

3. Third Degree (Complete) A–V Block

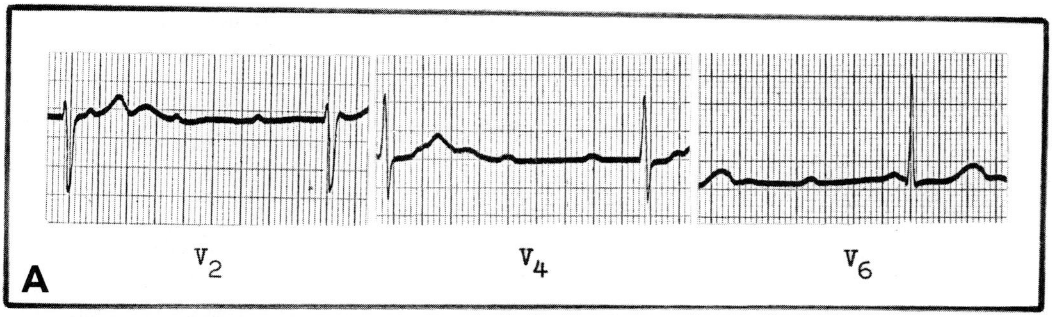

FIGURE 7–44. *A,* Third degree A–V block. The atria and ventricles beat independently in third degree (complete) A–V block. The atria beat at the usual sinus rate, whereas the ventricles beat much more slowly. An example of third degree A–V block was already seen in Figure 7–33. There is no constant relationship between the P waves and the QRS complexes. The patient, who had a previous electrocardiogram with normal A–V conduction (Fig. 7–44*B*), noted the sudden onset of the low heart rate; there was no accompanying chest pain and no evidence of myocardial infarction. What is the treatment of choice?
(Electrocardiogram reduced in size.)

Illustration continued on following page.

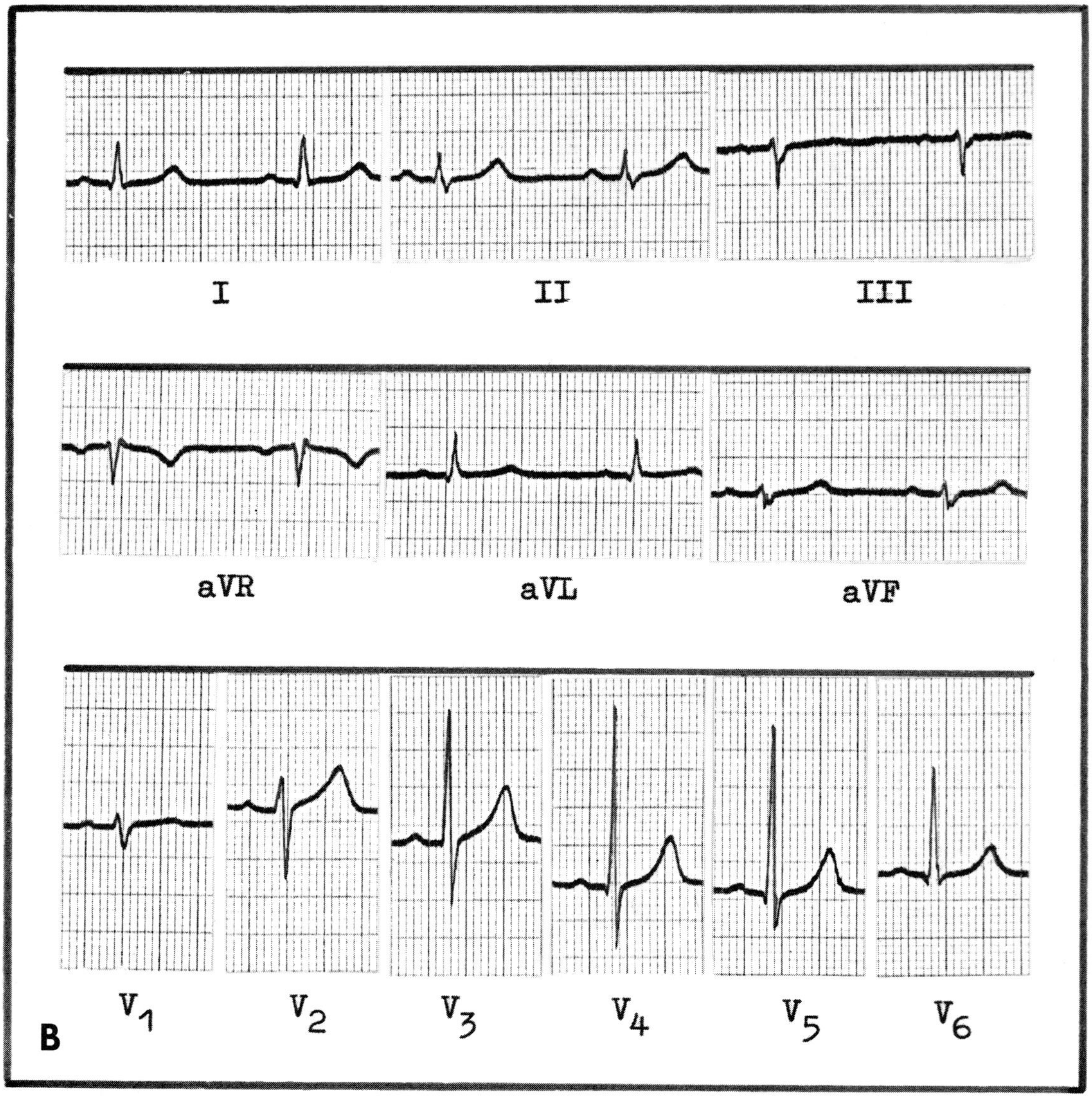

FIGURE 7–44 *Continued.* *B,* Prior electrocardiogram of patient who presented with complete A–V block described in Figure 7–44*A.*

Illustration continued on opposite page.

Pacemaker Therapy

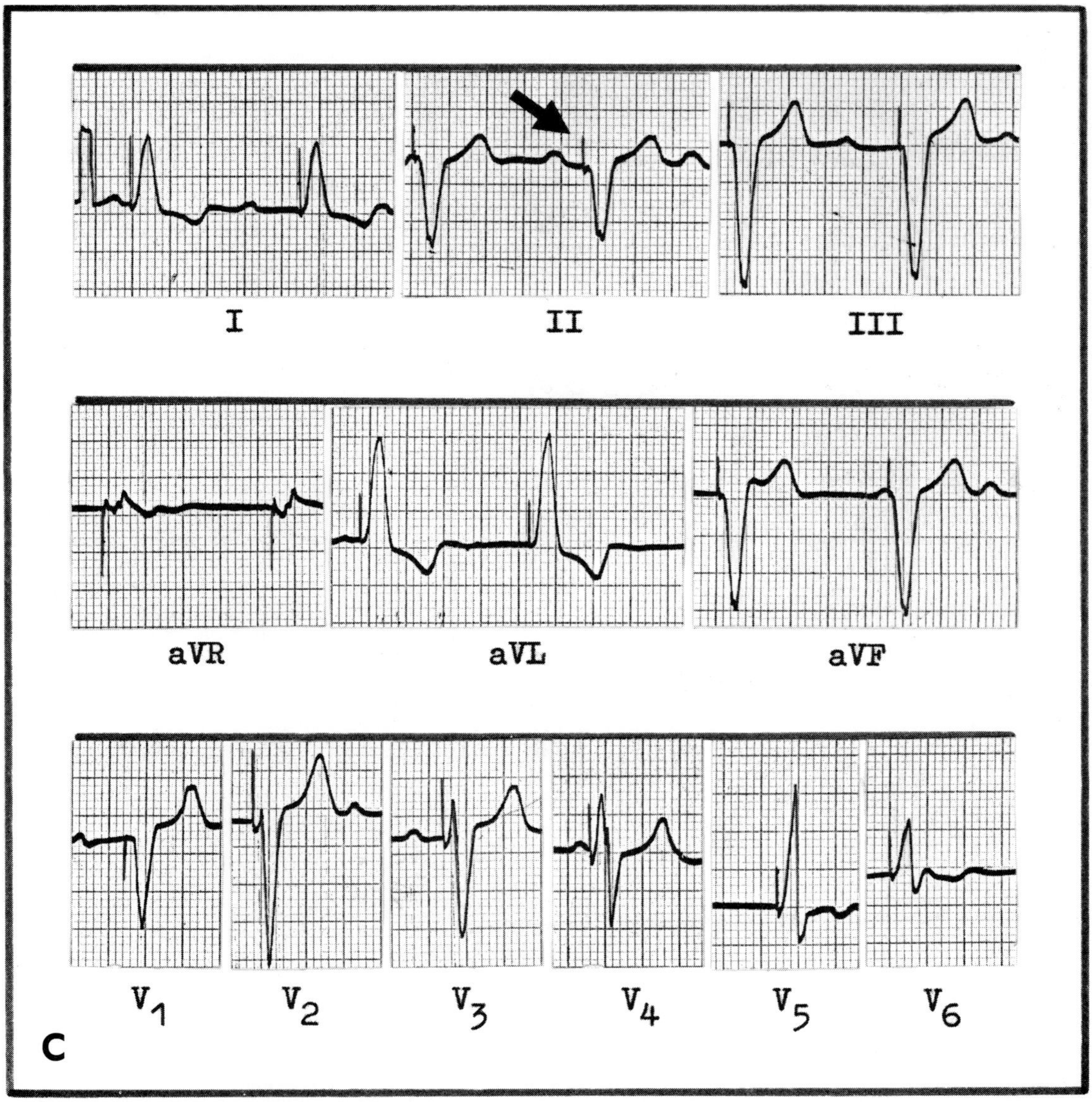

FIGURE 7–44 *Continued.* *C,* Following treatment with ventricular pacing. Note the pacer impulse preceding each ventricular deflection (indicated by an arrow in lead II).

In general, a patient with high grade A–V block, as seen here, may present with symptoms of cerebral insufficiency, such as dizziness or beclouded mentation, or may actually have lost consciousness due to the low rate and poor cardiac output, or to transient ventricular standstill or fibrillation. The present day treatment is electrical pacing to maintain a proper rate and good cardiac output.

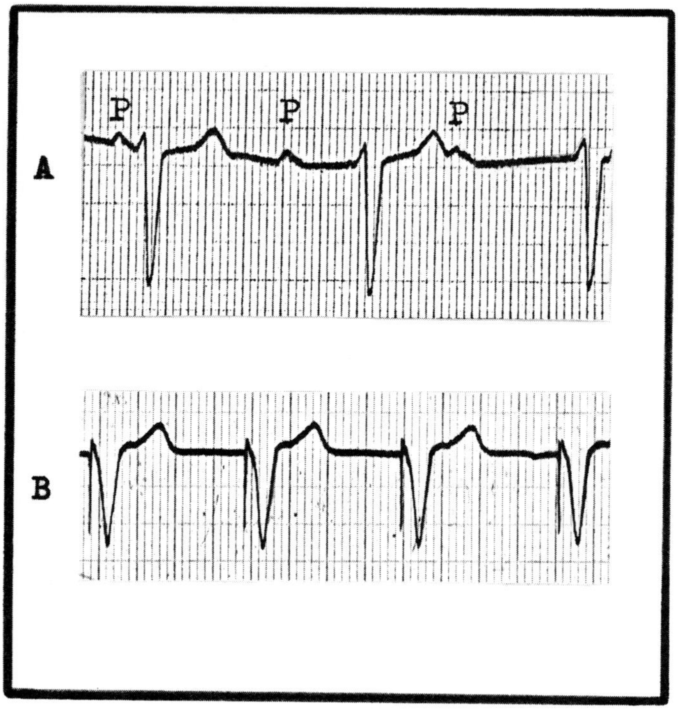

FIGURE 7–45. Third degree A–V block. The atria and ventricles are beating independently (*A*), the atria at the usual sinus rate and the ventricles more slowly. This rhythm followed open heart surgery and the patient was treated with permanent ventricular pacing (*B*).

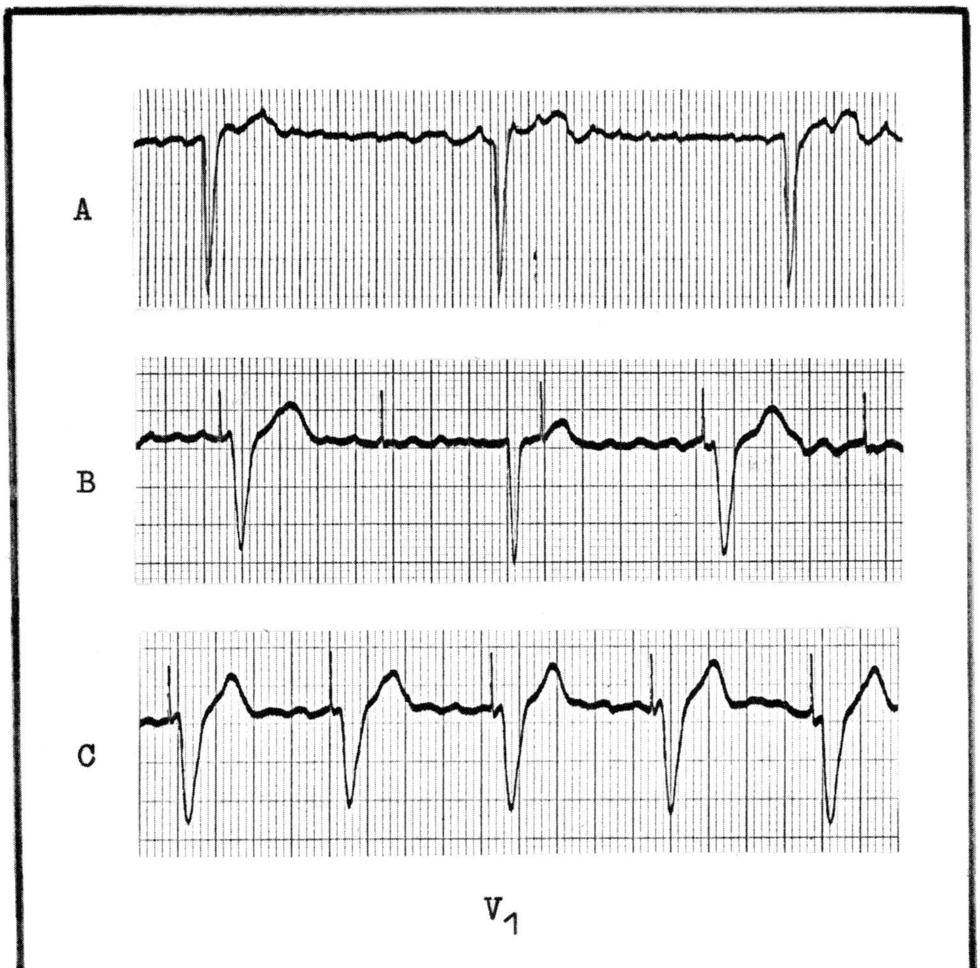

FIGURE 7–46. Complete A–V block in a patient with coarse atrial fibrillation (flutter-fibrillation) (*A*). During adjustment of the pacemaker (*B*), the pacemaker impulse is producing a response only erratically. 1:1 pacing is accomplished in *C*.

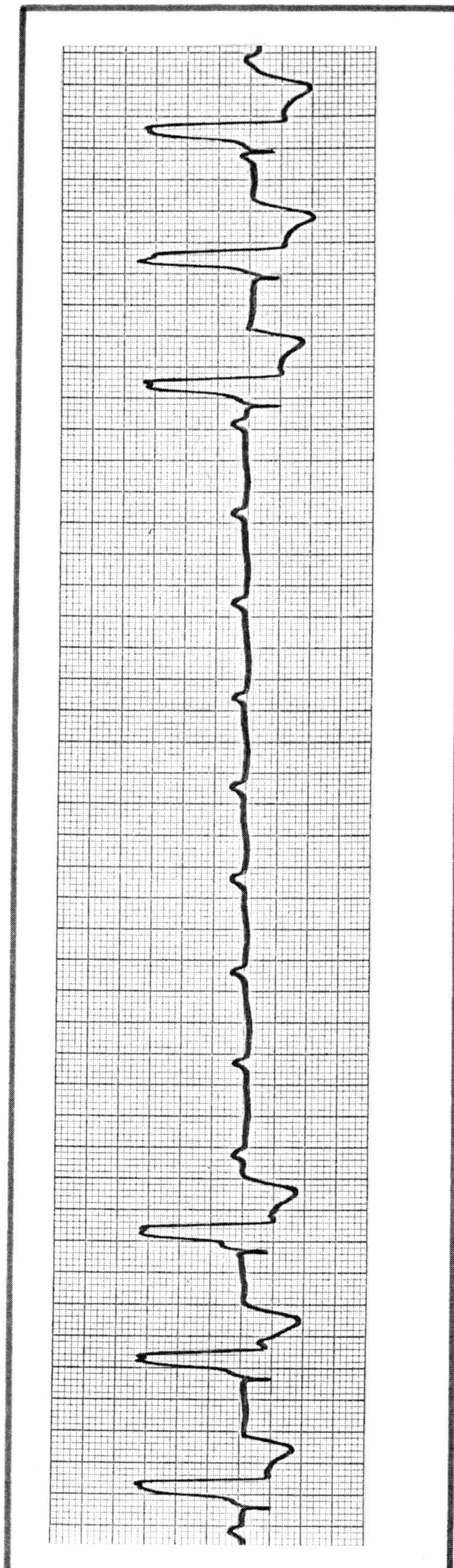

FIGURE 7–47. That ventricular pacing has improved many lives is dramatically illustrated above. During adjustment of the pacemaker only atrial depolarization (P waves) is seen, with complete standstill of the ventricles. With resumption of electrical pacing (indicated by the pacemaker impulses), ventricular complexes follow. (Electrocardiogram reduced in size.)

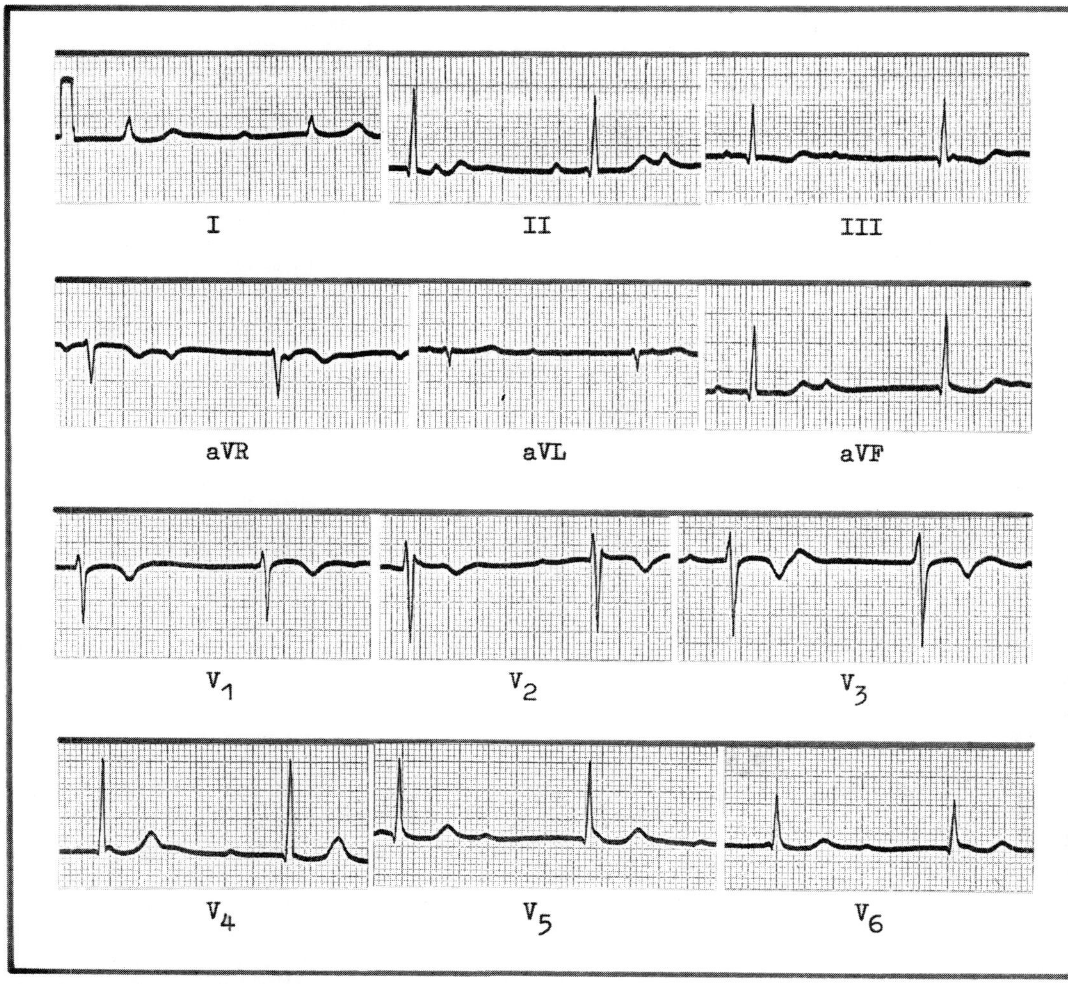

FIGURE 7–48. Congenital third degree (complete) A–V block in a young, asymptomatic patient. How would you treat this patient?
(Electrocardiogram reduced in size.)

The terms "atrioventricular block" and "atrioventricular dissociation" are often used interchangeably. *This is not correct.* You have just seen examples of third degree (complete) A–V block. A–V block is *not* synonymous with A–V dissociation. A–V dissociation merely means that the atria and ventricles are under separate control. A–V block is one category under A–V dissociation. Causes of A–V dissociation include:

1. Slowing or failure of the primary pacemaker (sinus), resulting in an escape rhythm (Fig. 7–9).
2. Acceleration of the subsidiary pacemaker (see Figs. 8–16 and 8–17, Chapter 8).
3. A–V block (complete) with slow idioventricular rhythm (Figs. 7–44A, 7–45A, 7–46A, 7–48).
4. Combination of Nos. 1, 2 and 3.

In closing this brief study of arrhythmias, remember that it is a very dynamic subject, and be ready to add new information to your foundation of knowledge.

8

DIGITALIS

Cassette Side 19

INTRODUCTION

In this chapter you will study some of the commonly seen electrocardiographic manifestations associated with digitalis *effects* and digitalis *toxicity*.

Although this is not a course in pharmacology and therapeutics, some salient features concerning this potent medication must be emphasized. It is a drug so often dispensed without much knowledge as to its effects and without recognition of specific evidence of toxicity. We occasionally hear of mistakes or drug accidents, such as reported in the *New York Times* several years ago (Fig. 8–1*A*). More recently, I received an urgent notice (Fig. 8–1*B*) from a drug house advising of a dosage error on a digitalis preparation. A physician who is familiar with the preparation and its dosage should recognize the typographical error immediately. The danger, however, arises when a physician who is unfamiliar with a preparation uses it according to the accompanying literature.

In a patient population, there is a spectrum response to an "average digitalizing" dose of a digitalis preparation. Each patient's treatment must be individualized and "tailored." Even the "average" dosage schedules represent a spectrum. At one end of the spectrum a certain number of patients will have digitalis toxicity, while at the other end a certain number will be underdigitalized (Fig. 8–1 *C*).

Because of the extent of the tragedy cited in Figure 8–1*A*, this example received worldwide attention, but it is not a rare nor isolated incident. Digitalis must not be used without thorough familiarity with its actions, its effects on the myocardium and on the periphery, its relationship to calcium and potassium metabolism and renal function, specific indications, contraindications and non-indications, preparations, dosage, absorption, excretion, interaction with concomitant medication, side effects and toxic manifestations. If you are not familiar with this information, even for the purpose of this course in electrocardiography, stop here and study the subject in one of the many good standard textbooks.

Digitalis can serve as the *prototype* for any medication in use today. A physician

THE NEW YORK TIMES, SUNDAY, JANUARY 8, 1967.

20 BELGIANS DEAD AFTER DRUG ERROR

Clerk Sent Wrong Substance to Clinic for Elderly

By CLYDE H. FARNSWORTH
Special to The New York Times

BRUSSELS, Jan. 7—An error made by a Brussels pharmaceutical house has resulted in the death of at least 20 elderly persons taking cancer treatment at a Belgian clinic.

It is one of the worst drug tragedies yet brought to public attention in Belgium and promises to stir new controversy in medicine. Belgium has had two doctor strikes in less than three years.

The drug house was identified in a brief announcement of the tragedy as the Arthur Gailly Clinic of Charleroi, an institution run by a Socialist insurance body.

An inexperienced stock clerk in the Brussels company substituted the drug Digitaline, a heart stimulant, for benzoate of estradiol, a hormone used in the treatment of cancer of the prostate.

The error was compounded, the clinic said, by the failure of pharmacists, both in the company and in the drug dispensary in the clinic, to take requisite control measures.

The clinic ordered 50 grams of the hormore in March, 1965, and instead of 50 grams of Digitaline.

The hormore can be admisistered in three daily doses of 10 milligrams each, while the maximum dosage for Digitaline is three milligrams daily.

After several of the patients died, doctors concluded that there was something wrong with the drug and asked the company to verify what it had delivered.

The company was unable to identify it. Last April a sample was sent to the drug control bureau of the Belgian Phammaceutical Association, which in a report last month said only that the product was not the hormone.

In the end a company pharmacist identified it as the heart drug. The long, involved process of identification came to a close with a letter from the company to the clinic saying that since digitaline is less expensive than the hormone, the clinic was being given a credit.

Of the 50 grams that the clinic received 23 grams were dispensed to patients. No one is sure how many patients died from the dosage.

There was public anger and bitterness. It was asked why it took so long to make the identification and bring the matter to public notice.

The law makes drug companies responsible for what they sell, but some of the blame is almost certain to fall on the clinic, especially since it is of the type that is already under heavy criticism from doctors.

The Socialist clinics pay their doctors a flat salary and have a reputation for mass production treatment in which individual patients get short shrift.

The doctors 'organizations believe the standards would rise if the doctors were paid according to the scale and kind of work they do.

A

FIGURE 8–1. *A*, © 1967 by the New York Times Company. Reprinted by permission.
Illustration continued on following page.

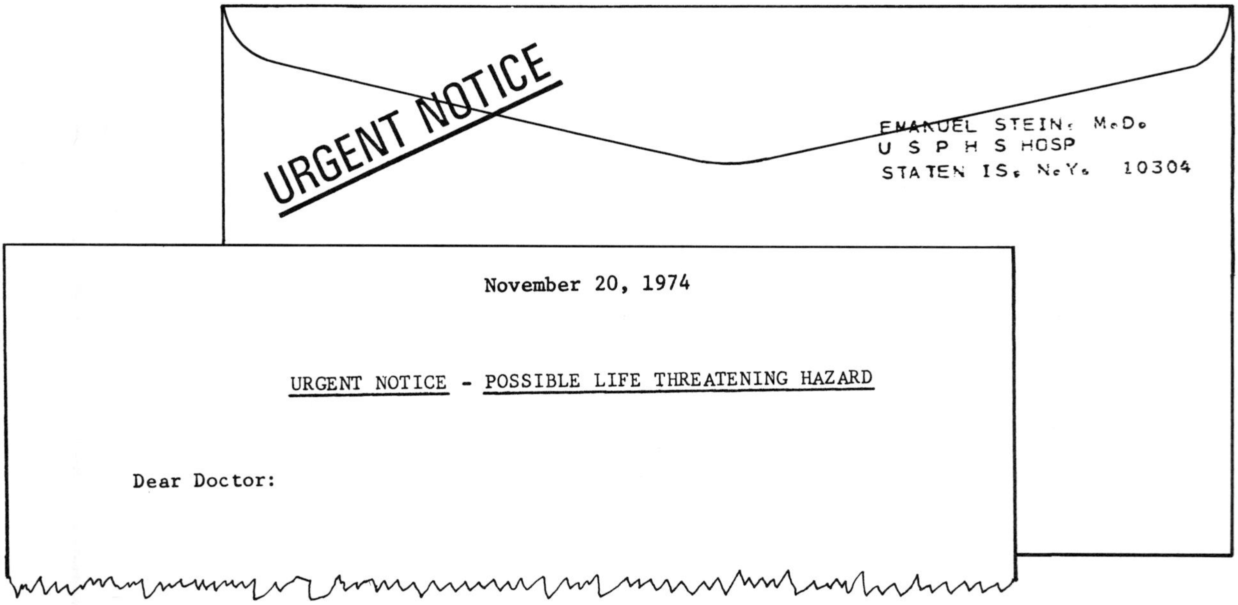
URGENT NOTICE

EMANUEL STEIN, M.D.
U S P H S HOSP
STATEN IS. N.Y. 10304

November 20, 1974

URGENT NOTICE - POSSIBLE LIFE THREATENING HAZARD

Dear Doctor:

FIGURE 8–1 *Continued. B,* Notification of a typographical dosage error in the literature accompanying a digitalis preparation.

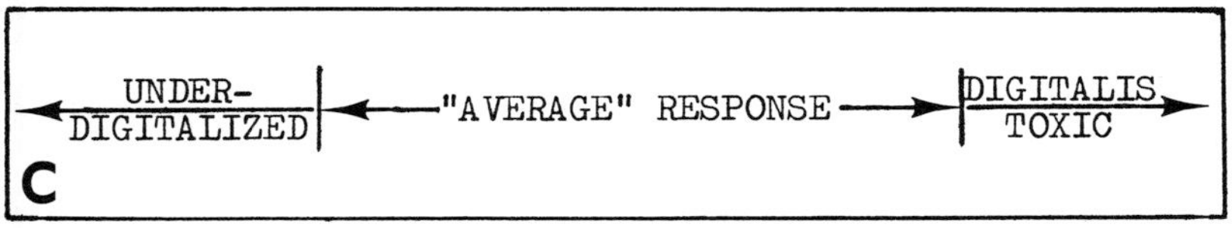

FIGURE 8–1 *Continued. C,* Response to an "average digitalizing" dose of a digitalis preparation.

must never affix his signature to a prescription or hand out samples without knowledge of the information listed above. How many times has the practicing cardiologist seen a patient in consultation who had been given digitalis and told to take the pills until the onset of nausea without a baseline electrocardiogram having been taken? Whether using digitalis to treat congestive heart failure or an arrhythmia, always keep the end points of the spectrum response in mind, relative to a given patient. Patients' responses may be quite variable and unpredictable, and careful follow-up is essential. How many times has the practicing cardiologist seen a patient who was given a digitalizing dose of a digitalis preparation for congestive heart failure, instructed about maintenance dosage and told to come back one month later? A sense of exhilaration is often prevalent in digitalized patients who feel better after having been in congestive heart failure. They remember the dramatic response to the digitalizing dose, and when they are not feeling well, even though it may be due to overdosage, they will take more tablets of digitalis, returning to the physician severely ill with digitalis toxicity. If this stage is missed, the next may be a complete halt of heart action—death caused by a "lifesaving" medicine. Patient instruction and understanding of the drug's actions are as vital as careful and frequent patient follow-up.

Perspectives must be kept in mind. However universal digitalis may be, it is used to treat certain signs and symptoms. What is presently needed is a way to prevent or remove the "cause" of these signs and symptoms. This is the subject of intensive investigation today.

William Withering, in the eighteenth

century, noted the beneficial effects of the foxglove plant on "dropsy." He wrote:

The Foxglove's leaves, with caution given,
Another proof of favouring Heav'n
    Will happily display;
The rapid pulse it can abate;
The hectic flush can moderate
And, blest by Him whose will is fate,
May give a lengthen'd day.*

Withering studied digitalis, the product of the foxglove plant and observed that "it has a power over the motion of the heart to a degree yet unobserved in any other medicine, and this power may be converted to salutory ends."†

Some of the electrocardiograms in this chapter have already been seen in previous chapters; the study of digitalis effects, and especially digitalis toxicity, is a study of *repolarization alterations, conduction disturbances* and *arrhythmias*. This chapter will serve as both a review and a reminder that digitalis, a most common medicine in cardiology today, may be both a blessing and a curse—a blessing for its "salutory" action on the heart and a curse in that it is so common a cause of devastating arrhythmias and drug toxicity.

*From L. S. Goodman and A. Gilman: The Pharmacological Basis of Therapeutics. New York, The Macmillan Company, 1956. Used by permission.
†Idem.

A. Electrocardiographic Manifestations of Digitalis

1. *Digitalis Effects on Ventricular Repolarization (S–T Segment and T Wave)*

Digitalis is commonly used to treat congestive heart failure as well as arrhythmias such as atrial fibrillation, atrial flutter and paroxysmal atrial tachycardia (when these arrhythmias are *not* caused by digitalis).

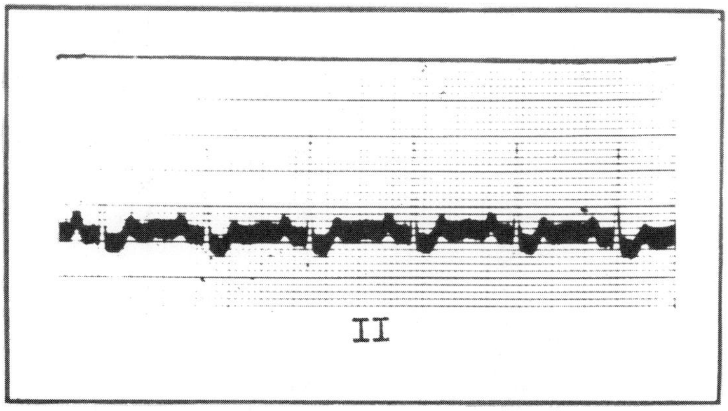

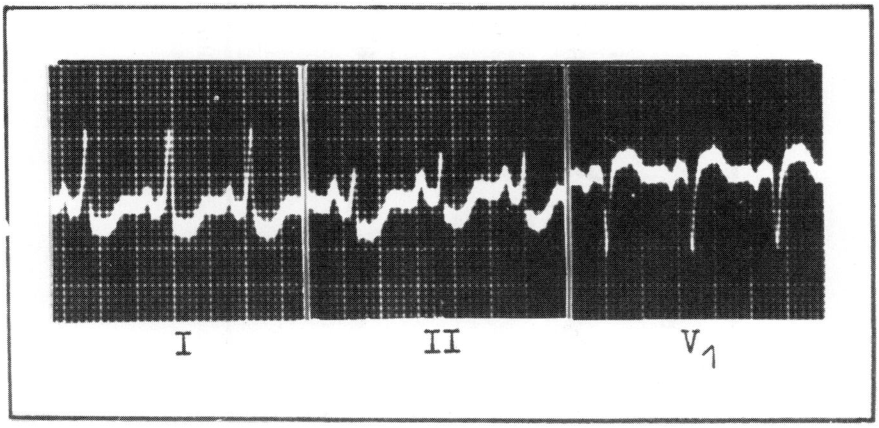

FIGURE 8–2. "Classical" alterations of the S–T segment caused by digitalis in two patients.
(Electrocardiograms reduced in size.)

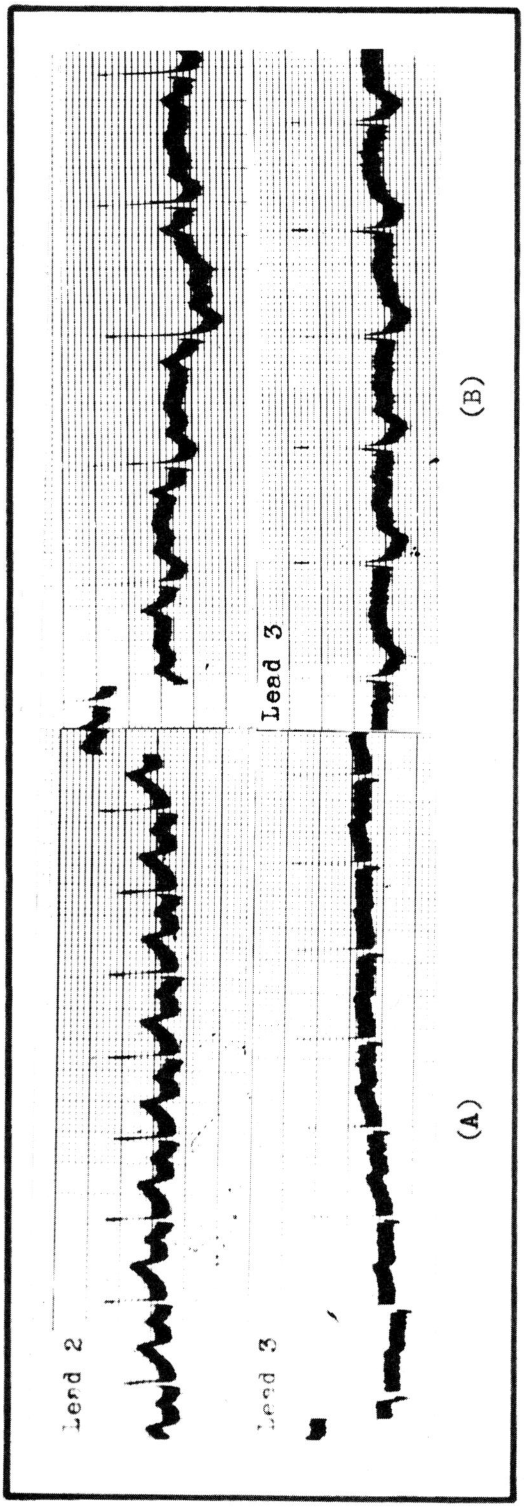

FIGURE 8–3. Before (*A*) and after (*B*) "digitalization." Describe these changes. (Electrocardiogram reduced in size.)

The electrocardiogram may be very helpful in following patients taking digitalis. Electrocardiographically, digitalis effects are seen in the ventricular repolarization phase affecting the S–T segment and the T wave. The whole repolarization phase may be accelerated, hence a shorter Q–T interval. The "classical" alterations of digitalis are described as a "fist-like" depression of the S–T segment (as if you were placing your fist in the S–T segment and depressing it), as "paint-brush" inscription (as if you were painting the S–T segment with gradual widening of the paint brush as you approach the S–T segment from the downslope of the R wave), or as "scooping" of the S–T segment. The elevation of the S–T segment in lead V_1 (Fig. 8–2) represents the same phenomenon as the S–T segment depression in leads I and II. With a good imagination you should have no difficulty with these descriptions. Figure 8–3 compares the electrocardiograms before and after digitalis administration.

As seen earlier, in our study of the S–T segment and T wave (Chapter 4), the repolarization phase of the ventricles is the energy consuming phase, the active phase, as compared with depolarization, and is therefore, more labile and more prone to alterations. It is best to study the repolarization phase as a unit, including both the S–T segment and the T wave, rather than trying to ascribe one set of rules to the S–T segment and another set to the T wave. Although early repolarization changes affecting the S–T segment are considered a classic sign of digitalis effect, late repolarization changes affecting the T wave may be seen even as the first, and often as the only, effect. This is well illustrated in our studies with digitalis. Review Figures 4–13 to 4–17 in Chapter 4. In a significant number of patients it was not possible to predict which part, or whether the entire phase (both the S–T segment and the T wave), of repolarization would be affected. This again stresses the need to follow each patient very closely without relying on "predictable" changes. Due to the increased lability of the repolarization phase in patients taking digitalis, a *positive* exercise test might not be reliable in these patients.

2. *Digitalis Effects on Atrio-Ventricular Conduction*

The question has frequently arisen as to whether prolongation of the P–R interval represents digitalis *effect* or digitalis *toxicity*. In our studies of effect of digitalis on atrioventricular conduction no significant differences were noted in the P–R interval at rest. As the rate of the heart was increased by atrial pacing, however, atrioventricular conduction time was prolonged as an effect of digitalis, resulting in a significant prolongation of the P–R interval. His bundle studies confirmed that the increase was within the interval from the atrial deflection to the His bundle deflection (A–H interval). Clinically, an increase in the *baseline* P–R interval, or advancement to higher degrees of A–V block, as seen in Figure 8–4 *A* and *B*, has been associated with *toxic* manifestations of digitalis. Although the subject of digitalis toxicity will be studied in a later section of this chapter, it is introduced here to emphasize the importance of close and careful patient follow-up.

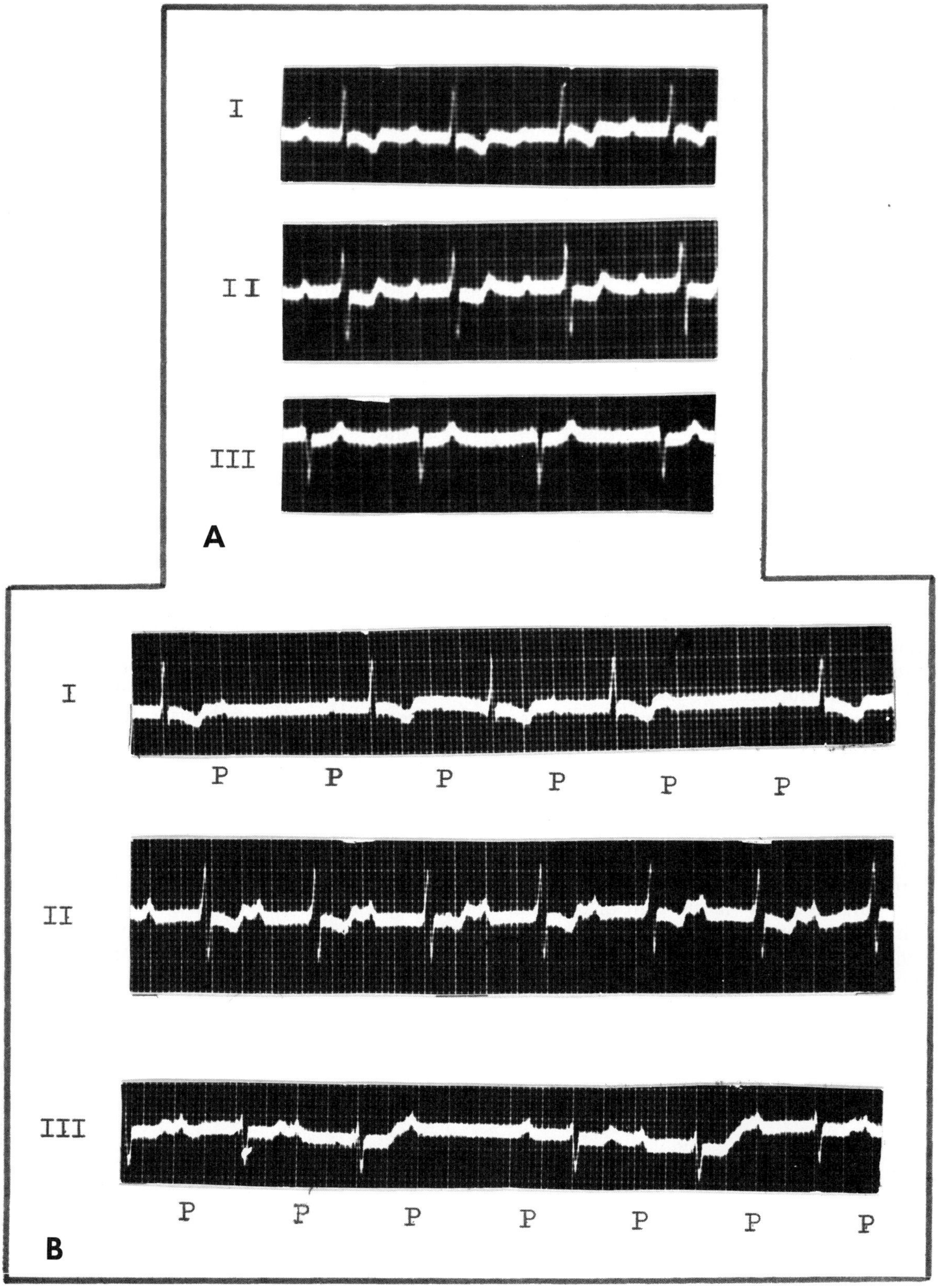

FIGURE 8–4. Progressive atrioventricular block due to digitalis, representing digitalis toxicity (see text above). *A,* First degree A–V block; *B,* progression of A–V block.

3. *Digitalis Effects on an Arrhythmia (Atrial Fibrillation with a Rapid Ventricular Response)*

Figure 8–5*A* and *B* illustrate an effect of digitalis on atrial fibrillation with a rapid ventricular response. The patient was a 35 year old man with mitral valve disease who presented with atrial fibrillation and a ventricular rate of approximately 125 beats per minute on an inadequate dose of digitalis. With proper adjustment of the dose the ventricular rate fell to approximately 75 beats per minute.

Atrial fibrillation with a rapid ventricular response is an excellent arrhythmia for the study of digitalis effects on heart rate. In normal sinus rhythm digitalis does not have much effect on the ventricular rate per se. In atrial fibrillation with, for instance, 500 atrial impulses per minute, the majority of these are blocked in the atrioventricular conduction system. However, if one impulse of every four reaches the ventricles in an irregular way, the average ventricular rate would be 125 beats per minute. Digitalis acts on the A–V conduction system and, by altering the

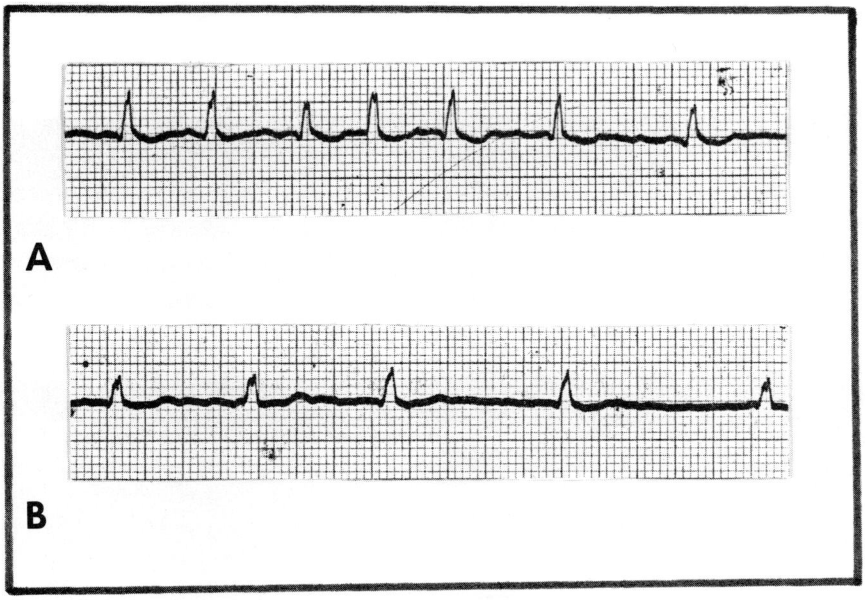

FIGURE 8–5. Digitalis effects on atrial fibrillation with rapid ventricular response (see text). *A*, Baseline; *B*, following increase in digitalis dosage.

effective refractory period, allows fewer impulses to get through. The atrial rate may increase—e.g., from 500 to 600 impulses per minute. The net effect of this would be that instead of an atrial rate of 500 per minute with a 4 : 1 ratio and a ventricular rate of 125 per minute, there would be an atrial rate of 600 per minute with an 8 : 1 ratio and a ventricular rate of 75 per minute. In atrial fibrillation (long-standing) the aim of digitalis therapy is not to convert to sinus rhythm but to slow the ventricular rate.

In spite of the good response with digitalis, the physician must use caution in treating a patient with this arrhythmia. Patients respond in different ways to overdosage of digitalis. As more and more digitalis is given, for instance to a patient with baseline atrial fibrillation or flutter-fibrillation, that patient may show no irritability of the heart whatever, no premature contractions and no tachycardia. The ventricular rate may, however, decrease from 125 to 85 to 75 to 60 to 50 to 40 and so on down to the point where the heart stops (see Fig. 8–6). Responses may not be predictable. This example of digitalis toxicity (Fig. 8–6) is introduced at this point to caution physicians treating patients with atrial fibrillation. Careful follow-up is essential.

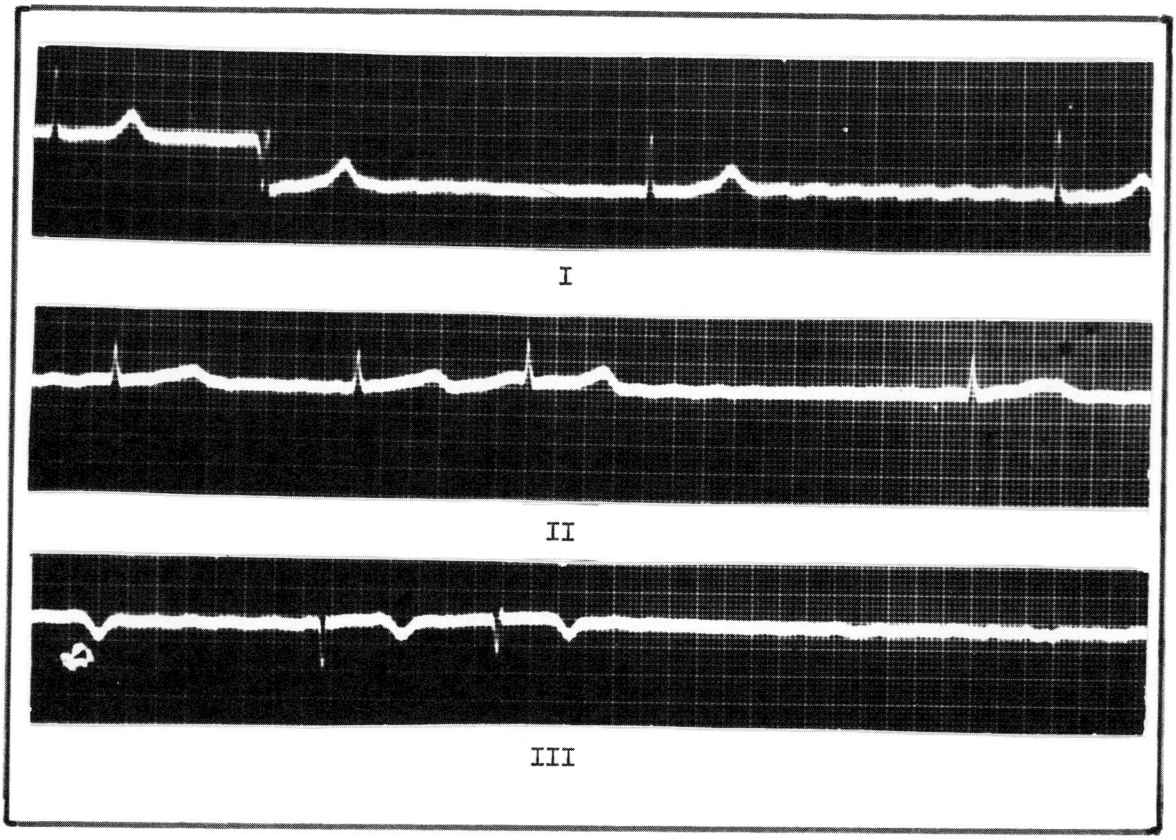

FIGURE 8–6. Digitalis toxicity. See text above. (Electrocardiogram reduced in size.)

Cassette Side 20

B. Electrocardiographic Manifestations of Digitalis Toxicity

The prevalence of digitalis toxicity must be continually emphasized and both the physician and the patient must be ever watchful—all the more so because toxic manifestations do not necessarily mean that the dose has been changed. The response may be altered by changes in absorption caused by gastrointestinal upset, by electrolyte imbalance due to diuretics, and so forth. Remember also that toxicity may be manifest before any therapeutic effects of digitalis are seen.

In a course in electrocardiography major emphasis must be placed on the electrocardiographic manifestations of digitalis, and it has often been stated that a study of digitalis includes a study of all of electrocardiography. A knowledge of digitalis, however, in all its facets, is vital; this has been emphasized. It is not possible to accurately predict which sign or signs of digitalis toxicity a given patient may develop. All the more care is necessary since, not infrequently, a patient may "feel better" while in digitalis toxicity. This has been seen many times, especially when a rapid heart rate is effectively reduced by alternate premature beats of the ventricle, or by alternate sinoatrial block. More than a cursory "How do you feel?" and quick pulse check are necessary in following a patient taking digitalis. Knowledge of the subject must be combined with knowledge of, and interest in, the patient.

1. Depressed Sinoatrial (S–A) Pacemaker Leading to:

a. Atrial Fibrillation. When the sinoatrial pacemaker is depressed by digitalis and sinus rhythm is no longer dominant, another rhythm must supervene for the patient to continue living. A most important rule to remember is that an arrhythmia or conduction disturbance developing in a patient on digitalis should be considered as resulting from digitalis.

Atrial fibrillation may replace sinus rhythm when the atria become disorganized upon suppression of the S–A node (Fig. 8–7). Note the electrocardiographic signs of digitalis effect. It is important to know the patient and to have baseline electrocardiograms available. The onset of atrial fibrillation in a patient with normal sinus rhythm may be paroxysmal and not necessarily related to the administration of digitalis.

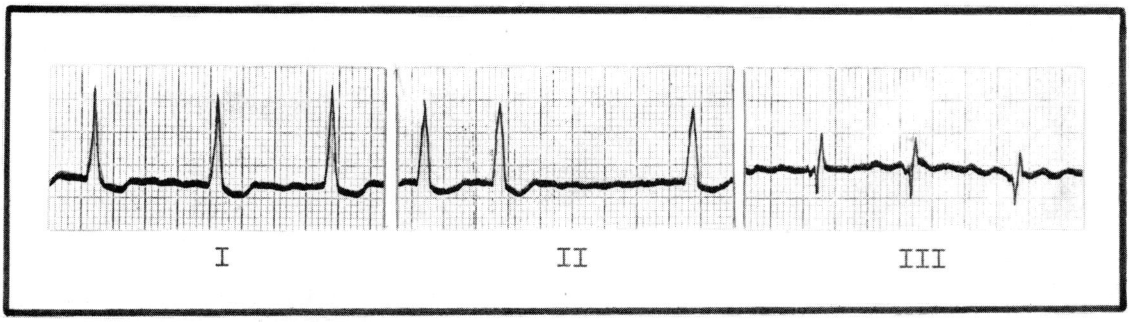

FIGURE 8–7. Atrial fibrillation in a patient with suppression of the S–A node due to digitalis. (Electrocardiogram reduced in size.)

b. Atrial Flutter. Atrial flutter is a rare arrhythmia in a patient with digitalis toxicity. It must be considered, however, lest the patient receive more digitalis in an attempt to "break" the flutter. The onset of atrial flutter, especially with a high degree of atrioventricular block, should arouse suspicion in a digitalized patient. Figures 8–8 and 8–9 are examples of atrial flutter with varying atrioventricular block.

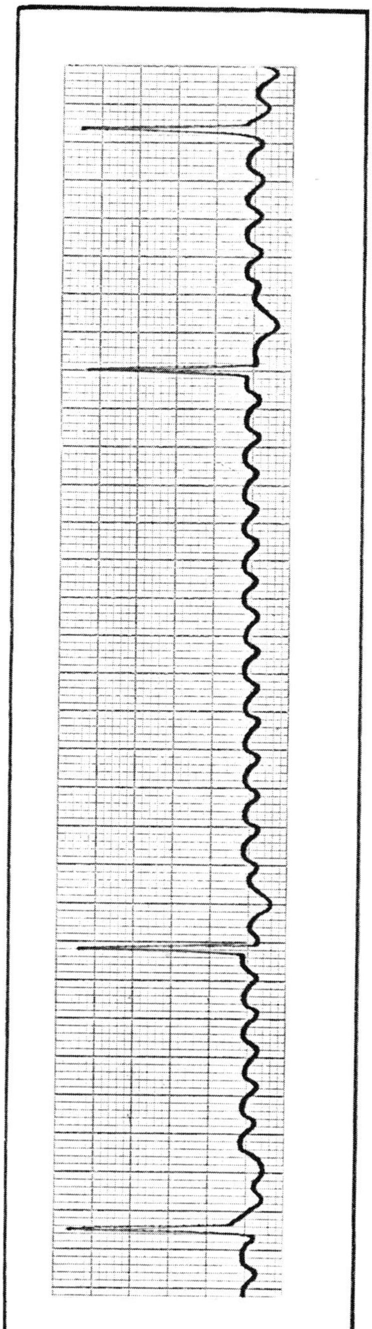

FIGURE 8–8. Atrial flutter with high degree of A–V block.

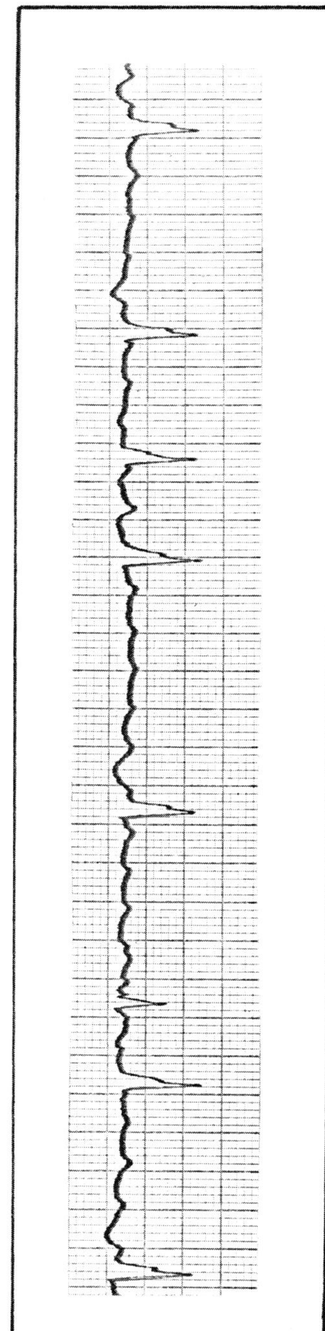

FIGURE 8–9. Atrial flutter with varying A–V block.

c. Paroxysmal Atrial Tachycardia. Paroxysmal atrial tachycardia with atrioventricular block is a common arrhythmia in digitalis toxicity. In fact, paroxysmal atrial tachycardia with atrioventricular block represents digitalis toxicity until proved otherwise (Fig. 8–10).

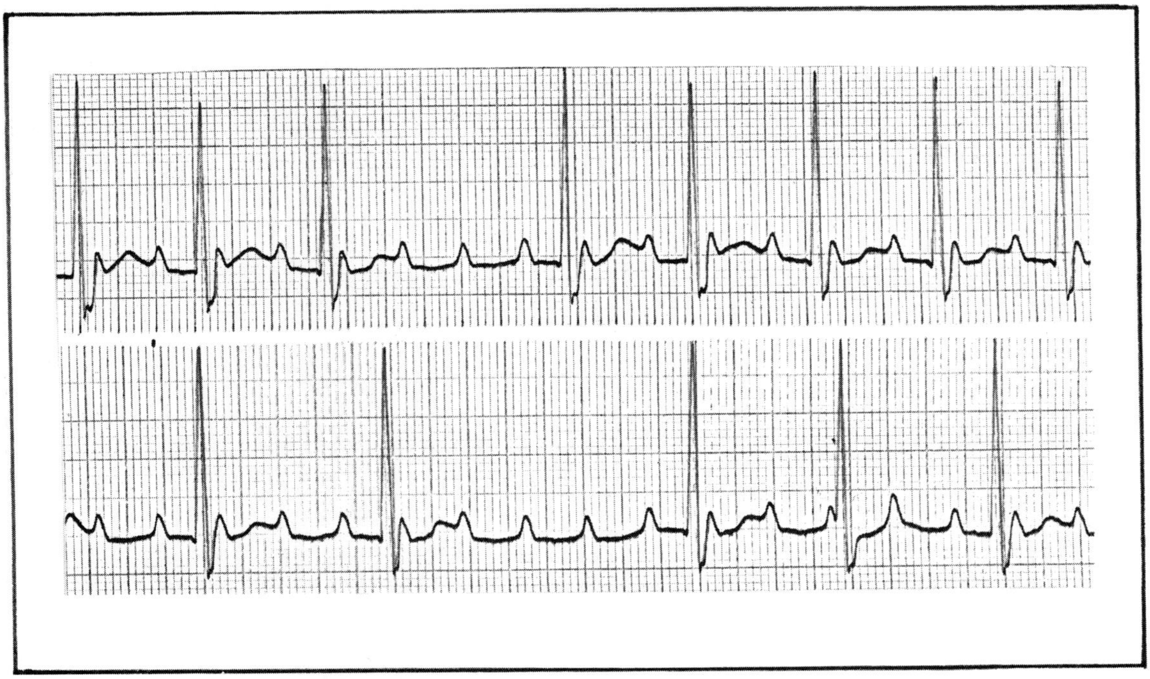

FIGURE 8–10. Paroxysmal atrial tachycardia with varying A–V block.

Atrial tachycardia with 1 : 1 atrioventricular conduction (no A–V block) is usually *not* due to digitalis toxicity (Fig. 8–11). An esophageal lead recording may help establish the diagnosis since P waves are not obvious. Digitalis was used to terminate the tachycardia.

The paroxysmal tachycardia with 1 : 1 atrioventricular conduction heralded by premature atrial contractions seen in Figure 8–12 is also *unlikely* to be due to digitalis toxicity. Digitalis was used to treat the arrhythmia.

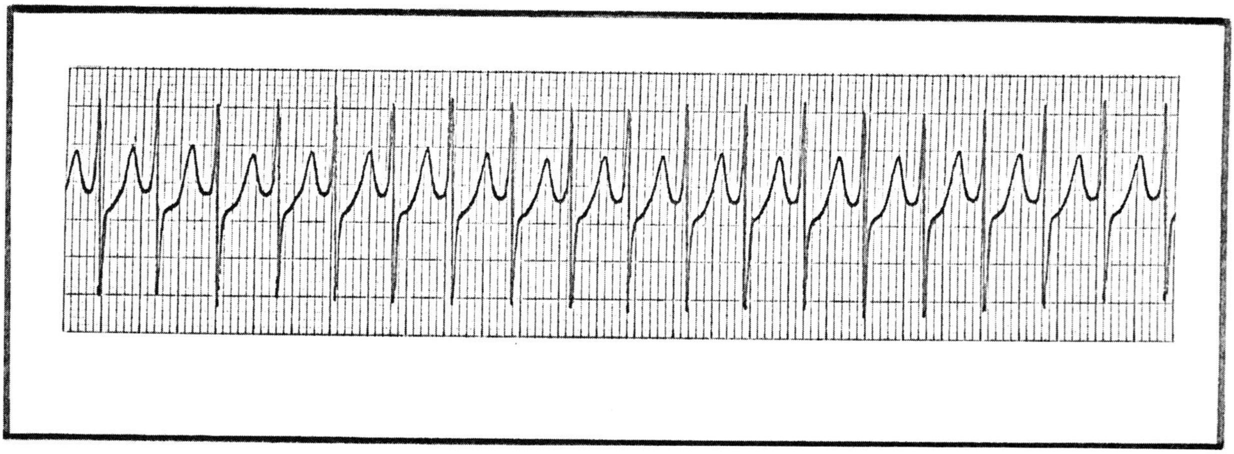

FIGURE 8–11. Paroxysmal atrial tachycardia with 1:1 A–V conduction (no A–V block).

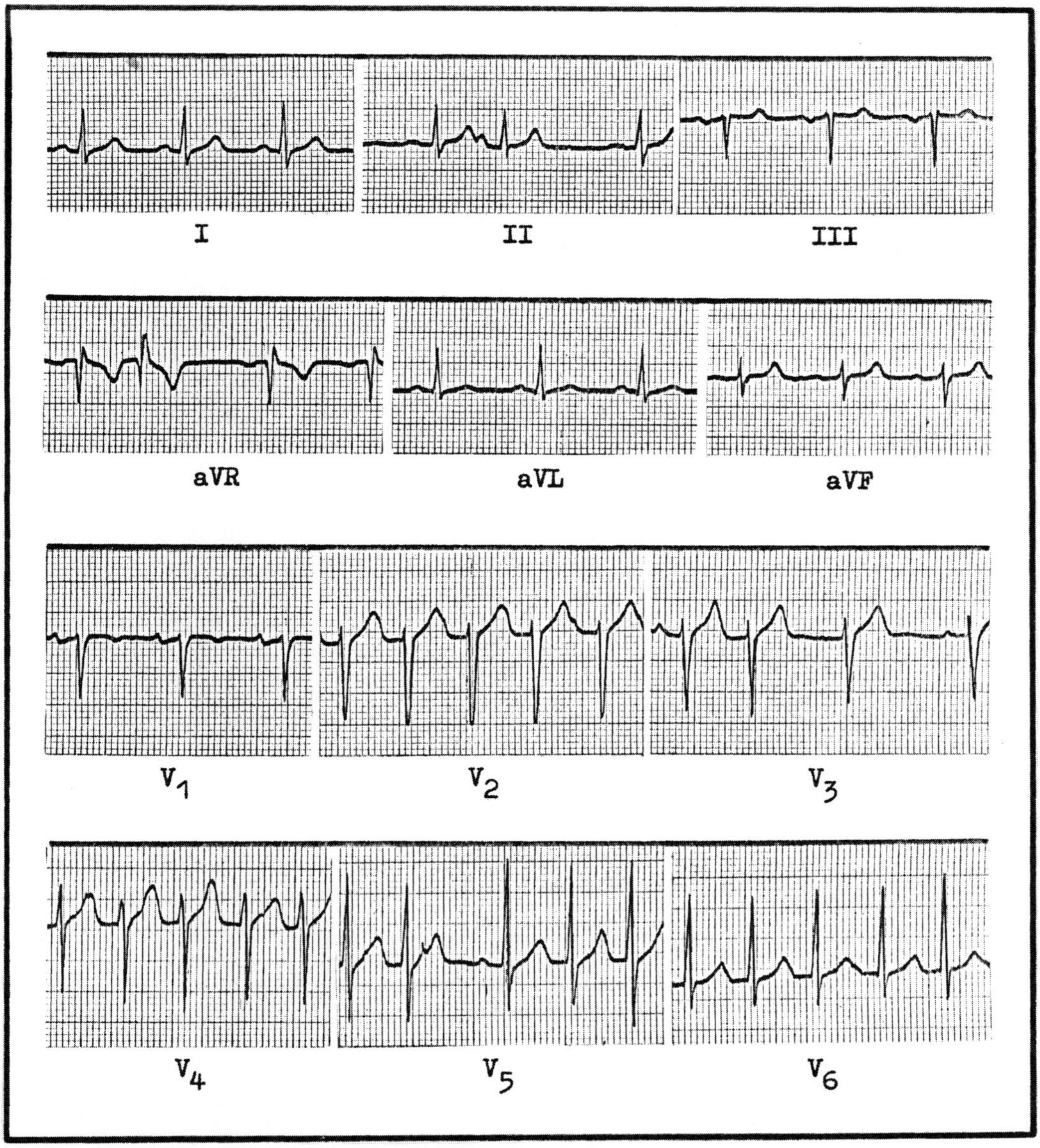

FIGURE 8–12. Premature beats of the atria and paroxysms of atrial tachycardia. (Electrocardiogram reduced in size.)

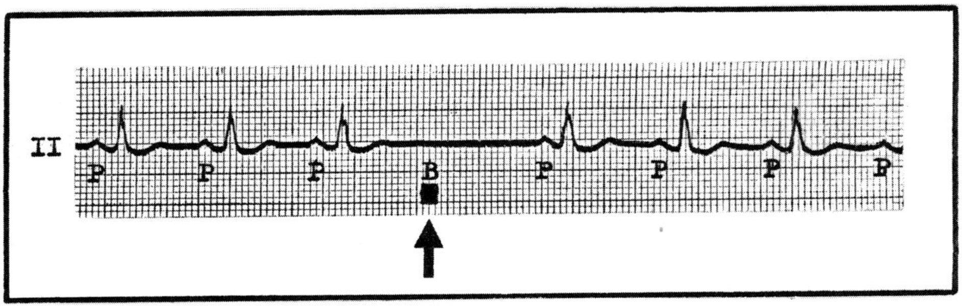

FIGURE 8–13. S–A block.
(Electrocardiogram reduced in size.)

d. Sinoatrial (S–A) Block. The sinoatrial node is believed to initiate the impulse but the propagation is blocked, so that the atria are not depolarized and hence, there is no P wave. The pause is a multiple of the regular cycle length. The block, represented by the letter *B* in Figure 8–13 is seen where the P wave should normally be. This may be an exceedingly dangerous arrhythmia in that every other beat may be blocked, with a resulting low rate. The physician may consider the patient well digitalized with a regular rhythm, instead of digitalis toxic. The next stage may be sinus arrest, with no other pacemaker taking over, and death of the patient.

e. Sinus Arrest. Sinus arrest is a sudden failure of the sinoatrial node to initiate an expected impulse (Fig. 8–14); it is a failure of impulse *formation,* rather than a failure of impulse propagation. If no other pacemaker becomes dominant at this point, death quickly follows.

f. Coronary Sinus Rhythm. Always beware of a change in rhythm in a digitalized patient; it may be an ominous sign. In Figure 8–15*B* we see the onset of coronary sinus rhythm without a significant change in heart rate. If the physician checks the pulse rate for 15 sec. and sends the patient on his way, this ectopic rhythm

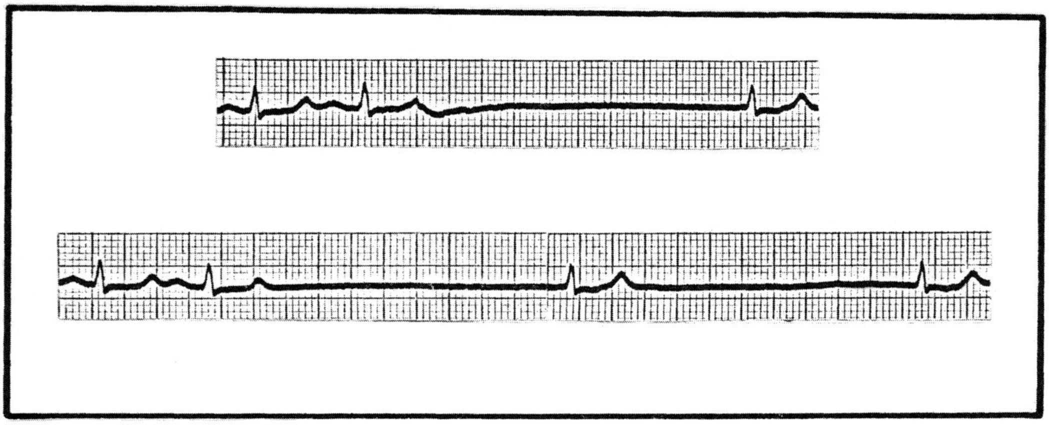

FIGURE 8–14. Sinus arrest with junctional escape.
(Electrocardiogram reduced in size.)

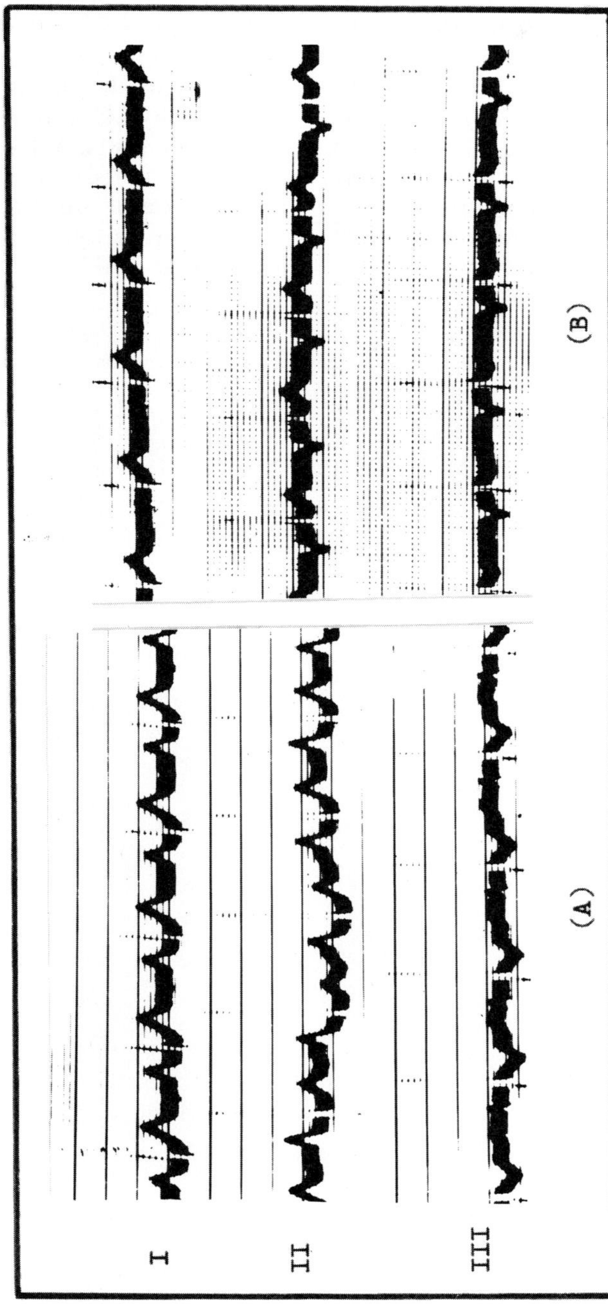

FIGURE 8–15. Onset of coronary sinus rhythm (*B*) in a patient taking digitalis; there is no significant change in heart rate.
(Electrocardiogram reduced in size.)

is missed, possibly forfeiting the only chance to detect digitalis toxicity.

2. *Junctional Rhythm*

Atrioventricular dissociation due to acceleration of the junctional pacemaker is frequently seen in digitalis toxicity. In Figure 8–16 the junctional rhythm of the atria, causing the P waves to "merge" with the QRS complexes. The junctional rhythm, although the rate is under 70 per minute, is really a *junctional tachycardia* because the junctional pacemaker is faster than its maximum inherent rate of 60 per minute.

Figure 8–17 is from a patient with more advanced digitalis toxicity. The rate of the junctional pacemaker is between 95 and 100 per minute, and the atrial rate, under sinus control, is between 80 and 90 per minute.

Review the "nodal" rhythms in Chapter 7. Although we use the term "junctional" rhythm you should be familiar with the terminology of "upper, middle and lower nodal" rhythms. What are some of the newer thoughts regarding the origin and propagation of these rhythms?

Another arrhythmia seen in digitalis toxicity is "bidirectional tachycardia,"

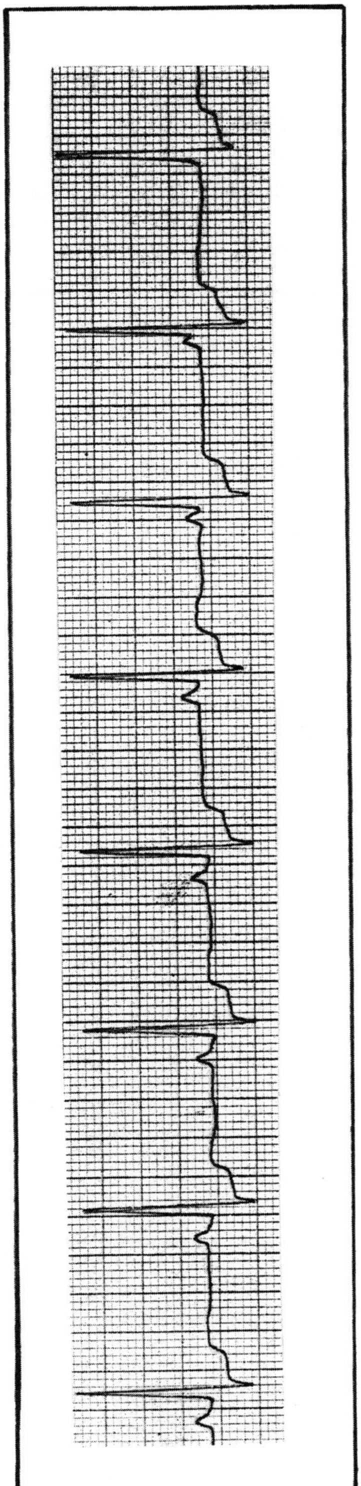

FIGURE 8–16. Acceleration of junctional pacemaker resulting in A–V dissociation in digitalis toxicity. The P waves "merge" with the QRS complexes.

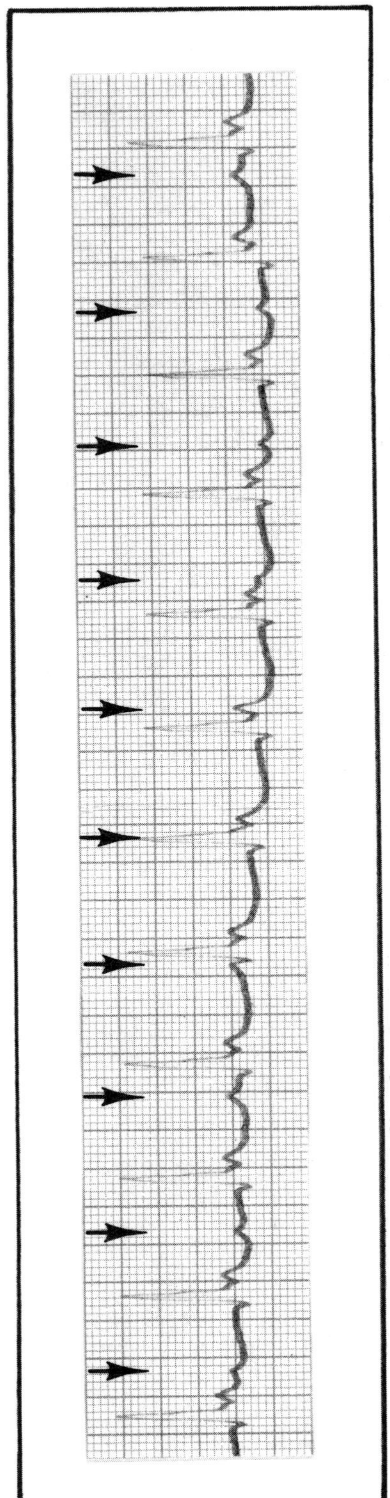

FIGURE 8–17. Junctional tachycardia with A–V dissociation in a digitalis toxic patient. The arrows point to the slower sinus P waves "marching through" the QRS complexes.

illustrated in Figure 8–18. Digitalis, although in low dose, may have added to the already irritable heart in this patient with a myocardial infarction. It is often not possible to determine the origin of impulse formation from the clinical electrocardiogram. We see a rightward and anterior vector alternating with a leftward and posterior vector. Is the pacemaker in the "nodal" or "junctional" area, with alternate block as the impulse passes down the anterior and posterior divisions of the left bundle? Are there two separate supraventricular sites of impulse formation, one in the atria and one in the "junctional" area, both in the atria or both in the "junctional" area? Is one pacemaker above the bundle of His and one below? Is this a bigeminal rhythm with alternate premature beats from a lower pacemaker? These remain important questions; hopefully, the answers will be forthcoming.

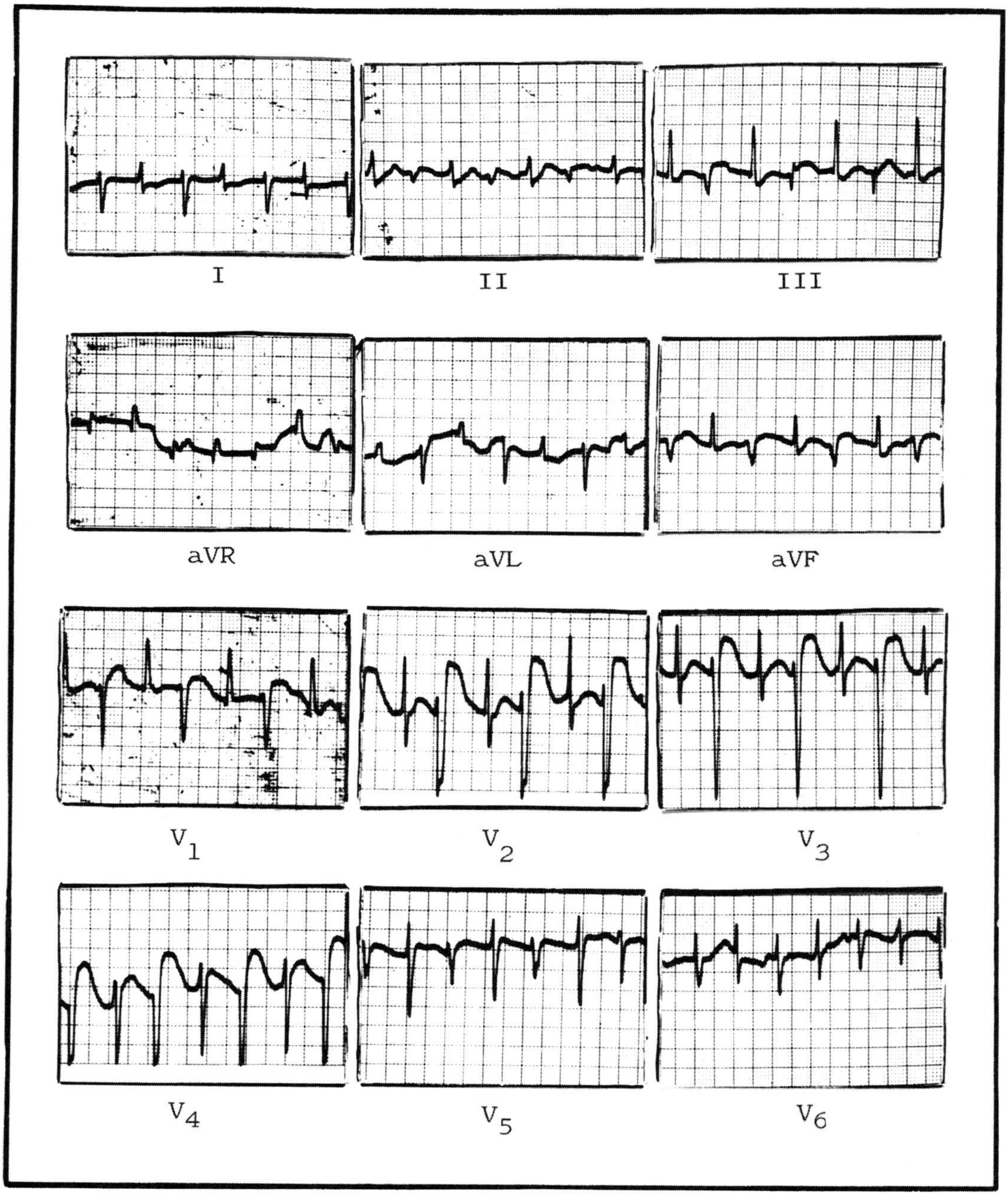

FIGURE 8–18. Bidirectional tachycardia. (Electrocardiogram reduced in size.)

3. *Increased Ventricular Irritability or Automaticity Leading to:*

a. Premature Beats of the Ventricle. Premature beats of the ventricle are common in digitalis toxicity. When they originate in more than one focus they are said to be multifocal, as seen in Figure 8–19. Note the different contours of the premature ventricular contractions. The multifocal origin of these beats is ominous, revealing an irritable heart. The next stages may be ventricular tachycardia, ventricular fibrillation and death.

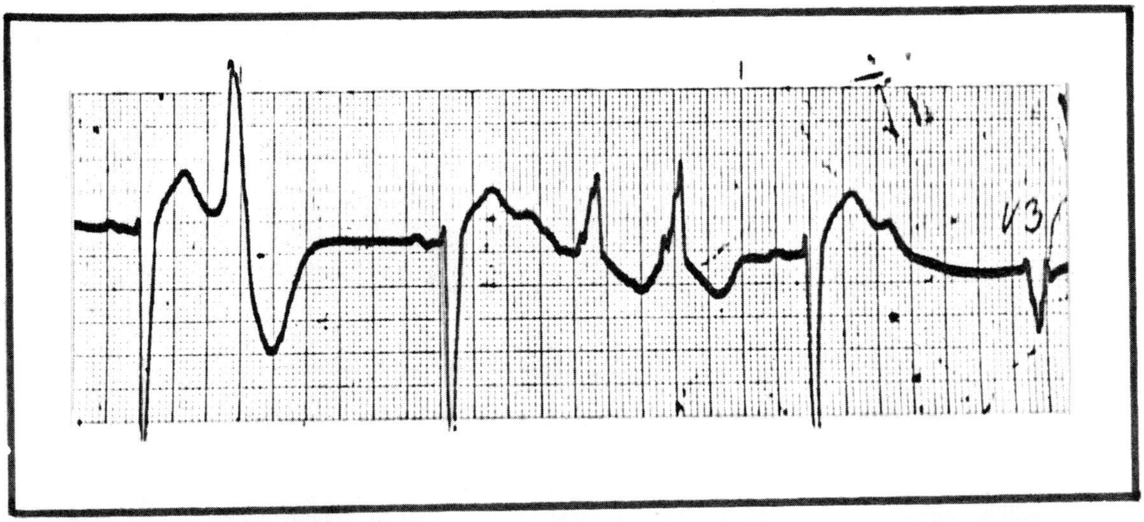

FIGURE 8–19. Multifocal premature ventricular contractions. In patients with chronic heart disease and premature ventricular contractions it may be extremely difficult to decide whether the premature ventricular contractions are secondary to the intrinsic heart disease or to the digitalis. This is also true of the high degree of atrioventricular block discussed at the end of this chapter. You must know your patient. (Electrocardiogram reduced in size.)

b. Group Beating (Bigeminy) Due to Alternate Premature Beats of the Ventricle. When the premature beats of the ventricle are of the same contour in any given lead they are said to be unifocal, from one ventricular focus. Figure 8–20 is from a patient with digitalis toxicity and is an example of bigeminy due to alternate premature beats of the ventricle. Note the fixed interval between the normal beat and the premature beat.

That physicians, like the rest of mankind, do not learn from history is well illustrated by the electrocardiographic tracings in Figure 8–21. On July 6 the patient arrived, digitalis toxic, with a very low effective heart rate and alternate premature beats of the ventricle (bigeminy). Digitalis was discontinued and the rate gradually increased until July 11, when digitalis treatment was restarted. On August 2 the patient was back to where he was on July 6. Although this sequence of events occurred decades ago, it is being repeated to this very day.

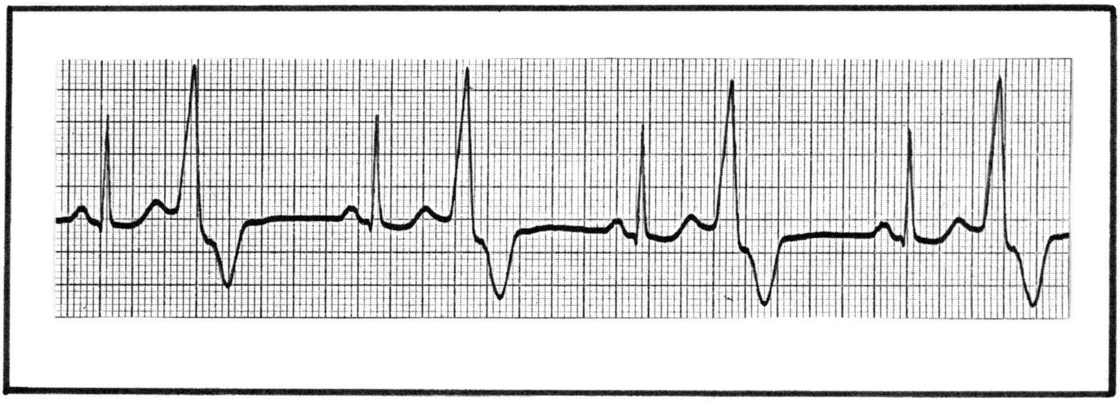

FIGURE 8–20. Bigeminy in a digitalis toxic patient. (Electrocardiogram reduced in size.)

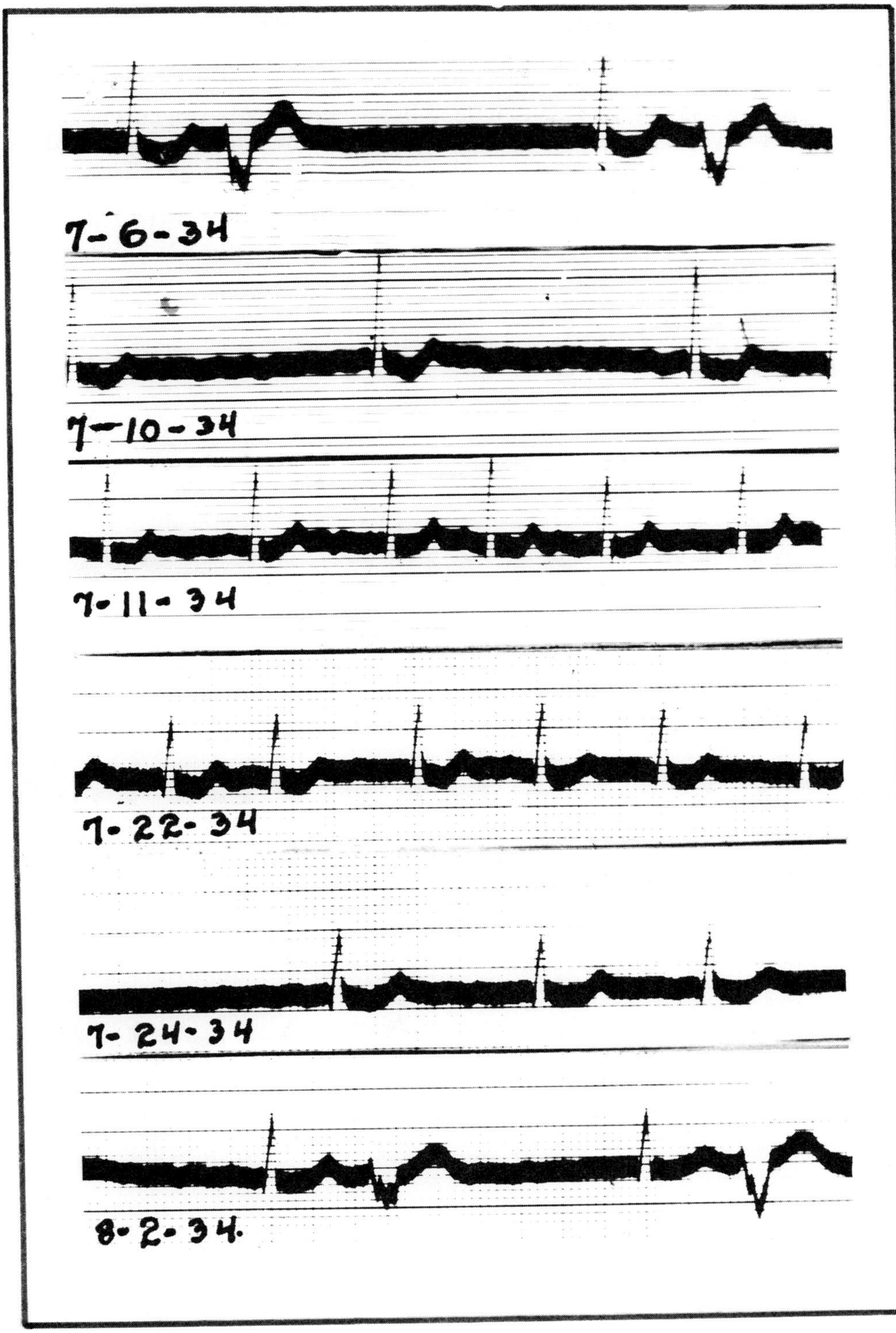

FIGURE 8–21. Patient with atrial fibrillation and digitalis toxicity (see text). (Electrocardiogram enlarged for clarity.)

4. *Atrioventricular (A–V) Conduction Disturbances Leading to:*

a. Marked First Degree A–V Block. As seen earlier (review discussion of digitalis effects on A–V conduction, also Figs. 8–4 *A* and *B*), clinically, an increase in the baseline P–R interval, or advancement to higher degrees of A–V block, has been associated with *toxic* manifestations of digitalis. This stage (Fig. 8–22) should not be missed, since it is a step along the path to disaster. An electrocardiographic rhythm tracing, at the very least, should be taken since the pulse rate may not change.

A patient may present with various rhythms during stages of digitalis toxicity. Figures 8–23*A* and *B* are from a digitalis toxic patient who had both first degree atrioventricular block and atrial flutter at different times. You must know your patient and have serial electrocardiograms to be sure that the atrial flutter is not merely a coincidental paroxysmal arrhythmia.

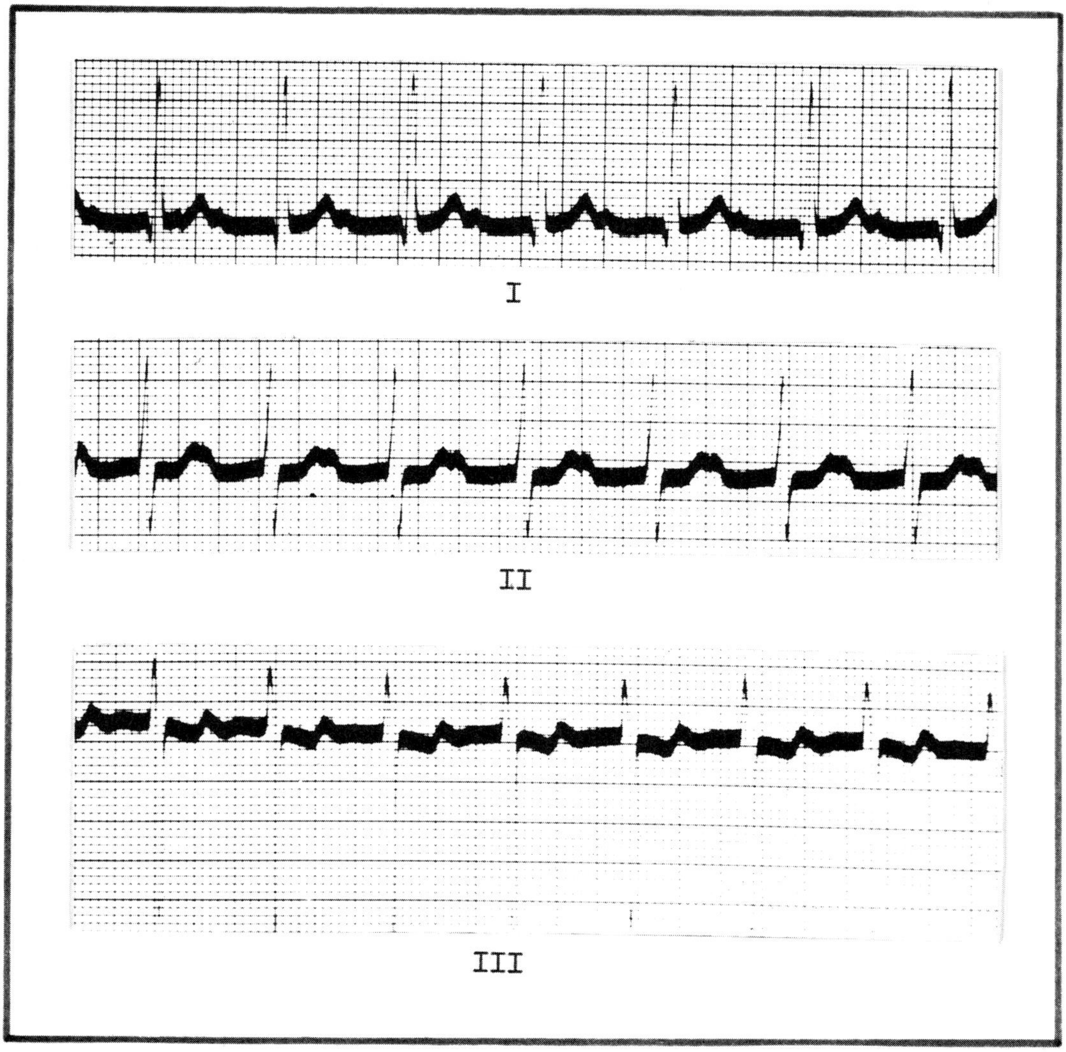

FIGURE 8–22. Marked first degree A–V block. (Electrocardiogram enlarged for clarity.)

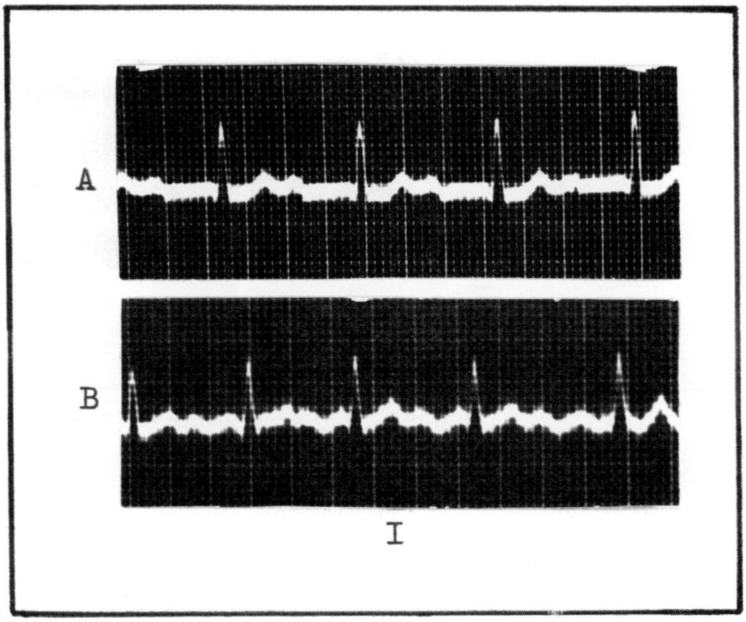

FIGURE 8–23. First degree A–V block (*A*) and atrial flutter (*B*) may be manifestations of digitalis toxicity. (Electrocardiogram enlarged for clarity.)

b. Second Degree A–V Block. A form of second degree A–V block is what is known as a Mobitz I block or the classical Wenckebach block. Ventricular beats are "dropped" in a cyclic manner. The P–R interval is less prolonged at first but becomes progressively longer until an atrial contraction no longer initiates a ventricular response. The cycle is then resumed. In Figure 8–24 the first P–R interval is shorter than the second and the third P wave does not conduct (first arrow). The fourth P wave starts the cycle again. The seventh P wave does not conduct (second arrow) and the cycle begins again with the eighth P wave. The block in Wenckebach periods has usually been shown to be above the bundle of His (by the use of His bundle recordings), presumably in the A–V node. Note that

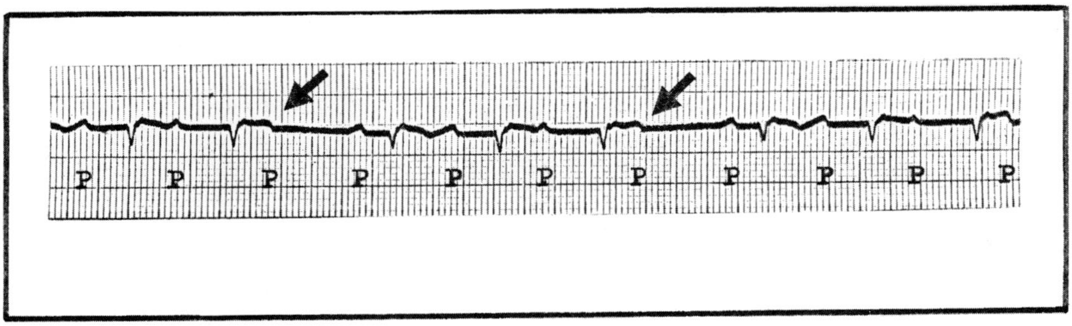

FIGURE 8–24. Mobitz I (Wenckebach) block. (Electrocardiogram reduced in size.)

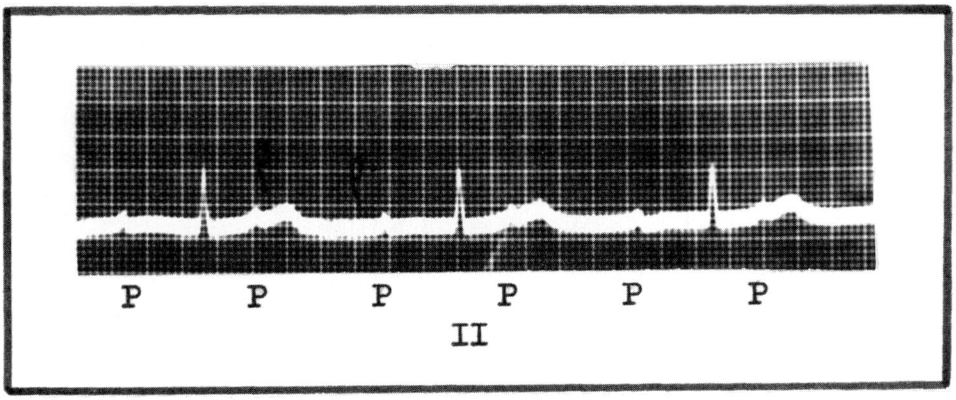

FIGURE 8–25. Second degree A–V block. (Electrocardiogram reduced in size.)

before the "dropped" ventricular beat, as the P–R intervals are progressively prolonged, the R–R intervals shorten.

Figure 8–25 is another example of second degree A–V block. Here only every second P wave conducts through to the ventricle. The ventricular rate is one half the atrial rate.

c. Third Degree (Complete) A–V Block. In third degree (complete) A–V block there is no constant relationship between the atria and the usually much slower ventricles. In Figure 8–26 the atria are beating at a rate of approximately 65 per minute and the ventricles at approximately 29 per minute.

Figure 8–27 is an example of complete A–V block in a patient with atrial fibrillation. The ventricular rate is low, with no clear evidence of atrial activity. The atrial activity is fine fibrillation, with no impulses entering the ventricular conduction system from the atria.

Figure 8–27 illustrates a principle of great importance. When the QRS complexes become regular in the presence of atrial fibrillation in a patient on digitalis, it usually means that atrioventricular block has supervened. When the ventricular rate is very low (35 per minute in Fig. 8–27 and 37 per minute in Fig. 8–28), the physician and the patient would generally become suspicious that all is not well. However, when a junctional rhythm becomes dominant and the regular rate is not very slow (Fig. 8–29), the patient may actually feel well in the presence of digitalis toxicity. If the physician examines the patient with a quick pulse check and congratulates himself on the regular rhythm, he may be sending his patient home to disaster. This stage,

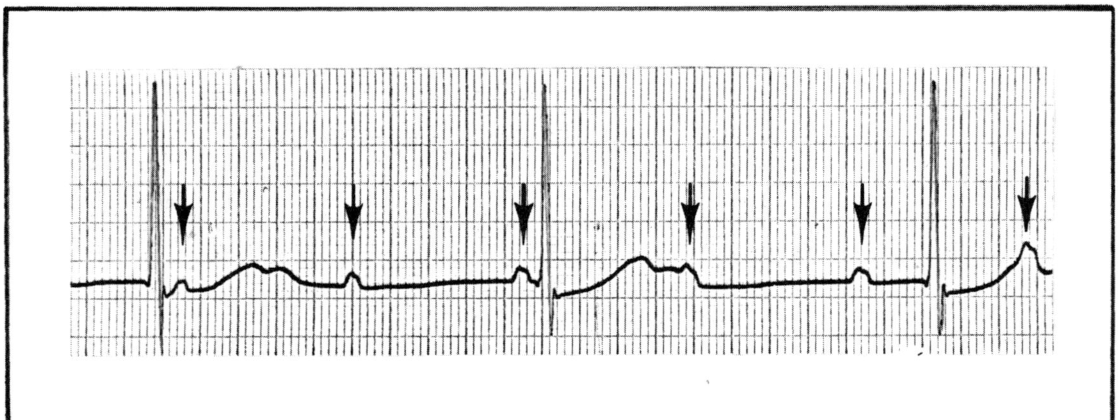

FIGURE 8–26. Third degree (complete) A–V block. The arrows point to the P waves, which are not related to the QRS complexes.

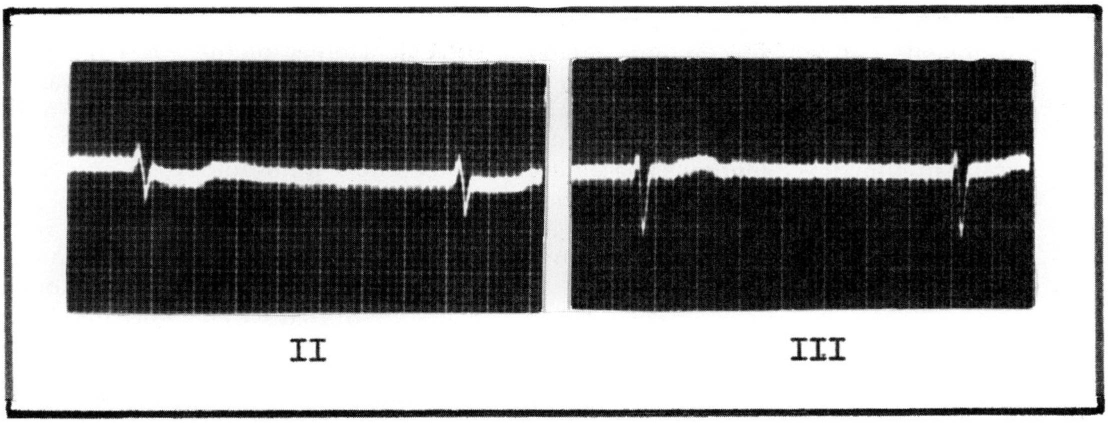

FIGURE 8–27. Complete A–V block in a patient with atrial fibrillation.

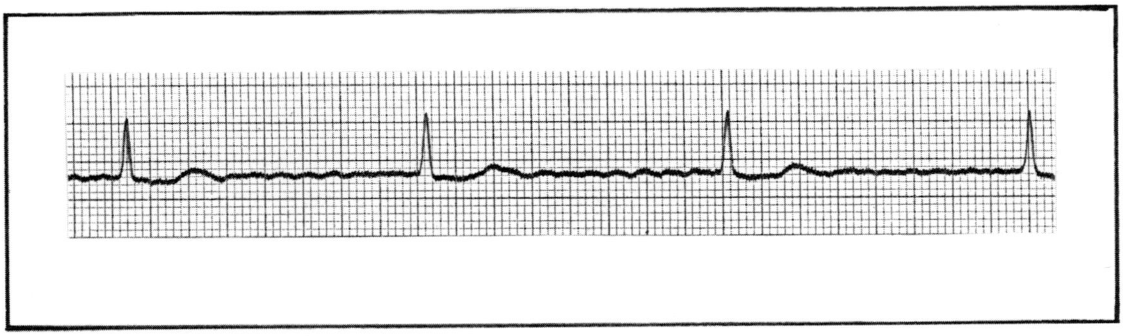

FIGURE 8–28. Complete A–V block in a patient with atrial fibrillation.

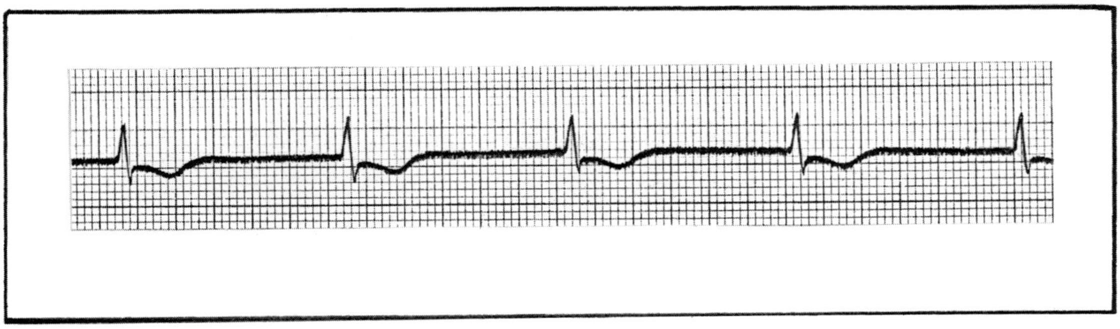

FIGURE 8–29. Junctional rhythm in a patient whose baseline rhythm was atrial fibrillation with an irregular ventricular response.

which already represents significant digitalis toxicity, is tragically common and too often missed. The important principle to remember is that if a patient on digitalis with known atrial fibrillation develops a regular rhythm, it is dangerous to assume, whatever the rate, that the new rhythm is sinus rhythm. At the very least, an electrocardiographic rhythm strip should be inspected.

EPILOGUE

We have now come to the end of our course. I want to express my thanks to all of you. I have done the best as I saw it to present a clear picture of a frequently misunderstood subject. My aim was clarity of presentation to facilitate understanding, to break through the quagmire of technical terminology, to present the concepts with a few basic rules.

I have had much satisfaction in the excellent grasp of the material among the people who were with us throughout the course. Within the framework of the time, the scope, the group and the subject, I have tried, to the best of my ability and experience, to shed some light. Thank you.

BIBLIOGRAPHY

Beckwith, J.: Grant's Clinical Electrocardiography. 2nd Ed. New York, McGraw-Hill Book Company, 1970.

Bellet, S.: Essentials of Cardiac Arrhythmias: Diagnosis and Management. Philadelphia, W. B. Saunders Company, 1972.

Fisch, C., and Surawicz, B. (Eds.): Digitalis. New York, Grune & Stratton, 1970.

Furman, S., and Escher, D. J. W.: Principles and Techniques of Cardiac Pacing. Hagerstown, Md., Harper & Row, 1970.

Harrison, T. R., and Reeves, T. J.: Principles and Problems of Ischemic Heart Disease. Chicago, Year Book Medical Publishers, 1968.

Hoffman, B. F., and Cranefield, P. S.: Electrophysiology of the Heart. New York, McGraw-Hill Book Company, 1960.

Hurst, J. W., and Logue, R. B.: The Heart. 3rd Ed. New York, McGraw-Hill Book Company, 1974.

Katz, L. N., and Pick, A.: Clinical Electrocardiography. Philadelphia, Lea & Febiger, 1956.

Lister, J. W., et al.: Arrhythmia Analysis by Intracardiac Electrocardiography. Springfield, Ill., Charles C Thomas, 1975.

Nadas, A. S., and Fyler, D. C.: Pediatric Cardiology. 3rd Ed. Philadelphia, W. B. Saunders Company, 1972.

Patton, R. D., Stein, E., Rosen, K. M., Lau, S. H., and Damato, A. N.: Bundle of His electrocardiograms: A new method for analyzing arrhythmias. Am. J. Cardiol. *26*:324, 1970.

Perloff, J. K.: The Clinical Recognition of Congenital Heart Disease. Philadelphia, W. B. Saunders Company, 1970.

Rosenbaum, M. B., et al.: The Hemiblocks. Oldsmar, Fla., Tampa Tracings, 1970.

Scherf, D., and Cohen, J.: The Atrioventricular Node and Selected Arrhythmias. New York, Grune & Stratton, 1964.

Schlant, R. C., and Hurst, J. W. (Eds.): Advances in Electrocardiography. New York, Grune & Stratton, 1972.

INDEX

Note: Page numbers in *italics* refer to illustrations. Page numbers followed by the letter "t" refer to tables.